MW00681830

Diagnosis in Paediatric Haematology

For Churchill Livingstone

Commissioning Editor: Gavin Smith
Copy Editor: Ruth Swan
Project Controller: Sarah Lowe
Text Design: Sarah Cape
Cover Design: Andrea Purdie

Diagnosis in Paediatric Haematology

Harry Smith MD FRCPA

Paediatric Haematologist, Department of Pathology, Royal Brisbane Hospital
Clinical Professor in Child Health, University of Queensland

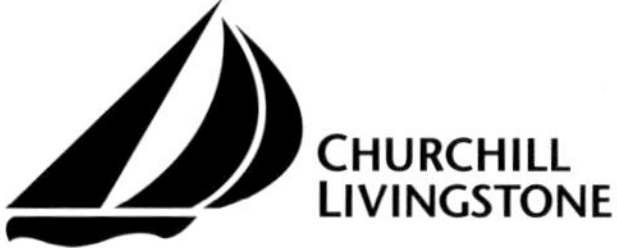

NEW YORK EDINBURGH LONDON MADRID MELBOURNE SAN FRANCISCO
TOKYO 1996

CHURCHILL LIVINGSTONE
Medical Division of Pearson Professional Limited

Distributed in the United States of America by Churchill Livingstone Inc., 650 Avenue of the Americas, New York, N.Y. 10011, and by associated companies, branches and representatives throughout the world.

First published 1996

ISBN 0 443 05106 2

British Library Cataloguing in Publication Data
A catalogue record for this book is available from the British Library.

Library of Congress Cataloging in Publication Data
A catalog record for this book is available from the Library of Congress.

The publisher's policy is to use **paper manufactured from sustainable forests**

Printed in Hong Kong

Contents

A summary of contents is given at the head of each chapter.

1. Normal values and appearances **1**
2. Microcytic and macrocytic anaemias **13**
3. Normocytic anaemias **61**
4. Lymphocytic leukaemias **113**
5. Myeloid leukaemias. Non-haemopoietic malignancies in marrow **143**
6. Anomalies of leucocyte structure **201**
7. Benign change in leucocytes: leucocytosis, leucopenia, infection **239**
8. Disorders of haemostasis **273**

Preface

My hope for this manual of diagnosis is that it will give guidance in 'front-line' interpretation of blood/marrow abnormalities of childhood as they present to a routine department of laboratory haematology. Emphasis has been given to problems and the potential for error.

To keep within the confines of this remit, several aspects of the subject have accordingly been omitted or given only minor consideration — methods and procedures are not given consideration as such, comprehensive accounts of clinical manifestations are not given, 'sophisticated' procedures are not given prominence and treatment is considered only if its efficacy (or otherwise) is of value in diagnosis.

I have, however, gone beyond these confines, I hope justifiably, in certain areas; firstly, some electron micrographs have been included which help to explain light microscopic appearances or assist significantly in diagnosis; secondly, summaries and/or clinical photographs are given of uncommon conditions — paediatricians expect the pathologist to offer the most likely explanation/s for abnormalities of blood and marrow, and pathologists are asked on occasion to see patients or may wish to do so themselves.

While intended primarily for medical and scientific staff concerned with laboratory diagnosis, the manual may be useful to paediatricians who wish to be involved in the process of laboratory diagnosis.

Acknowledgements

I am indebted to many for their expertise and time in reviewing parts of the text — Dr B Bain (London, anaemias, leukaemias), Prof A Bellingham (London, erythrocyte enzyme defects), Prof P Castaldi (Sydney, haemostasis), Dr R Collins (Brisbane, leukaemia immunophenotyping), Prof B Lake (London, leucocyte anomalies, storage diseases), Prof M Levin (London, infection), Dr Y W Liew (Brisbane, erythrocyte serology), H Miller (Brisbane, drug effects), Dr R Minchinton (Brisbane, leucocyte and platelet serology), Dr C Morgan (Brisbane, haemostasis), C McCarthy (Brisbane, cytogenetics), Dr J Rowell (Brisbane, haemostasis), Dr V Siskind (Brisbane, statistical analysis), Dr G Tauro (Melbourne, leukaemia, erythrocyte enzymes), Prof R Trent (Sydney, haemoglobinopathies), and Prof J Wiley (Melbourne, disorders of erythrocyte electrolyte flux). I thank the staff of the haematology division (Head, A Cooney) and ancillary departments for expert and cheerful support over the years — electron microscopy (Head, N Hudson), photography (B Stewart, J Warner, R Johnston and his staff) and Herston Medical Library (Head, R Boot). Colleagues who have kindly sent material for photography are acknowledged in the captions to the illustrations.

Photomicrographic equipment was generously donated by the Royal Childrens Hospital Foundation.

I am much indebted to my wife, Jan, for the expert and grinding tasks of word processing, deciphering of the illegible and coping with innumerable changes of text. Judy Waters and Lowri Daniels of Churchill Livingstone gave welcome encouragement in bleak periods, with Judy Waters also providing the title. Sarah Lowe and Gavin Smith of Churchill Livingstone have artfully overseen the blending together of text, tables and photographs.

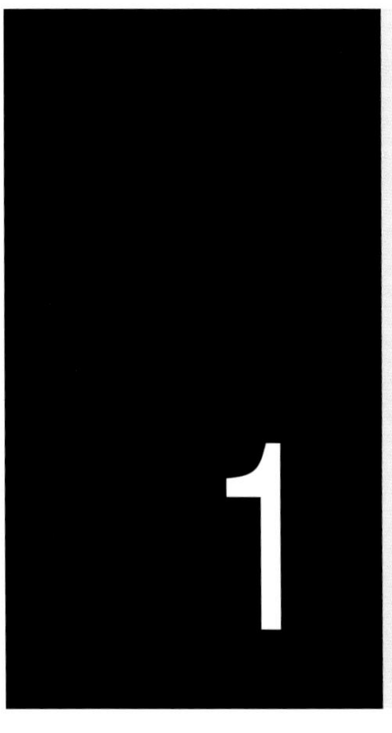

1 Normal values and appearances

A summary of peculiarities of blood and marrow in childhood, except for haemostasis (Ch. 8).

Erythrocytes 2
Hb, MCV, hct, MCH 2
Immature erythrocytes 2
Macrocytosis 4
Pyknocytosis 4
Spherocytosis 4
Howell-Jolly bodies 4
Pitted (pocked) erythrocytes 4
Hb chain types 4
Blood group serology 4
Enzymes 6
Iron status 6
Folate, B_{12} 6

Serum haptoglobin 8

Leucocytes 8
Granulocytes 8
Lymphocytes 8
Eosinophils 8
Monocytes 8

Bone marrow 10
Cellularity 10
Lymphocytes 10
Immature lymphocytes 10
Plasma cells 10
M/E ratio 10
Iron stores 10

Erythrocytes (Table 1.1)

Hb, MCV, hct, MCH

The polycythaemia of the newborn (Table 1.2) is due to erythropoietin excess caused by hypoxia in utero. The Hb fall after birth results from: (i) erythropoietin switchoff by the higher ambient oxygen tension, (ii) red cell destruction (life span of neonatal cells about 90 days, compared with 120 for older children). Lowest values are reached at about 2 months. An Hb of < 10.0 g/dl is abnormal for a full-term infant of any age. The slight differences in the sexes at puberty are due to differences in androgen production.

Hb values for prematures at birth are approximately the same as for full-term infants, but the post-natal decline is steeper and lower (Table 1.3). This is due in part to shorter cell survival (half life approx 15 days vs 29 for full term, Kaplan & Hsu 1961).

Fetal red cells are macrocytic (Tables 1.2, 1.4), the MCV (and MCH) falling after birth as fetal cells are replaced. Reduction in cell size in late pregnancy is accompanied by increase in cell count, as a result of which Hb and hct remain constant (Table 1.4). An MCV of < 70 fl is abnormal at any stage of childhood.

The polycythaemia of the neonate is accompanied by high red cell and blood volume — average cell volume in the term neonate is 39 ml/kg, and blood volume 85 ml/kg (90 ml in prematures). After rising in the first week (to about 105 ml/kg blood volume), values decline to reach stability at about 6 months, with average values in childhood of 25 ml/kg for red cell and 75 ml/kg for blood volume.

Immature erythrocytes

Reticulocytes and erythroblasts are conspicuous in fetal life and in the first days after birth (Table 1.5), numbers declining with erythropoietin switchoff. Persistence of raised values after 5–7 days is abnormal. A temporary, slight increase in reticulocytes to upper normal occurs at about 2 months when erythropoietin production returns.

Immature erythrocytes are more numerous in pre-term infants (Table 1.6), but the pattern of post-natal decline is similar to that for term infants.

Table 1.1 Red cell peculiarities in the normal neonate

Values
Polycythaemia
High red cell, blood volume
Reticulocytosis
Erythroblastosis
Form
Macrocytosis
Pyknocytosis
Spherocytosis
Howell-Jolly bodies
'Pocked' cells
Heinz bodies
Other
Hb chain types
Blood group serology
Haemopoietic factors
Iron
Folate, B_{12}
Erythropoietin
Enzymes

Table 1.2 Ranges (mean ± 2 SD) for erythrocytes in normal, full-term iron-sufficient children[1]

		Hb g/dl	MCV fl	Count × 10^{12}/l	MCH pg	hct
Birth		14.5–22.0	95–125	3.9–5.5	31–37	0.46–0.60
0–1 week		14.0–22.0	90–120	3.9–6.3	31–37	0.42–0.64
2 weeks		12.5–20.0	86–120	3.6–6.2	28–40	0.39–0.63
1 month		11.0–18.0	85–120	3.0–5.4	28–40	0.35–0.55
2 months		10.0–13.5	80–115	2.7–4.9	26–34	0.30–0.42
3–6 months		10.0–13.5	75–105	3.1–4.5	25–35	0.30–0.42
0.5–2 yr		10.5–13.5	70–86	3.7–5.3	23–31	0.30–0.42
2–6 yr		11.0–14.0	73–85	3.9–5.3	24–30	0.33–0.42
6–12 yr		11.5–15.5	77–95	4.0–5.2	25–33	0.35–0.45
12–18 yr	F	12.0–16.0	78–100	4.1–5.1	25–35	0.36–0.46
	M	13.0–16.0	78–98	4.5–5.3	25–35	0.37–0.49

Note: MCHC through childhood is 32–36 g/dl
[1] From electronic counters. Data adapted from various sources, mainly Dallman 1977

Table 1.3 Hb (median and 95% range) in the first 6 months of life in iron-sufficient pre-term infants[1,2]

	Birth weight 1000–1500 g	1501–2000 g
2 weeks	16.3, 11.7–18.4	14.8, 11.8–19.6
1 month	10.9, 8.7–15.2	11.5, 8.2–15.0
2 months	8.8, 7.1–11.5	9.4, 8.0–11.4
3 months	9.8, 8.9–11.2	10.2, 9.3–11.8
4 months	11.3, 9.1–13.1	11.3, 9.1–13.1
5 months	11.6, 10.2–14.3	11.8, 10.4–13.0
6 months	12.0, 9.4–13.8	11.8, 10.7–12.6

[1] Serum ferritin ≥ 10 μg/l
[2] From Lundström et al 1977

Table 1.4 Erythrocyte values (mean ± 1 SD) for first natal day from 24 weeks gestation onwards[1]

Weeks gestation	Hb g/dl	MCV fl	Count × 10^{12}/l	hct
24–25	19.4 ± 1.5	135 ± 0.2	4.65 ± 0.43	0.63 ± 0.04
26–27	19.0 ± 2.5	132 ± 14.4	4.73 ± 0.45	0.62 ± 0.08
28–29	19.3 ± 1.8	131 ± 13.5	4.62 ± 0.75	0.60 ± 0.07
30–31	19.1 ± 2.2	127 ± 12.7	4.79 ± 0.74	0.60 ± 0.08
32–33	18.5 ± 2.0	123 ± 15.7	5.00 ± 0.76	0.60 ± 0.08
34–35	19.6 ± 2.1	122 ± 10.0	5.09 ± 0.5	0.61 ± 0.07
36–37	19.2 ± 1.7	121 ± 12.5	5.27 ± 0.68	0.64 ± 0.07

[1] From Zaizov & Matoth 1976

Table 1.5 Immature erythrocytes in blood in full-term infants

	Reticulocytes %	×10^9/l	Erythroblasts ×10^9/l
Cord	3–7	110–450	0–1.0
Day 1	3–7	110–450	0–0.5
3	1–3	50–150	0–0.01
7	0.1–2	10–100	0
4 weeks	0.1–2	10–100	0
>4 weeks	0.1–2	10–100	0

Table 1.6 Immature erythrocytes on the first natal day after various periods of gestation

Weeks gestation	Reticulocytes % of erythrocytes	Erythroblasts × 10^9/l
23–25	5–10	2.8 ± 1.6[1]
26–30	5–10	1.8 ± 1.6[1]
31–35	3–10	
36–37	3–7	0–2.0
Term	3–7	0–1.0

[1] Mean ± SD. Derived from Forestier et al 1986

Peculiarities of form (Table 1.1)

In general, peculiarities are more pronounced in pre-term infants.

- Macrocytosis (Tables 1.2, 1.3)

- Pyknocytosis

Pyknocytes are irregularly contracted, whole erythrocytes. Projections are few (< 5), irregularly distributed, short and broad-based (Fig. 1.1). In normal infants, numbers vary up to about 2% for term, and 6% for pre-term infants, in the first 6 months of life. Values peak at about 3 months. After 6 months, the upper limit of normal is about 0.5%.

- Spherocytosis

Small numbers (< 1%) of spherocytes are not uncommon in normal infants in the first weeks (Fig. 1.1). Their significance is unknown. Occurrence in larger numbers or after 2 weeks is abnormal.

- Howell-Jolly bodies

Occasional Howell-Jolly bodies are normal in the first month, especially in prematures (Fig. 1.1), and are an indication of (physiologic) hypofunction of the spleen.

- Pitted (pocked) erythrocytes (Figs. 2.8, 3.27, Table 1.7)

Pits are openings of subsurface vacuoles, containing material discarded during cell maturation (ferritin, haemoglobin, mitochondria and membranous structures, Schnitzer et al 1971). The vacuoles are removed without detriment to the cell by the spleen (pitting function). Pits may be observed by differential interference phase-contrast in dried, unstained blood films or (for precise quantitation) glutaraldehyde-fixed wet preparations (Holroyde et al 1969). Minute 'holes' in cells in routinely stained films (Fig. 3.27) correspond to pits visible by differential interference phase-contrast.

Table 1.7 Pitted erythrocytes in wet, fixed preparations[1]

	% of erythrocytes
Pre-term, at birth	
Birth weight: < 1500 g	60–87
1500–2500 g	25–70
Term, birth weight > 2500 g	
At birth	12–36
1 month	5–28
2 months	2–12
3–6 months	0.4–4.8
6 months onwards	0.4–3.5

[1] After Holroyde et al 1969

Note 1. When pit counts are high, pits are also more numerous per cell and are larger

2. Mature values are reached by 3 months in term, and by 4 months in pre-term infants

3. In some infants with asplenia, counts may be normal at birth but do not diminish (or may increase) over ensuing months

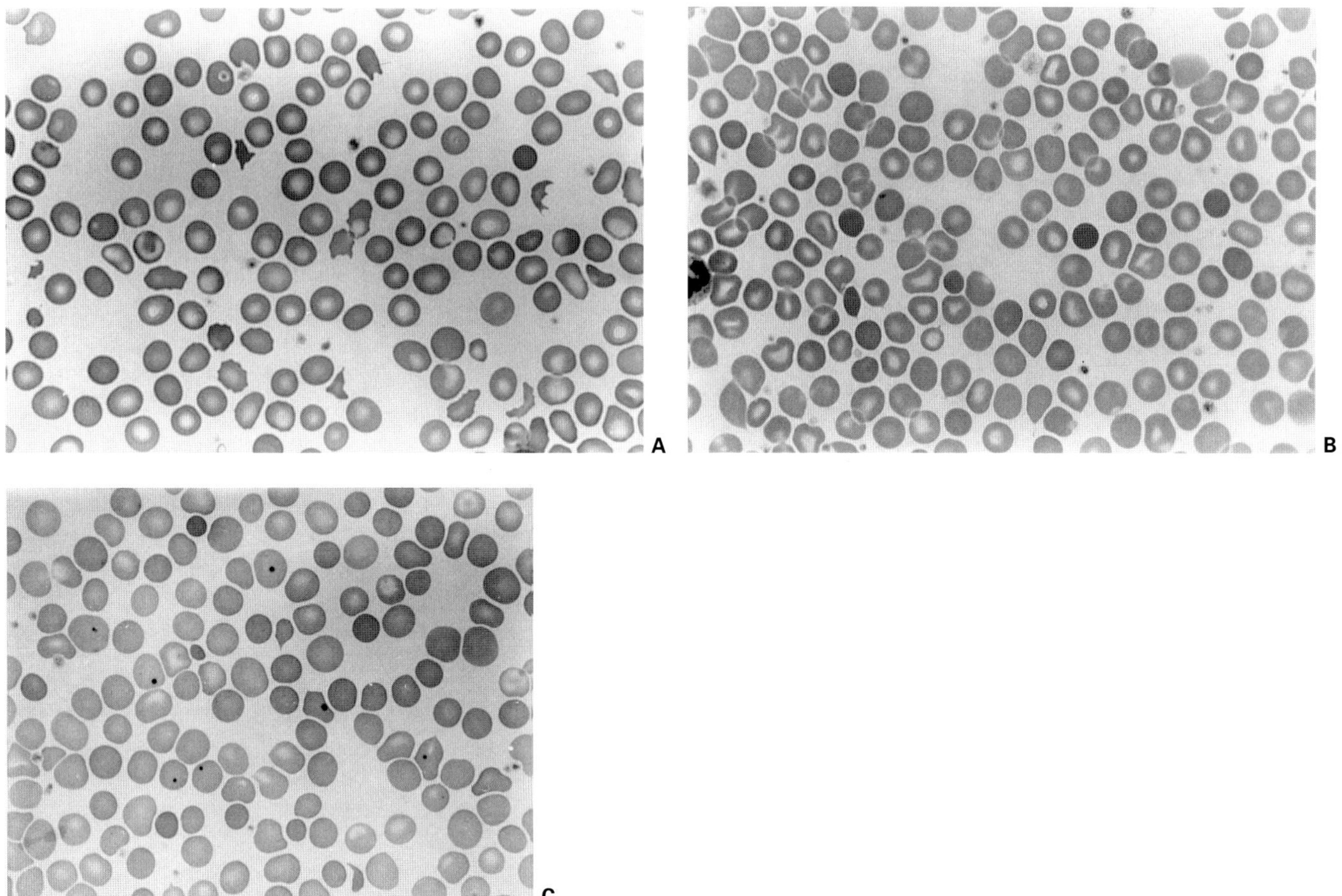

Fig. 1.1 Temporary peculiarities of erythrocytes in normal neonates: **a** pyknocytosis; **b** spherocytosis; **c** Howell-Jolly bodies. All × 480

Other erythrocyte characteristics

- Hb chain types

Changes from fetal life onwards are summarized in Tables 1.8 and 1.9.

HbF reaches a minimum at 12–18 months. The small amounts (< 1%) in older children are best assessed by Kleihauer or immunologic technique (Zago et al 1979; alkali denaturation suitable for values > 2%). HbF is unevenly distributed, being confined to a population of 'F cells'.

HbA_2 rises slowly after birth to its final level at 12–18 months.

- Blood group serology

Expression of i and deficiency of I antigens are characteristic of early childhood. Adult characteristics are attained by the end of the first year.

Expression of ABH antigens is deficient in the first year, as is expression of Lewis antigen in the first 2 years. AB isoagglutinins (IgM) are rarely detectable in cord blood, any isoagglutinins being most likely maternal IgG. Normal values (mean 1/128, range 1/16–1/512) are reached usually by 2–3 years (rarely 5 years).

- Enzymes (Table 1.10)

The deficit of protective enzymes such as glutathione peroxidase may contribute to the vulnerability of neonatal erythrocytes to Heinz body formation (p. 84).

Haemopoietic factors

- Iron status (Table 1.11)

Serum iron and ferritin are high at birth because of haemolysis and erythropoietin switchoff. Lowest levels are reached at 0.5–4 years and remain low, compared with adults, throughout childhood. Iron-binding capacity rises progressively through childhood.

- Folate, B_{12}

The normal range for red cell folate in childhood is 100–750 μg/l. In the first 3 months values are somewhat lower (50–400) in prematures, because of curtailment of storage in the last trimester and more rapid post-natal growth. The serum level is a less reliable index of stores than erythrocyte content. A range of 5–30 μg/l is applicable to childhood in general, although values may be slightly lower in the second half of the first year (3–30 μg/l), and may be lower in prematures in the first 3 months (2–15 μg/l) for the reasons noted above (Vanier & Tyas 1966, 1967).

The normal range for serum B_{12} is 145–700 ng/l.

Table 1.8 Haemoglobin synthesis in fetal and post-natal life

	Inception of synthesis	Reaches maximum synthesis		Duration
ζ chain	early fetal			< 3 months fetal
ϵ chain	early fetal			< 3 months fetal
α chain	early fetal	approx 3 months fetal		life
β chain	5–6 weeks fetal	3–6 months fetal		life
γ chain	approx 1 month fetal	3–7 months fetal		declines after approx 30 weeks fetal
δ chain	approx 7 months fetal	about 12 months post-natal		life
Embryonic haemoglobins		Gower 1	$\zeta 2\epsilon 2$	
		Gower 2	$\alpha 2\epsilon 2$	
		Portland	$\zeta 2\gamma 2$	
Haemoglobins in normal cord blood		F	$\alpha 2\gamma 2$	60–85%
		A	$\alpha 2\beta 2$	15–40%
		A_2	$\alpha 2\delta 2$	< 1.8%
		Barts	$\gamma 4$	< 0.5%
		Portland	$\zeta 2\gamma 2$	trace in some cords only

Table 1.9 Normal values for HbF and HbA_2

	HbF (%)[1] mean	HbF (%)[1] ± 2 SD	HbA_2 (%)[2] mean	HbA_2 (%)[2] ± 2 SD
1–7 days	75	61–80		
2 weeks	75	66–81		
1 month	60	46–67	0.8	0.4–1.3
2 months	46	29–61	1.3	0.4–1.9
3 months	27	15–56	2.2	1.0–3.0
4 months	18	9.4–29	2.4	2.0–2.8
5 months	10	2.3–22	2.5	2.1–3.1
6 months	7	2.7–13	2.5	2.1–3.1
8 months	5	2.3–12	2.7	1.9–3.5
10 months	2.1	1.5–3.5	2.7	2.0–3.3
12 months	2.0	1.3–5.0	2.7	2.0–3.3
13–16 months	0.6	0.2–1.0	2.6	1.6–3.3
17–20 months	0.6	0.2–1.0	2.9	2.1–3.5
21–24 months	0.6	0.2–1.0	2.8	2.1–3.5

[1] From Schröter & Nafz 1981
[2] From Metaxotou-Mavromati et al 1982

Table 1.10 Enzyme activities in neonatal vs adult erythrocytes[1]

Lower	Approx equal	Increased
Glutathione peroxidase	Triosephosphate isomerase	Aldolase
Glutathione synthetase	Glyceraldehyde-3-phosphate dehydrogenase	Enolase
Phosphofructokinase		Glucose-phosphate isomerase
Catalase		Glucose-6-phosphate dehydrogenase
Adenylate kinase		Hexokinase
NADP-metHb reductase		Phosphoglycerate kinase
		Pyruvate kinase

[1] From Oski 1993

Table 1.11 Reference ranges (95% limits) for serum iron status in iron-sufficient children[1]

	Iron µmol/l median	Iron µmol/l range	Iron-binding capacity µmol/l mean	Iron-binding capacity µmol/l range	Transferrin saturation % median	Transferrin saturation % range	Ferritin µg/l median	Ferritin µg/l range
0.5 month	22	11–36	34	18–50	68	30–39	101	25–200
1 month	22	10–31	36	20–52	63	35–94	356	200–600
2 months	16	3–29	44	24–64	34	21–63	180	50–200
4 months	15	3–29	54	40–68	27	7–53	80	20–200
6 months	14	5–24	58	40–76	23	10–43	30	7–142
0.5–4 yr	14	5–25	64	48–79	18	10–40	30	7–142
5–10 yr	16	5–30	67	43–91	22	10–45	30	7–142
11–15 yr	17	5–30	76	52–100	24	11–45	30	7–142

[1] Adapted from Siimes et al 1974, Milman & Cohn 1984, Meites 1989

Serum haptoglobin

Haptoglobin is virtually absent at birth (low synthesis in liver), and rises to its permanent level at 6–12 months (Table 1.12). Low values in infancy therefore cannot be taken as evidence of haemolysis.

Table 1.12 Reference ranges for serum haptoglobin[1]

	Haemoglobin binding capacity mg/dl mean	range (95%)
Cord blood	0	0
1–7 days	10	0–41
1–4 weeks	28	0–45
1–3 months	59	41–95
3–6 months	91	64–134
6–12 months	115	43–160
1–5 yr	109	51–160
5–10 yr	107	62–186
> 10 yr	110	41–165

[1] Khalil et al 1967

Leucocytes

Granulocytes

Neutrophilia is normal in the first 3 days, as is some degree of shift to the left in the first months (Table 1.13). Sessile tags on neutrophil nuclei (Fig. 6.14) are common in infancy (2 or more tags in up to 10% of cells).

Table 1.13 Reference ranges (95% confidence limits) for neutrophils[1]

		$\times 10^9$/l
Total neutrophils	0–60 h	2.9–14.5
	61–120 h	1.8–7.2
	5–28 days	1.8–5.4
	1–6 months	1.0–8.5
	0.5–8 yr	1.5–8.0
	8–16 yr	1.8–8.0
Immature neutrophils	0–60 h	0–1.4
	61–120 h	0–0.6
	5–28 days	0–0.5
Immature/total neutrophils	0–60 h	< 0.16
	61–120 h	< 0.13
	5–28 days	< 0.12
Immature/mature ratio	0–1 month	≤ 0.3

Immature neutrophils = band + less mature forms. Band = neutrophil in which width of narrowest segment of nucleus is not < $\frac{1}{3}$ of width of broadest segment

[1] Data for neonates are for full-term and pre-term, from Manroe et al 1979. Other data from Dallman 1977

Lymphocytes

Lymphocytosis is outstanding in blood (and marrow) in childhood (Table 1.14). The excess is of small dark lymphocytes; larger, pale, granulated cells (natural killer cells) remain at fairly constant levels through childhood (Fig. 1.2). The granules have a distinctive ultrastructure of parallel tubular arrays.

Lymphoblasts resembling those in acute lymphoblastic leukaemia may occur in children with no evidence of leukaemia, especially in the first 5 years (Fig. 1.2). An acceptable upper limit is 2 cells in a film. Larger numbers, especially if associated with abnormal blood values or with clinical features suggesting leukaemia, should be taken seriously. In our experience, no child with normal numbers of lymphoblasts as so defined, and normal blood values has re-presented with leukaemia.

Atypical ('reactive') lymphocytes may occur in small numbers in apparently healthy children, especially in the first 3 years, as an indication probably of subclinical viral infection.

Eosinophils, monocytes

Eosinophils are slightly more numerous in children under 5 years and monocytes in children under 2 years (Table 1.14).

Table 1.14 Reference ranges (95% confidence limits) for leucocytes[1]

		$\times 10^9$/l
Lymphocytes	birth	2.0–11.0
	12 h	2.0–11.0
	24 h	2.0–11.5
	1–2 weeks	2.0–17.0
	1 month	2.5–16.5
	6 months	4.0–13.5
	1 yr	4.0–10.5
	2 yr	3.0–9.5
	4 yr	2.0–8.0
	6 yr	1.5–7.0
	8 yr	1.5–6.8
	10 yr	1.5–6.5
	16 yr	1.2–5.2
Monocytes	0–60 h	0–1.9
	2–5 days	0–1.7
	5–30 days	0.1–1.7
	1 month–2 yr	0.1–1.2
	2–14 yr	0.1–0.8
Eosinophils	0–30 days	0–0.8
	1 month–5 yr	0–0.7
	5–15 yr	0–0.5

[1] From Dallman 1977, Weinberg et al 1985

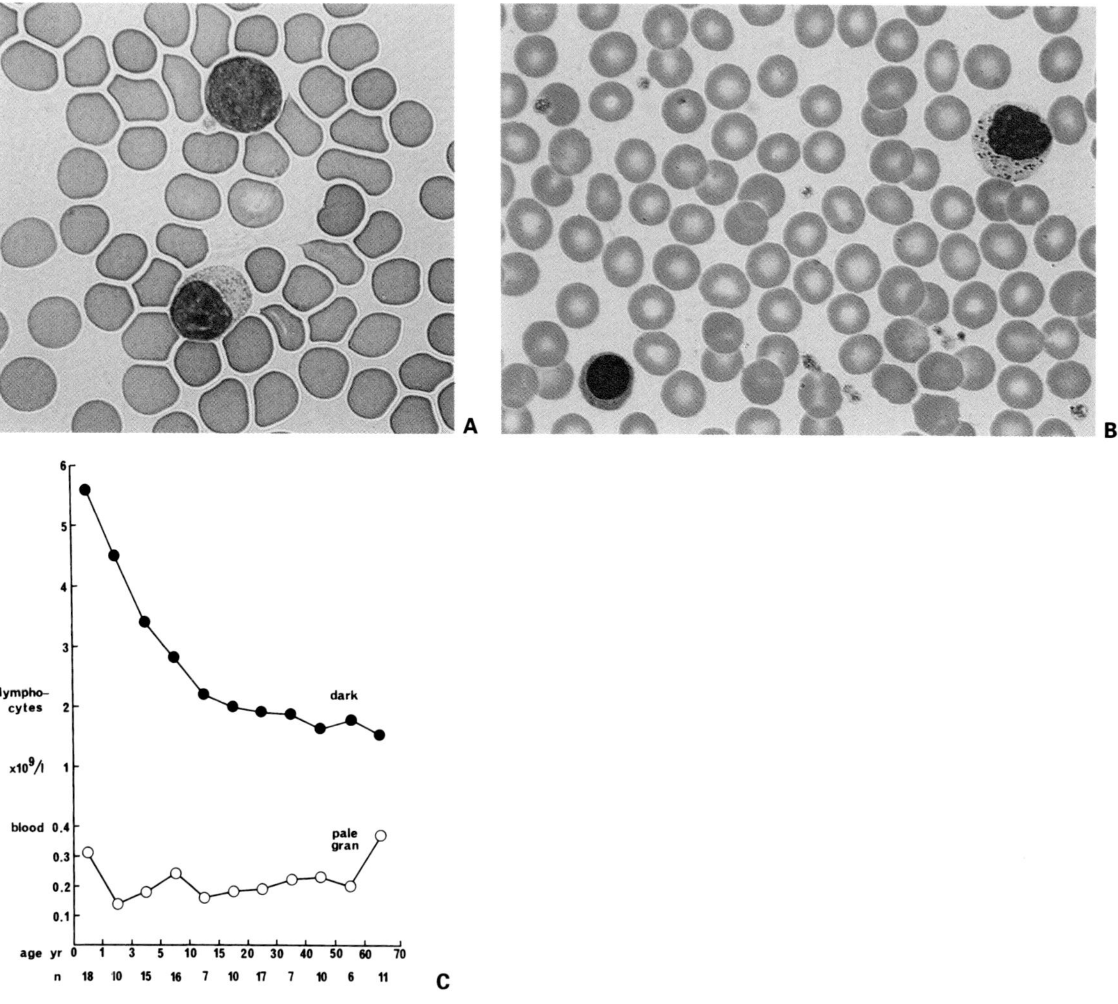

Fig. 1.2 Lymphocytes in blood of normal children. **a** Lymphoblast and lymphocyte. **b** Small basophilic lymphocyte and large granular lymphocyte. **c** Concentration of lymphocytes in normal children; n = number examined, 'dark' = small basophilic lymphocytes, 'pale gran' = pale (large) granulated lymphocytes. The decline in count with age is due to decline in small basophilic lymphocytes. **a,b** × 750

Bone marrow (Table 1.15)

Distinctive characteristics include:

- Haemopoietic cellularity (Fig. 1.3)

Cellularity (trephine biopsies of iliac marrow) declines from a range of 59–95% (mean 79%) in the first decade, to 42–87% (mean 64%) in the second (Hartsock et al 1965).

- Lymphocytosis

Peak values occur at about 1 month.

- Immature lymphocytes (Fig. 1.3)

In the first years especially, lymphoblasts may be noted in increased numbers, as well as immature cells with scant cytoplasm and homogeneous, smooth chromatin with no or indistinct nucleoli ('haematogones', Longacre et al 1989). Fluorescent cell sorting may show substantial expansion of populations with 'common' to mature Ig-positive phenotypes. These characteristics should not be confused with genuine leukaemia (p. 136).

- Plasma cells

Their sparseness in the first years limits the value of marrow examination for assessment of immune deficiency.

- Myeloid/erythroid ratio

This peaks at about 1 month and reaches a stable level at about 1 year.

- Iron stores

In the first month storage is demonstrable (haemolysis, underutilization from erythropoietin switchoff). Otherwise, there is usually no stainable storage iron in normal children in the first 5 years (Smith et al 1955) and erythroblast iron is sparse (< 10% of cells). Deficiency of marrow iron in this period cannot therefore be taken as evidence of iron deficiency.

Table 1.15 Marrow composition (% of nucleated cells) in childhood[1]

	0–1 month	1 month–1 yr	1–7 yr	7–14 yr
Leucoblasts	0–4	0–4	0–3	0–3
Neutrophils				
Promyelocytes	0–4.5	0–4.5	0–4.5	0.5–4.5
Myelocytes	8–25	8–25	8–25	8–25
Metamyelocytes + stabs	15–35	15–35	15–35	10–30
Segmented	5–30	5–30	5–30	5–30
Eosinophils, all stages	0–7	0–5	1–9	1–9
Basophils, all stages	0–0.8	0–0.8	0–0.8	0–0.8
Erythroblasts	6–38	6–38	6–38	6–38
M/E ratio	1.2–11.8	2.5–10.0	2.5–8.0	2.5–8.0
Lymphocytes	5–60	15–45	5–35	5–30
Plasma cells	0–0.05	0.02–0.16	0.16–0.54	0.22–0.52

[1] Modified from Glaser et al 1950

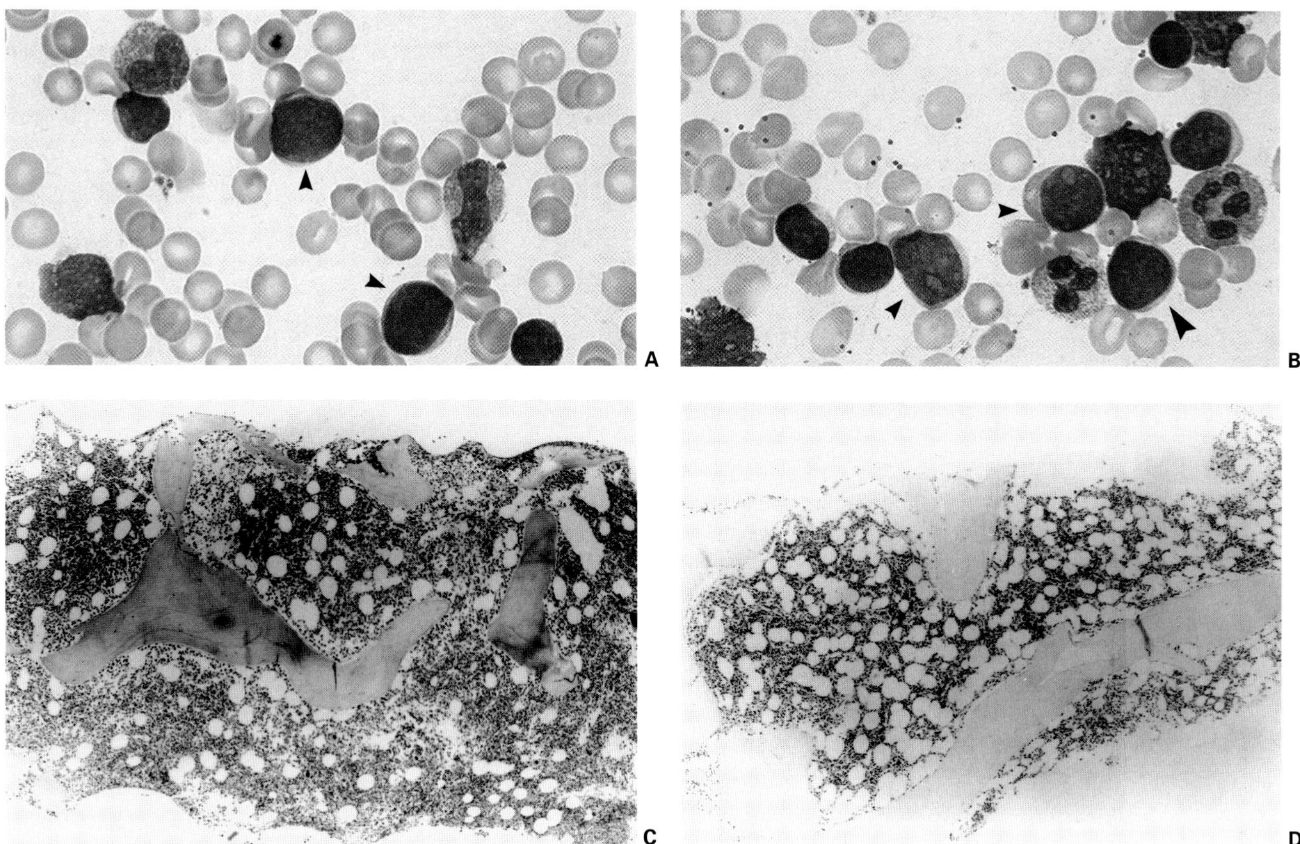

Fig. 1.3 Normal marrow in childhood. **a,b** Immature lymphocytes in a 3-month-old infant. **a** Shows 2 haematogones (arrows) and 2 mature lymphocytes. **b** Shows one haematogone (large arrow), 2 nucleolated lymphoblasts (small arrows) and 3 mature lymphocytes. **c,d** Decline in cellularity with age: **c** at 2 years, **d** at 13 years. **a,b** × 750; **c,d** × 40

REFERENCES

Dallman P R 1977 Blood and blood forming tissues. In: Rudolph A M, Barnett H L, Einhorn A H (eds) Pediatrics, 16th edn. Appleton-Century-Crofts, New York, ch 24

Forestier F, Daffos F, Galactéros F et al 1986 Hematological values of 163 normal fetuses between 18 and 30 weeks of gestation. Pediatric Research 20: 342–346

Glaser K, Limarzi L R, Poncher H G 1950 Cellular composition of the bone marrow in normal infants and children. Pediatrics 6: 789–824

Hartsock R J, Smith E B, Petty C S 1965 Normal variations with aging of the amount of hematopoietic tissue in bone marrow from the anterior iliac crest. American Journal of Clinical Pathology 43: 326–331

Holroyde C P, Oski F A, Gardner F H 1969 The "pocked" erythrocyte. Red-cell surface alterations in reticuloendothelial immaturity of the neonate. New England Journal of Medicine 281: 516–520

Kaplan E, Hsu K S 1961 Determination of erythrocyte survival in newborn infants by means of Cr-labelled erythrocytes. Pediatrics 27: 354–361

Khalil M, Badr-El-Din M K, Kassem A S 1967 Haptoglobin level in normal infants and children. Alexandria Medical Journal 13: 1–9

Longacre T A, Foucar K, Crago S et al 1989 Hematogones: a multiparameter analysis of bone marrow precursor cells. Blood 73: 543–552

Lundström U, Siimes M A, Dallman P R 1977 At what age does iron supplementation become necessary in low-birth-weight infants? Journal of Pediatrics 91: 878–883

Manroe B L, Weinberg A G, Rosenfeld C R, Browne R 1979 The neonatal blood count in health and disease. I. Reference values for neutrophilic cells. Journal of Pediatrics 95: 89–98

Meites S (ed) 1989 Pediatric clinical chemistry. Reference (normal) values, 3rd edn. AACC Press, Washington

Metaxotou-Mavromati A D, Antonopoulou H K, Laskari S S et al 1982 Developmental changes in hemoglobin F levels during the first two years of life in normal and heterozygous ß-thalassemia infants. Pediatrics 69: 734–738

Milman N, Cohn J 1984 Serum iron, serum transferrin and transferrin saturation in healthy children without iron deficiency. European Journal of Pediatrics 143: 96–98

Oski F A 1993 The erythrocyte and its disorders. In: Nathan D G, Oski F A (eds) Hematology of infancy and childhood, 4th edn. Saunders, Philadelphia, ch 2

Schnitzer B, Rucknagel D L, Spencer H H, Aikawa M 1971 Erythrocytes: pits and vacuoles as seen with transmission and scanning electron microscopy. Science 173: 251–252

Schröter W, Nafz C 1981 Diagnostic significance of hemoglobin F and A_2 levels in homo- and heterozygous ß-thalassemia during infancy. Helvetia Paediatrica Acta 36: 519–525

Siimes M A, Addiego J E, Dallman P R 1974 Ferritin in serum: diagnosis of iron deficiency and iron overload in infants and children. Blood 43: 581–590

Smith N J, Rosello S, Say M B, Yeya K 1955 Iron storage in the first five years of life. Pediatrics 16: 166–173

Vanier T M, Tyas J F 1966 Folic acid status in normal infants during the first year of life. Archives of Disease in Childhood 41: 658–665

Vanier T M, Tyas J F 1967 Folic acid status in premature infants. Archives of Disease in Childhood 42: 57–61

Weinberg A G, Rosenfeld C R, Manroe B L, Browne R 1985 Neonatal blood cell count in health and disease. II. Values for lymphocytes, monocytes and eosinophils. Journal of Pediatrics 106: 462–466

Zago M A, Wood W G, Clegg J B et al 1979 Genetic control of F cells in human adults. Blood 53: 977–986

Zaizov R, Matoth Y 1976 Red cell values on the first postnatal day during the last 16 weeks of gestation. American Journal of Hematology 1: 275–278

2 Microcytic and macrocytic anaemias

Though not consistently satisfactory, the MCV is a practical starting point for classification of anaemias.

Microcytosis 14
Iron deficiency anaemia 14
Congenital atransferrinaemia 18
Anaemia of chronic disease 18
Antibody to transferrin receptor 18
Sideroblastic anaemias 20
Congenital erythropoietic protoporphyria 22
Congenital microcytic anaemia with iron overload 22
Haemoglobinopathies 22

Macrocytosis 32
Cobalamin deficiency 34
Folate deficiency 38
Hypothyroidism 40
Vitamin C deficiency 40
Thiamine deficiency 40
Copper deficiency 40
Congenital dyserythropoietic anaemias 40
Chromosomal disorders, liver disease 42
Marrow hypoplasia 44
Erythroblastopenia 53
Osteopetrosis 56
Other marrow pathology 56
Drugs and macrocytosis 56
Pearson's syndrome 56
Hereditary orotic aciduria 56
Lesch-Nyhan syndrome 58
Other causes of macrocytosis 58

Abbreviations and notes

cbl: cobalamin; CDA: congenital dyserythropoietic anaemia/s; DAT: direct antiglobulin (Coombs) test; DEB: diepoxybutane; hct: haematocrit; HE: hereditary elliptocytosis; HPFH: hereditary persistence of fetal Hb; IF: intrinsic factor; LDH: lactate dehydrogenase; PNH: paroxysmal nocturnal haemoglobinuria; TC: transcobalamin; TEC: transient erythroblastopenia of childhood; thal: thalassaemia/ic.

Photomicrographs: blood films are × 480 unless otherwise stated.

Electrophoretic patterns in figures are at pH 8.6.

Microcytic anaemias, microcytosis

Microcytosis (Table 2.1) is almost always due to impaired formation of haem or of globin and is usually associated with hypochromia. Causes will be considered in their order of listing in the table.

Table 2.1 Red cell microcytosis in childhood

Impaired formation of Hb
Haem
Fe
Deficit of total body Fe (Table 2.2)
Defective transport of Fe to marrow
Congenital atransferrinaemia
Defective utilization by erythroblasts
Chronic disease
Antibody to transferrin receptor
Expanded red cell mass
Protoporphyrin
Hereditary sideroblastic anaemias
Ferrochelatase
Plumbism
Erythropoietic protoporphyria
Congenital microcytic anaemia with iron overload
Globin
Haemoglobinopathies
Thalassaemias
Structural variants[1]
Fragmentation[1]

[1] Rarely associated with low MCV

IRON DEFICIENCY ANAEMIA

The commonest anaemia of childhood.

Blood changes (Fig. 2.1)

Anaemia of a degree (to 1.5 g/dl) which would be fatal if due to recent blood loss is not rare and may be surprisingly well tolerated as a result of effective haemodynamic adjustment.

In addition to the MCV, the MCH and MCHC (less sensitive) may be low. Some distortion of shape is common — elliptocytosis, target cells and minor fragmentation. The severity of these changes is roughly proportional to the severity of the anaemia (compare thalassaemia, p. 24).

A population of normal cells indicates evolving disease or the early stages of recovery. Polychromasia and basophilic stippling may be noted in recovery. Reticulocytes may appear increased, but not when corrected for hct (reticulocytes % × actual hct/normal hct for age). Erythroblasts are sparse in blood films and may be small and show irregular haemoglobinization (Fig. 2.1), nuclear budding and fragmentation, and multinuclearity.

Thrombocytosis (to $> 1000 \times 10^9/l$) is not uncommon and may last for some weeks after the start of treatment. Thrombocytopenia (mild to moderate only) is rare, and recovers with treatment. Hypersegmentation of neutrophil nuclei suggests accompanying covert folate lack (Das et al 1978).

Combination with other features will produce unusual appearances:

- With macrocytosis and pyknocytosis in the neonate, (Fig. 2.1).
- With HE. Elliptocytosis is excessive for the anaemia and microcytosis; HE will be found in parent/s.
- With thalassaemia minor. Iron status should be assessed routinely in work-up for suspected thalassaemia (p. 32).
- With polycythaemia in cyanotic congenital heart disease (Fig. 3.4).
- Other associations are occasionally seen (Fig. 2.1).

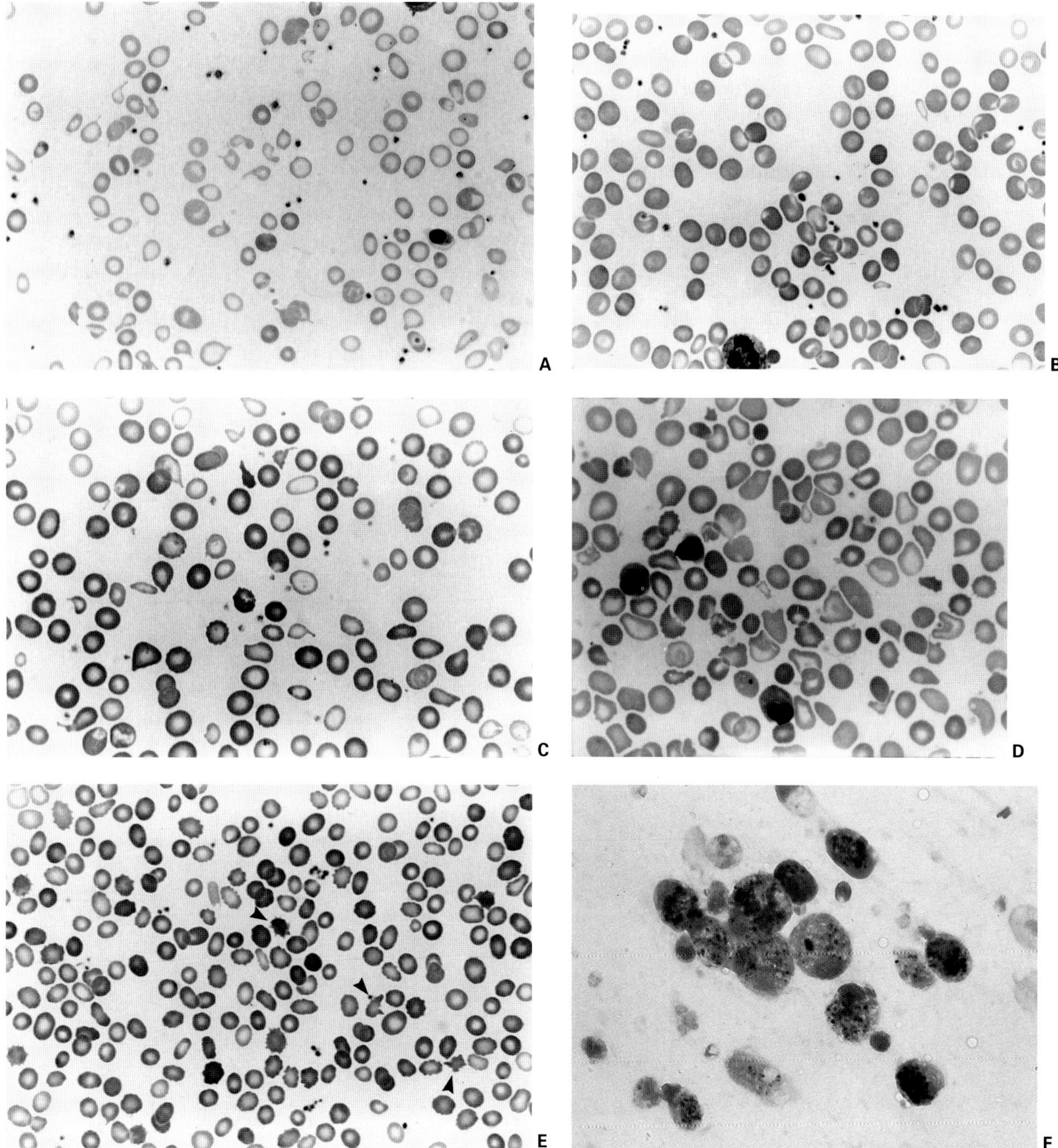

Fig. 2.1 Iron deficiency anaemia. **a** 9-month-old child, Hb 4.0 g/dl, MCV 49 fl, cow's milk colitis. Erythroblast shows defective haemoglobinization. **b** 9-year-old child with bouts of vomiting (causing gastritis and bleeding), somnolence and self-mutilation, ?diencephalic syndrome; note dimorphism. Hb 8.2 g/dl, MCV 62 fl. **c,d** 2 neonates with low normal MCV and a population of microcytic cells from chronic fetomaternal blood loss. **c** 8 days old, Hb 7.9 g/dl; maternal HbF at 10 days 2.5%. **d** 2 days old, Hb 10.8 g/dl, reticulocytes 27%; note also cell distortion, erythroblastosis and spherocytosis. **e** Acanthocytosis (examples arrowed) with a microcytic, hypochromic population in a 2-year-old boy with hypo-β–lipoproteinaemia and iron deficiency from malabsorption, t(14;18) associated; Hb 8.2 g/dl, MCV 63 fl. **f** Iron-laden macrophages in sputum, idiopathic pulmonary haemosiderosis (Perls × 500).
d Courtesy of Dr J O'Duffy

Clinical history (Table 2.2)

Diet

The commonest cause is failure to introduce iron-containing foods at the time (5–6 months for full-term infants) when the endowment of iron in the last trimester has been exhausted. This timing also coincides with onset of a 2–3 year period of rapid growth. Anaemia may occur before 6 months in premature infants because of curtailment of iron endowment in pregnancy, and anaemia after 2 years should arouse suspicion of causes other than dietary deficiency (Fig. 2.1).

Pica is a significant factor if material ingested has an affinity for iron, e.g. clay. Pica itself may be ameliorated by correction of iron deficiency (McDonald & Marshall 1964). Lead poisoning may be associated with iron deficiency (Yip et al 1981). Absorption of lead may be increased in iron deficiency, as lead and iron share a common absorptive mechanism whose activity is enhanced in iron deficiency.

Malabsorption

Malabsorption is a cause of (treatment-unresponsive) iron deficiency anaemia, but anaemia is usually not severe.

Malabsorption in cystic fibrosis is rarely associated with iron deficiency anaemia, though treatment with iron increases Hb in some patients (Shepherd et al 1984).

A microcytic anaemia may occur in scurvy, requiring both iron and vitamin C for correction; however, the characteristic though uncommon anaemia of scurvy is normocytic normochromic and responds to ascorbic acid alone (Oski 1990).

A specific malabsorption for iron has been proposed (Buchanan & Sheehan 1981).

Blood/iron loss

Cow's milk enteropathy causes bleeding which stops usually within 3–4 days of withdrawal of milk. Enteropathy does not occur if introduction of milk is delayed until after 5 months.

In coeliac disease, iron deficiency is due predominantly to blood loss from inflamed mucosa and, to a lesser extent, to anorexia. Malabsorption does not appear to be important — orally administered iron is absorbed. In inflammatory bowel disease iron deficiency anaemia may be associated with the anaemia of chronic disease (p. 18). In Meckel's diverticulum, blood loss is due to erosion of gastric mucosa in the diverticulum and may be sudden or chronic.

Frequent blood taking is an important cause of anaemia in infants. In the newborn with iron deficiency (Fig. 2.1) there may be a history of an obstetric procedure such as fetal version in early pregnancy, and an increase in HbF may be demonstrable in maternal blood; a satisfactory explanation, however, is often not found. In idiopathic pulmonary haemosiderosis, iron-containing macrophages may be demonstrated in sputum (Fig. 2.1) or gastric aspirate (macrophages originating in lung); anaemia occurs because the pulmonary macrophages do not re-enter the circulation.

Loss in urine of iron (carried with transferrin) may occur in nephrosis (Ellis 1977), and haemoglobinuria and haemosiderinuria are notable in prosthetic heart valve surgery and PNH.

Table 2.2 Iron deficiency in childhood

Deficient intake
Diet
Malabsorption
Pica
Gastric resection
Lymphoma of bowel
Scurvy (?)
Specific malabsorption for Fe
Excessive loss
Gastrointestinal blood loss
Cow's milk enteropathy
Coeliac disease
Inflammatory bowel disease — Crohn's, ulcerative colitis
Meckel's diverticulum
Drugs — aspirin, steroids, indomethacin (erosion, platelet dysfunction)
Peptic ulcer
Hookworm
Tumour — lymphoma
Hereditary telangiectasia (rarely a problem before puberty)
Other
Frequent blood taking
Fetomaternal, feto-fetal
Idiopathic pulmonary haemosiderosis
Menstruation
Bleeding into tumours, cysts
Haemodialysis
Urine
Nephrosis
Haemoglobinuria, haemosiderinuria
Expansion of red cell mass — polycythaemia

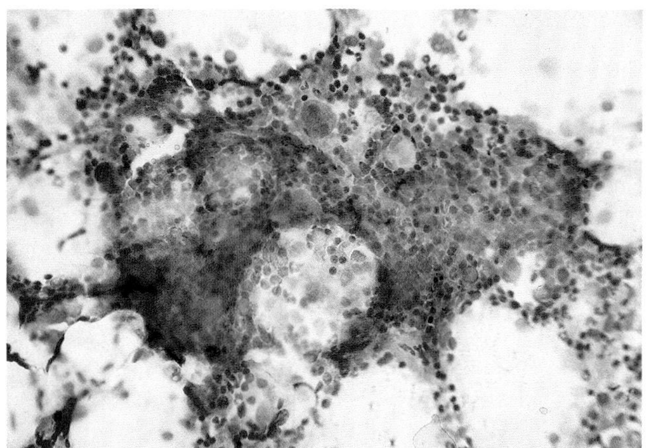

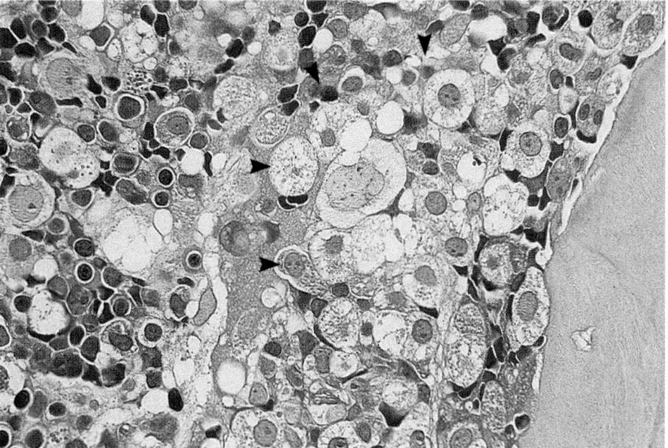

Fig. 2.2 Microcytic anaemia with excess storage iron of undetermined cause in a 23-month-old child: Hb 8.7 g/dl, MCV 52 fl, serum Fe 3 μmol/l, normal ferritin and iron-binding capacity. **a** Marrow fragment with iron-containing macrophages (normally absent at this age), no sideroblasts. **b** Trephine biopsy: group of histiocyte-like cells (arrows, probably reactive) adjacent to normal marrow. The iron pattern is that of anaemia of chronic disease, but there is no clinical evidence of this (well child) and C reactive protein is normal. **a** Perls × 200; **b** H & E × 480

Confirmation of diagnosis (Table 2.3)

A satisfactory response to oral iron (5 mg/kg/day) is indicated by:

- increase in Hb — 1–2 g/dl within 3–4 weeks, and Hb normal in about 2 months (irrespective of severity)
- reticulocytosis — peak at 5–10 days, up to 10% in severe anaemia, minimal rise in mild anaemia
- reappearance of normal cells in blood.

Marrow examination for iron is of no value in proving deficiency in the first years (absence of stores normal), but may be useful for diagnosis of conditions with increased stores, e.g. chronic disease (Fig. 2.2).

Differential diagnosis

Inadequate response to oral iron may be due to:

- failure to take medication, or discontinuance because of gastric irritation
- persisting blood loss
- infection
- missed diagnosis (Table 2.1, 2.3), e.g. occult malabsorption or chronic disease.

CONGENITAL ATRANSFERRINAEMIA

A rare, iron-unresponsive, microcytic anaemia (Table 2.7). Iron is absorbed normally from bowel and deposited in liver and other tissues, but not in marrow. Transferrin deficiency may be confirmed by immunologic methods. Inheritance is autosomal recessive.

ANAEMIA OF CHRONIC DISEASE (Tables 2.3, 2.4, Fig. 2.2)

A common anaemia. Important clues are evidence of active disease (increased C reactive protein, ESR, Igs) and (usually) normal to increased iron stores in marrow.

Anaemia is attributed to subnormal synthesis of transferrin, impaired mobilization of iron from macrophages by transferrin, and subnormal erythropoietin response (Baer et al 1987). Anaemia may be aggravated by circumstances peculiar to individual disorders, e.g. treatment-induced gastric erosion in rheumatoid disorders.

Iron deficiency may be combined with anaemia of chronic disease in, for example, rheumatoid arthritis and inflammatory bowel disease, and may be difficult to diagnose. Serum ferritin is a guide to the likely effectiveness of oral iron — a trial is worthwhile with values < 50 ng/ml, with a good chance of response if < 25 ng/ml (Koerper et al 1978).

ANTIBODY TO TRANSFERRIN RECEPTOR (Table 2.7)

A rare disorder due to inhibition by antibody of incorporation of Fe into erythroblasts. Azathiaprine and steroids are effective.

Table 2.3 Red cell microcytosis in childhood

	Fe deficiency	Chronic disease	Thal minor
Hb, g/dl	down to ~ 2.0	usu > 7	usu > 9
MCV, fl	often < 50	usu > 50 (may be n)	usu > 50
rbc changes*	∝ anaemia	∝ anaemia	excessive for anaemia
Dimorphic rbc	often	often	0
Stippling	unusual	variable	variable
RCC	∝ anaemia	∝ anaemia	n to ↑
MCV/RCC	usu > 13		usu < 13
s ferritin	↓	n to ↑	n
Fe	↓	↓	n
Tf (TIBC)	↑	↓	n
Tf satn	↓	n to ↓	n
CRP	n	↑	n
Response to oral Fe	good	0 to poor	0
HbF, EPP	n	n	see text
FEP	↑	↑	n
Marrow			
Storage Fe	↓	n to ↑	n to ↑
Sideroblasts	↓	↓	n

* Poikilocytosis, elliptocytosis, targets
CRP = C reactive protein; FEP = free erythrocyte protoporphyrin; n = normal; RCC = red cell count; s = serum; satn = saturation; Tf = transferrin; TIBC = transferrin (total) iron binding capacity

Table 2.4 Chronic disease and anaemia in childhood

Infection
- Chronic bacterial/viral, including TB

Inflammation
- Inflammatory bowel disease
  - Crohn's
  - Ulcerative colitis
- Rheumatoid and like disorders
- Castleman's (Keller et al 1972)

Tumour/hyperplasia
- Langerhans cell histiocytosis
- Hodgkin's disease
- Non-Hodgkin lymphoma[1]

[1] Rare chronic lymphomas or in lead-up (may be years) to overt disease

Table 2.5 Sideroblastic anaemias of childhood

Hereditary	
X-linked	Pyridoxine responsive
	Pyridoxine refractory
Autosomal recessive	Pyridoxine responsive
	Pyridoxine refractory
	Thiamine-responsive megaloblastosis (Wolfram's syndrome)
Mitochondrial	Pearson's syndrome
Acquired	
Toxins	Lead
Drugs	Isoniazid
	Chloramphenicol
	Cyclophosphamide
Other	Rheumatoid arthritis
	Antibody-induced
	Pre myeloid leukaemia
	Copper deficiency

SIDEROBLASTIC ANAEMIAS

Sideroblastic anaemias are identified by an excess in marrow (> 10% of nucleated cells) of ringed sideroblasts, with ≥ 4 siderotic, perinuclear granules (iron-laden mitochondria, Fig. 2.3). Sideroblastic marrows usually show some erythroid hyperplasia and megaloblastosis.

Important sideroblastic anaemias of childhood (Table 2.5) are the acquired (especially plumbism), hereditary proper and Pearson's syndrome.

Hereditary sideroblastic anaemia (Fig. 2.3, Table 2.6)

Usually a proportion of cells is microcytic. The MCV however may be normal because some cells are mildly macrocytic. Pappenheimer bodies may occur, especially after splenectomy. Female carriers of the usual (X-linked) form may show a double population of cells, depending on the degree of lyonization. Neutropenia, neutrophil dysfunction, thrombocytopenia and platelet dysfunction occur in some cases, suggesting a broad stem cell defect.

Diagnosis requires marrow examination, and identification as hereditary requires exclusion of acquired causes (Table 2.5).

Anaemia is due to impaired production of haem, with a component of ineffective erythropoiesis from iron loading of mitochondria. ALA synthase deficiency is consistent but non-specific, and ferrochelatase also is deficient in some cases.

The disorder may be subdivided (Table 2.5) according to inheritance and response to pyridoxine (cofactor for ALA synthase). Anaemia manifests at any age from a few months to 7–8 years. Manifestations are indistinguishable for X-linked (the most common) and other types of inheritance.

Thiamine-responsive megaloblastosis (Wolfram's syndrome)

See page 40.

Pearson's syndrome

See page 216.

Table 2.6 Hereditary sideroblastic anaemia vs iron deficiency

	Hereditary sideroblastic anaemia	Iron deficiency
MCV	n to ↓	↓
Blood film: siderocytes	often	0
Reticulocytes	n to ↓	n to slight ↑
Serum		
Fe	↑	↓
Iron-binding capacity	↓	↑
Transferrin saturation	↑	↓
Free erythrocyte protoporphyrin	n	↑
Haptoglobin	↓	n
Marrow		
Sideroblasts	↑, ringed	↓
Storage iron	n to ↑	↓

Table 2.7 Rare microcytic anaemias

	Serum Fe	Serum Fe-binding capacity	Marrow Fe	Liver Fe	Reference
Congenital atransferrinaemia	↓	↓↓	↓	↑	Goya et al 1972
Congenital microcytic anaemia with iron overload	↑	↓	↓	↑	Stavem et al 1985
Antibody (IgM) to transferrin receptor[2]	↑	n	0	↑[1]	Larrick & Hyman 1984

[1] Inferred from ferrokinetics
[2] Described in an adult

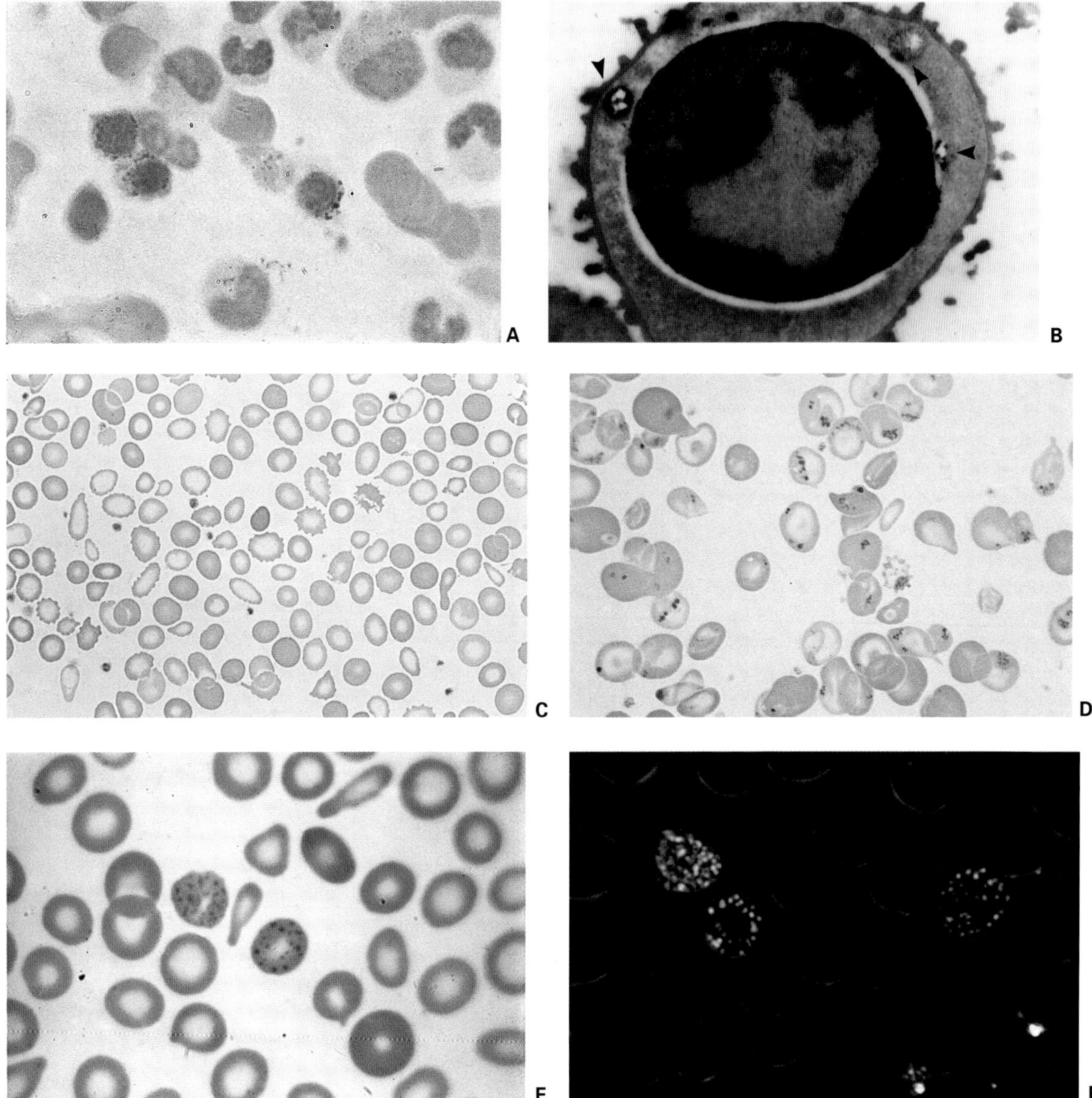

Fig. 2.3 Sideroblastic anaemias. **a–d** hereditary; **e,f** plumbism. **a** Marrow (Perls), ringed sideroblasts. **b** Erythroblast containing iron in perinuclear mitochondria (arrows). **c** blood film, dimorphic population of hypochromic and normal cells. **d** Another boy, post-splenectomy; numerous cells contain Pappenheimer bodies. **e** Stippled and hypochromic cells, Hb 8.6 g/dl. **f** Same child, stippled cells in dark-field illumination. **a** × 1200; **b** × 7000; **c** × 480; **d** × 630; **e,f** × 1200

Acquired sideroblastic anaemias

Plumbism (Piomelli 1993)

Chronic intake of a substantial burden of lead is a cause of ringed sideroblastosis. A low intake (e.g. petrol) does not produce haematologic effects, while acute industrial exposure, which is likely to produce haemolysis, is not a childhood risk.

Plumbism may be combined with, and enhanced by, iron deficiency in children with pica (p. 16). Microcytic anaemia in lead poisoning appears to be due more to coexistent iron deficiency than to lead (Clark et al 1988). Plumbism (including neurologic effects) can occur without microcytosis or anaemia.

Haematologic features useful in distinction from iron deficiency include erythrocyte stippling (often coarse; ribosomal aggregation, Fig. 2.3), poor response to iron treatment and ringed sideroblastosis in marrow. Definitive diagnosis requires estimation of blood lead.

Some of the effects of plumbism may be attributed to inhibition of ferrochelatase, which, effecting the chelation of iron into the protoporphyrin ring, could explain the excess of both protoporphyrin and iron and, being mitochondrial, could also explain the disposition of the excess iron. However, the disposition of the iron may be due rather to interference with transmitochondrial movement (Labbé 1990). Inhibition of pyrimidine-5'-nucleotidase, which cleaves nucleotides remaining after nuclear extrusion, is an explanation for the coarse stippling (ribosomal RNA and mitochondrial fragments) comparable to that in the genetic deficiency (p. 97).

Drugs

Sideroblastosis in patients receiving isoniazid is attributed to impairment in haem synthesis by pyridoxine antagonism (pyridoxine being the cofactor for ALA synthase). Sideroblastosis occurring in (rare) patients receiving chloramphenicol is attributed to diminished synthesis of mitochondrial proteins, including ferrochelatase.

Other causes of sideroblastosis

Ringed sideroblastosis occurs in occasional patients with rheumatoid arthritis (Harvey et al 1987). An (IgG) antibody-induced sideroblastosis is described (Ritchey et al 1979); there was no response to pyridoxine, but cure was achieved with cyclophosphamide.

Pre-leukaemic sideroblastosis is common in adults but rare in childhood. The marrow is likely to show granulocyte/megakaryocyte dysplasia and to have an abnormal karyotype.

For copper deficiency see page 247.

CONGENITAL ERYTHROPOIETIC PROTOPORPHYRIA

A slight microcytosis is common but anaemia is usually minimal, and frank haemolysis, curable by splenectomy, rare (Porter & Lowe 1963). Gallstones may form in childhood. Impairment of haem formation and the more important accumulation of free protoporphyrin in red cells are due to ferrochelatase deficiency. Inheritance is autosomal dominant.

CONGENITAL MICROCYTIC ANAEMIA WITH IRON OVERLOAD

A rare disorder, attributed to ferrochelatase deficiency in marrow erythroblasts. See also Table 2.7.

HAEMOGLOBINOPATHIES (Higgs & Weatherall 1993)

The term 'haemoglobinopathy' is used here in the wide sense for the two major types of haemoglobin pathology — rate of production (thalassaemias) and structure (Hb variants). There is some overlap — for example some structural variants such as HbE are thalassaemic in that production is subnormal.

Investigation for haemoglobinopathy might be considered for:

- microcytosis and hypochromia, especially with 'thalassaemic' changes (see below)
- work-up of a family with an affected member
- origin from an area with known high incidence, e.g. HbC, S in Africans
- unexplained haemolysis
- familial polycythaemia
- unexplained cyanosis.

A suggested schema is given in Table 2.8. In a good 90% of cases, diagnosis can be made with routinely available procedures. Specialized techniques are required for e.g. 'silent' thalassaemia carriers, complex co-inheritance of abnormal genes, 'difficult' minor cases of α thal, antenatal diagnosis and familial polycythaemia.

Only the more common disorders diagnosable by routine procedures are considered here (Tables 2.9–2.14). Some clinical aspects are considered first and then laboratory features, in the order in Table 2.8.

Clinical features

- Age at clinical onset

α chain disorders are manifest at birth and persist through life; γ chain abnormalities are manifest at birth and decline thereafter; β chain anomalies (e.g. thalassaemias, HbS) do not manifest till 4–6 months, when β chain production normally peaks (Fig. 2.8e).

- Ethnic background

Examples include the dominance of β thalassaemias in the Mediterranean, α thalassaemias in SE Asia, and HbC, S in Africa.

- Association with other genetic syndromes

The only consistent association is of HbH disease and a mental retardation/dysmorphism syndrome (Wilkie et al 1990a,b); in some of these cases there is a micro-deletion at the α gene locus (16p13.3).

Table 2.8 Laboratory investigations for suspected haemoglobinopathy

Red cell indices
Stained blood film
Reticulocytes (new methylene blue, brilliant cresyl blue)
HbA_2 (column chromatography, elution post-electrophoresis)
HbF (Kleihauer, alkali denaturation)
Hb electrophoresis, pH 8.6, 6.2; 7.0 (HbMs)
Sickle cell prep or dithionite solubility
HbH inclusions (new methylene blue)
Heinz bodies (methyl violet, rhodanile blue)
If spleen intact, incubate 24–48 h or use acetylphenylhydrazine provocation
Unstable Hb (heat denaturation, isopropanol precipitation)
Iron status, + acute phase reactant, e.g. C reactive protein
Pit count (splenic hypofunction)
Hb spectroscopy (methaemoglobin)
Family study
Specialized procedures
Oxygen dissociation
Globin chain synthesis
Globin chain structure
Gene analysis

Table 2.9 β thalassaemias

	Thalassaemic changes in rbc	HbA_2	HbF	HbEPP	Other
β^0					
Heterozygous	mild; from 4–6 months	3.5–7.0%	↑ to 2–5% in some cases	↑A_2; F band may be visible	A_2 may be lowered by severe Fe deficiency or coexistent α thal
Homozygous	severe; from 4–6 months	~2%	~98%	almost all F; some A_2	thal major
β^+					
Heterozygous	mild; from 4–6 months	3.5–7.0%	↑ to 2–5% in some cases	↑A_2; F band may be visible	
Homozygous					
Medit	severe; from 4–6 months	variable	70–95%	mostly F; some A;A_2	thal major or intermedia[1]
Other[2]	mod to severe; from 4–6 months	2.2–5%	20–40%	F,A,A_2	thal intermedia[1]
Heterozygous					
Silent carrier	none	n	n	n	needs globin chain synthesis or gene analysis
'Quiet' carrier	mild	n	n	n	needs globin chain synthesis or gene analysis

Medit = Mediterranean; n = normal; ~ = approximately
[1] Moderate to severe haematologic changes but not requiring regular transfusions
[2] e.g. Negro

Erythrocyte values and morphology

In thalassaemias, in contrast to iron deficiency, red cell changes are excessive for the degree of anaemia and are evident in the absence of anaemia — hypochromia, elliptocytosis, target cell formation, stippling and fragmentation (Table 2.6, Fig. 2.4). Although the MCV is characteristically reduced in thalassaemias, it may be low normal in thalassaemia major because of the presence of large thin cells containing irregular clumps of Hb (leptocytes, Fig. 2.5).

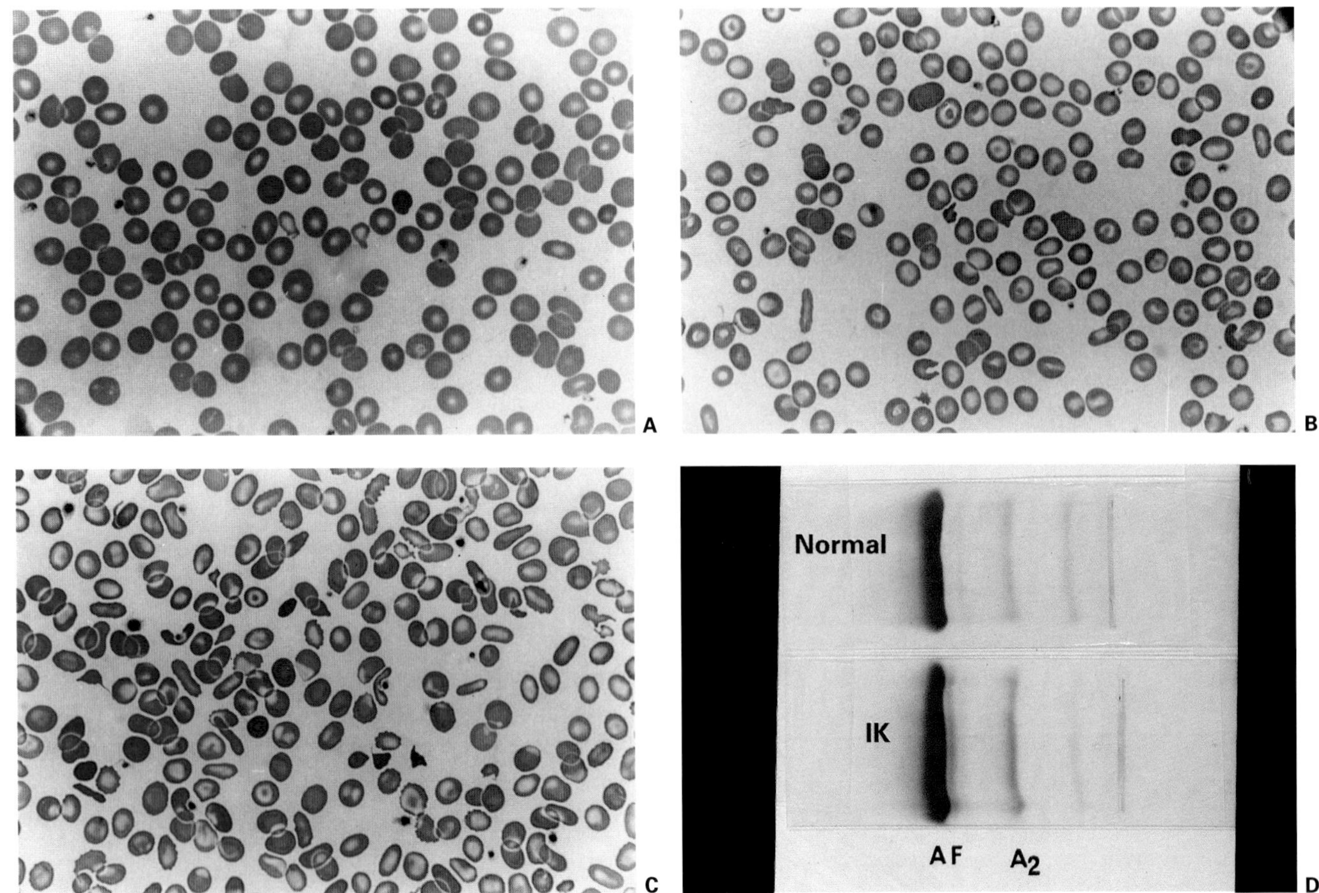

Fig. 2.4 β thal minor, changes from slight to moderate. **a** 12 years, Hb 12.6 g/dl, MCV 74 fl, HbF < 1%, HbA_2 4.9%. **b** 6 years, Hb 9.8 g/dl, MCV 56 fl, HbA_2 5.5%, F < 1%. **c** 12 months, Hb 10.2 g/dl, MCV 51 fl, HbF 2.6%, HbA_2 5.5%. **d** Pattern from a 3-year-old (IK) with HbA_2 6.5% and unusually high F (10%).

Table 2.10 α thalassaemias

	Thalassaemic changes in rbc	HbA_2	HbF	HbEPP	Other
α-thal 2	0 to minimal	n	n	1–3% Bart's (γ4) at birth	trace of Bart's at birth in some normal infants
α-thal 1	mild; from birth	n	n	H < 2%; 2–10% Bart's at birth	
HbH disease	severe; from birth	< 2%	n	H 5–40%, Bart's usually < 5%. At birth, H 10–40%, Bart's 15–25%. In SE Asia, CS band common	
Hb Bart's hydrops	severe; at birth	< 2%	0	Bart's 70–80%, Portland ($\zeta_2\gamma_2$) 10–15%, H < 5%. No or trace F,A	death in utero or within hours of (usually) premature birth

CS = Hb Constant Spring; n = normal

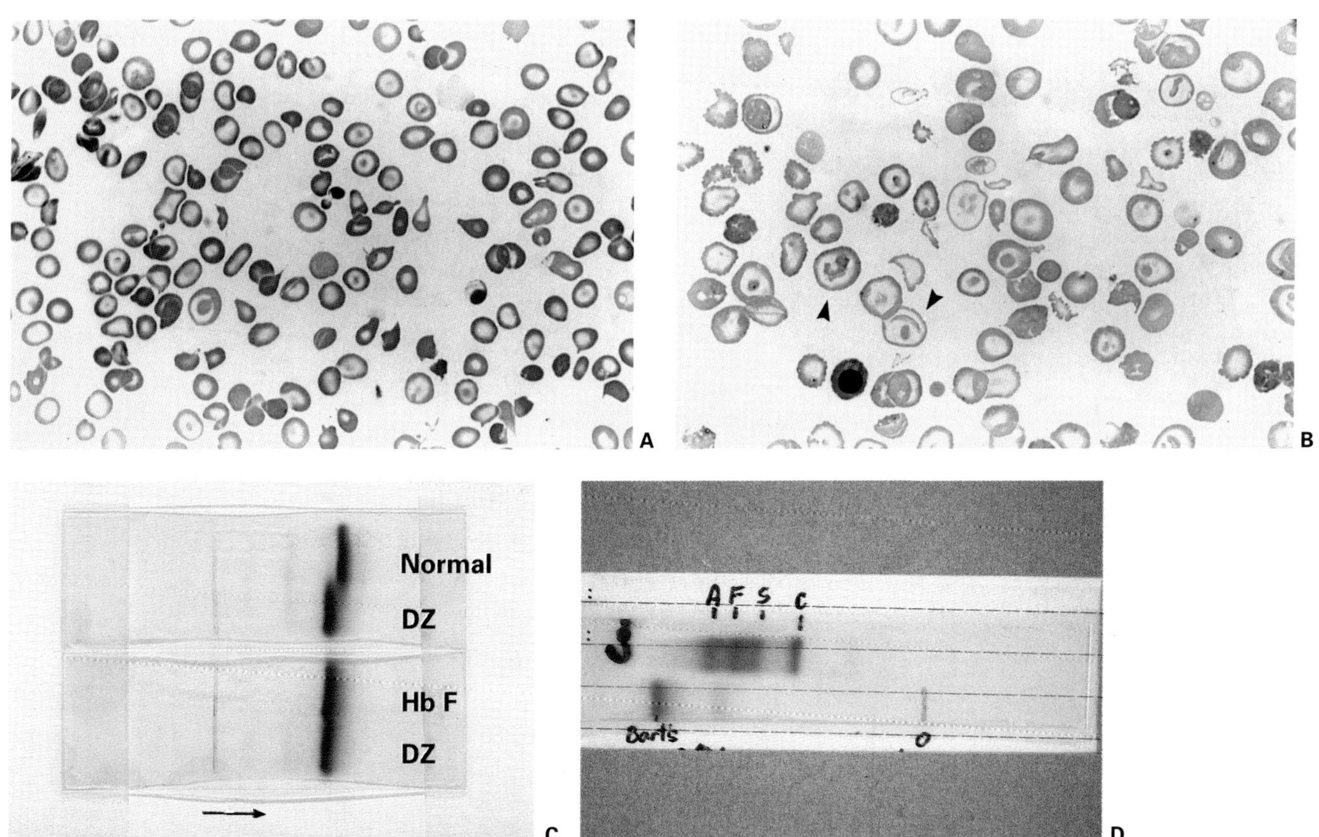

Fig. 2.5 Major thalassaemias. **a** Dβ° thal, 11 years, Hb 8.2 g/dl, MCV 62 fl, HbD 94%, A_2 4.2%, F 1.5%, no A. **b** Hb Bart's hydrops, death hours after premature (31 weeks) birth; Hb 4.2 g/dl, MCV 101 fl (n > 106); leptocytes (arrows). **c** β°β° thal, 10 months (DZ); Hb is almost entirely F. **d** Hb Bart's hydrops, showing Bart's and a faint unidentified band between A and F; O = origin. **a** Courtesy of Dr D Gill. **b** Courtesy of Dr R Rodwell

Thalassaemias may coexist with other common disorders such as hereditary elliptocytosis (Figs 2.6, 3.6), G6PD deficiency (Fig. 3.16) or iron deficiency. Assessment of iron status should be routine in the work-up for haemoglobinopathy.

Target cells occur in most thalassaemias and are conspicuous in some structural variants (especially homozygous), e.g. C and E (Fig. 2.7).

Sickle cells (Fig. 2.8) occur in sickle cell anaemia (SS), and to a lesser degree the double heterozygote with, for example, β thal, C, D, δβ thal.

Fig. 2.6 (facing page) α thalassaemia. **a** (new methylene blue × 1200), HbH inclusions (large arrow), reticulocyte (small arrow). **b** 1-day-old infant with α thal -2, showing 7% Hb Bart's. **c** 3-year-old (BT) with HbH disease, showing a fast H band; ca = carbonic anhydrase, O = origin. **d** double heterozygote for α thal (from father, --/αα), and hereditary elliptocytosis (from mother), 7 years, Hb 11.7 g/dl, MCV 61 fl.

Table 2.11 Less common thalassaemias

	Thalassaemic changes in rbc	HbA_2	HbF	HbEPP	Other
δβ (high F thal)					
Heterozygous	mild; from 4–6 months	n or ↓	5–15%, heterogeneous distribution	F band	
Homozygous	mod; from 4–6 months	↓	100%	F only	thal intermedia
δβ fusion (Lepore)					
Heterozygous	mild; from 4–6 months	n	↑ to 2–3%, in most cases	Lepore 8–20%	
Homozygous	mod to severe; from 4–6 months	↓	~ 80%	Lepore ~ 20%, F ~ 80%	thal intermedia
CS					
Heterozygous	0 to minimal	n	n	CS 0.5–0.8%. At birth 1–2% Bart's	+ 2 deleted α genes → HbH disease
γδβ					
Heterozygous	mild, from birth; ↓ with age but do not disappear	n or ↓	↓ in neonate	↓F; no Bart's (γ4) or H(β4)	neonatal haemolysis; evolves to nA_2F β thal; homozygote not observed (probably non-viable)

CS = Constant Spring; n = normal; ~ = approximately

Table 2.12 Common structural variants of haemoglobin

	Anaemia	MCV	rbc morphology	HbA_2	HbF	HbEPP	Other
SA	no	n	n or a few targets	n	n	S 30–45%*	pos HbS tests
SS	mod to severe; from 4–6 months	n	sickle cells; targets+; often autosplenectomy	usu n; occ sl ↑	5–20%, heterogeneous distribution	S 80–95%; F 5–20%	pos HbS tests
EA	n	sl ↓	1–10% target cells	n	n	E(+A_2) 20–35%	E is mildly unstable
EE	sl	↓	many targets		n	E(+A_2) > 90%; rest = F	
CA	0 to sl	↓	10–30% targets			C ~ 40%, A ~ 60%	
CC	sl	↓	many targets; irregularly contracted cells; crystals, esp post-splenectomy			C ~ 95%; F	

* Proportion of HbS is lower if α thal is co-inherited
esp = especially; mod = moderate; n = normal; occ = occasionally; sl = slight; usu = usually; ~ = approximately

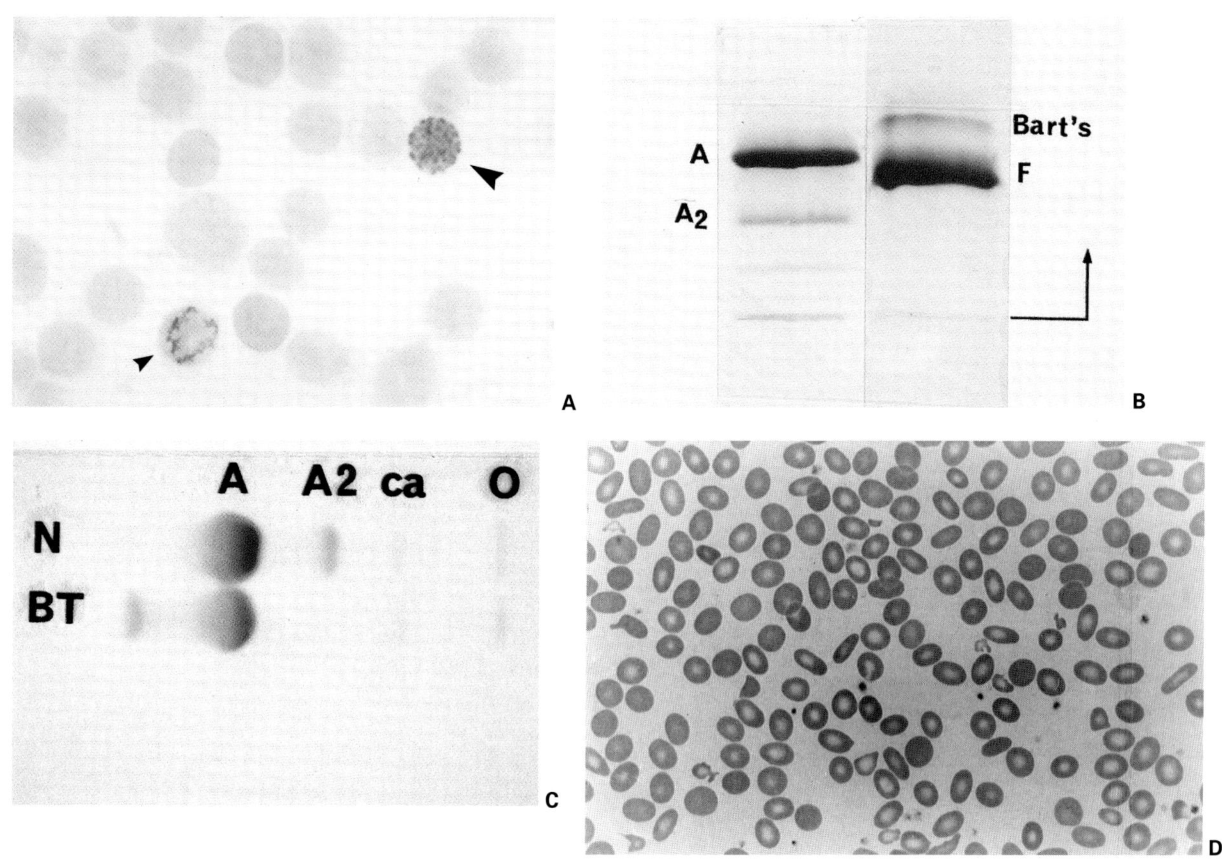

Table 2.13 Some doubly heterozygous haemoglobinopathies

	Anaemia	MCV	rbc morphology	HbA_2	HbF	HbEPP	Other
$S\beta^0$ thal	usu severe; from 4–6 months	↓	severe thal; many targets (more than in SS); occ sickles	↑, to 5%	↑, to 10%	S 85%, A 0, A_2 5%, F 10%	sickle cell anaemia
$S\beta^+$ thal, Medit	usu severe; from 4–6 months	↓	as above	↑, to 5%	↑, to 5%	S 80%, A 10%, A_2 5%, F 5%	sickle cell anaemia
$S\beta^+$ thal, Negro	mild	↓	mild thal	↑, to 5%	↑, to 5%	S 65%, A 25%, A_2 5%, F 5%	
SC	mild to mod; from 4–6 months	sl ↓	many targets (about 50% of cells); SC poikilocytes with bent crystals; occ sickles; occ autosplenectomy			S ~ 50%, C ~ 50%	
$E\beta$ thal	severe; from 4–6 months	↓	severe thal	A_2 ~ 5% by HPLC		E(+A_2) 60–70%; F 30–40%; some A in $E\beta^+$ thal	thal major or (less often) intermedia
$C\beta$ thal	mod to severe; from 4–6 months	↓	many targets			C 65–95%, F 5–35%; lower values for C and some A if thal is β^+	

HPLC = high pressure liquid chromatography; Medit = Mediterranean; mod = moderate; occ = occasional; sl = slight; usu = usually; ~ = approximately

Splenic hypofunction is common in sickle cell disorders: Howell-Jolly bodies appear and 'pocked' erythrocytes increase (Fig. 2.8b). Hypofunction is early and severe in SS and Sβ^0 thal (at 6 months to 3 years, when the spleen is anatomically enlarged). After 6–8 years the spleen commonly becomes shrunken from infarction and fibrosis ('autosplenectomy'). Hypofunction is later in onset and less frequent in SC and Sβ^+ thal (Pearson et al 1985).

Angular crystals, which may distort cell shape, are characteristic of HbC disorders: CC, and to a lesser extent SC and C thal (Fig. 2.7, Bain 1993). They are more numerous after dehydration of cells for a few hours in 3% NaCl (Ringelhann & Khorsandi 1972), and after splenectomy.

Shrunken cells, sometimes bitten-out, may occur in unstable haemoglobinopathies (Fig. 2.9). Coarse inclusions of precipitated Hb (coarser than stippling and Pappenheimer bodies) occur in some unstable haemoglobinopathies (e.g. Bristol, Hammersmith) and rare 'inclusion-body' thalassaemias (Beris et al 1988). They increase strikingly after splenectomy.

Table 2.14 Thalassaemia intermedia; some possible origins

β thal
$\beta^0\beta^+$, some cases
$\beta^+\beta^+$, some cases
$\beta^+\beta^+$ with coexisting α thal or HPFH
β^0 + triplicated α thal
$E\beta^+$ or $E\beta^0$
δβ thal
Homozygous
$\delta\beta$-β^0
Lepore
Homozygous

In HPFH there are no or minimal changes in erythrocyte indices and morphology. There are no haematologic changes in the congenital methaemoglobinaemias (lack of polycythaemia is attributed to segregation of the metHb in a subpopulation of the oldest cells).

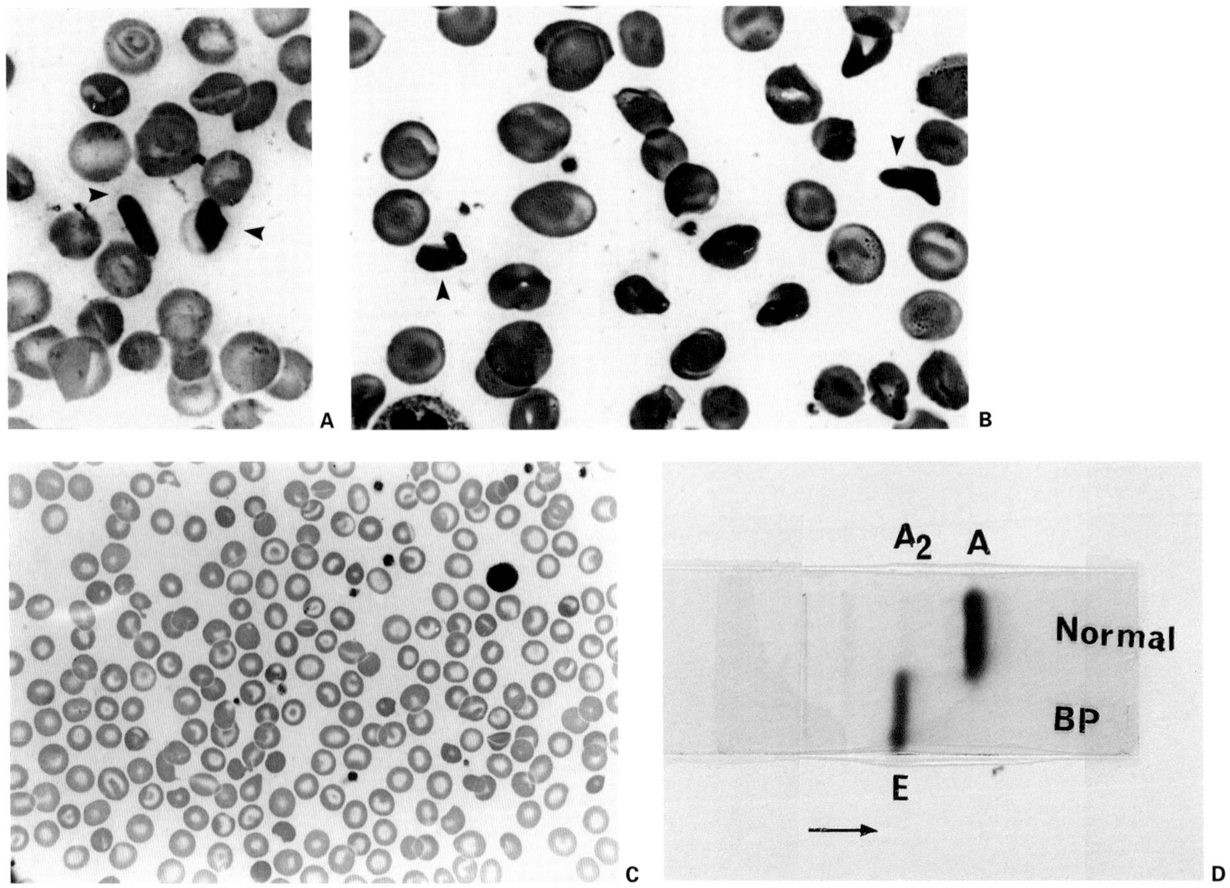

Fig. 2.7 C and E haemoglobinopathies. Crystals (arrows) in CC (**a**) and SC (**b**). Crystals in **b** are 'bent'. **c,d** EE, microcytosis and target cells, Hb 10.7 g/dl, MCV 59 fl, no HbA on electrophoresis. **a,b** × 950

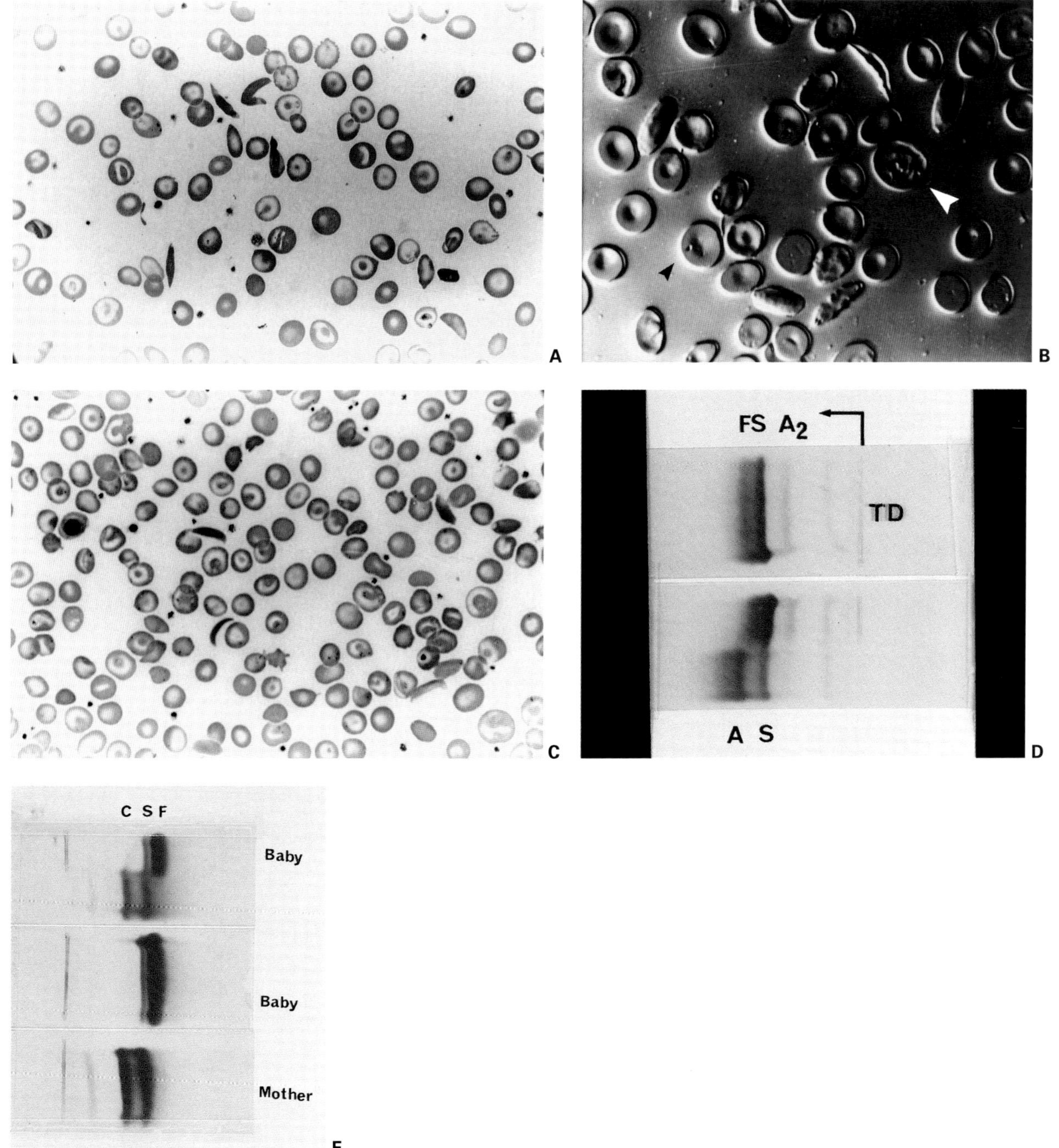

Fig. 2.8 HbS disorders. **a,b** Sβ^+ thal (African), 7 years, Hb 7.1 g/dl, MCV 83 fl, HbS 54%, A 36%, A_2 8.9%, F 0.5%. **a** Target and sickle cells. **b** (Normaski optics × 750): sickles and cells with pits (arrows); pit count 16% (n < 3.5%), suggesting splenic hypofunction. **c** Sβ° (Mediterranean), 3 years, Hb 8.2 g/dl, MCV 67 fl, HbS 71%, F 25%, no A; film shows targets and sickles. **d** Sβ° thal, 4 years (TD); S 69, F 27, A_2 4%, no A. **e** S trait in a 1-day-old infant (mother SC); HbS 10%, F 90%; S had increased to 17% 2 weeks later. **c** Courtesy of Dr D Gill

Reticulocytes in β thal major are low for the anaemia because of damage to erythroblasts by insoluble α chains. In α thalassaemias, reticulocytes are higher because erythroblasts are little affected, anaemia being due mainly to damage by the more soluble β and γ chains to mature erythrocytes. With structural variants also (e.g. S and C), counts tend to be high because anaemia is predominantly haemolytic. A brisk drop in reticulocyte count with worsening of anaemia should raise a suspicion of parvovirus. These episodes usually turn off spontaneously after about 10 days.

HbF

An increase in HbF occurs in haemoglobinopathies (Tables 2.9–2.13), and HPFH.

In HPFH pancellular type, HbF is 15–35% in the heterozygote and 100% in the homozygote. In the heterocellular form, which may be regarded as an expansion of the normal, small population of HbF-containing (F) cells, HbF is lower — in the homozygote, to 30%. The trait has, in some families, X-linked dominant inheritance (Miyoshi et al 1988).

HbA_2

Increase is characteristic of β thalassaemias (Table 2.9). Increase may occur in folate and B_{12} deficiency (to 6.0%, Alperin et al 1977). In β thal heterozygotes, iron deficiency may diminish the level to mask the diagnosis; this however appears to be significant only in severe deficiency. HbA_2 is low in HbH disease and HPFH.

Hb electrophoresis

Mobilities of common haemoglobins are shown in Figures 2.4–2.10.

Less than half of unstable haemoglobins have abnormal mobility. Separation of HbMs from HbA requires special treatment (Table 2.15, compare acquired methaemoglobinaemia, Fig. 3.11e).

HbH inclusions (Fig. 2.6)

Assiduous search is required in the 2α gene deletion, while inclusions cannot usually be detected in the one gene deletion.

Table 2.15 Some causes of cyanosis

	HbMs	**Reductase deficiency**[1]	**Underoxygenation**
Cause of cyanosis	metHb	metHb	↑ de-oxyHb
Clinical effects of cyanosis	minimal	minimal	anoxaemic distress
Haematologic effects	sl ↑ retics in some types	0	0
Defect	globin aminoacid substitution	cytochrome b reductase	underoxygenation
Blood colour	brown	brown	blue-purple
Effect of oxygenation (shake with air)	no change	no change	becomes pink
Absorption spectrum	2 peaks, wavelengths shorter than normal	normal (peaks at 502, 632 nm)	normal
+KCN	little or no change	632 nm peak abolished	632 nm peak abolished
Electrophoresis			
pH 8.6	most are normal	normal	normal
pH 7.1 after conversion to metHb by ferricyanide	most are abnormal — slower than normal metHb	normal (metHb slower than oxyHb)	normal
Amount of metHb	α chain: 20–30% of Hb β: 40–50%	genetic: 10–40% acquired: often > 40%	
Oxidant chemicals	rarely relevant	important precipitant (Table 2.16)	not relevant
Inheritance	aut dominant	genetic type aut recessive	normal

[1] Genetic deficiency or transient physiologic deficiency in the neonate

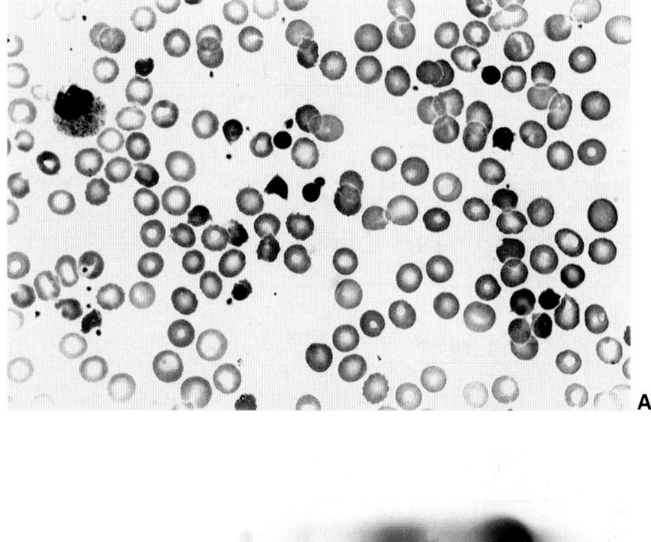

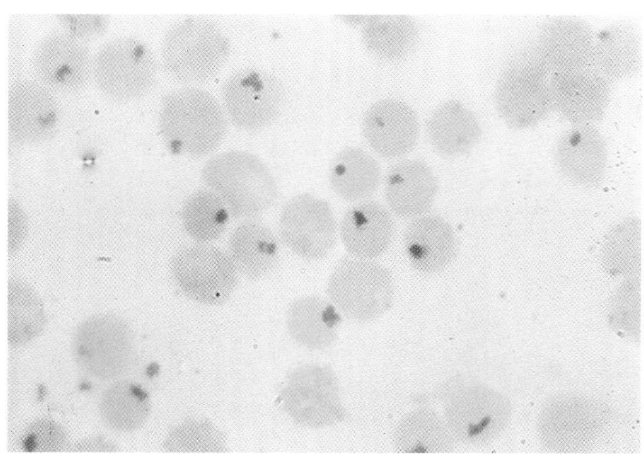

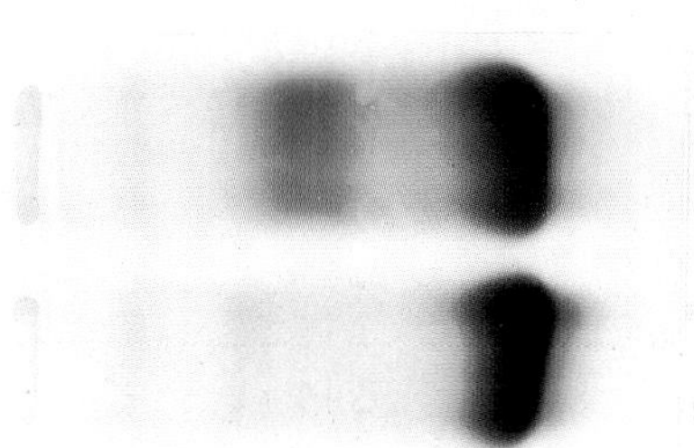

Fig. 2.9 Hb Köln. **a** Irregularly contracted cells and occasional spherocyte. **b** Post splenectomy: numerous Heinz bodies (methyl violet × 950). **c** Showing abnormal band (normal below) (naphthalene black).

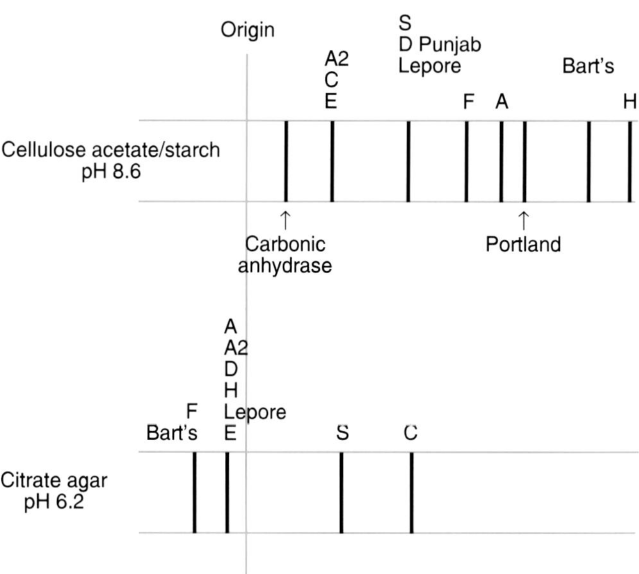

Fig. 2.10 Relative mobilities of the more common haemoglobins.

Heinz bodies

Excessive numbers are an important sign of unstable Hb. The count may be increased by prolonged incubation or by provocation with acetylphenylhydrazine. Numbers may be spectacular (and size larger) after splenectomy (Fig. 2.16), or in some types (Hb Köln) after ingestion of sulphonamides.

Unstable haemoglobins

Some haemoglobins not ordinarily classified as unstable, e.g. E, F, H, give a slight deposit in precipitation tests. Some rare variants (e.g. Geneva) are so unstable that little of the abnormal Hb can be detected.

An increase in Heinz bodies is common, but may be equivocal in unsplenectomized subjects. An abnormal band (10–30% of Hb) is noted on electrophoresis in about half the cases (Fig. 2.9); the abnormal Hb is more conspicuous after splenectomy or if there is co-inheritance of β thal to reduce the amount of HbA.

Morphologic changes are usually mild and include shrinkage, bites, slight microcytosis attributed to loss of membrane and Hb by splenic culling of Hb precipitates, prominent stippling and coarse inclusions (in Hb Bristol, Hammersmith, Geneva). In rare β chain variants (Indiannapolis, Geneva), considerable instability results in a thalassaemic phenotype, with increased A_2 and inclusions of α chains (Beris et al 1988).

Haemolysis is mild in some types (Köln) and severe in others (Hammersmith, Bristol). Haemolysis is evident in the neonate in the α and γ chain anomalies; in γ chain variants haemolysis is transient and mild (3 normal γ genes to compensate). In the (more common) β chain anomalies, e.g. Köln, haemolysis does not manifest until 4–6 months. Haemolysis may be worsened by fever and, in Hb Köln, ingestion of sulphonamides.

Some types have altered oxygen affinity, more often increased than decreased. In high affinity variants (e.g. Köln), anaemia tends to be mild as a result of erythropoietin stimulation.

Autosomal dominant inheritance is evident in about two thirds of cases, with the remainder, especially those with high O_2 affinity, attributed to spontaneous mutation. The homozygous state is presumed, in most instances at least, to be incompatible with life.

Iron status

Assessment is important for distinguishing thalassaemia from iron deficiency and for recognition of co-occurrence.

Pitted (pocked) cell count

A useful confirmation of splenic hypofunction (p. 108 and Fig. 2.8b).

Hb spectroscopy

This is the most reliable method for recognition of HbMs, a rare cause of cyanosis. Characteristics which distinguish HbMs from more common causes of cyanosis are given in Table 2.15. Drugs/chemicals which may induce methaemoglobinaemia are listed in Table 2.16.

Family history

The haemoglobinopathies, with a few exceptions (some unstable haemoglobinopathies), have negligible mutation rates and can be traced through the generations. Compound abnormalities with similar phenotypes, e.g. SS and $S\beta^0$ thal, can be clarified by examination of parents and sibs. In addition, the silent carrier (no lab abnormality by routine methods) or quiet carrier (minimal abnormality) can be inferred in a parent whose child is more severely affected than the other parent.

Macrocytic anaemias, macrocytosis

Spurious macrocytosis may be due to:

- cold agglutination
- uncontrolled diabetes mellitus (ingress of water faster than egress of glucose in hypotonic medium of the measuring system).

Genuine macrocytosis may be due to:

- reticulocytosis (greater volume of young erythrocytes)
- fetal erythropoiesis, either appropriate for age, or as a pathological persistence or reactivation
- overhydration, e.g. hereditary hydrocytosis
- defective synthesis of DNA.

Causes of macrocytosis will be discussed in the order set out in Table 2.17.

Table 2.16 Drugs/chemicals which may induce methaemoglobinaemia

Analgesics
  Acetoaminophen (paracetamol)
  Phenacetin
  Antipyrine
  Phenazopyridine (pyridium)
Anaesthetics
  Nitrous oxide
  Local anaesthetics — lignocaine, prilocaine, benzocaine
Antibacterials
  Sulphanilamide
  p-aminosalicylic acid
  Dapsone
  Cetrimide
Antimalarials
  Primaquine
  Pamaquine
  Maloprim
Antihelminthic
  Piperazine
Anticonvulsants
  Phenytoin
Nitrates/nitrites
  Fertilizer-contaminated drinking water
  Preserved meats
  Vasodilators: nitroprusside, nitroglycerol
  'Recreational' drugs: amyl nitrate/nitrite, butyl/isobutyl nitrite
Dyes, solvents or agents used in their manufacture (e.g. for laundry inks, wax crayons)
  Aniline derivatives
  Benzene derivatives
  Phenetidin
  Phenylenediamine
  Phenylhydroxylamine
Other
  Apricot kernels (cyanide)
  Carrots } reductases converting
  Spinach } nitrates to nitrites
  Vitamin K_3 (menadione)
  Methylene blue
  Resorcinol (keratolytic)

Note 1. These agents are more likely to induce oxidant damage if cytochrome b reductase is deficient, either as a temporary physiologic deficiency in the normal neonate, or as the permanent, genetic defect
2. Haemolysis is unusual with these exposures

Table 2.17 Red cell macrocytosis in childhood

Spurious	Cold agglutination Uncontrolled diabetes mellitus
Overhydration	Hereditary hydrocytosis
Expected	Reticulocytosis Normal for age (fetal erythropoiesis)
Deficiency	Cobalamin[1] (Tables 2.20, 2.21) Folate[1] (Table 2.22) Thyroid Vitamin C[1] Thiamine[1] (?) Copper[1]

Other	Dyserythropoiesis
	  Congenital: types I[1], III
	  Acquired
	    Myeloid leukaemias[2]
	      AML M6[1]
	      MDS[1]
	      Monosomy 7 MPD
	      Juvenile CML
	    Drugs[1,3]
	    Post marrow transplant
	    Parvovirus
	Chromosomal disorder
	  Trisomy 21
	  Triploidy
	Liver disease
	Marrow
	  Hypoplasia
	    Panhypoplasia[4]
	    Erythroblastopenia, congenital
	  Osteopetrosis
	  Other replacement
	Drugs[1,3] (Table 2.35)
	Pearson's syndrome
	Hereditary orotic aciduria[1]
	Lesch-Nyhan[1]
	Other

[1] Megaloblastic or likely to be megaloblastic
[2] Macrocytosis may antedate overt manifestations by months to years
[3] Noted in two places as dyserythropoiesis is outstanding with only some drugs
[4] Megaloblastoid dyserythropoiesis is a feature of some syndromes, e.g. Fanconi, in the period preceding frank aplasia

COBALAMIN DEFICIENCY (Cooper et al 1993)

'Cobalamin deficiency' is used here in the broad sense for either total body deficiency or purely cellular starvation. In the total deficiency a fall in serum level precedes anaemia and morphologic changes in blood. A decrease may occur, for obscure reasons, in folate deficiency — cbl rises within 7 days after folate treatment (but will not in true cbl deficiency); a decrease also occurs in the rare genetic TCI deficiency, but is of no pathologic significance as TCI does not transport cbl into cells. Conversely, tissue deficiency may occur with normal serum levels in TCII deficiency and cellular defects of cbl handling.

Cbl deficiencies (Table 2.20, Fig. 2.11) are rare, apart from the infant of the strict vegan nursing mother. The genetic defects are autosomal recessive. Investigations which may be required for megaloblastosis are summarized in Table 2.18.

Disorders of supply/absorption manifest later than disorders of transport to or handling of cbl in cells (Table 2.21), because cbl from general body tissues (e.g. liver) is usable in the first but not the second.

In megaloblastosis of any causation, associated leucopenia and thrombocytopenia may raise a clinical suspicion of leukaemia or aplastic anaemia (Fig. 2.12). Hypersegmentation of neutrophil nuclei ($>2\%$ with 6 lobes or $>5\%$ with ≥ 5 lobes) is common. Increase in serum LDH results from degeneration of erythroblasts in marrow. The sequence of reversal of blood changes after successful treatment is shown in Table 2.19.

Table 2.18 Investigations which may be required for megaloblastosis in childhood

History
- e.g. age at onset, diet, drugs, maternal cobalamin status

Blood
- Serum
  - Cobalamin
  - Folate
  - Antibodies to intrinsic factor, parietal cells
  - Antinuclear factor
  - Transcobalamin II
- Red cell folate
- Lymphoblasts: TCII production

Marrow
- Morphology (marrow may not be required if megaloblasts in blood)

Urine
- Protein
- Formiminoglutamic acid
- Methylmalonic acid
- Homocystine
- Orotic acid

Schilling (urinary excretion) test
- In infants preferably with total body counter to avoid errors from incomplete urine collection, contamination of urine with unabsorbed cobalamin in faeces

Response to treatment
- Folate, cobalamin (Table 2.19)

Fibroblasts
- For defects of cobalamin metabolism

Other tests
- As appropriate for diagnosis of disorders in Table 2.17
- If mother breast-feeding:
  - maternal diet, serum B_{12}, parietal cell and intrinsic factor antibodies

Table 2.19 Reversal of megaloblastosis, sequence of changes

Effacement of megaloblastic change in erythroblasts	<2 days
↑ reticulocyte count	5–10 days
↓ in MCV by >5 fl	<2 weeks
Correction of:	
thrombocytopenia	<2 weeks
neutropenia	<2 weeks
hypersegmentation	<4 weeks
anaemia	3–6 weeks

Table 2.20 Cobalamin deficiency in childhood

Inadequate intake
Breast-fed infant of mother who:
is strict vegan[1]
has pernicious anaemia (untreated or inadequately treated)[2]
Strict veganism
Deficiency or abnormality of intrinsic factor (parietal cells)
Selective (inherited)[1]
Global mucosal deficiency
Gastric atrophy
Juvenile pernicious anaemia[1]
Gastrectomy
Malabsorption (terminal ileum)
Specific
Imerslund-Gräsbeck[1]
Global
Regional ileitis, ileal resection or bypass, coeliac disease[3]
HIV infection
Competition for cobalamin in small intestine
Bacterial overgrowth (diverticulum, blind pouches, anastomoses, fistulae, antibiotics, e.g. neomycin)
Fish tapeworm (*Diphyllobothrium latum*) infestation (eating raw fish)
Defective transport
TCII deficiency[1]
Cellular defects in cobalamin metabolism[1]
Inherited[1]
Prolonged nitrous oxide anaesthesia

[1] Summarized in Table 2.21
[2] Intake may be further impaired by malabsorption due to placentally-transferred anti-IF antibody
[3] Since the lesion is more severe in the upper small bowel, this is more likely to be associated with folate than with cobalamin deficiency

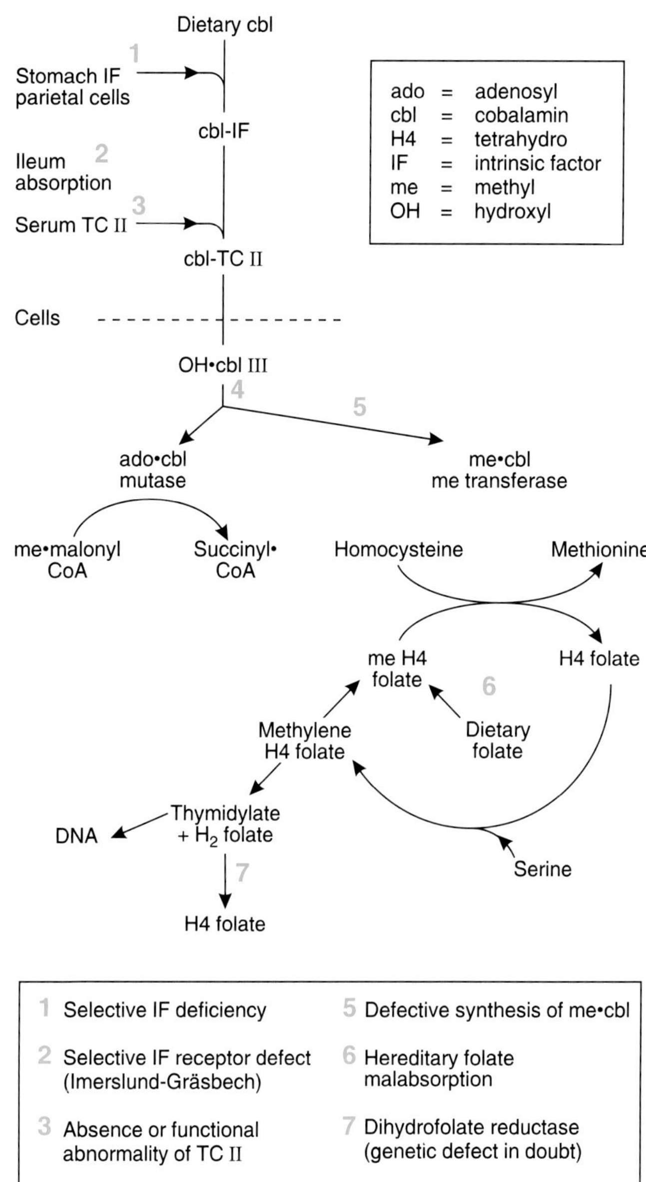

Fig. 2.11 Genetic defects of cobalamin/folate transport and metabolism associated with megaloblastosis.

Breast-fed infant of strict vegan mother (Fig. 2.12, Table 2.21)

Meat, fish and dairy products are the most important sources of cbl, which is derived eventually and exclusively from bacteria (cbl synthesized by colonic flora is not absorbed).

Anaemia is usually severe. Neurologic dysfunction (irritability, convulsions, regression of milestones) may manifest before anaemia. The mother may appear dull or obfuscated, with low or low normal serum cbl.

Juvenile pernicious anaemia (Table 2.21)

The basic lesion (autoimmune gastric atrophy) is similar to that in adults. Autoimmune dysfunction of other tissues (thyroid, parathyroid, adrenal; immune deficiency) may antedate megaloblastosis by some years. The Schilling test is abnormal and correctable by IF.

Congenital absence of or non-functioning IF (Table 2.21)

The stomach mucosa is normal in structure and function except for IF production. The Schilling test is abnormal, with correction by IF.

Selective IF receptor defect (specific cbl malabsorption, Imerslund-Gräsbeck syndrome) (Table 2.21)

The terminal ileum, the site of cbl-IF absorption, is histologically normal. Accompanying (and unexplained) proteinuria and aminoaciduria persist after correction of cbl deficiency. The Schilling test is abnormal, with no correction by IF.

Ileal disease

Malabsorption in HIV infection (Harriman et al 1989) is due to opportunistic infection of the small bowel with microsporidia (Field et al 1993).

Table 2.21 Some cobalamin deficiency states in childhood associated with megaloblastosis

	Age at clinical onset	**Serum cbl**	**Antibodies**		**Homo-cystine, plasma, urine**	**Methyl-malonic acid, plasma, urine**	**Other**	**Response to cbl injections**
			IF	**PC**				
Breast-fed infant of strict vegan	3–18 months	$\downarrow\downarrow$	0	0	+/–	+/–		pharmacologic doses OH or CNcbl
Juvenile PA (gastric atrophy)	> 10 yr	$\downarrow\downarrow$	+	+	+/–	+/–	polyglandular failure (rare < 20 yr)	pharmacologic doses OH or CNcbl
Selective IF deficiency	1–5 yr	$\downarrow\downarrow$	0	0	+/–	+/–		pharmacologic doses OH or CNcbl
Selective IF receptor defect (Imerslund-Gräsbeck)	usu 0.5–3 yr, occ to 15 yr	$\downarrow\downarrow$	0	0	+/–	+/–	proteinuria	ditto; but proteinuria not corrected
TCII deficiency[1]	< 3 months	usu n, occ $\downarrow$	0	0	+/–	+/–	immune deficiency (T,B, granulocytes)	high dose OH or CNcbl
Defective mecbl synthesis (cblE,G defects)	usu < 3 months, occ to 21 yr	n	0	0	++	0	developmental delay	high dose OHcbl; neurologic abnormalities difficult to reverse
Defective synthesis of mecbl + adocbl (cblC, D,F defects)	usu < 3 months, some older (to 14 yr)	n to $\uparrow$	0	0	++	++	variable psychomotor retardation	high dose OHcbl; neurologic abnormalities difficult to reverse

ado = adenosyl; IF = intrinsic factor; me = methyl; n = normal; PA = pernicious anaemia; PC = parietal cells
[1] May present with erythroid hypoplasia rather than megaloblastosis

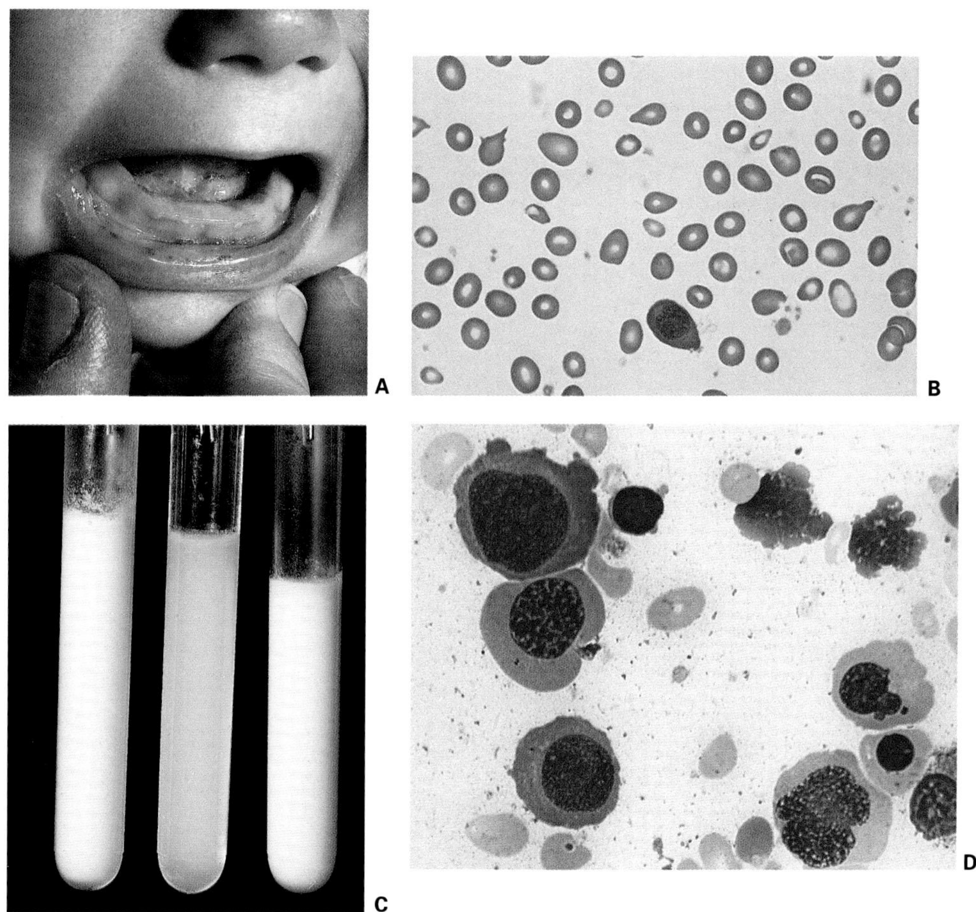

Fig. 2.12 Megaloblastosis in infancy. **a** Petechiae (thrombocytopenia) from folate deficiency in one of prematurely-born twins 3 months old; the clinical appearance led to an initial suspicion of leukaemia. **b** B_{12} deficiency in infant of strict vegan nursing mother, showing oval macrocytes and a megaloblast. **c** Milk from mother of infant in (**b**), between 2 normals; thinness is due to low fat; it contained no measurable B_{12}. **d** Marrow of another infant of strict vegan mother, showing megaloblasts; serum B_{12} unmeasurable.

TCII deficiency (Table 2.21)

Deficiency of TCII (unlike TCI) causes severe megaloblastosis, which, like cellular cbl defects in general, presents early in life with developmental delay and failure to thrive. It may be associated with immunodeficiency — hypogammaglobulinaemia (pneumocystis pneumonia, chronic diarrhoea), and deficiency of specific granulation of neutrophils (staphylococcal infection). Hypogammaglobulinaemia improves somewhat with cbl replacement. Diagnosis may be made by radioimmunoassay or chromatography.

Defects of cellular utilization/metabolism (cbl defects)

Some of these are associated with megaloblastosis (Table 2.21). Diagnosis requires examination of cultured fibroblasts for cbl uptake, synthesis of adenosyl- and methyl-cbl, and genetic complementation analyses between patient fibroblasts and fibroblasts with known defects. The E/G defects are likely to be associated with cerebral atrophy (Watkins & Rosenblatt 1989, Fig. 2.13).

FOLATE DEFICIENCY (Table 2.22, Fig. 2.11)

Folate deficiency is more common but is usually less severe in its effects than B_{12} deficiency. Haematologic effects are similar. Homocysteine is usually in excess but not methylmalonic acid (compare cbl deficiency). A low cell folate (polyglutamate) may occur in cbl deficiency (cbl is required for generation of intracellular polyglutamates); conversely, red cell folate values may be normal in true deficiency when the reticulocyte count is raised.

Folate deficiency may coexist with iron deficiency, e.g. from suboptimal intake or malabsorption; iron deficiency may not be obvious until red cell mass is expanded by folate treatment.

Success of treatment is signalled by a reticulocytosis peaking at 7–10 days, with return of Hb to normal in 3–6 weeks (Table 2.19).

Table 2.22 Folate deficiency in childhood

Folate deficiency in childhood
Suboptimal intake
Special diets, e.g. goat's milk
Malnutrition, kwashiorkor
Malabsorption (upper small intestine)
Global
Coeliac disease
Crohn's disease
Dermatitis herpetiformis
Specific
Drugs — anticonvulsants
Hereditary folate malabsorption
Increased requirement
Prematurity
Chronic haemolysis
Exfoliative dermatitis
Some inflammations, malignancies
Pregnancy
Excess loss
Dialysis
Skin: some dermatoses
Enzyme inhibition — dihydrofolate reductase
Drugs (Table 2.35)
Impaired cellular uptake (?)

Suboptimal intake

Folates are of vegetable origin (best sources: liver, kidney, fruit juices, spinach). Because of the ubiquitous distribution of good sources, deficient intake in affluent countries is more likely to result from special diets (e.g. goat's milk for allergy) than dietary lack. Because storage (liver) is less than for cbl, deficiency manifests in weeks rather than months.

Absorption defects

Global malabsorptions are a common cause of folate deficiency. Malabsorption may also contribute to the folate deficiency in some exfoliative skin disorders (loss from skin also).

Hereditary folate malabsorption is the only genetic defect of folate transport/metabolism associated with megaloblastosis (Rosenblatt 1989). There are no other features of malabsorption. The CNS is affected (defective transport of folate), with ataxia, convulsions, mental retardation and calcification of basal ganglia. Megaloblastic anaemia manifests in the first months. A standard oral test dose (5 mg) gives a subnormal (< 100 μg/l) rise in serum folate. Haematologic abnormalities are reversed by small doses, but CSF levels (and neurologic damage) require high oral dosage or parenteral or intrathecal administration or other forms of folate, e.g. folinic acid or methyltetrahydrofolate. All but one of the cases reported have been girls. Inheritance is autosomal recessive.

Some anticonvulsants interfere with absorption.

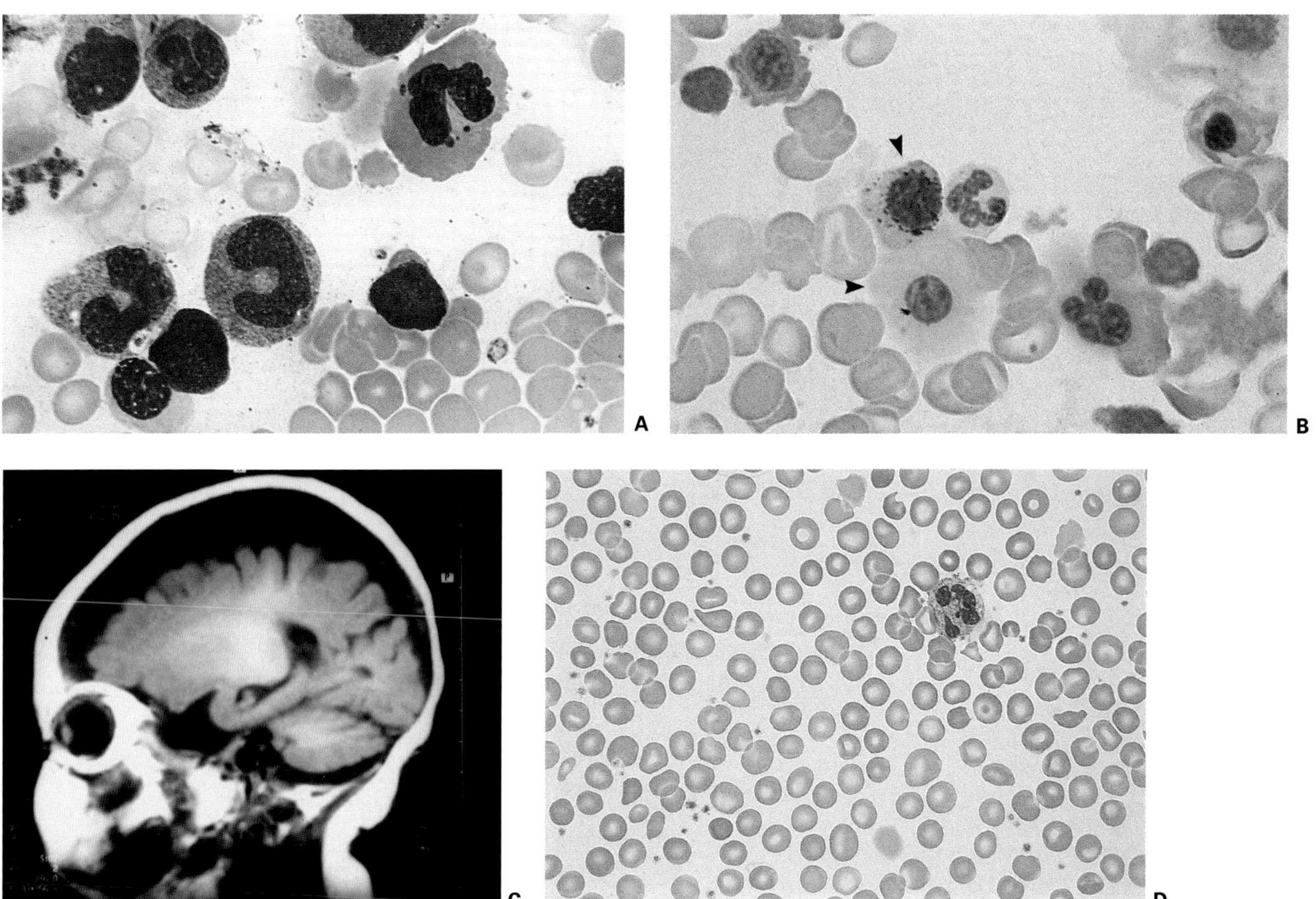

Fig. 2.13 Probable cbl E or G defect in a 6-month-old girl with cerebral atrophy; Hb 6.7 g/dl, MCV 101 fl. **a** Marrow, showing a megaloblast and 2 large stab neutrophils. **b** Marrow (Perls × 950): ringed sideroblast and a siderocyte (arrows). **c** MRI showing cerebral atrophy. **d** Blood at 1 month of age, showing some oval macrocytes and a hypersegmented neutrophil, though Hb (10.5 g/dl) and MCV (97 fl) are within normal limits. High dose OHcbl has given good haematologic and some neurologic improvement.

Increased requirement

Rapid growth and a poor endowment of liver stores at birth render premature infants susceptible to folate deficiency (Fig. 2.12a).

Cellular deficiency may result from increased cell activity, (though serum and red cell folate are usually not diminished), in chronic haemolytic anaemias and in some inflammations (rheumatoid arthritis, Crohn's disease) and malignancies.

Excessive loss

In exfoliative skin disorders folate deficiency is due to mitotic activity of regenerating skin cells, loss by desquamation and, in some, associated malabsorption.

Interference with folate metabolism

In patients originally described as having genetic dihydrofolate reductase deficiency (better response to folinic than folic acid), the basic defect appears to lie elsewhere, although the low levels of enzyme in liver biopsies are unexplained. Enzyme deficiency is most often due to drugs (below).

Syndromes of impaired cellular uptake of methyltetrahydrofolate may manifest as marrow hypoplasia (p. 50) or as dyserythropoiesis resembling CDA type III (Howe et al 1979).

HYPOTHYROIDISM (Erslev 1990)

Macrocytosis may occur in hypothyroidism; cbl and folate levels are normal. More commonly, however, anaemia is normocytic or microcytic (iron deficiency is demonstrable in some cases). Acanthocytosis occurs in some cases (Fig. 3.14).

VITAMIN C DEFICIENCY (Oski 1990)

Megaloblastosis occurs in about 10%, effective treatment requiring folic acid as well as vitamin C (maintains dihydrofolate reductase in reduced form). Iron-deficient microcytosis may also occur (bleeding, impaired absorption of iron). The 'characteristic' but uncommon anaemia is normocytic normochromic, responding to ascorbic acid only.

THIAMINE DEFICIENCY

Megaloblastosis responsive only to high dose (25–100 mg daily) thiamine is associated with the 'DIDMOAD' constellation (diabetes insipidus, diabetes mellitus, optic atrophy, deafness) in the rare Wolfram's syndrome (Borgna-Pignatti et al 1989). The diabetes mellitus (or abnormal glucose tolerance) is insulin-dependent; deafness is sensorineural. The disorder is attributed to a defect in thiamine phosphokinase. Inheritance is autosomal recessive.

Both the haematologic changes and the signs of beriberi (rarely present) improve with thiamine treatment. There was some improvement in deafness and diabetes mellitus in one infant (Mandel et al 1984). Ringed sideroblasts may be noted in small numbers in marrow.

COPPER DEFICIENCY

Megaloblastosis and sideroblastosis may occur in copper deficiency. See neutropenia (p. 247).

CONGENITAL DYSERYTHROPOIETIC ANAEMIAS

Macrocytosis occurs in some types of CDA, considered together here for comparison (Table 2.23, Fig. 2.14). Impaired synthesis of β globin chains occurs in several types and manifests as a deposition of α chains in erythroblasts (Wickramasinghe & Pippard 1986, Fig. 2.14). Other ultrastructural changes include duplications of plasma membrane (type II) and 'Swiss-cheese' nuclear degeneration (type I, Fig. 2.14). Macrophages containing effete erythroblasts and PAS-positive crystalline material (Gaucher-like) are further evidence of poor quality of erythroblasts.

Fig. 2.14 (facing page) Congenital dyserythropoietic anaemias. **a,b** Type II in a 6-year-old girl; multinucleated erythroblasts and erythrocyte distortion. Hb 8.0 g/dl, MCV 93 fl. **c–f** Probable type I in a 10-month-old girl needing frequent transfusions since birth (cord Hb 12.1 g/dl). Arrows in **c** show degenerate erythroblasts, and in **d**, inclusions. **e** 'Swiss-cheese' degeneration of erythroblast nuclei. **f** Inclusion, unenclosed, probably of α globin chains. **a** × 750; **b** × 480; **c,d** × 750; **e** × 5000; **f** × 20 000. **a,b** Courtesy of Dr G Tauro

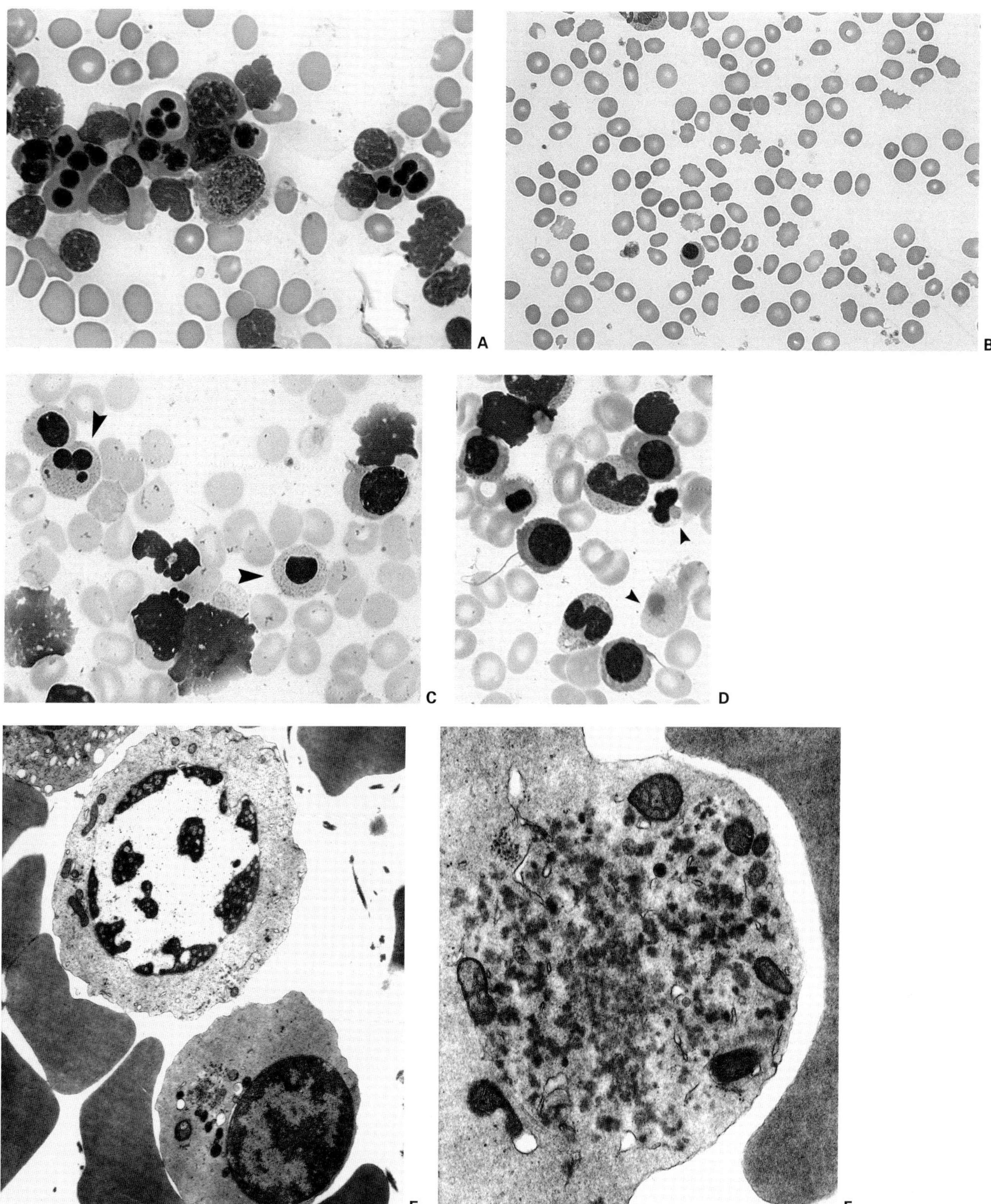
A
B
C
D
E
F

Electron microscopy is required to detect erythroblast abnormality in some cases (Fig. 2.15).

Although these disorders are genetic, age at clinical onset varies from infancy to adulthood.

In type II, underglycosylation of membrane glycoproteins appears to be the basis for the structural abnormality of the membrane and the generation of HEMPAS antigen. The defect in other types is unknown.

Fig. 2.15 (facing page) Congenital dyserythropoietic anaemia of unclassified type in a 6-month-old boy with chronic normocytic anaemia (lowest Hb 6.3 g/dl), erythroblasts normal by light microscopy. **a** Lifting of nuclear membrane (small arrows), which has formed an apparently free-lying vesicle (large arrow) (× 17 000). **b** Continuity between cytoplasm and nucleoplasm at sites of loss of nuclear membrane (arrows) (× 15 000). Courtesy of Dr P Kanowski

Differential diagnosis

1. Other causes of dyserythropoiesis
A degree of dyserythropoiesis is common in iron-deficiency, megaloblastic and aplastic anaemias. Dyserythropoiesis is outstanding in:

- AML M6, myelodysplasias. Dyserythropoiesis is not confined to the erythron (Figs 5.13, 5.20, 5.21)
- some children receiving cytotoxic drugs (Fig. 2.16)
- post marrow transplantation
- parvovirus — transplacental infection may cause anaemia in the neonate resembling CDA type II (Brown et al 1994).

2. Disorders with similar serology
PNH resembles type II CDA in showing haemolysis in acidified sera (Ham's test); but in PNH lysis occurs in the patient's own acidified serum and sugar lysis is positive.

CHROMOSOMAL DISORDERS, LIVER DISEASE

Macrocytosis of obscure origin occurs in trisomies (21,18 triploidy, Sipes et al 1991) and in some patients with liver disease.

Table 2.23 Congenital dyserythropoietic anaemias

	I	II (HEMPAS[1])	III	IV
Approx %	25	55	15	5
Erythrocytes				
Size	macro	usu normo, occ macro	macro	normo
Distortion[2]	++	+	++	+
Erythroblasts	megaloblastoid; 2–5% binuclear, ~2% with chromatin bridges	10–40% bi- and multinuclear; pluripolar mitoses; karyorrhexis	10–40% 'gigantoblasts' (up to 12 nuclei)	similar to II
Serology				
Acid haemolysis	neg	pos[3]	neg	neg
Sugar lysis	neg	neg	neg	neg
Anti I	weak	strong	weak	weak
Anti i	weak	strong	weak	weak
Other	evidence of haemolysis[4]	haemolysis usually more severe than in I, with more severe anaemia. Gaucher-like cells in marrow		
Inheritance[5]	AR	AR	AD	AD in some

[1] Hereditary erythroblastic multinuclearity with positive acidified serum (test)
[2] Ovals, fragments, odd shapes, stippling, Cabot rings
[3] Lysis by approx $\frac{1}{3}$ of acidified normal sera, due to IgM antibody against HEMPAS antigen; no lysis in patient's own acidified serum
[4] Mild increase in bilirubin, increased lactate dehydrogenase, decreased haptoglobin
[5] AD = autosomal dominant; AR = autosomal recessive

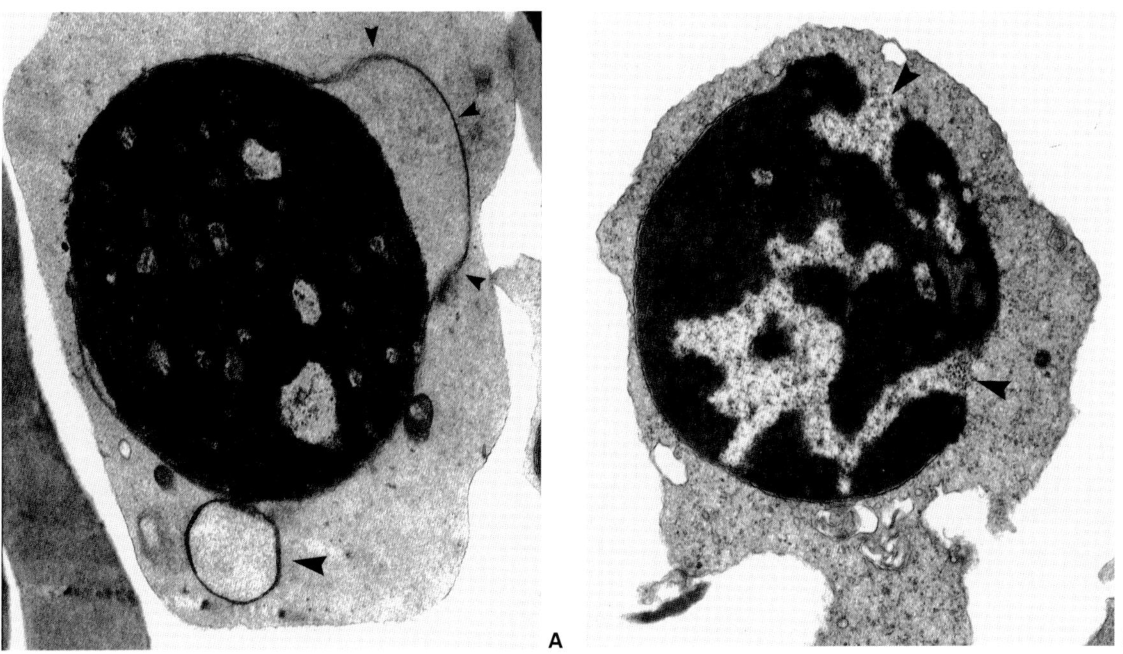

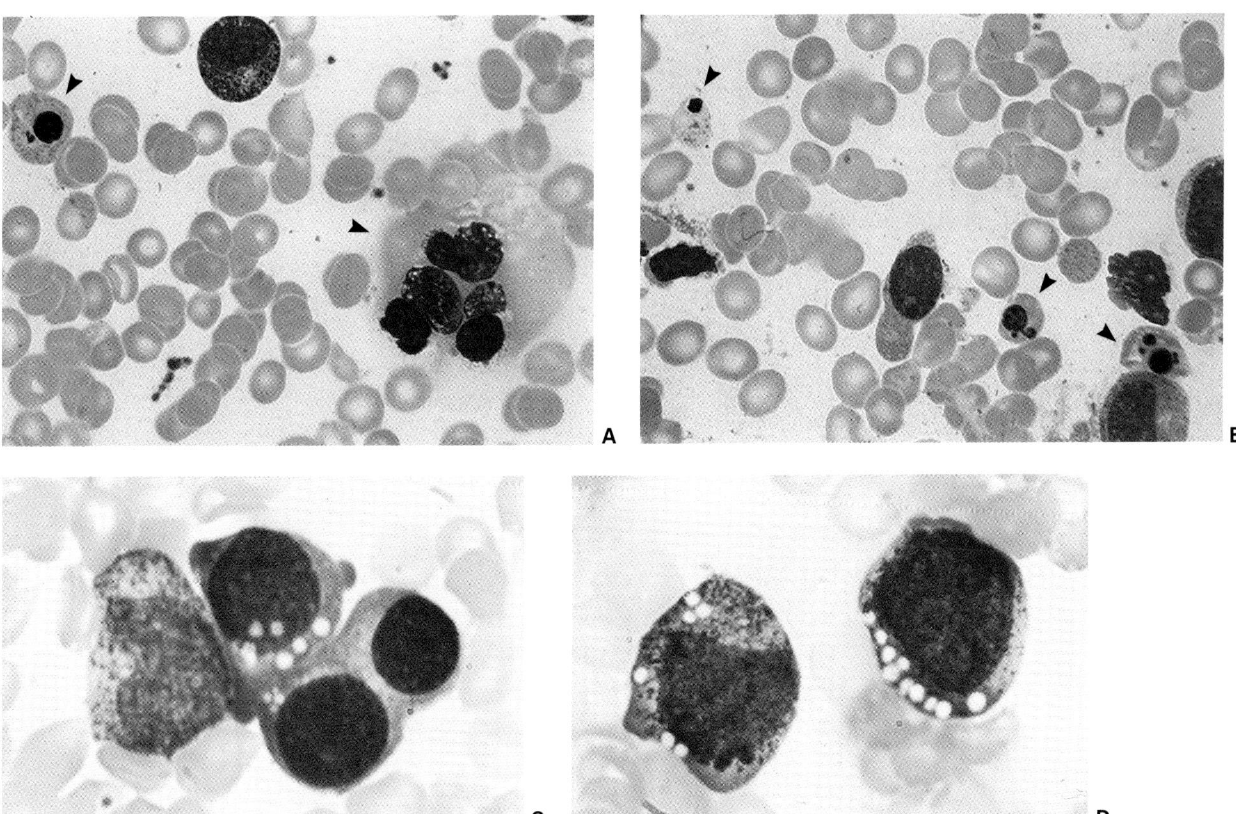

Fig. 2.16 Marrow damage from drugs. **a,b** Severe dyserythropoiesis (arrows) in ALL treated with vincristine, methotrexate and 6-mercaptopurine; Hb 9.5 g/dl, MCV 101 fl (n < 90). **c,d** Vacuolation of erythroblasts and neutrophil myelocytes from high-dose chloramphenicol. **a,b** × 750; **c,d** × 1200

MARROW HYPOPLASIA

Macrocytosis is characteristic of congenital but not acquired erythroblastopenia and occurs in a proportion of patients with panhypoplasia.

Panhypoplasia (aplasia) of marrow

Pancytopenia without leukaemic cells in the blood is most likely due to aplasia, but diagnosis requires aspirate and trephine biopsy of marrow. Causes of pancytopenia are listed in Table 2.24.

Blood

Pancytopenia is usually severe (Hb to about 3 g/dl). In about 40% of cases erythrocytes are macrocytic. Reticulocytes are usually decreased, but occasionally are inexplicably excessive for the anaemia. HbF may be increased, especially in genetic types and those with macrocytosis, to about 15% of the total, with heterogeneous distribution.

As a result of diminution in the erythron, serum iron and transferrin saturation are increased; B_{12} and folate may be increased. Erythrocyte i (and in some cases I) antigen may be increased. Lymphocytes are normal to decreased. Platelet size is not increased (cf immune thrombocytopenias).

The first sign of recovery is a rise in reticulocyte count, followed by increase in Hb, then neutrophils, with platelets slowest to recover, if at all.

Marrow (Fig. 2.17)

Hypoplasia may be patchy, especially early in the disease. Marrow consists of little more than fat, stromal cells, lymphocytes and plasma cells; mast cells may be prominent. There may be mild dyserythropoiesis. Because of diminution in the erythron, storage iron and sideroblasts may be increased; ring sideroblasts are not seen, except in rare specific syndromes, e.g. Pearson's (p. 216).

Criteria for severe disease are summarized in Table 2.25.

Table 2.24 Pancytopenia in childhood

Artefact: clot in sample
Genuine (by dominant mechanism)
Destruction of mature elements
Infection, most commonly viral
Immune
Infection
SLE
Complement — PNH
Marrow failure (stem cells, mature elements)
Infiltration
Leukaemia
Other malignancies
Panhypoplasia (Table 2.26)
Myelosclerosis
Osteopetrosis
Severe megaloblastosis
Sequestration
Hypersplenism (most common cause portal hypertension)
Mechanism obscure
Organic acidaemias

Table 2.25 Criteria for severe aplastic anaemia[1]

Blood	neutrophils	$< 0.5 \times 10^9/l$
	platelets	$< 20 \times 10^9/l$
	reticulocytes	< 1% (corrected for hct[2])
Marrow	severe hypocellularity	
	moderate hypocellularity with < 30% residual cells haemopoietic	

[1] Camitta et al 1982. Severe is defined as at least 2 blood criteria + either marrow criterion

[2] $\frac{\text{hct}}{\text{normal hct for age}} \times$ reticulocytes %

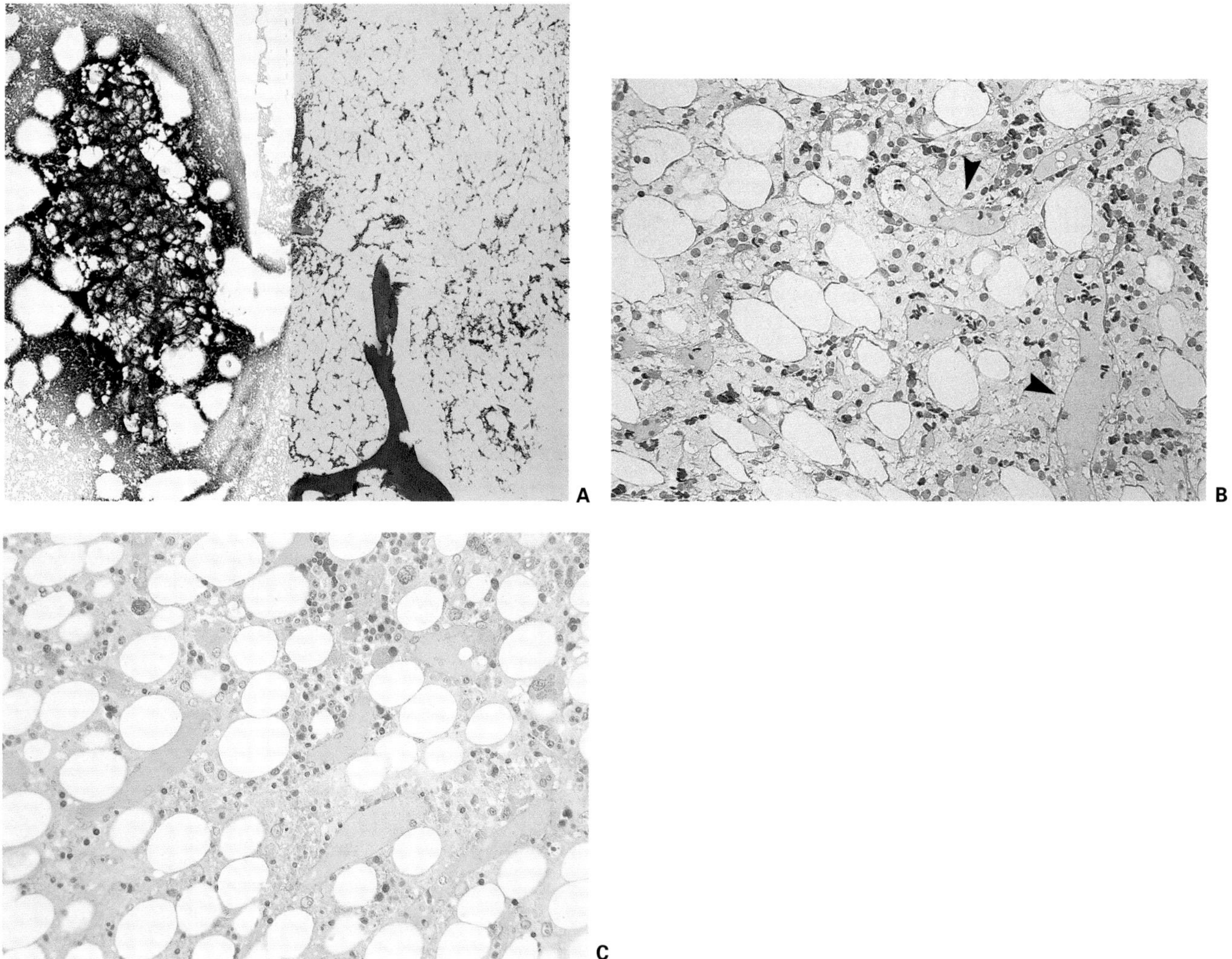

Fig. 2.17 Marrow aplasia/destruction. **a** Aplasia in a 12-year-old girl, cause undetermined, aspirate vs trephine biopsy. **b** 10-year-old, 4 weeks after presumed viral hepatitis (non-A,B,C). Arrows show lymph vessel. Amorphous pink interstitial material is oedema (oedema generalized though serum albumin normal) (H & E). **c** (PAS): marrow destruction, with abundance of PAS-positive material, 13-year-old girl with severe varicella, 12 days after onset of rash; no virus particles seen by electron microscopy. Death occurred 4 days later from Pseudomonas septicaemia. **a** × 32; **b,c** × 200

Recognized causes (Table 2.26)

Drugs (Miller & O'Reilly 1989)
Drugs may cause (a) predictable, dose-related, reversible marrow suppression, and (b) unpredictable, dose-unrelated, idiosyncratic, usually irreversible damage.

The sequence of changes in reversible suppression is shown in Table 2.27. Vacuolation is non-specific — vacuolation of granulocytes may occur in copper deficiency and of erythroblasts in patients on phenylalanine-restricted diets (Sherman et al 1964). Suppression is attributed to a variety of mechanisms, including impairment of DNA synthesis (cytotoxics) and inhibition of ferrochelatase (chloramphenicol).

Drugs which can seriously damage marrow usually do so in unpredictable and devastating fashion and in only a minuscule proportion of those exposed. Susceptibility is presumably genetic. This effect usually does not occur until after cessation of the drug — with chloramphenicol at least 6–10 weeks, and up to 12 months later.

Some drugs, e.g. chloramphenicol, have both dose-related and idiosyncratic effect, rarely one following the other (Daum et al 1979).

Paediatric drugs and toxins with, or with suspected capacity to cause marrow aplasia are listed in Table 2.28. Some (e.g. benzol) have a potential for causing leukaemia, which usually does not occur until many years after exposure.

Infection (Kurtzman & Young 1989, Hibbs & Young 1992)
1. Viral infection
As with idiosyncratic reaction to drugs, hypoplasia occurs in only a minuscule proportion of those exposed. However, viral infection is probably an underdiagnosed cause: EBV for example may be demonstrable in patients without the typical clinical features of infective mononucleosis (Lau et al 1994), and acyclovir may produce haematologic improvement when a virus aetiology cannot be proven (Gómez-Almaguer et al 1988). The destructive effect of virus may be due to direct action or an immune effect such as T-lymphocyte mediated suppression.

- The best known association is with viral hepatitis — usually non-A, -B, -C (Fig. 2.17). Hypoplasia is usually severe, though the preceding hepatitis may not be, and manifests at a mean of 9–10 weeks after onset of hepatitis.
- Hypoplasia occurs in isolated instances of infection with EBV, HIV, varicella (Fig. 2.17), CMV, dengue-type viruses, measles, mumps and parvovirus. Hypoplasia is more likely if there is associated immunodeficiency either drug-induced or natural, e.g. EBV in X-linked lymphoproliferative disorder (p. 252). Although the effect of parvovirus is ordinarily restricted to the erythron, panhypoplasia occasionally occurs in apparently normal persons (Hamon et al 1988).

2. Transient hypoplasia may occur in rickettsial infection, e.g. Q fever (Hitchins et al 1986) and ehrlichiosis (Pearce et al 1988).

Table 2.26 Panhypoplasia of marrow in childhood: recognized causes[1]

Drugs and chemicals (Table 2.28)
Infection, especially viral
Inherited (Tables 2.30, 2.31)
Malignancy
Pre-ALL
Myelodysplasia, e.g. monosomy 7 MPD
Immune
Graft vs host disease
PNH
SLE
Chronic mucocutaneous candidiasis
Thymoma
Severe megaloblastosis
Ionizing radiation
Other
Anorexia nervosa
Preceded by acquired amegakaryocytic thrombocytopenia

[1] A cause is not identified in 30–50% of cases

Table 2.27 Dose-related effects of chloramphenicol[1]

	Timing
Reticulocytopenia, increase in serum Fe	2–5 days
Marrow	
Erythroblast depletion	3–7 days
Vacuolation of precursor cells	
Anaemia	5–10 days
Thrombocytopenia (mild)	10–14 days
Neutropenia[2]	10–21 days

[1] From Oski 1979
[2] Neutropenia is an indication for cessation of treatment

Table 2.28 Paediatric drugs and chemicals which may cause marrow aplasia

Cytotoxics	
Antibacterial	Chloramphenicol (more often oral than intravenous) Sulphonamides (some)
Antimalarial	Mepacrine* Quinacrine Chloroquine Trimethoprim* Pyrimethamine*
Antihistamine	Cimetidine Ranitidine Chlorpheniramine
Anticonvulsant	Phenytoin, other hydantoins
Tranquillizer	Promazine* Chlorpromazine* Carbamazepine
Anti-inflammatory	Indomethacin Diclophenac Gold
Antipurines	Azathiaprine*
Antidiabetic	Chlorpropamide Tolbutamide
Antithyroid	Propylthiouracil Methimazole
Other drugs	Allopurinol* Quinidine* Acetazolamide Penicillamine
Solvents	Benzol White spirit (benzine, naphtha and other synonyms) Carbon tetrachloride Kerosene Glue (sniffing)* Model aeroplane 'dope'* Hair dyes*
Insecticides	DDT Lindane Chlordane Organophosphates

With the exception of those marked*, agents listed regularly produce marrow depression or have an accepted relation to marrow aplasia

Genetic syndromes and panhypoplasia
(Tables 2.29, 2.30)

1. *Fanconi's syndrome* (Fig. 2.18)
Diagnosis is most reliably made by quantitation of chromosomal breaks (cultured blood lymphocytes) induced by the DNA cross-linking agent, diepoxybutane (DEB, Auerbach et al 1989). Abnormal fragility appears to be specific for Fanconi's anaemia and is detectable from birth and before onset of cytopenias. A scoring system for diagnosis, using other characteristics, has been devised (Table 2.30).

Approximately 7% of patients do not have malformations; malformation-free subjects in sibships which also contain classic cases were once thought to have a separate disorder (Estren & Dameshek 1947). The DEB procedure is therefore recommended for all cases of panhypoplasia, whether associated with malformations or not. The DEB procedure does not reliably detect the carrier state (autosomal recessive). Sibs and parents may share some of the somatic anomalies but do not have blood changes. Heterogeneity (Alter 1993) is in part explicable by the existence of at least 2 genes for the disorder (chromosomes 9 and 20).

Blood abnormalities are rare before 18 months and may not manifest till about 20 years. Average age at onset of pancytopenia is about 6½ years for boys and about 8½ years for girls. Thrombocytopenia is usually the first sign, and may be misdiagnosed as idiopathic if the association with somatic anomalies is not recognized; granulocytopenia and then anaemia follow, evolving over months to years. Fetal features, e.g. macrocytosis and increased HbF (heterogeneous distribution) and i antigen are common, even before onset of anaemia.

Dyserythropoiesis is common, with megaloblastosis, internuclear bridges, karyorrhexis and defective haemoglobinization. In the presymptomatic period the marrow may appear normal or show hyperplasia.

There is a risk (about 20%) of malignancy, especially AML M4 and squamous cell carcinoma. Malignancy is occasionally the presenting feature.

2. *Dyskeratosis congenita* (Jacobs et al 1984)
Ectodermal dysplasia is characteristic — in skin, nails and teeth (Fig. 2.18) and in hair (loss and premature greying); leukoplakia of squamous surfaces may produce stricture of hollow viscera (e.g. oesophagus) and is a risk (about 10%) for malignancy. Growth retardation is common.

Table 2.29 Genetic syndromes and marrow panhypoplasia

DNA repair defect
Fanconi
Dyskeratosis congenita
Pancreas-marrow syndromes
Shwachman
Pearson
Atypical cystic fibrosis
Other
Defective cellular uptake of folate
Aplasia preceded by congenital amegakaryocytic thrombocytopenia
Other rare defects (Table 2.31)

Table 2.30 Assessment of likelihood of Fanconi's syndrome*

Characteristic	Score	
Growth retardation	+1	
Skin		
Pigmentation (café au lait spots) ± hypopigmented areas	+1	
Thumb and radius		
Absent or triphalangeal thumb, hypoplasia of 1st metacarpal, absent radius one or both sides with absence of corresponding thumb	+1	
Microphthalmia	+1	
Kidney, urinary tract		
Absence of one kidney, horseshoe kidney, double ureters	+1	
Thrombocytopenia	+1	
Other skeletal defects	−1	
Learning difficulties	−1	
Total score	−1	Probability of Fanconi's: 0.00
	0	0.20
	1	0.31
	2	0.75
	3	0.92
	4	0.98

*Adapted from Auerbach et al 1989

Cytopenias occur in up to half the patients, presenting usually in the second to third decade. Thrombocytopenia or anaemia usually precedes pancytopenia. Rarely, isolated thrombocytopenia precedes skin changes by several years. Fetal characteristics (macrocytosis, increased HbF) are common. Chromosomal fragility (as indicated by DEB) is normal.

Most cases are X-linked recessive; some are autosomal recessive (these tend to be severe) or autosomal dominant.

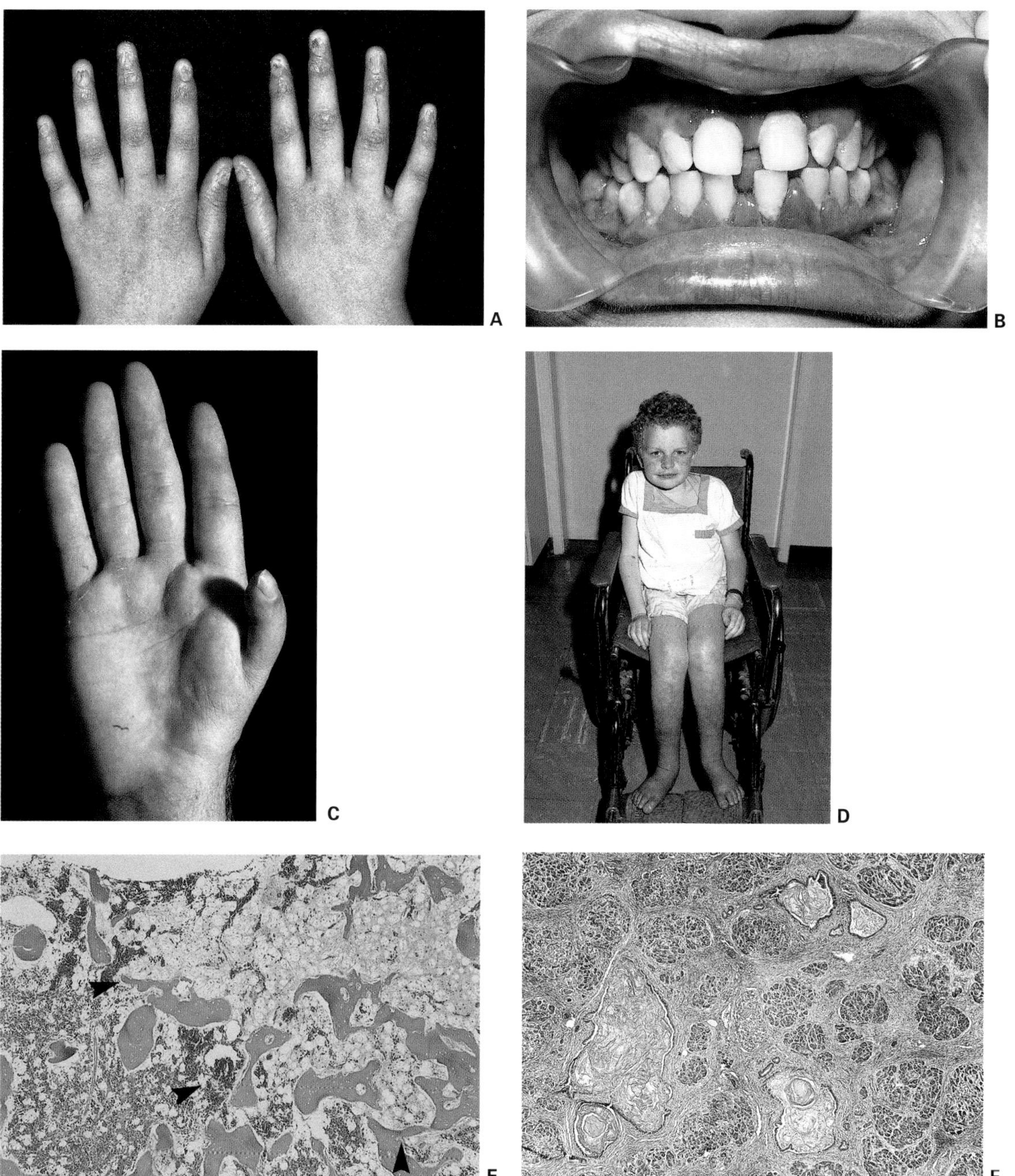

Fig. 2.18 Syndromes associated with marrow hypoplasia. **a,b** Dyskeratosis congenita, dystrophy of nails and surrounding skin, dystrophy of teeth. **c** Fanconi's syndrome, short mispositioned thumb (hypoplasia of metacarpal on X-ray). **d–f** 11-year-old boy with patchy marrow hypoplasia (**e**, arrows, × 25) and exocrine pancreatic fibrosis (**f** × 20). Main symptoms were diarrhoea and chest infections from infancy, anaemia, thrombocytopenia and dysautonomia (hypothermia, erythroderma [**d**], day/night sleep reversal, hyponatraemia). **c** Courtesy of Dr I Bunce

3. *Shwachman's syndrome* (Aggett et al 1980)
Exocrine pancreatic insufficiency (fatty replacement), neutropenia, metaphyseal dyschondroplasia and growth retardation.

Neutropenia is intermittent rather than constant and may be cyclic, though not with the same predictability as true cyclic neutropenia. The neutrophil count may rise with infection, and is responsive to administration of GCSF (Moore 1991). Monocytes are usually not increased.

About 50% of patients have anaemia; however this is persistent in only a minority. Increase in HbF is common even without anaemia, but substantial increase (to 30%) is unusual. About 70% have thrombocytopenia, which varies independently of the neutrophil count and may be severe ($< 60 \times 10^9/l$). About 10% have pancytopenia.

Marrow hypoplasia of varying degree is common, even without pancytopenia. Maturation arrest in myeloid cells or sparsity of myeloid precursors may be noted. The erythron is normal or hyperplastic. Occasionally the marrow appears normal (patchy disease). Rare Gaucher-like cells may be noted (Fig. 6.36b).

The relation of pancreatic insufficiency to the cytopenias is not clear; pancreatectomy does not produce cytopenias.

Inheritance is thought to be autosomal recessive; defective neutrophil mobility may be demonstrable in parents.

There is a risk (about 5%) of leukaemia (ALL, AML, juvenile CML).

Differential diagnosis is from other pancreas-marrow syndromes:

- Pearson's syndrome — vacuolation of granulocyte precursors and erythroblasts is characteristic (p. 216)
- atypical cystic fibrosis — see below
- other syndromes of neutropenia and pancreatic pathology (Fig. 7.2).

4. *Pearson's syndrome*
Transfusion-dependent macrocytic anaemia with other abnormalities (p. 216).

5. *Atypical cystic fibrosis*
Patchy marrow hypoplasia (anaemia, thrombocytopenia) may be associated with pancreatic fibrosis and features of dysautonomia (Fig. 2.18).

6. *Defective cellular uptake of folate*
Reversible marrow depletion may occur in severe megaloblastosis of any cause. An autosomal dominant syndrome of permanent hypoplasia with megaloblastosis of surviving elements, attributed to a defect in cellular uptake of methyltetrahydrofolate, is described by Branda et al (1978). Presentation was in adulthood. High dose folate produced striking improvement, but macrocytosis and marrow hypocellularity persisted. Other members of the kindred had impaired cellular uptake of folate, leukaemia or neutropenia.

Another syndrome of impaired membrane transport of folate manifests as dyserythropoiesis (p. 40).

7. *Aplasia preceded by congenital amegakaryocytic thrombocytopenia* (Freedman & Estrov 1990)
A rare disorder. Severe diminution in megakaryocytes in marrow, attributed to stem cell defect, occurs without associated physical defects or abnormal chromosome fragility. About 80% evolve, at a median age of about 3 years, into aplastic anaemia.

8. *Other rare genetic defects*
Pancytopenia due to or likely to be due to marrow aplasia may occur in other rare genetic disorders (Table 2.31).

Malignancy and marrow hypoplasia

Transient marrow aplasia is an uncommon but important prodrome for ALL (p. 134, Fig. 4.17). Hypoplasia with fibrosis is significant in myelodysplasias, especially monosomy 7 MPD (Fig. 5.19).

Immune destruction of marrow

1. *Graft vs host disease*
Marrow destruction is severe, with high mortality. Transfused, unirradiated lymphocytes are a high risk if an immunocompetent (or incompetent) recipient shares an HLA haplotype with an HLA-homozygous donor (facilitates engraftment of viable donor lymphocytes, Shivdasani et al 1993).

2. *PNH* (Rotoli & Luzzatto 1989)
Exceptionally rare in childhood. A variety of cells is abnormally sensitive to lysis by complement, due to a defect in the glycosyl-phosphatidyl-inositol anchor which binds proteins to the cell membrane (including those which protect against complement).

Table 2.31 Rare hereditary aplasias of marrow which may present in childhood

Name of syndrome if given	Main features	Inheritance[1]	References
WT	radio-ulnar and thumb anomalies; short clinodactylous 5th fingers; risk of leukaemia	AD	Gonzalez et al 1977
Ataxia-pancytopenia-monosomy 7	cerebellar ataxia (atrophy), monosomy 7, AML	AD	Daghistani et al 1989
—	Friedreich's (spino-cerebellar) ataxia, short stature, hypogonadism	AR	Samad et al 1973
—	immune deficiency (IgA decrease), cutaneous malignancies	AR	Abels & Reed 1973
Sekel	growth retardation (prenatal onset), mental deficiency, microcephaly, prominent beaked nose, receding chin; hypoplastic anaemia in ~10%	AR	Butler et al 1987
Dubowitz	growth retardation (prenatal onset), microcephaly, hoarse high-pitched voice, eczema, mild mental retardation, peculiar facies; hypoplastic anaemia in ~10%	AR	Walters & Desposito 1985
—	microcephaly, cerebral, esp cerebellar, hypoplasia, growth retardation (prenatal onset); isolated thrombocytopenia (megakaryocyte deficiency) at birth proceeding to pancytopenia at about 1 yr	AR	Hreidarsson et al 1988
—	small for age; short webbed neck, broad nasal bridge, prominent epicanthic folds, large ears, proximally located thumbs; no mental retardation	AR	Sackey et al 1985

[1] Or most likely inheritance
AD = autosomal dominant; AR = autosomal recessive; ~ = approx

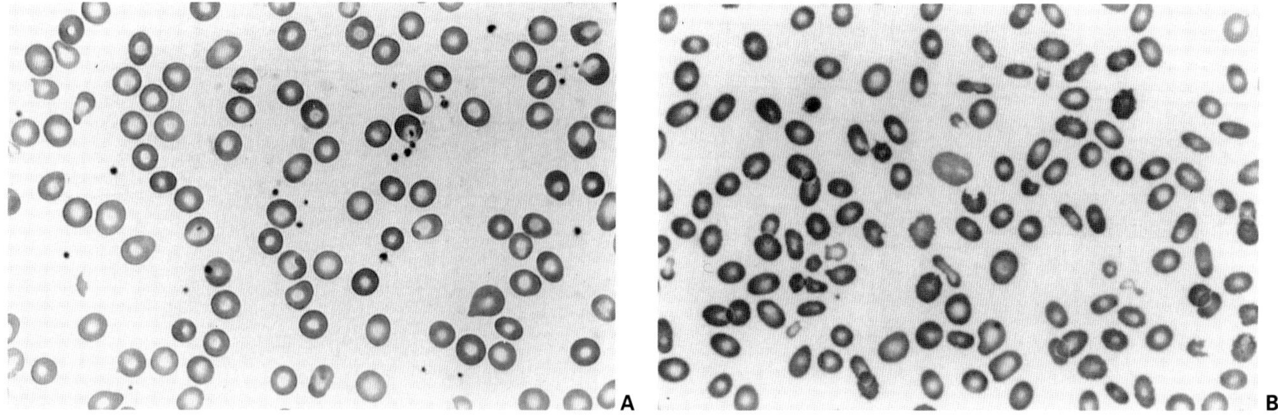

Fig. 2.19 Diamond-Blackfan anaemia. **a** At 6 weeks, Hb 4.6 g/dl, MCV 102 fl (normal). **b** At 5 years, Hb 7.9 g/dl, MCV 91 fl (n < 86).

Diagnosis might be considered for:

- Haemolysis of obscure origin

Chronic haemolysis is more common than sleep-induced haemoglobinuria, and haemosiderinuria is constant. The DAT is negative. Reticulocytes may be inappropriately low (marrow hypoplasia, ineffective erythropoiesis, iron deficiency from haemosiderinuria). The MCV is often high for the reticulocyte count, but microcytosis may result from iron deficiency. Haemolysis may be exacerbated by exercise, infection, vaccination and blood transfusion (increase in blood temperature or acidity, infusion of complement).

- Unexplained pancytopenia/marrow hypoplasia

About 25% of patients with PNH proceed over a period of years to marrow aplasia (5–10% of patients with various aplasias, e.g. drug-induced, Fanconi, evolve to PNH). Marrow storage iron may be subnormal from haemosiderinuria, in contrast to the excess usual in aplasia. Dyserythropoiesis is not conspicuous.

- Unexplained venous thrombosis

Thrombosis has a predilection for abdominal, especially hepatic veins (Budd-Chiari syndrome), and is attributed to release of thromboplastins from granulocytes and platelets by complement.

The sucrose lysis test, based on enhanced binding of complement in solutions of low ionic strength, is reliable for screening, though a single normal result does not exclude the diagnosis. A positive result should be confirmed by a formal Ham's acid lysis test; lysis also occurs in the patient's own acidified serum. Haemosiderinuria and decrease in neutrophil alkaline phosphatase and red cell acetylcholinesterase are useful supporting features.

The Ham's test is positive also in CDA type II (Table 2.23), but lysis does not occur in the patient's own acidified serum, sugar lysis is negative and dyserythropoiesis is conspicuous.

3. SLE and marrow hypoplasia

Marrow depletion is rare in SLE and may be global or affect only the erythron. Maternal SLE is a cause of marrow depletion in the neonate.

4. Chronic mucocutaneous candidiasis

Aplasia occurs in some patients. Aplasia, T-cell dysfunction in handling of candida and endocrinopathy (parathyroid) are attributed to autoimmune effect.

5. Thymoma

Association with hypoplasia (erythroblastopenia or panhypoplasia) is very rare in childhood. Talerman & Amigo (1968) described a 5-year-old child with anaemia which evolved to marrow aplasia 4 weeks after thymectomy.

Other aplasias

- Anorexia nervosa

Hypoplasia with 'gelatinous' transformation and necrosis is described (Smith & Spivak 1985); in spite of this, cytopenias are mild or absent. The commonest blood abnormality is acanthocytosis (p. 88).

- Preceded by acquired amegakaryocytic thrombocytopenia

'Acquired amegakaryocytic' thrombocytopenia is a rare precursor to aplasia (Scarlett et al 1992). Thrombocytopenia is severe but anaemia and leucopenia are mild to moderate. There are no associated physical anomalies and chromosomal fragility is not increased. In addition to virtual absence of megakaryocytes, the erythron is dysplastic (macrocytosis, mild increase in HbF) and hyperplastic. About 20% evolve to frank aplasia. Diagnosis requires exclusion of other thrombocytopenias with subnormal megakaryocyte numbers in marrow (Table 8.25), especially Fanconi's anaemia.

ERYTHROBLASTOPENIA (Tables 2.32–2.34)

Macrocytosis occurs in only some types. The commonest erythroblastopenias in childhood are Diamond-Blackfan anaemia and TEC.

Congenital erythroblastopenia (Diamond-Blackfan) (Table 2.33, Freedman 1993)

The defect is thought to lie in receptors for growth-promoting factors such as erythropoietin (increased in serum), interleukin-3 and Steel factor.

Age at onset

Approximately one quarter are anaemic at birth, 65% are manifest by 6 months and 90% by 1 year. Onset after 1 year should suggest other causes until proven otherwise.

Blood

Erythrocytes characteristically have fetal attributes (Table 2.33). HbF is heterogeneously distributed. The DAT is negative unless antibodies develop from transfusion. Increase in erythrocyte adenosine deaminase is common but of uncertain significance and non-specific. Neutropenia and thrombocytopenia may occur from hyperplenism. Karyotype and chromosomal fragility are normal.

Marrow

Overall cellularity is normal though erythroblasts are deficient. Surviving erythroblasts are mainly basophilic forms; they may show dyspoiesis and rarely vacuolation. In about 5%, erythroblasts are normal to increased in numbers and show maturation arrest. In another 5% a single aspirate is normal (? sampling of isolated erythroblast island).

Somatic abnormalities

Anomalies are noted in about one quarter. Most common are retarded growth and abnormalities of head, face and eyes, with the 'Cathie' facies regarded as typical: 'tow-coloured hair, snub nose, wide-set eyes, thick upper lip and an intelligent expression' (Cathie 1950).

Inheritance

About 80% are sporadic. Most of the remainder have autosomal recessive inheritance (these may be the mildest). In autosomal dominant kindreds the carrier parent usually shows macrocytosis and increase in HbF, with minimal or no anaemia.

Table 2.32 Erythroblastopenia in childhood

Genetic
- Diamond-Blackfan

Acquired
- TEC
- Virus
- Drugs (Table 2.34)
- Malignancy
  - Pre-ALL
  - Hodgkin's disease
- Immune
  - SLE
  - Rheumatoid arthritis
  - Thymoma
  - Without associated disease
- Other

Table 2.33 Diamond-Blackfan anaemia vs TEC

	Diamond-Blackfan	TEC
Age at onset	90% < 1 yr	85% 1–4 yr, rarely to 16 yr
Preceding viral illness	no	often
Failure to thrive	+	0
Neurologic disturbance	0	occasional
Somatic abnormalities	in about 30%	no
Fetal characteristics		
↑ MCV, ↑ HbF, ↑ i antigen	characteristic; persistent	may show mild ↑ in recovery
Natural history	most need treatment; spontaneous improvement in about 15%; risk of leukaemia	spontaneous recovery

Table 2.34 Drugs and isolated erythroblastopenia in childhood

Cytotoxics

Anti-epileptic
- Diphenylhydantoin
- Carbamazepine
- Sodium valproate
- Phenobarbital

Antibacterial
- Chloramphenicol
- Co-trimoxazole
- Sulphasalazine
- Isoniazid

Antithyroid
- Carbimazole

Immunosuppressant
- Azathiaprine
- Gold*

Anaesthetic
- Procainamide
- Halothane*

*Relationship to erythroblastopenia uncertain

Natural history
Some cases show a measure of spontaneous improvement after puberty; a normal Hb and MCV however are usually not achieved. There is a small risk of leukaemia, usually AML.

Differential diagnosis
From TEC (Table 2.33) and transplacental parvovirus infection (see below).

Transient erythroblastopenia of childhood

(Table 2.33, Freedman 1993)

The commonest spontaneous erythroblastopenia of childhood.

Essential for diagnosis
- Normocytic anaemia, reticulocytopenia and erythroblastopenia occurring de novo in a previously healthy child
- Exclusion of other causes of erythroblastopenia (Table 2.32).

Other features
- Clinical features

Usually minimal, apart from pallor. Occasional children have transient neurologic disturbance of uncertain significance (hemiparesis, seizures, unsteady gait, disturbed eye movements, Michelson & Marshall 1987).

- Blood

Anaemia (to about 2.5 g/dl), develops over some weeks — slower than for acute haemolysis but more rapid than for marrow panhypoplasia. The DAT is positive (weak, complement) in some cases. Red cell adenosine deaminase is not increased (compare Diamond-Blackfan). Neutropenia and thrombocytopenia occur in some cases (Hanada et al 1989).

- Marrow

Erythroblasts are absent or deficient (< 8% of cells), the residuum being early forms (Fig. 2.20). Degenerate forms may be noted. Overall cellularity may be mildly diminished. Storage iron may be increased (reduced erythron). If marrow is sampled in the recovery phase, appearances are likely to be normal.

- Natural history

Spontaneous recovery occurs usually within 2 weeks, but occasionally not for 2 months or rarely 8 months (these cases may be different from the usual). Rarely there is recurrence within a year.

Nature of the disorder
A virus is an attractive explanation for the destruction of mature erythrocytes, reticulocytes and erythroblasts. The significance of a history of viral illness or immunization is uncertain because of their frequency in childhood. An immune component is likely. Parvovirus is a cause in a few cases (Hanada et al 1989). TEC has been reported occasionally in more than one family member, not necessarily at the same time.

Differential diagnosis
- Diamond-Blackfan anaemia and other erythroblastopenias (Tables 2.32–2.34).
- If the child is seen first in the recovery phase, an erroneous diagnosis of haemolytic anaemia may be made.
- (Rare) cases of ALL with anaemia as the only blood manifestation (no blast cells) may be misdiagnosed as TEC if marrow is not examined.

Viruses and erythroblastopenia

- Parvovirus (Harris 1992)

B19 parvovirus is a cause of transient (1–2 weeks) erythroblastopenia ('aplastic' crisis) in patients with genetic haematologic disorders, e.g. hereditary spherocytosis, pyruvate kinase deficiency, sickle cell anaemia, and occasionally in previously normal persons. Anaemia in the neonate may result from transplacental infection (Brown et al 1994).

Giant pronormoblasts (Fig. 2.20) are characteristic. In the neonate marrow appearances may resemble type II CDA. The DAT is mildly positive (complement) in some cases. Thrombocytopenia and/or neutropenia may occur (Fig. 2.20). Marrow may be erythroblastopenic when there is little or no reduction in Hb. The P antigen is the cell receptor for the virus (Brown et al 1993).

Parvovirus may be a significant cause of chronic benign neutropenia of childhood (p. 245), and the cause of erythema infectiosum (fifth disease) in previously normal children and of a polyarthralgia syndrome in adults. Infection in the first or second trimester of pregnancy may cause non-immunologic fetal hydrops. Infection may become chronic (years) if antibody production is impaired, as in leukaemia, HIV infection and genetic immunodeficiency.

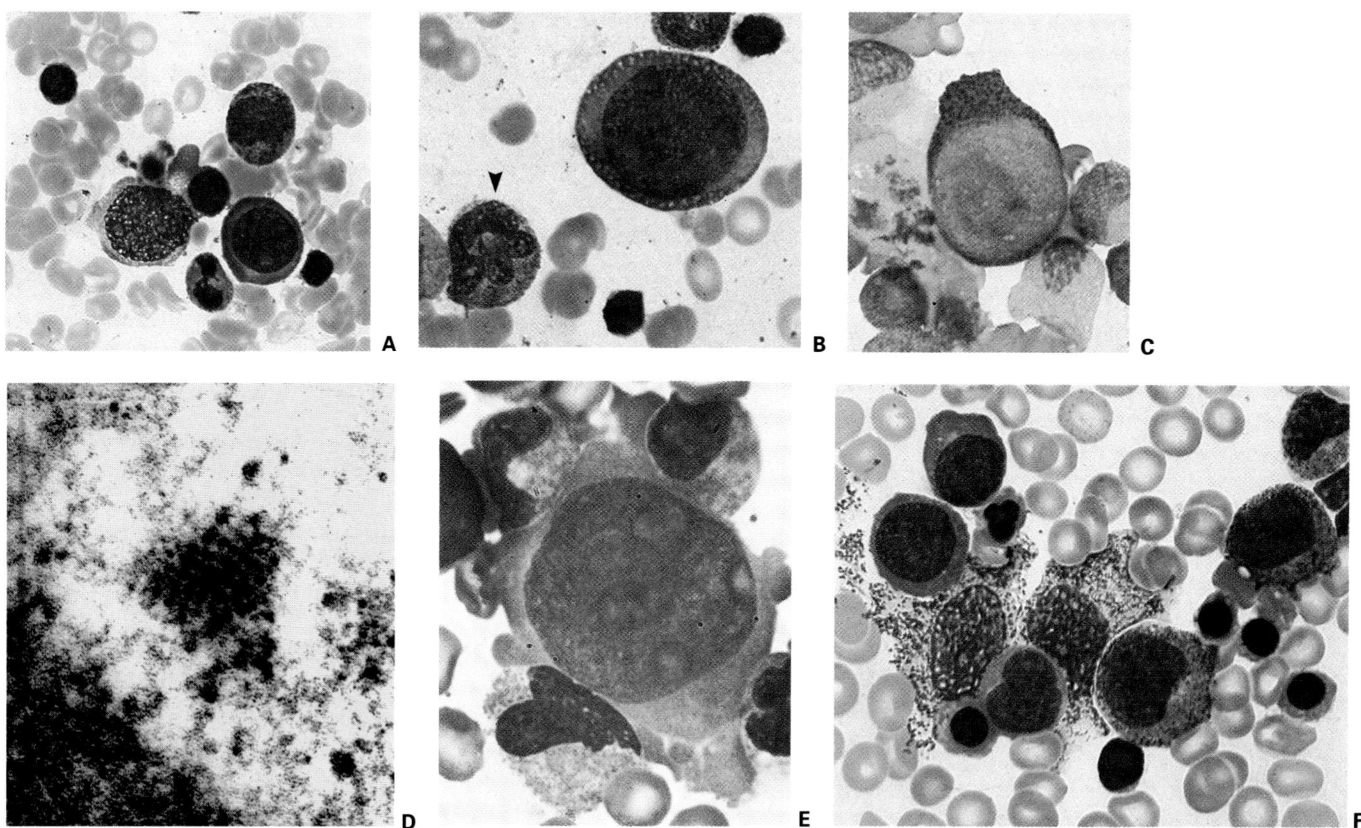

Fig. 2.20 Large and giant erythroblasts in marrow, compared with normal (**f**). **a** Large erythroblasts (the only kind seen in this marrow), TEC. **b–d** Giant erythroblasts in parvovirus infection. **b** Field also contains a large, dysplastic neutrophil (arrow). **c** PAS-positive granulation. **d** Array of 12–15 nm virus particles in nucleus of degenerate erythroblast. 16-month-old child, Hb 3.8 g/dl, MCV 88 fl ($n < 85$), neutrophils 0.9, platelets 129×10^9/l; all the changes were attributed to viral effect as there was no evidence for megaloblastosis (normal B_{12}, folate, LDH). **e** Giant erythroblast with prominent nucleoli, parvovirus infection. All × 750 except **d** × 105 000, **e** × 1000

- EBV (Hibbs & Young 1992)

EBV has been implicated in some patients with erythroblastopenia, either previously normal haematologically or with genetic disorders such as Diamond-Blackfan syndrome or sickle cell anaemia.

- Other viruses

A viral cause may be suggested by recovery following treatment with immunoglobulin (Domeyer et al 1991).

Malignancy and erythroblastopenia

Erythroblastopenia may be a prodrome, by some months, of ALL (p. 134), and is a rare spontaneous occurrence in Hodgkin's disease.

Immune erythroblastopenia

This may occur with or without recognized immune disorder (Table 2.32, Freedman 1993). The antibody (IgG, occasionally IgM) may be directed against erythroid cells or erythropoietin. Treatment with anti-lymphocyte globulin is sometimes effective (Corcione et al 1991).

Anti-D from fetomaternal incompatibility may destroy erythroblasts in neonatal marrow (Giblett et al 1956).

In one child (Talerman & Amigo 1968) possible erythroblastopenia (marrow not examined) evolved to marrow aplasia 4 weeks after thymectomy for thymoma.

Other causes of erythroblastopenia

Drugs are an uncommon cause (Table 2.34). Erythroblastopenia has been noted in rare genetic defects such as TCII deficiency (Niebrugge et al 1982) and purine nucleoside phosphorylase deficiency (Giblett et al 1975).

OSTEOPETROSIS (MARBLE-BONE DISEASE, ALBERS-SCHÖNBERG) (Fig. 2.21)

Haematologic changes occur in the severe (recessive) but not the mild (dominant) form.

A leucoerythroblastic anaemia occurs, with macrocytosis (reticulocytosis, increase in F cells) and immature myeloid cells. Extramedullary haemopoiesis results in enlargement of liver and spleen (and hypersplenism). Blindness and cranial nerve palsies manifest in infancy or childhood. Marrow transplantation is effective (replaces the defective osteoclasts, Moore 1991).

OTHER MARROW PATHOLOGY

Lymphangiectasia of marrow may be associated with normocytic anaemia (Fig. 2.21). The significance of the association is uncertain, as extensive bone disease may not be associated with anaemia (Cohen & Craig 1955).

DRUGS AND MACROCYTOSIS

Drugs may cause macrocytosis by a variety of mechanisms, usually with a final common effect of interference with DNA synthesis (Table 2.35). Marrow aplasia (Table 2.28) may contribute.

About half of patients taking anticonvulsants have decreased blood folate, attributed at least in part to impairment of absorption. Macrocytosis and megaloblastosis are common but anaemia is rare.

Cytotoxic drugs frequently cause macrocytosis/megaloblastosis, sometimes with severe dyserythropoiesis (Fig. 2.16). In general, antipurines have a less severe effect than other cytotoxics. Of the folate antagonists, methotrexate regularly causes changes; other antifolates are likely to cause megaloblastosis only if folate stores are suboptimal.

PEARSON'S SYNDROME

See page 216.

HEREDITARY OROTIC ACIDURIA (Suttle et al 1989)

Impairment in synthesis of uridine-5-monophosphate (UMP) from orotic acid via orotidine-5-monophosphate is due to a defect in UMP synthase. Clinical features manifest usually before 3 months (up to 7 years), with megaloblastic anaemia (folate and B_{12} normal), orotic acid crystalluria (often with urinary obstruction), physical and mental retardation and fine, sparse hair.

A proportion of the macrocytes may be hypochromic. In urine an abundant white flocculent deposit of microscopic needle-shaped crystals forms after standing for a few hours, especially in the cold. Precise identification of the crystals may be made by chromatography or isotope dilution. Diagnosis may be confirmed by enzyme assay of erythrocytes or cultured fibroblasts. Inheritance is autosomal recessive. High dose uridine (150 mg/kg/day) bypasses the enzyme block; folate and B_{12} are ineffective.

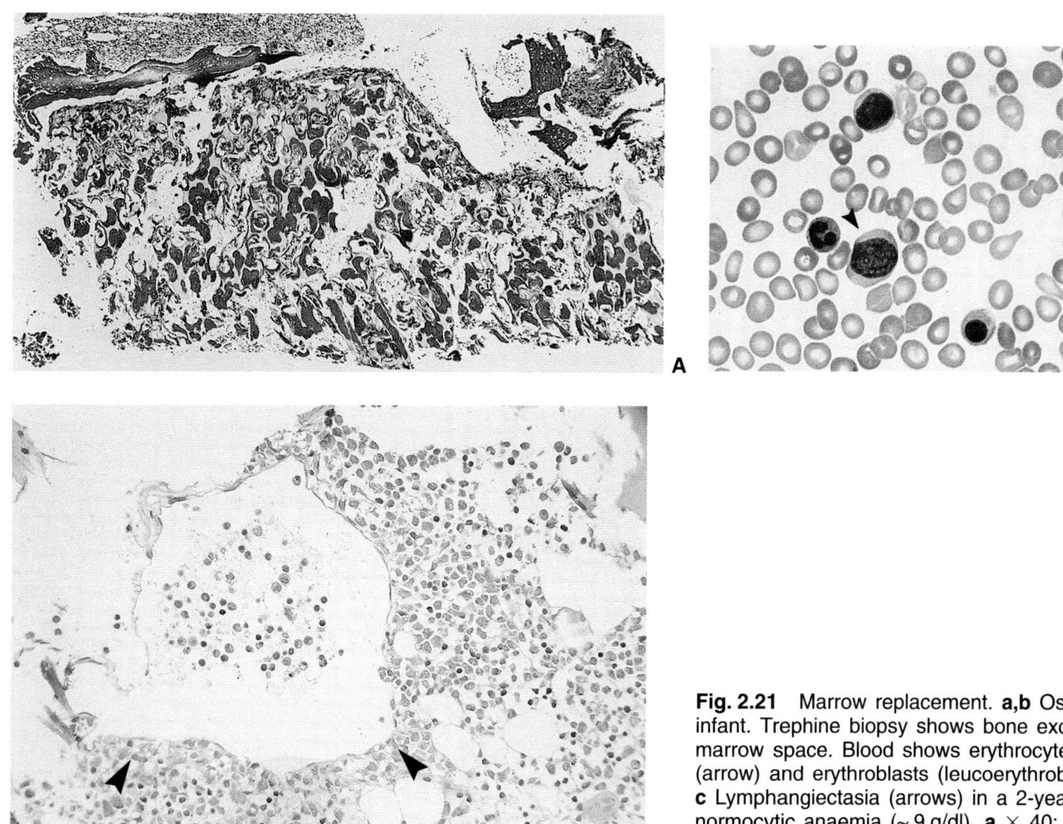

Fig. 2.21 Marrow replacement. **a,b** Osteopetrosis in a 2-month-old infant. Trephine biopsy shows bone excess and restriction of marrow space. Blood shows erythrocyte distortion, myeloblast (arrow) and erythroblasts (leucoerythroblastic anaemia). **c** Lymphangiectasia (arrows) in a 2-year-old boy with chronic normocytic anaemia (~ 9 g/dl). **a** × 40; **b** × 480; **c** × 200. **a,b** Courtesy Dr P O'Regan

Table 2.35 Paediatric drugs which may cause macrocytosis/megaloblastosis

		Action
Anticonvulsants	diphenylhydantoin	interference with folate absorption and DNA synthesis
	primidone	
	sodium valproate	
	phenobarbital	
	imipramine	
Cytotoxics		
Antipyrimidines	cytosine arabinoside	↓ DNA polymerase
	5 fluorouracil	↓ thymidylate synthetase
	azauridine	↓ orotidylic decarboxylase
	hydroxyurea	↓ ribonucleotide reductase
	azacytidine	cytidine analogue
Folate antagonists	methotrexate	
	pyrimethamine	inhibition of dihydrofolate reductase
	trimethoprim	
	pentamidine	multiple effects
Antipurines	6MP	
	thioguanine	
	azathiaprine	
Other	para-aminosalicylic acid	malabsorption of folate, B_{12}
	azidothymidine	thymidine analogue
	colchicine	inhibition of mitotic spindle

↓ = inhibition

LESCH-NYHAN SYNDROME

Megaloblastic anaemia (?deficient nucleic acid synthesis) is inconstant in this rare X-linked syndrome of mental retardation, choreoathetosis, self-mutilation and hyperuricaemia. Megaloblastosis, but not the other manifestations, may respond to high dose (1.5 g daily) adenine.

OTHER CAUSES OF MACROCYTOSIS

Macrocytosis may be noted in congenital haemolytic anaemias (e.g. pyruvate kinase deficiency) in the absence of anaemia or significant reticulocytosis.

Macrocytosis may rarely be attributed to 'freezing' of development in fetal life (Fig. 2.22).

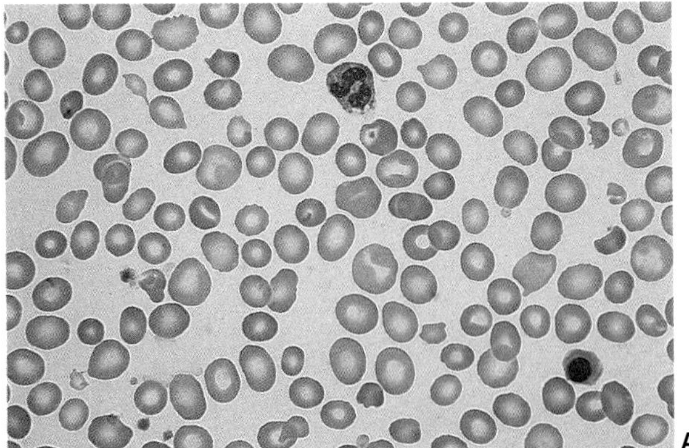

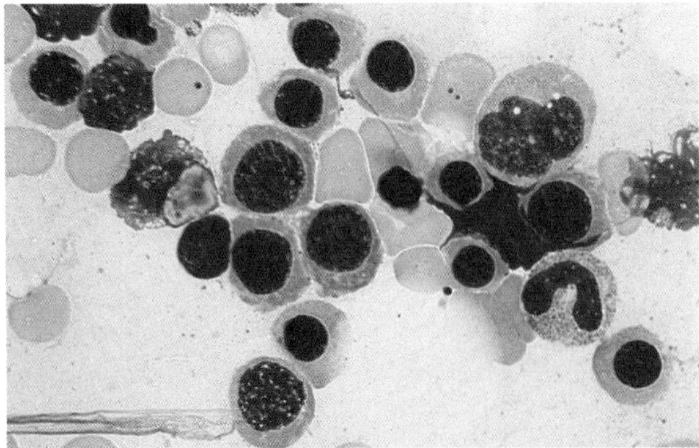

Fig. 2.22 Macrocytosis, normoblastic hyperplasia and thrombocytopenia in a 10-month-old infant with severe failure to thrive. Hb 9.2 g/dl, MCV 122 fl (n < 85), HbF 33%, reticulocytes 14%, platelets 80 × 10^9/l. Death occurred at 11 months, weight 2.4 kilos (normal 3rd centile > 7.3). The fetal erythropoiesis and failure to thrive were attributed to 'freezing' of development at the 6th month of pregnancy, when the mother had a severe flu-like illness. Courtesy of Dr J O'Duffy

REFERENCES

Abels D, Reed W B 1973 Fanconi-like syndrome. Immunologic deficiency, pancytopenia, and cutaneous malignancies. Archives of Dermatology 107: 419–423

Aggett P J, Cavanagh N P C, Matthew D J et al 1980 Shwachman's syndrome. A review of 21 cases. Archives of Disease in Childhood 55: 331–347

Alperin J B, Dow P A, Petteway M B 1977 Hemoglobin A_2 levels in health and various hematologic disorders. American Journal of Clinical Pathology 67: 219–226

Alter B P 1993 Fanconi's anaemia and its variability. British Journal of Haematology 85: 9–14

Auerbach A D, Rogatko A, Schroeder-Kurth T M 1989 International Fanconi anemia registry: relation of clinical symptoms to diepoxybutane sensitivity. Blood 73: 391–396

Baer A N, Dessypris E N, Goldwasser E, Krantz S B 1987 Blunted erythropoietin response to anaemia in rheumatoid arthritis. British Journal of Haematology 66: 559–564

Bain B J 1993 Blood film features of sickle cell-haemoglobin C disease. British Journal of Haematology 83: 516–518

Beris Ph, Miescher P A, Diaz-Chico J C et al 1988 Inclusion body β-thalassemia trait in a Swiss family is caused by an abnormal hemoglobin (Geneva) with an altered and extended β chain carboxy-terminus due to a modification in codon β114. Blood 72: 801–805

Borgna-Pignatti C, Marradi P, Pinelli L et al 1989 Thiamine-responsive anemia in DIDMOAD syndrome. Journal of Pediatrics 114: 405–410

Branda R F, Moldow C F, MacArthur J R et al 1978 Folate-induced remission in aplastic anemia with familial defect of cellular folate uptake. New England Journal of Medicine 298: 469–475

Brown K E, Anderson S M, Young N S 1993 Erythrocyte P antigen: cellular receptor for B19 parvovirus. Science 262: 114–117

Brown K E, Green S W, de Mayolo J A et al 1994 Congenital anaemia after transplacental B19 parvovirus infection. Lancet 343: 895–896

Buchanan G R, Sheehan R G 1981 Malabsorption and defective utilization of iron in three siblings. Journal of Pediatrics 98: 723–728

Butler M G, Hall B D, Maclean R N, Lozzio C B 1987 Do some patients with Seckel syndrome have hematological problems and/ or chromosome breakage? American Journal of Medical Genetics 27: 645–649

Camitta B M, Storb R, Thomas E D 1982 Aplastic anemia. Pathogenesis, diagnosis, treatment, and prognosis. New England Journal of Medicine 306: 645–652, 712–718

Cathie I A B 1950 Erythrogenesis imperfecta. Archives of Disease in Childhood 25: 313–324

Clark M, Royal J, Seeler R 1988 Interaction of iron deficiency and lead and the hematologic findings in children with severe lead poisoning. Pediatrics 81: 247–254

Cohen J, Craig J M 1955 Multiple lymphangiectases of bone. Journal of Bone and Joint Surgery 37-A: 585–596

Cooper B A, Rosenblatt D S, Whitehead V M 1993 Megaloblastic anemia. In: Nathan D G, Oski F A (eds) Hematology of infancy and childhood, 4th edn. Saunders, Philadelphia, ch 10

Corcione A, Pasino M, Molinari A C et al 1991 A pediatric case of pure red cell aplasia: successful treatment with anti-lymphocyte globulin and correlation with in vitro T cell-mediated inhibition of erythropoiesis. British Journal of Haematology 79: 129–130

Daghistani D, Curless R, Toledano S R, Ayyar D R 1989 Ataxia-pancytopenia and monosomy 7 syndrome. Journal of Pediatrics 115: 108–110

Das K C, Herbert V, Colman N, Longo D L 1978 Unmasking covert folate deficiency in iron-deficient subjects with neutrophil hypersegmentation: dU suppression tests on lymphocytes and bone marrow. British Journal of Haematology 39: 357–375

Daum R S, Cohen D L, Smith A L 1979 Fatal aplastic anemia following apparent 'dose-related' chloramphenicol toxicity. Journal of Pediatrics 94: 403–406

Domeyer C, Schulte-Overberg U, Boll I et al 1991 Erythroblastopenia in two patients after splenectomy and polychemotherapy. American Journal of Pediatric Hematology/Oncology 13: 320–325

Ellis D 1977 Anemia in the course of the nephrotic syndrome secondary to transferrin depletion. Journal of Pediatrics 90: 953–955

Erslev A J 1990 Anemia of endocrine disorders. In: Williams W J, Beutler E, Erslev A J, Lichtman M A (eds) Hematology, 4th edn. McGraw-Hill, New York, pp 444–445

Estren S, Dameshek W 1947 Familial hypoplastic anemia of childhood. Report of eight cases in two families with beneficial effect of splenectomy in one case. American Journal of Diseases of Children 73: 671–687

Field A S, Hing M C, Milliken S T, Marriott D J 1993 Microsporidia in the small intestine of HIV-infected patients. A new diagnostic technique and a new species. Medical Journal of Australia 158: 390–394.

Freedman M H 1993 Pure red cell aplasia in childhood and adolescence: pathogenesis and approaches to diagnosis. British Journal of Haematology 85: 246–253

Freedman M H, Estrov Z 1990 Congenital amegakaryocytic thrombocytopenia: an intrinsic hematopoietic stem cell defect. American Journal of Pediatric Hematology/Oncology 12: 225–230

Giblett E R, Varela J E, Finch C A 1956 Damage of bone marrow due to Rh antibody. Pediatrics 17: 37–44

Giblett E R, Ammann A J, Wara D W et al 1975 Nucleoside-phosphorylase deficiency in a child with severely defective T-cell immunity and normal B-cell immunity. Lancet 1: 1010–1013

Gómez-Almaguer D, Marfil-Rivera J, Kudish-Wersh A 1988 Acyclovir in the treatment of aplastic anemia. American Journal of Hematology 29: 172–173

Gonzalez C H, Durkin-Stamm M V, Geimer N F et al 1977 The WT syndrome — a 'new' autosomal dominant pleiotropic trait of radial/ulnar hypoplasia with high risk of bone marrow failure and/or leukemia. Birth Defects: Original Article Series 13, 3B: 31–38

Goya N, Miyazaki S, Kodate S, Ushio B 1972 A family of congenital atransferrinemia. Blood 40: 239–245

Hamon M D, Newland A C, Anderson M J 1988 Severe aplastic anaemia after parvovirus infection in the absence of underlying haemolytic anaemia. Journal of Clinical Pathology 41: 1242

Hanada T, Koike K, Hirano C, Takeya T, Suzuki T, Matsunaga Y, Takita H 1989 Childhood transient erythroblastopenia complicated by thrombocytopenia and neutropenia. European Journal of Haematology 42: 77–80

Harriman G R, Smith P D, Horne McD K et al 1989 Vitamin B12 malabsorption in patients with acquired immunodeficiency syndrome. Archives of Internal Medicine 149: 2039–2041

Harris J W 1992 Parvovirus B19 for the hematologist. American Journal of Hematology 39: 119–130

Harvey A R, Pippard M J, Ansell B M 1987 Microcytic anaemia in juvenile chronic arthritis. Scandinavian Journal of Rheumatology 16: 53–59

Hibbs J R, Young N S 1992 Viruses and the blood. Baillière's Clinical Haematology 5: 245–271

Higgs D R, Weatherall D J 1993 The haemoglobinopathies. Baillière's Clinical Haematology 6: 1–331

Hitchins R, Cobcroft R G, Hocker G 1986 Transient severe hypoplastic anemia in Q fever. Pathology 18: 254–255

Howe R B, Branda R F, Douglas S D, Brunning R D 1979 Hereditary dyserythropoiesis with abnormal membrane folate transport. Blood 54: 1080–1090

Hreidarsson S, Kristjansson K, Johannsson G, Johannsson J H 1988 A syndrome of progressive pancytopenia with microcephaly, cerebellar hypoplasia and growth failure. Acta Paediatrica Scandinavica 77: 773–775

Jacobs P, Saxe N, Gordon W, Nelson M 1984 Dyskeratosis congenita. Haematologic, cytogenetic and dermatologic studies. Scandinavian Journal of Haematology 32: 461–468

Keller A R, Hochholzer L, Castleman B 1972 Hyaline-vascular and plasma-cell types of giant lymph node hyperplasia of the mediastinum and other locations. Cancer 29: 670–683

Koerper M A, Stempel D A, Dallman P R 1978 Anemia in patients with juvenile rheumatoid arthritis. Journal of Pediatrics 92: 930–933

Kurtzman G, Young N 1989 Viruses and bone marrow failure. Baillière's Clinical Haematology 2: 51–67

Labbé R F 1990 Lead poisoning mechanisms. Clinical Chemistry 36: 1870

Larrick J W, Hyman E S 1984 Acquired iron-deficiency anemia caused by an antibody against the transferrin receptor. New England Journal of Medicine 311: 214–218

Lau Y-L, Srivastava G, Lee C-W et al 1994 Epstein-Barr virus associated aplastic anaemia and hepatitis. Journal of Paediatrics and Child Health 30: 74–76

McDonald R, Marshall S R 1964 The value of iron therapy in pica. Pediatrics 34: 558–562

Mandel H, Berant M, Hazani A, Naveh Y 1984 Thiamine-dependent beriberi in the 'thiamine-responsive anemia syndrome'. New England Journal of Medicine 311: 836–838

Michelson A D, Marshall P C 1987 Transient neurological disorder associated with transient erythroblastopenia of childhood. American Journal of Pediatric Hematology/Oncology 9: 161–163

Miller D R, O'Reilly R J 1989 Aplastic anemia. In: Miller D R, Baehner R L (eds) Blood diseases of infancy and childhood, 6th edn. Mosby, St Louis, pp 465–469

Miyoshi K, Kaneto Y, Kawai H et al 1988 X-linked dominant control of F-cells in normal adult life: characterization of the Swiss type as hereditary persistence of fetal hemoglobin regulated dominantly by gene(s) on X chromosome. Blood 72: 1854–1860

Moore M A S 1991 Clinical implications of positive and negative hematopoietic stem cell regulators. Blood 78: 1–19

Niebrugge D J, Benjamin D R, Christie D, Scott C R 1982 Hereditary transcobalamin II deficiency presenting as red cell hypoplasia. Journal of Pediatrics 101: 732–735

Oski F A 1979 Hematologic consequences of chloramphenicol therapy. Journal of Pediatrics 94: 515–516

Oski F A 1990 Anemia related to nutritional deficiencies other than vitamin B12 and folic acid. In: Williams W J, Beutler E, Erslev A J, Lichtman M A (eds) Hematology, 4th edn. McGraw-Hill, New York, ch 53

Pearce C J, Conrad M E, Nolan P E et al 1988 Ehrlichiosis: a cause of bone marrow hypoplasia in humans. American Journal of Hematology 28: 53–55

Pearson H A, Gallagher D, Chilcote R et al 1985 Developmental pattern of splenic dysfunction in sickle cell disorders. Pediatrics 76: 392–397

Piomelli S 1993 Lead poisoning. In: Nathan D G, Oski F A (eds) Hematology of infancy and childhood, 4th edn. Saunders, Philadelphia, ch 14

Porter F S, Lowe B A 1963 Congenital erythropoietic protoporphyria I. Case reports, clinical studies and porphyrin analyses in two brothers. Blood 22: 521–531

Ringelhann B, Khorsandi M 1972 Hemoglobin crystallization test to differentiate cells with Hb SC and CC genotype from SS cells without electrophoresis. American Journal of Clinical Pathology 57: 467–470

Ritchey A K, Hoffman R, Dainiak N et al 1979 Antibody-mediated acquired sideroblastic anemia: response to cytotoxic therapy. Blood 54: 734–741

Rosenblatt D S 1989 Inherited disorders of folate transport and metabolism. In: Scriver C R, Beaudet A L, Sly W S, Valle D (eds) The metabolic basis of inherited disease, 6th edn. McGraw-Hill, New York, ch 81

Rotoli B, Luzzatto L 1989 Paroxysmal nocturnal haemoglobinuria. Baillière's Clinical Haematology 2: 113–138

Sackey K, Sakati N, Aur R J A et al 1985 Multiple dysmorphic features and pancytopenia: a new syndrome? Clinical Genetics 27: 606–610

Samad F U, Engel E, Hartmann R C 1973 Hypoplastic anemia, Friedreich's ataxia and chromosomal breakage: case report and review of similar disorders. Southern Medical Journal 66: 135–140

Scarlett J D, Williams N T, McKellar W J D 1992 Acquired amegakaryocytic thrombocytopenia in a child. Journal of Paediatrics and Child Health 28: 263–266

Shepherd R W, Holt T L, Thomas B J et al 1984 Malnutrition in cystic fibrosis: the nature of the nutritional deficit and optimal management. Nutrition Abstracts and Reviews 54: 1009–1022

Sherman J D, Greenfield J B, Ingall D 1964 Reversible bone-marrow vacuolizations in phenylketonuria. New England Journal of Medicine 270: 810–814

Shivdasani R A, Haluska F G, Dock N L et al 1993 Brief report: graft-versus-host disease associated with transfusion of blood from unrelated HLA-homozygous donors. New England Journal of Medicine 328: 766–769

Sipes S L, Weiner C P, Wenstrom K D et al 1991 The association between fetal karyotype and mean corpuscular volume. American Journal of Obstetrics and Gynecology 165: 1371–1376

Smith R R L, Spivak J L 1985 Marrow cell necrosis in anorexia nervosa and involuntary starvation. British Journal of Haematology 60: 525–530

Stavem P, Romslo I, Hovig T et al 1985 Ferrochelatase deficiency in the bone marrow in a syndrome of congenital hypochromic microcytic anemia, hyperferremia, and iron overload of the liver. Scandinavian Journal of Gastroenterology 20 (suppl 107): 73–81

Suttle D P, Becroft D M O, Webster D R 1989 Hereditary orotic aciduria and other disorders of pyrimidine metabolism. In: Scriver C R, Beaudet A L, Sly W S, Valle D (eds) The metabolic basis of inherited disease, 6th edn. McGraw-Hill, New York, ch 43

Talerman A, Amigo A 1968 Thymoma associated with aregenerative and aplastic anemia in a five-year-old child. Cancer 21: 1212–1218

Walters T R, Desposito F 1985 Aplastic anemia in Dubowitz syndrome. Journal of Pediatrics 106: 622–623

Watkins D, Rosenblatt D S 1989 Functional methionine synthase deficiency (cblE and cblG): clinical and biochemical heterogeneity. American Journal of Medical Genetics 34: 427–434

Wickramasinghe S N, Pippard M J 1986 Studies of erythroblast function in congenital dyserythropoietic anaemia, type I: evidence of impaired DNA, RNA, and protein synthesis and unbalanced globin chain synthesis in ultrastructurally abnormal cells. Journal of Clinical Pathology 39: 881–890

Wilkie A O M, Buckle V J, Harris P C et al 1990a Clinical features and molecular analysis of the α thalassemia/mental retardation syndromes. I. Cases due to deletions involving chromosome band 16p13.3. American Journal of Human Genetics 46: 1112–1126

Wilkie A O M, Zeitlin H C, Lindenbaum R H et al 1990b Clinical features and molecular analysis of the α thalassemia/mental retardation syndromes. II. Cases without detectable abnormality of the α globin complex. American Journal of Human Genetics 46: 1127–1140

Yip R, Norris T N, Anderson A S 1981 Iron status of children with elevated blood lead concentrations. Journal of Pediatrics 98: 922–925

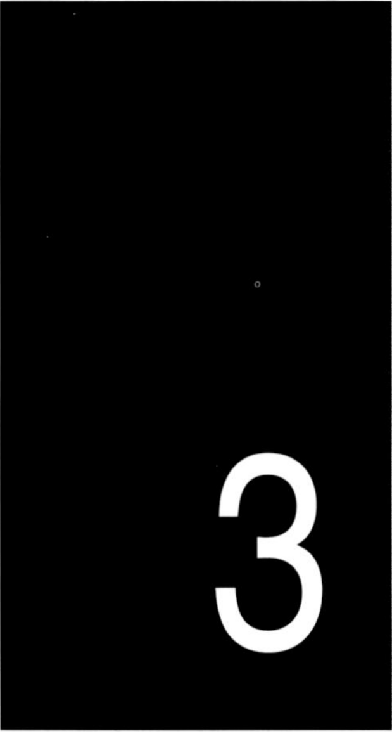

3 Normocytic anaemias

Recent blood loss 62

Impaired production 64

Haemolytic disorders 64

With distinctive morphology
- Spherocytosis 64
- Elliptocytosis 76
- Fragmentation 80
- Target cells 82
- Pyknocytosis 82
- Bite cells 86
- Acanthocytosis 86
- Crenation 90
- Spiculated (spur) cells 90
- Blister cells 92
- Puddled Hb 92
- Stomatocytosis 94
- Prominent basophilic stippling 97
- Bizarre poikilocytosis 97

Without distinctive morphology 98
- Infection 98
- Alloimmune haemolysis 98
- Renal disease 98
- Vitamin deficiency/excess, trace element deficiency, hyperlipidaemia 100
- Enzyme defects 102
- Congenital erythropoietic porphyria 107

Asplenia, splenic atrophy/hypofunction 108

Abbreviations and notes

ADA: adenosine deaminase; C: complement; DAT: direct antiglobulin (Coombs) test; EPO: erythropoietin; hct: haematocrit; HE: hereditary elliptocytosis; HS: hereditary spherocytosis; HUS: haemolytic-uraemic syndrome; IAT: indirect antiglobulin test; PK: pyruvate kinase; TEC: transient erythroblastopenia of childhood; thal: thalassaemia; TTP: thrombotic thrombocytopenic purpura; vWF: von Willebrand factor.

Photomicrographs: blood films are × 480 unless otherwise stated.

Discussion of these anaemias will follow the order in Table 3.1

Recent blood loss

Typical features are normocytic anaemia and reticulocytosis; there is no jaundice, though internal bleeds may give a mild hyperbilirubinaemia after a few days as a result of absorption from degenerating blood.

In the neonate (Table 3.2), when a source of blood loss cannot be identified, fetomaternal or feto-fetal loss is to be considered. Some fetomaternal traffic in cells is normal; however, transfer of significant volumes (> 40 ml) is uncommon (about 1%), with loss of > 100 ml being rare and sometimes fatal.

Transfer occurs usually at delivery, though the tear in the placenta is not always obvious. Transfer of substantial amounts over a period before delivery is likely to be associated with exceptionally high levels of HbF in maternal blood (Fig. 3.1, Willis & Foreman 1988) and/or appearances of iron deficiency in the blood film (Fig. 2.1). Losses may follow obstetric procedures such as amniocentesis or external version, but often a cause is not found.

Diagnosis is most easily made by the Kleihauer procedure (Fig. 3.1); in interpretation of high values, pre-existing conditions such as β thalassaemia are to be excluded. Low levels (< 1%), which may be due to pregnancy itself, can be clarified if needed by an immunofluorescent procedure (Popat et al 1977) or serologic detection of D-positive fetal cells in the mother (if D-negative, Mollison et al 1993). Fetomaternal transfer of D-positive cells is a cause of apparent change in maternal group from D-negative to weak D-positive or D^u.

If there is group incompatibility, fetal cells will not survive for more than a few hours in the maternal circulation. In this event, examination of maternal buffy coats for erythrophagocytosis and of serum for rise in immune anti-A, anti-B may be useful.

Significant feto-fetal transfer (> 5 g/dl difference, Fig. 3.1) occurs in up to one third of identical twin (single placenta) births.

Table 3.1 Normocytic anaemias of childhood

- Recent blood loss
- Impaired production
  - Erythroblast deficiency
    - Global marrow deficiency[1,2]
    - Pure erythroblastopenia[2]
  - Dyserythropoiesis
    - Genetic
    - Acquired
  - Deficiency of erythroblast stimulants
    - Erythropoietin
    - Thyroid
    - Vitamin C
    - Protein (?)
- Haemolysis
  - With distinctive red cell morphology
  - Without distinctive red cell morphology
- Sequestration
  - Hypersplenism[1]
- Haemodilution
  - Acute glomerulonephritis
  - Overhydration
  - Water immersion

[1] Anaemia is part of pancytopenia
[2] In some types anaemia is macrocytic

Table 3.2 Blood loss anaemia in the neonate

- Prenatal
  - Fetomaternal
    - Spontaneous
    - Cephalic version
    - Amniocentesis
  - Twin-to-twin
- At birth
  - External
    - Obstetric accidents/pathology
      - Rupture of normal or abnormal cord (varices, anomalous insertion)
      - Placenta praevia, abruptio placentae
      - Incision of placenta at caesarean section
    - Excessive blood taking for tests
  - Internal
    - Scalp haemorrhage
    - Intracranial
    - Ruptured abdominal viscus

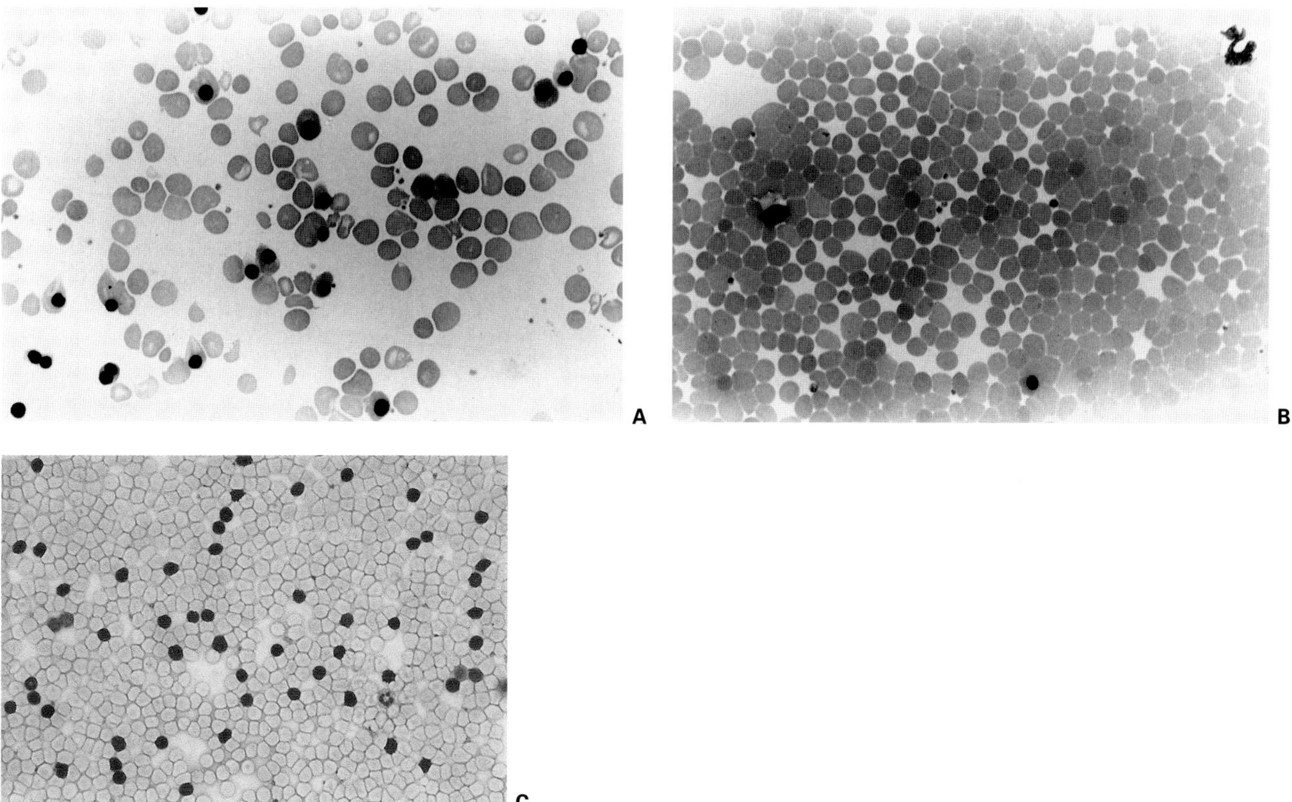

Fig. 3.1 Feto-fetal (**a,b**) and fetomaternal (**c**) transfusion. **a,b** Infants 1 day old; anaemia (Hb 8.6 g/dl) and erythroblastosis in **a**, polycythaemia (Hb 25.3 g/dl) in **b**. Maternal Kleihauer in **c** 6.3%, = approximately 300 ml fetal blood. The magnitude of the loss (approx whole fetal blood volume) and the fact that the infant survived indicate that loss was occurring over a period before delivery. **a,b** × 310; **c** × 200

Normocytic anaemias due to impaired production

Erythroblast deficiency as part of global marrow deficiency

These disorders, summarized in Table 3.3, are discussed elsewhere — panhypoplasia (p. 44), leukaemias (Chs 4 and 5), storage diseases (Ch. 6), osteopetrosis (p. 56).

Erythroblastopenias

These are considered together for comparison in Chapter 2 (p. 53, Table 2.32).

Dyserythropoiesis

The dyserythropoieses are considered together in Chapter 2 (p. 40, Table 2.34).

Deficiency of erythroblast stimulants

Erythropoietin (EPO)
EPO deficiency is significant in:

- Anaemia of prematurity

In addition to the normal post-natal switchoff of EPO, there is muted EPO response to anaemia in the newborn and fetus, because fetal EPO (mainly from liver) is less sensitive to hypoxia than the renal EPO of later life. Other factors in the anaemia of prematurity are post-natal haemolysis and, if relevant, excessive blood taking. Iron deficiency is not a factor. After about 2 months, however, when EPO production (and reticulocytosis) resumes, iron supplementation is beneficial (and necessary for the EPO to be fully effective).

- Anaemia of renal failure; haemolysis of uncertain origin (p. 98) also participates.

- Some other anaemias, e.g. chronic disease (p. 18).

Thyroid, vitamin C
See page 40.

Protein
The hypoproteinaemia of severe neonatal cystic fibrosis may be associated with a normocytic anaemia with cell distortion and evidence of membrane damage (Fig. 3.14).

Haemolytic anaemias

The recognition of haemolysis per se is rarely a problem in childhood. A suggested basic laboratory work-up is given in Table 3.4. Care is needed in interpretation; for example the reticulocyte count may be decreased in the crises of parvovirus infection, and a low serum haptoglobin is normal in the first months of life (Table 1.12), in liver disease (decreased production) and in congenital ahaptoglobinaemia. On the other hand, a rise (acute phase response) in inflammation and malignancy may mask reduction from haemolysis.

Haemosiderinuria (Fig. 3.26) is an inconstant feature of chronic haemolysis, occurring, for example, in PK deficiency, PNH and with prosthetic heart valves; but it may also result from resorption of haematomas (Reeve 1971).

As a practical starting point, haemolytic disorders may be classified into those with and those without morphologic changes in erythrocytes (Table 3.5). Morphologic abnormality is not necessarily associated with anaemia.

SPHEROCYTOSIS (Table 3.6)

Genuine spherocytosis is to be distinguished from:

- artefact (excessive heat during drying of film); cells are fuzzy, distribution in film patchy, not demonstrable on repeat testing
- 'whiskered' spherocytes' (Figs 3.15, 3.26)
- normal finding (neonate, Fig. 1.1).

Table 3.3 Global marrow insufficiency

Panhypoplasia
Infiltration
- Leukaemia
- Other
  - Histiocytosis
  - Storage disease

Fibrosis
- Malignancy
  - Leukaemia
    - AML, especially M7
    - Myelodysplasia, e.g. monosomy 7 MPD
    - ALL (minority)
  - Other
    - Neuroblastoma
- Histiocytosis
- Idiopathic[1]

Osteopetrosis

[1] In most of these, myelosclerosis is a precursor to, or an early manifestation of malignancy which does not become overt until some months later

Table 3.4 Initial investigation for suspected haemolysis

Blood values, reticulocytes
Stained blood film
Heinz bodies
Direct antiglobulin (Coombs) test
Serum
- Bilirubin total, conjugated
- Haptoglobin
- Lactate dehydrogenase

Red cell enzymes
- G6PD screen, assay
- Pyruvate kinase screen

Urine
- Haemosiderin
- Erythrocytes
- Haemoglobin
- Myoglobin

In neonate
- Blood groups of infant and mother
- Specificity of heat eluate of infant cells

In selected cases
- Hb electrophoresis
- Unstable Hb — isopropanol precipitation
- Sugar lysis

Table 3.5 Red cell morphology of value in diagnosis of haemolysis

Spherocytosis
Elliptocytosis
Fragmentation
Target cells
Pyknocytosis
Bitten-out cells
Acanthocytosis
Crenation (echinocytosis)
Spiculated (spur) cells
Blister cells
Puddling of Hb
Stomatocytosis
Sickle cells
Crystals
Coarse stippling
Bizarre poikilocytosis
Parasites (malaria, babesia, bartonella)

Table 3.6 Spherocytosis in childhood

Artefact
Normal: neonate[1]
Non-immune
- Hereditary
- Burns
- Infection
  - Clostridial
  - Other
- Envenomation
- Cyanotic congenital heart disease
- Enzyme deficiency[1,2]
- Total parenteral nutrition[1]
- Copper intoxication
- Obstructive jaundice/liver failure[1]
- Hypophosphataemia

Immune
- Alloimmune
  - Fetomaternal — ABO
  - Organ transplantation
  - Incompatible transfusion
- Autoimmune
  - Infection
    - Virus, mycoplasma
    - Neuraminidase-producers — pneumococcus, clostridium[3]
  - Autoimmune disease[4,5]
  - Some drugs
  - Idiopathic[4]
- Infusion of anti-A/B/D-containing material
- Drug-immune

[1] Spherocytosis minor
[2] Spherocytosis may be notable in glutathione peroxidase, phosphoglycerate kinase and glucose phosphate isomerase deficiencies
[3] T activation; often with fragmentation; DAT negative with monoclonal reagents (older type sera may give positive reaction due to presence of anti-T, Seger et al 1980)
[4] In the neonate, may be associated with maternal autoimmune disease
[5] Spherocytosis inconspicuous or absent in some cases with strong positive DAT

Hereditary spherocytosis

In most cases spectrin is deficient in quantity or defective at sites of binding to integral proteins such as 4.1 (Becker & Lux 1993, Fig. 3.2). Binders themselves, e.g. ankyrin, are deficient or defective in some cases. Instability of structure of spectrin or in its binding to the lipoprotein envelope may induce spot weaknesses, which could explain the membrane loss which is the anatomic basis of spherocytosis. Excessive blebbing following exposure to oxidants has been shown (Malorni et al 1993).

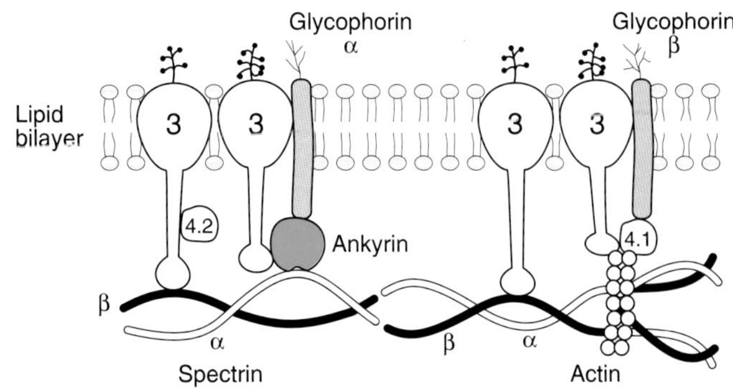

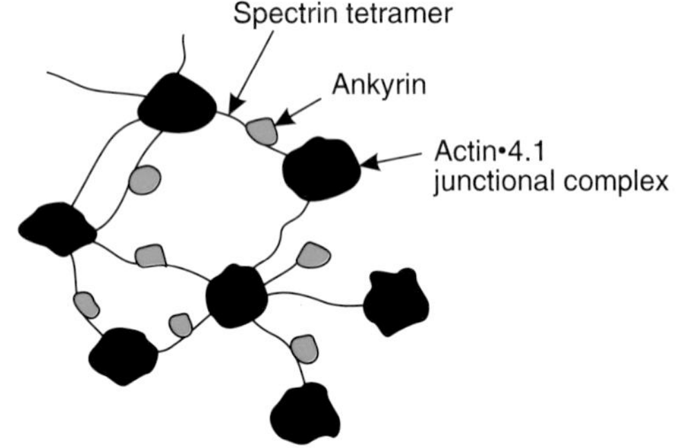

Fig. 3.2 Proteins of the erythrocyte skeleton, simplified.

Identification of spherocytosis as hereditary
Acquired conditions (Table 3.6) will as a rule be associated with appropriate clinical background. However, in some cases of autoimmune disease (e.g. SLE), this is subtle, and spherocytosis may be misinterpreted as hereditary if a DAT is not done. HS may coexist with other common types of spherocytosis — if, for example, combination with fetomaternal ABO incompatibility is suspected, follow-up for at least 3 months is helpful (features of ABO incompatibility will have waned).

Erythrocyte morphology (Figs 3.4–3.7)
Features tend to be uniform in affected members of the one kindred, though exceptions occur.

Spherocytes may be sparse or absent:

- In crisis. Preferential destruction of spherocytes, together with suboptimal morphology (thin films) and reticulocytopenia may cause uncertainty in diagnosis.
- In about 1% (Krueger & Burgert 1966) spherocytosis is minimal in the neonatal period, becoming typical at about 3 months (Fig. 3.3).
- In rare cases spherocytosis is evident only after splenectomy or after cholecystectomy for gallstones (Becker & Lux 1993). Fragility is usually abnormal in these cases.
- In severe cases needing frequent transfusion, spherocytes may be sparse if only post-transfusion samples are available.

Morphology may be atypical in certain infrequent circumstances:

- Acanthocytosis may be noted in some severe cases, in the neonatal period (Fig. 3.3) and after splenectomy.
- In occasional kindreds bottle-shaped or 'pincer' cells are notable (Fig. 3.3).
- After splenectomy spherocytosis is not as evident.
- Associated disease — increase in surface/volume ratio in megaloblastosis, iron deficiency, thalassaemia and obstructive jaundice will tend to normalize the shape.
- Oval spherocytosis or association with elliptocytosis suggests a diagnosis of haemolytic HE with spherocytosis (p. 78).

Other features of red cell morphology
Howell-Jolly bodies in unsplenectomized patients suggest splenic hypofunction, attributable to reticuloendothelial blockade. This is more likely in children > 5 years old. Because of impaired removal, spherocytes in these cases are likely to be profuse, with longer survival in patients than in normals (Wiley 1970).

The pitted cell count (Fig. 3.27) is unreliable for diagnosis of splenic hypofunction in HS, as the abnormal membrane impedes the formation of subsurface vacuoles, the anatomic basis of pits visible by interference microscopy (O'Grady et al 1984).

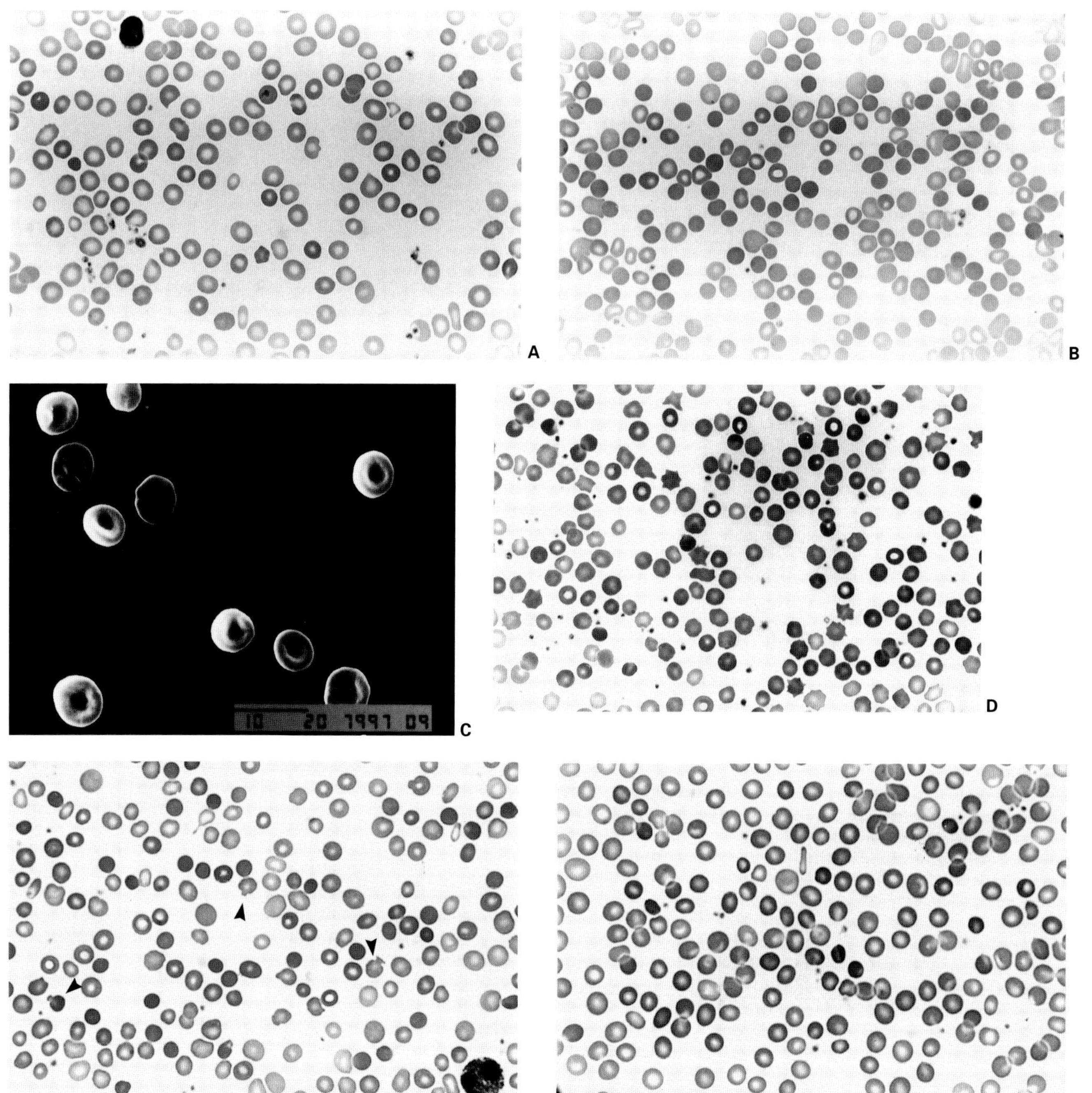

Fig. 3.3 Hereditary spherocytosis. **a,b** Evolution with age. **a** 3 months, minimal abnormality, Hb 7.5 g/dl. **b** 5 years, developed abnormality, Hb 12.6 g/dl. Appearances became typical at 4–6 months. **c** Scanning microscopy — spherocytes are not completely spherical. **d** With acanthocytosis in a 6-month child; at 13 months acanthocytosis was still present but less marked. **e** 'Pincer-cell' variant (arrows) in a 6-year-old. **f** Possible minimal disease in a 2-year-old, hypertonic cryohaemolysis 25% (n $<20\%$). **c** $\times$ 1200

Erythrocyte values

In up to 30% there is no anaemia. The MCHC tends to be high as a result of cellular dehydration from loss of cell K^+ and water. The MCH is normal.

Worsening of anaemia and reticulocytosis during common infections is attributed to reticuloendothelial stimulation. The DAT may become transiently and mildly positive (C3d) in these episodes. 'Aplastic' crisis (anaemia, reticulocytopenia, erythroblastopenia) is due in most cases to parvovirus infection (p. 54) and may be the presenting manifestation. Megaloblastic crises, from folate intake insufficient for the hyperplastic erythron, are rare in childhood.

Confirmation of diagnosis

Autohaemolysis with improvement by added glucose (Dacie & Lewis 1991) is sensitive, but results are abnormal also in immune spherocytosis and in some apparently normal persons. Again, though added glucose usually does not cause improvement in immune spherocytosis, there may be no correction in severe HS.

Traditionally, confirmation is made with an osmotic fragility procedure. Use of unincubated blood is insensitive but will detect the tail of more fragile cells which have been conditioned by the adverse conditions of glucose supply and pH in the spleen. Incubated (24 h) fragility is more sensitive but does not differentiate the fragile tail, as all the cells have been conditioned to greater fragility by the incubation.

In neonates, autohaemolysis and osmotic fragility (fresh or incubated) are abnormal even without spherocytosis (Schröter & Kahsnitz 1983). Reliable interpretation requires use of neonates as controls and of venous rather than cord blood, in which the spread of values is too wide.

Other osmotic fragility procedures are less cumbersome to perform and need less blood than the classic procedure. In glycerol-based procedures glycerol in the hypotonic saline medium slows entry of water sufficiently to allow precise quantitation of rate and degree of haemolysis, e.g. acidified glycerol lysis time (Bucx et al 1988) and the 'Pink' test (Balari et al 1989).

The procedures above depend on the poor tolerance of the spherocyte for increase in volume on account of its diminished surface area/volume ratio. In contrast, the hypertonic cryohaemolysis procedure (Streichman et al 1990) is thought to depend on the instability in relation of the spectrin-actin mesh to the phospholipid envelope. It uses only small volumes of blood and is more sensitive than osmotic fragilities, detecting a proportion of carrier parents with normal blood films and values (Fig. 3.3). However, abnormal results are obtained in a minority with autoimmune haemolysis (Streichman et al 1990) and in haemolytic-uraemic syndrome. A comparison of the cryohaemolysis procedure with the acidified glycerol lysis time (stored 24 h) and the Pink test (stored 24 h) gave these results for sensitivity: 100% for cryohaemolysis, 42% for acidified glycerol and 67% for the Pink (Kempin 1993).

Laser light scattering, by giving precise determinations of MCV, allows reliable recognition of spherocytes (Pati et al 1989).

Association with other anomalies

In kindreds with chromosome defects at gene sites for membrane proteins, HS may be associated with somatic abnormalities such as psychomotor retardation and dysmorphism, e.g. 8q deletion (ankyrin gene, Chilcote et al 1987).

Associations with progressive neurologic disease (McCann & Jacob 1976) and with cardiomyopathy (Moiseyev et al 1987) are attributed to the fact that proteins of the red cell skeleton such as spectrin, ankyrin and 4.1 occur also in brain and heart. An association with neonatal giant cell hepatitis has been suggested (Fraga et al 1968).

Inheritance

In about three quarters of cases inheritance is autosomal dominant. The other quarter, which tend to be more severe, are attributed to spontaneous mutation or recessive inheritance. Homozygosity for dominant spherocytosis appears to be incompatible with life, with some exceptions (Duru et al 1992).

Burns

Spherocytosis (often microspherocytosis) from thermal damage to spectrin and other proteins is likely with > 15% burns, and lasts up to 3 days. There may be some budding or fragmentation (Fig. 3.4).

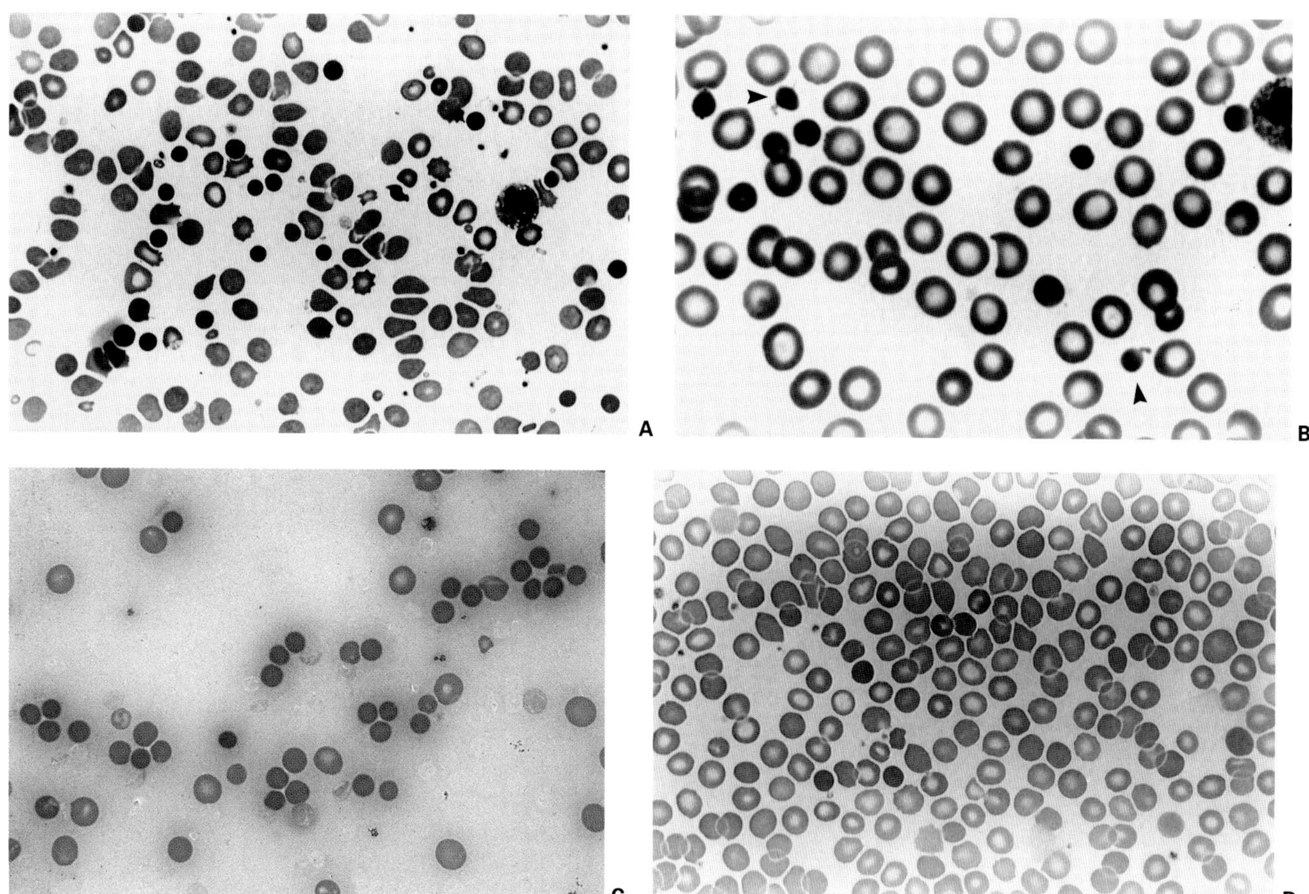

Fig. 3.4 Spherocytosis, non-immune, non-hereditary. **a,b** 2 children with burns; arrows in **b** show budding. **c** *Cl. welchii* septicaemia, spherocytosis and 'poached egg' leakage of Hb. **d** Spherocytosis with population of microcytic cells, 8-month-old child with cyanotic congenital heart disease, Hb 13.7 g/dl, MCV 66 fl (n > 70). **b** x 750

Infection

- Clostridial

Spherocytosis, often with a 'poached egg' appearance, may be a dramatic occurrence in *Clostridium welchii* sepsis (Fig. 3.4). Virtually the entire red cell mass may be destroyed (Dean et al 1967). Damage to spectrin by protease appears to be more important than damage to the envelope by phospholipase (Simpkins et al 1971). Haemolysis in clostridial infection may also result from T activation (p. 74).

- Other

Spherocytosis in viral infection is usually immune (p. 75). However, non-immune spherocytosis, usually minor, may be noted in viral and other infections (CMV, congenital syphilis).

Other non-immune spherocytoses (see also Table 3.6)

Spherocytosis may occur in:

- Envenomation (snakes, spiders, bees, wasps, jellyfish). Infrequent. Due to direct membrane damage, intravascular coagulation or rarely immune effect (Eichner 1984).
- Cyanotic congenital heart disease. Minor and of obscure origin (Fig. 3.4, Hughes & Lovric 1962).
- Total parenteral nutrition, if administered rapidly (McGrath et al 1982). See also chylomicronaemia (p. 230).
- Copper intoxication. May follow debridement of burns with copper sulphate (Holtzman et al 1966).
- Obstructive jaundice/liver failure. Spherocytes in most cases are an evolution by membrane loss from 'spiculated spherocytes' (Fig. 3.15, p. 90).
- Hypophosphataemia (< 0.5 mg/dl). Spherocytosis with decreased cell ATP and 2,3 DPG noted after prolonged vomiting and diarrhoea, or in pancreatitis with starvation (Klock et al 1974).

Immune spherocytosis

A positive DAT (Table 3.7) is not necessarily associated with haemolysis or spherocytosis — neither occurs in some patients with autoimmune disease, and spherocytosis does not occur in Rh disease of the newborn.

Alloimmune haemolysis

A suggested schema for initial investigation is given in Table 3.8.

The DAT may rarely be negative:

- IgG on cell surface too sparse to be detected by routine methods
- in some patients with anti-C, the presence of antibody being inferred from haemolysis of transfused C-positive, and normal survival of C-negative blood, or from shortened survival of labelled erythrocytes (Harrison et al 1986).

In some cases the nature of a presumed fetomaternal incompatibility is obscure (Fig. 3.15) — maternal and infant groups are apparently compatible, eluate of infant cells cannot be shown to have group specificity, and there is no clinical or serologic evidence (DAT, antinuclear factor) of autoimmune disease in the mother. These cases may be due to: (a) incompatibility for a rare paternal antigen (e.g. Wr^a, Vw), (b) HLA immunization, or (c) a drug or infection in the mother causing an immune effect in fetus but not in mother. The DAT is usually weak IgG, transient, and with some exceptions (Fig. 3.15) not associated with significant haemolysis.

Fetomaternal

ABO incompatibility
The most frequent type, consistently associated with spherocytosis.

The problem is almost restricted to group A or B babies of O mothers, who are more likely to have or to produce IgG (placenta-crossing) antibody than A or B mothers; IgG anti-A and to a lesser extent anti-B occur spontaneously together with the IgM antibodies in a high proportion of O persons, the titre of IgG anti-A being stimulated by exposure to A or A-like substances in blood or blood products and some vaccines. Because of pre-existing antibody, ABO incompatibility is more likely to cause haemolysis in a first pregnancy than Rh disease.

Although about 15% of pregnancies are at risk for ABO incompatibility, significant haemolysis occurs in only 1–2%, and severe anaemia (< 10 g/dl) is rare (about 1/3000, Letsky 1991). The mildness of haemolysis is due to sparseness of A and B sites on fetal erythrocytes and diversion of antibody to A and B sites widely distributed in other tissues. Jaundice is more common than anaemia and, as for any pathologic haemolysis, occurs usually in the first 24 hours. Jaundice is usually not obvious at birth because of clearing of bilirubin by the placenta. In some infants there is, for unexplained reasons, a significant increase in conjugated bilirubin (Sivan et al 1983).

Osmotic fragility and autohaemolysis are increased but do not add useful diagnostic information. The DAT (IgG) is usually not strongly positive. Because of the sparseness of antibody binding, complement is not activated and intravascular haemolysis does not occur.

Diagnosis is best made by testing heat eluate of infant cells with monospecific IgG anti-A, anti-B (Issitt 1985). Samples should be taken promptly, as the antibodies disappear within days. The IAT using infant plasma is also usually positive.

Co-occurrence with other common causes of anaemia or jaundice, e.g. HS, should be suspected if anaemia is severe (< 10 g/dl). To resolve uncertainty, review should be made at 3–6 months, when evidence of ABO incompatibility will have disappeared.

Table 3.7 Positive DAT in childhood

Alloimmune haemolysis
Autoimmune haemolysis
Infused anti-A/B/D-containing material
Drug-immune haemolysis
Unexplained

Table 3.8 Recognition of alloimmune haemolysis: initial investigation

Direct antiglobulin test
Broad spectrum
Monospecific — IgG, C3, C3d
If negative, indirect antiglobulin test with:
Eluate from cells
Infant plasma
Blood group specificity of eluate from cells
Blood grouping and, if neonate, of mother also[1]
Blood values, reticulocytes
Blood film
Spherocytosis
Agglutination
Erythrophagocytosis
If relevant, procedures for detecting incompatible transfusion

[1] Antenatal screening will have detected most antibodies before birth

Incompatibility other than ABO
Although any antigen with the capacity to produce IgG antibody may cause haemolytic disease, the problem is virtually restricted to D, ABO, and in < 5%, c, Kell, E and Fy^a. Anaemia is most severe with D, c and Kell (in approximately this order), the others rarely causing severe disease. Spherocytosis is consistent in ABO disease but is not a feature of Rh (Fig. 3.21), and is rare in other incompatibilities (Fig. 3.5). Diagnosis is best made by testing eluate of infant cells for specificity. Anti-D may affect erythroblasts and reticulocytes as well as erythrocytes (Giblett et al 1956).

Haemolysis from Kell incompatibility is uncommon, mainly because of the infrequency of Kell positivity (about 5% in Caucasian populations). Jaundice is less of a problem than anaemia, and erythroblastosis and reticulocytosis are restrained, because the antibody has affinity for erythroblasts as well as erythrocytes (Letsky 1991).

Organ transplantation
ABO incompatibility in organ transplants may induce spherocytosis, agglutination and a positive DAT.

- With liver transplants, antibody originates from donor lymphocytes, is first detectable 8–16 days after transplant and remains for 10–40 days (Ramsey et al 1984). Though donors are ABO matched, there is a potential for incompatibility as testing for subgroups A1 and A2 is usually not done. Though both are detected by anti-A serum, A2 is qualitatively different from A1, and a proportion of A2 and A2B subjects have naturally occurring anti-A1 (about 3% and 25% respectively).
- Antibody of recipient origin may target erythrocytes in transplanted tissue such as marrow. Recipient antibody usually phases out as the graft takes, but may remain if recipient lymphocytes survive as a form of chimaerism.

Incompatible transfusion
Spherocytosis with a positive DAT (IgG + C3d) and often agglutination and erythrophagocytosis occurs in incompatible transfusion, especially of delayed types (3–14 days after transfusion). About one third of delayed reactions are due to Kidd (Jk^a) and another third to Rh, the corresponding figures for immediate reactions being 9% and 42% (Mollison et al 1993). Kidd antibody has the unusual property of decay to levels which are undetectable in routine pre-transfusion compatibility testing, re-exposure to positive cells (about 70% of population) producing a rapid return to potent levels. Incompatibility is identified by standard procedures (Issitt 1985).

Other causes of spherocytosis which may be operating in these patients include infection (p. 98) and use of high dose intravenous immunoglobulin (p. 75).

Autoimmune haemolysis (Sokol et al 1984)

Investigations are considered here in the order of listing in Table 3.9.

Blood values
Autoagglutination will result in spurious values — MCV (high), cell count and hct (low) and MCHC (high). The degree of correction by pre-warming the sample depends on the thermal range of the antibody.

Reticulocytopenia rather than reticulocytosis occurs occasionally (Greenberg et al 1980), because of affinity of antibody for immature as well as mature erythrocytes, or because of parvovirus infection.

Transient thrombocytopenia and/or neutropenia may accompany anaemia. The antibodies are different from those against the erythrocytes (cf Evans syndrome, p. 308).

Table 3.9 Investigation of suspected autoimmune haemolysis in childhood

Blood values, reticulocyte count
Blood film
• Spherocytosis, agglutination, erythrophagocytosis
• Evidence of viral infection, malaria
DAT
• Broad spectrum
• Monospecific: IgG, IgM, IgA, C3, C3d, C4 (DAT may be positive only at 4°C)
Donath-Landsteiner antibody; ensure adequate amount of complement
Blood group specificity
• Cell panel at 4°C, room temp, 37°C
• IAT with same panel at 37°C (to exclude additional antibodies); use monospecific anti-IgG
• Reactivity for papainized vs untreated cells (Pr specificity)
Cold agglutinin titre
Tests for associated infection, disease (Table 3.10)

DAT = direct antiglobulin test; IAT = indirect antiglobulin test

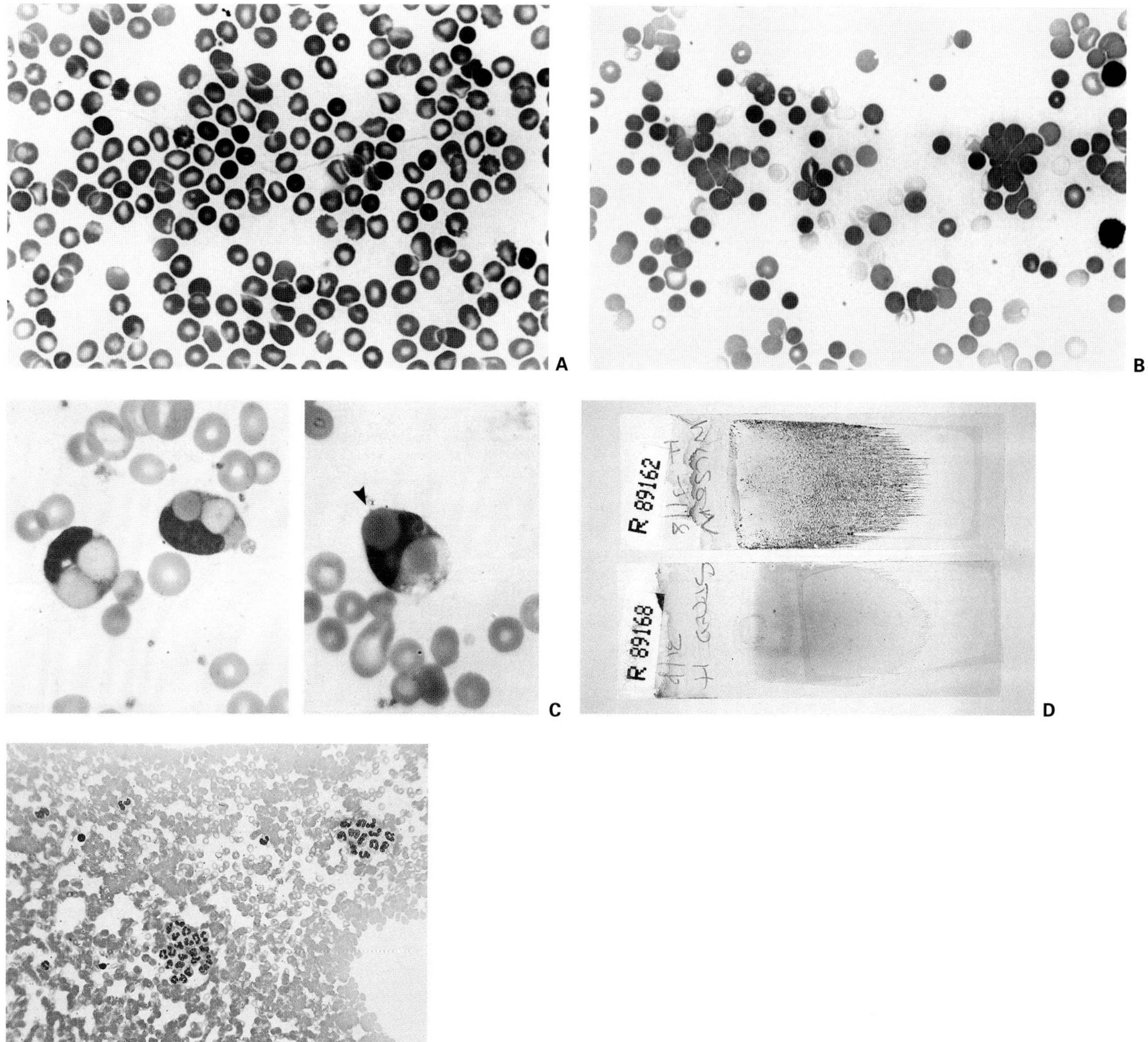

Fig. 3.5 Immune spherocytosis. **a** With IgG-positive DAT in a 3-day-old infant, Hb 15.0 g/dl and jaundice requiring 2 exchange transfusions; no blood group incompatibility detected. At 9 weeks spherocytosis had virtually disappeared and DAT was negative. The most likely explanation is fetomaternal incompatibility for a rare private antigen inherited from the father. **b** Severe haemolysis due to anti-Pr — spherocytosis, agglutination and erythrocyte ghosts. **c** Erythrophagocytosis (plain blood film) in transient IgG haemolysis, probably infection-related. Arrow shows phagocytosed polychromatic cell. **d** Erythrocyte agglutination (above, normal below), mycoplasma infection, Hb 2.9 g/dl. **e** Neutrophil agglutination, plain blood film, mycoplasma infection, Hb normal. Erythrocyte agglutination was noted in other parts of the film. **c** × 800; **e** × 160

Blood film (Fig. 3.5)
With IgG antibodies, sphering of cells is due predominantly to splenic macrophages (receptors for IgG and C3); with IgM antibodies, sphering occurs predominantly in the liver (macrophage receptors for C3 but not IgM). Spherocytosis may be absent, for unknown reasons, in occasional cases of autoimmune disease with strong IgG DAT. Fragmentation due to T activation (below) may accompany immune spherocytosis (Fig. 3.8).

Agglutination is a feature mainly of IgM antibodies. Leucoagglutination is uncommon.

Erythrophagocytosis, which requires both Ig and C3 on the red cell, is more obvious in smears of buffy coat made after incubation at 37°C for 2–3 hours. Phagocytosis by neutrophils rather than monocytes may be characteristic of paroxysmal cold haemoglobinuria (Hernandez & Steane 1984).

An increase in reactive lymphocytes is an indication of associated viral infection. Malaria may be associated with a positive DAT, but Hb and reticulocytes are not different from those with a negative DAT (Abdalla & Weatherall 1982).

The DAT
The polyspecific reagent often lacks antibodies potent enough to detect molecules such as C3d and IgA, which alone are occasionally present in autoimmune haemolysis. If suspicion is strong, a negative result should be followed with monospecific reagents. In IgM haemolysis, for example, the polyspecific DAT is often negative, partly because cold IgM will not remain attached at room temperature, the standard temperature for testing, and partly because accompanying C3d is often of weak intensity.

Causes of negative polyspecific and monospecific DAT in immune haemolysis include:

- unsatisfactory technique (Dacie & Lewis 1991)
- some cold antibodies, e.g. anti-Pr (Curtis et al 1990); a clue may be given by differences in results obtained over a range of temperatures — 4°C, room temperature, 37°C
- T activation.

T activation (cryptantigen exposure, Novak 1990) is an uncommon but serious haemolysis due to exposure of T antigen by neuraminidase produced by some organisms (*Pneumococcus, Clostridium*). Haemolysis is due to binding of anti-T occurring naturally in serum after the age of about 6 months (IgM, does not cross placenta), and is aggravated by anti-T introduced in plasmas containing high levels of anti-T. T antigen exposure by pneumococcus may be associated with HUS due to neuraminidase damage to glomerular endothelium (p. 80). Clostridial infection is a significant cause in neonatal necrotizing enterocolitis and occasionally other bowel disorders; haemolysis however may not be a problem (because of absence of anti-T in early life) unless anti-T is introduced by transfusion.

Th and Tn activation occur rarely as temporary (months) phenomena in the neonate, most likely due to delay in maturation of glycosyl transferases. Haemolysis and polyagglutination are not significant problems. In adults Tn activation is usually a pre-leukaemic change.

Diagnosis requires examination with appropriate lectins.

Donath-Landsteiner antibody (Bird et al 1976)
This biphasic (bithermic) Ig antibody attaches with complement in the cold, lysis occurring at body temperature from complement which remains attached (paroxysmal cold haemoglobinuria). Diagnosis requires a 2-sample technique (Dacie & Lewis 1991).

The DAT is positive usually for C3d only. Anaemia may be severe, with variable spherocytosis, fragmentation and agglutination. Haemoglobinuria is common (uncommon in warm antibody haemolysis).

Viral infection is a common association — nondescript upper respiratory infection, varicella, measles, mumps and influenza, and measles immunization. Haemolysis in these cases is likely to be transient (1–6 weeks). Syphilis was once a common association; in these cases the antibody is likely to persist. Specificity is usually for P, occasionally I.

Blood group specificity
The procedures in Table 3.9 are recommended to:

- determine the thermal amplitude of the antibody
- detect possible additional antibodies (important if transfusion is contemplated)
- detect cold antibodies such as anti-Pr which may be negative by all routine methods and yet cause severe haemolysis (Curtis et al 1990).

Specificity is usually for I, P or Rh (Table 3.10), rarely others, e.g. Vel (Becton & Kinney 1986).

Cold agglutinin titre

The titre is usually not increased in cold antibody haemolysis. However, in puzzling cases with negative DAT, a raised titre may be a clue to the presence of antibody (Curtis et al 1990).

Associated disease

The commonest association is with viral infection, either nondescript respiratory or specific (Table 3.10). Spherocytosis, often with fragmentation, may occur in infection by neuraminidase-producing organisms (T activation, above), e.g. pneumococcus (pneumonia, meningitis, often with HUS) and clostridium spp (necrotizing enterocolitis). Mixed infections may occur (Fig. 3.8e).

Warm IgG haemolysis is likely to be associated with systemic disease rather than with viral infection; occasionally haemolysis precedes overt clinical expression of the disease (e.g. SLE). In the neonate IgG antibody may be passively acquired from a mother with autoimmune disorder (Sokol et al 1982).

Evans syndrome is a combination of severe ($< 50 \times 10^9/l$) thrombocytopenia (and often neutropenia) with warm antibody haemolysis without detectable underlying disorder. The several antibodies do not cross react (Pegels et al 1982).

Although up to one third of patients on α methyl dopa become DAT positive, haemolytic anaemia is rare (< 1%). Antibodies (Table 3.10) are evident usually only after a lag of 3–6 months and may remain positive for weeks to months after cessation.

Severe IgG haemolysis unaccompanied by recognizable immune disease is not rare in the first year (or weeks) of life.

Infused anti-A/B/D-containing material

A positive DAT (IgG, C3d, occasionally IgA), often with spherocytosis, may follow infusion of anti-A/B/D in immunoglobulin (Guillain-Barré syndrome, prophylaxis for immunosuppressed patients), plasma and Factor VIII and IX concentrates (Mollison et al 1993). The effect may last for some weeks after infusion.

Table 3.10 Autoimmune haemolysis in childhood

Type of antibody	DAT	Specificity	Associated disease
Cold IgM	C3d	I	mycoplasma viral infection, e.g. CMV
		i	viral infection, infective mononucleosis
Cold IgG (Donath-Landsteiner)	C3d	P, occ I	viral infection measles vaccination syphilis now rare cause
Cold IgM or IgG	C3d or neg	Pr[1]	idiopathic viral infection
Warm IgG	IgG[2] ± C3	broad: often within Rh system, e.g. c,e	idiopathic SLE rheumatoid arthritis inflammatory bowel disease[3] Hodgkin's disease non-Hodgkin lymphoma ovarian cyst Evans syndrome genetic immunodeficiency[4] viral infection methyl dopa[5]

[1] Destroyed by proteases
[2] Occasionally +IgA or rarely IgA only or complement only
[3] Ulcerative colitis, Crohn's disease; DAT may become negative after colectomy
[4] X-linked hypogammaglobulinaemia, Wiskott-Aldrich, IgA deficiency, hyper IgM syndrome, purine nucleoside phosphorylase deficiency
[5] True autoimmune, no drug specificity

Table 3.11 Drug-immune haemolysis[1]

Mechanism	Drugs	DAT	IAT	Other
Drug-dependent drug fixation	penicillin cephalosporins tetracycline	IgG, occ +C, IgM	neg	serum and eluates give pos IAT only with drug-treated cells
Immune complex adsorption	quinine quinidine phenacetin PAS rifampicin	C, occ +IgG	neg	serum but not eluate[2] gives pos IAT with drug-treated cells
True autoantibody	methyl dopa indomethacin	IgG	neg	usually Rh specific (c,e)

[1] After Dacie & Lewis 1991
[2] Because eluate does not contain drug

Drug-immune haemolysis (Table 3.11)

This is rare in childhood. In most cases the antibody has drug specificity (cf methyl dopa). Penicillin produces immune haemolysis only if given in high dose for several weeks.

Unexplained positive DAT

This is rare in childhood, but not uncommon in adults without haemolysis or relevant symptoms (Dacie & Lewis 1991).

Table 3.12 Elliptocytosis in childhood

Normal
- < 5% usually but not necessarily normal

Associated with other anaemias/disease
- Iron deficiency anaemia
- Megaloblastic anaemias
- Thalassaemias
- Cytotoxics
- Myelosclerosis
- Congenital dyserythropoiesis

Hereditary elliptocytosis (HE)
- Mild HE
- Spherocytic HE (haemolytic HE with spherocytosis)
- Stomatocytic (Melanesian, SE Asian) HE
- Hereditary pyropoikilocytosis

ELLIPTOCYTOSIS

Elliptocytosis is common and usually secondary in a variety of anaemias (Table 3.12). In general, elliptocytosis affecting > 30% of cells is likely to be genetic rather than acquired.

Hereditary elliptocytoses (Becker & Lux 1993)

In all types (Table 3.12), elliptocytosis affects only mature cells, precursor cells being normal in shape. A variety of molecular defects is known, the usual end result being impairment of spectrin self-association or a defect in the spectrin-actin-protein 4.1 junctional complex (Fig. 3.3), i.e. impairment of horizontal stability of skeleton (cf defect in vertical stability in HS). Many defects are silent, especially in the heterozygous state.

Mild ('common') HE (Fig. 3.6)

This is the commonest form, designated mild because of the absence of significant haemolysis. In some cases a mild reticulocytosis and decrease in serum haptoglobin are an indication of haemolysis (no consistent relation between proportion of elliptocytes and degree of haemolysis).

Significant haemolysis, with or without a degree of anaemia, fragmentation and poikilocytosis, may occur in viral or bacterial infection, malaria and transplant rejection. Small numbers of elliptocytes (of the order of 5%), ordinarily regarded as normal, are an indication of HE if inheritance can be demonstrated and acquired causes (Table 3.12) excluded.

Inheritance is autosomal dominant. The homozygous state produces severe anaemia, with poikilocytosis, budding, fragmentation, spherocytosis, and increased osmotic fragility; response to splenectomy is consistently satisfactory.

Atypical manifestations:

- Infancy

The proportion of elliptocytes may not reach their final level till about 3–4 months. A component of irregularity in shape also may be noted in the first months (Fig. 3.6b).

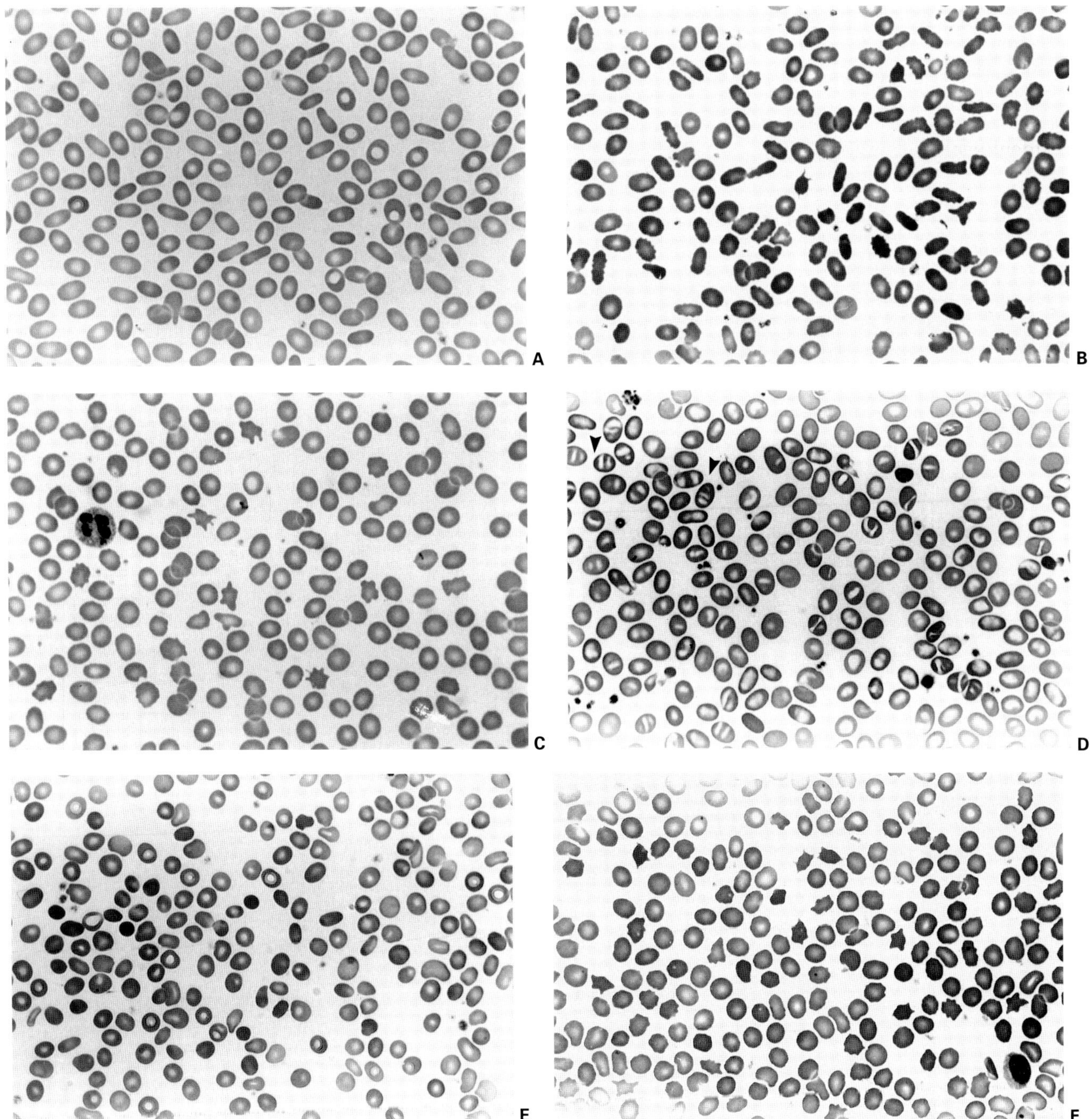

Fig. 3.6 Hereditary elliptocytosis. **a–c** Mild type. **a** Typical appearances, some rod-shaped cells. **b** 15-week-old infant, Hb 11.2 g/dl; superimposed irregularities were not present after 9 months. **c** Combined elliptocytosis and acanthocytosis, inherited from mother in a 13-year-old. **d** Melanesian ovalostomatocytosis, 13-year-old. Some cells (arrows) contain 1 or 2 transverse bars of Hb. A low normal Hb (12.2 g/dl) and microcytosis (69 fl) were due to associated α thal trait. **e,f** Haemolytic HE with spherocytosis in child (**e**) and mother (**f**, post-splenectomy). Most of the acanthocytes in (**f**) are elliptic.

In Negro infants especially, pyknocytosis, fragmentation and haemolysis (of obscure origin) may so dominate as to be misidentified as infantile pyknocytosis (Carpentieri et al 1977). The dense cells are rich in HbF. Pyknocytosis persists for 6 months to 2 years. Identification as a form of HE is confirmed by finding typical HE in one parent.

- Association with acanthocytosis

A not uncommon association (Fig. 3.6) of uncertain significance. As for HE in general, transmission is autosomal dominant, though abnormality may be less obvious in the affected parent. A similar appearance occurs in anorexia nervosa (p. 88), disappearing as the clinical state improves.

- Association with other diseases

Other common disorders, e.g. iron deficiency, thalassaemia, may be randomly associated (Fig. 3.6).

- Association with dyserythropoiesis

In this variant(?), apparently confined to parts of Italy, erythrocytes are oval rather than elliptic, erythroblasts show dyspoiesis and there is an element of ineffective erythropoiesis. Anaemia and dyserythropoiesis manifest in adolescence or early adulthood. Response to splenectomy is only partial (Torlontano et al 1979).

Haemolytic HE with spherocytosis (Fig. 3.6)

About 5% of cases of HE. Elliptocytes tend to be less elongated than in mild HE and some are small. The ratio of elliptocytes to spherocytes varies from family to family and among members of the same family. Osmotic fragility (especially incubated), autohaemolysis and hypertonic cryohaemolysis are abnormal; autohaemolysis is glucose-responsive. This type differs from mild HE also in being usually associated with splenomegaly and overt haemolysis. In differential diagnosis double heterozygosity for HS and mild HE is to be excluded. Inheritance is autosomal dominant, but abnormality may vary in degree within the one kindred. Response to splenectomy is satisfactory.

Melanesian (South-East Asian) elliptocytosis (Fig. 3.6)

Oval stomatocytosis, with some cells containing 1 or 2 transverse bars of Hb, is diagnostic. It is confined to aboriginal inhabitants of Melanesia, Indonesia and other parts of SE Asia.

An extension of the N-terminal end of the anion-transport protein 3 (Jones et al 1990) renders the membrane rigid; cells are resistant to osmotic lysis, heat fragmentation and malarial parasitization. Autohaemolysis, however, is increased. A range of surface antigens is poorly expressed (Booth et al 1977) because the rigid membrane inhibits expression or detectability by conventional (agglutination) techniques. Haemolysis is mild or absent.

In those with numerous ovalocytes (> 80%) inheritance is autosomal dominant (homozygosity is probably lethal). In those with fewer ovalocytes, inheritance may not be demonstrable and may be recessive.

Hereditary pyropoikilocytosis (HPP) (Fig. 3.7)

This rare variant of HE is characterized by severe haemolysis and bizarre poikilocytosis (elliptocytosis, budding, fragmentation, spherocytosis). The MCV is low because of fragmentation, osmotic fragility and autohaemolysis are grossly increased and the cells are sensitive to thermal damage — fragmentation occurs after heating for 10–15 minutes at 45–46°C (normal = 49°C), and with prolonged incubation (> 6 h) occurs at lower temperatures or even at body temperature.

HPP appears to be the homozygous or doubly heterozygous state for a variety of silent or mild HE genes. In about 30% of kindreds a parent or sib has mild HE or mild HE with poikilocytosis.

In diagnosis, other causes of bizarre poikilocytosis are to be excluded (Table 3.21). Splenectomy greatly diminishes but does not eliminate haemolysis.

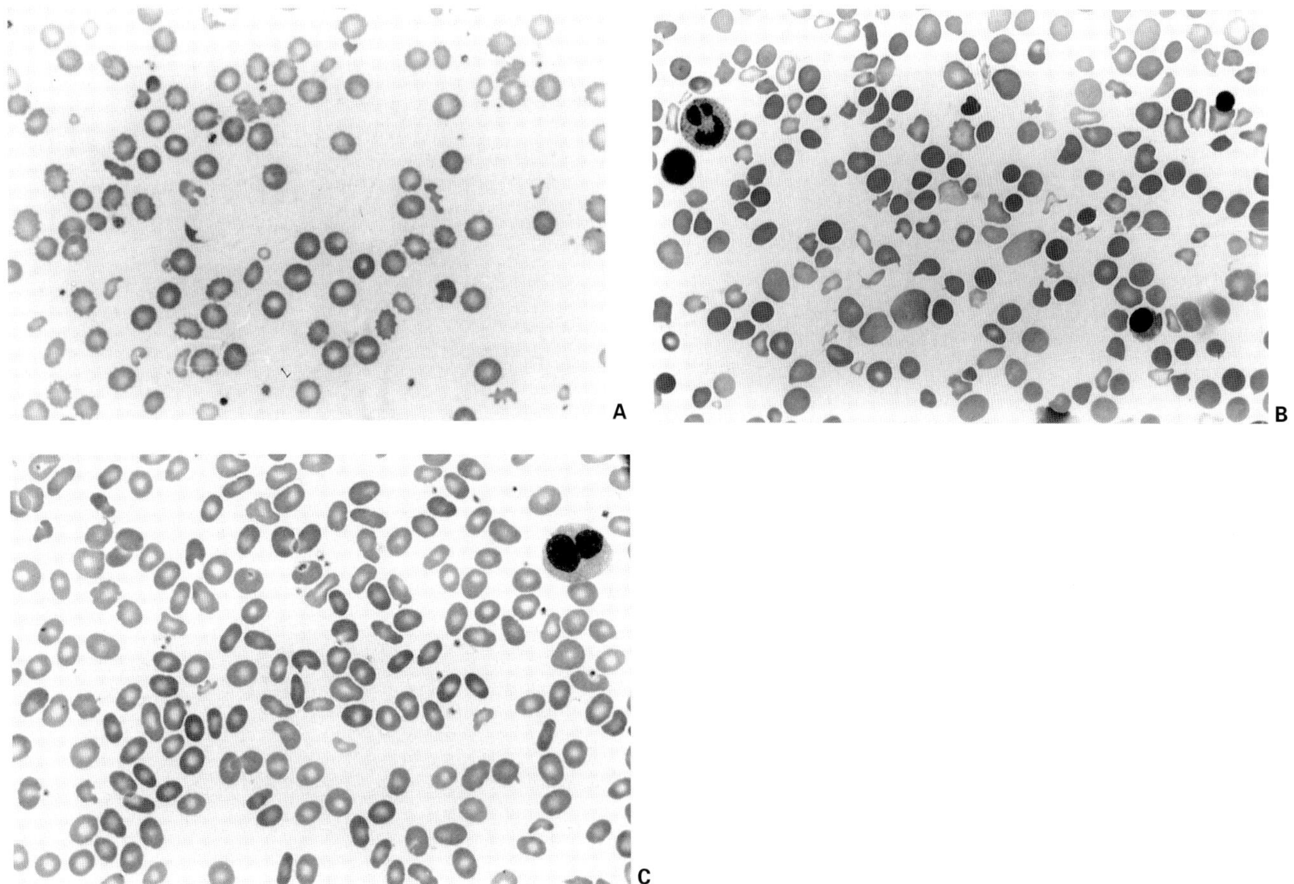

Fig. 3.7 Hereditary pyropoikilocytosis. **a** 13-day-old infant, Hb 4.9 g/dl, MCV 64 fl (n > 85). Some of the microcytosis and anaemia were possibly due to associated α thal trait. **b,c** Haemolytic anaemia resembling pyropoikilocytosis. **b** 1 day, Hb 11.2 g/dl. **c** Same child, 4 years, elliptocytosis more conspicuous; inheritance autosomal dominant with variable penetrance; splenectomy in affected members of kindred curative when performed. **a** Courtesy of Dr B Williams

FRAGMENTATION HAEMOLYSIS

Fragmentation is a component in a variety of haemolytic disorders, but dominant in only a few (Table 3.13).

- Haemolytic-uraemic syndrome (Fig. 3.8, Kaplan et al 1992, Moake 1994)

Fragmentation is a requirement for diagnosis, though some nephrologists will diagnose HUS in the absence of fragmentation if clinical features are typical. Occasionally appearances are not convincing until some days after onset of symptoms. Fragmentation is traditionally attributed to slicing of cells as they push through (renal) vessels encumbered by thrombus. However, shearing of cells bound to endothelium by large vWF multimers is another possibility. 'Fragments' identified by light microscopy are, in some cases at least, punctured and shrunken whole cells (Fig. 3.8). A few spherocytes are common, but immune spherocytosis from infection may be added (Fig. 3.8e).

In the most common (diarrhoea-associated) form, thrombosis is attributed to exotoxin-induced endothelial damage (p. 292). In pneumococcus-induced HUS, endothelial damage is due to neuraminidase produced by the organism and is usually associated with neuraminidase-induced damage (T activation, cryptantigen exposure) in other tissues, especially erythrocytes (p. 74) and platelets. Haemolysis and thrombocytopenia are aggravated by anti-T occurring naturally in plasma of most persons after 6 months of age (in patient per se or introduced in plasmas, Novak 1990). Rarer types of HUS are considered on page 292.

For haemostatic changes see page 292 and Table 8.21.

- Thrombotic thrombocytopenic purpura

TTP may be regarded as a more widespread expression (including the brain in particular) of the platelet thrombosis which is predominantly renal in HUS (Moake 1994). It is very rare in childhood. Onset in the neonate is described (Murphy et al 1987a). Plasma infusions commonly produce improvement, attributed to dilution of a platelet-aggregating factor (Murphy et al 1987b). The course may be chronic (decades) and overt manifestations may be preceded by a long lead-in period of isolated thrombocytopenia. Upshaw (1978) described an infant with recurrent, plasma-responsive episodes of thrombocytopenia and fragmentation haemolysis who, over a follow-up of 11 years, did not evolve to clinically recognizable TTP.

Table 3.13 Fragmentation haemolysis in childhood

Intravascular coagulation/thrombosis
Endothelial damage
Organisms or their endotoxins/enzymes
HUS[1]
Septicaemias[2]
Haemangioma, if extensive[2]
TTP
SLE renal disease[2]
Release of thromboplastin into circulation
Neoplasm[2]
AML M3
Disseminated neuroblastoma
Envenomation[2]
Dead tissue[2]
Necrotizing enterocolitis[1]
Deficit of natural anticoagulants (ATIII, proteins C,S)
Purpura fulminans[2]
Liver disease[2]
Membrane defect/damage
Burns[2]
Hereditary pyropoikilocytosis
Selenium deficiency
Turbulence-induced damage
Mechanical heart valves

[1] T activation may contribute to haemolysis
[2] Fragmentation in minority of cases only

- Cardiac valve disease

Haemolysis and fragmentation from valve implantation occur with mechanical rather than tissue valves (Wheeler & Pettigrew 1986). Fragmentation is rare in stenosis of cardiac or aortic valves before operation (Ravenel et al 1969).

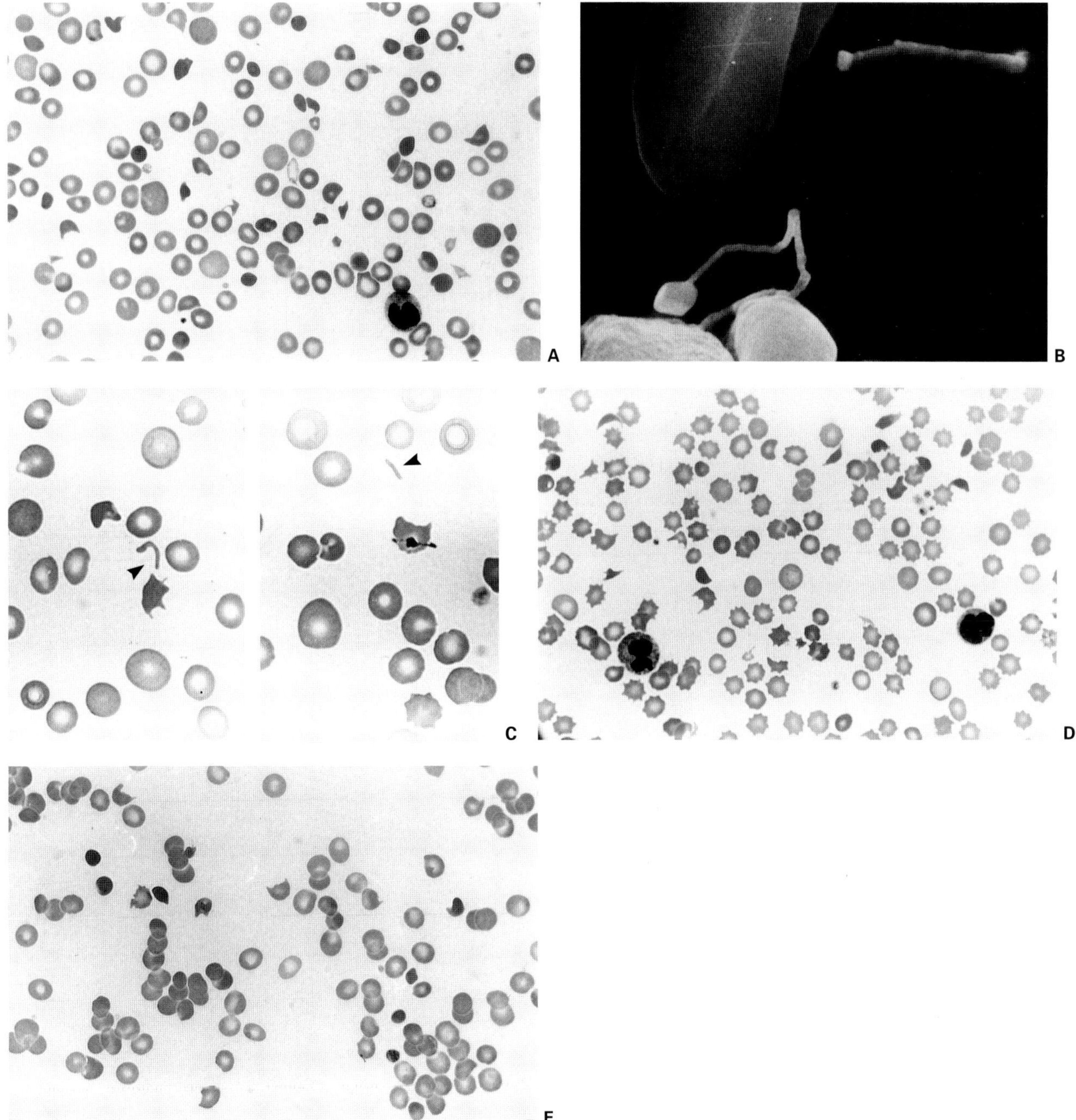

Fig. 3.8 Haemolytic-uraemic syndrome. **a–d** Diarrhoea-associated, **e** pneumococcus associated (T activation). **a** Typical appearance with fragments, contracted cells and occasional spherocytes. **b** Scanning micrograph, showing 2 shrunken whole erythrocytes, the probable counterpart of 'splinters' seen by light microscopy (**c**, arrows). **d** Superimposed, transient (1 day) crenation, attributed to hyponatraemia and hypoalbuminaemia. **e** Additional spherocytosis and agglutination (C3d positive), due to associated parainfluenza infection. **b** × 2500; **c** × 750

TARGET CELLS (Fig. 3.9, Table 3.14)

Artefact should be suspected if target cells are unevenly distributed in the film, are not present on repeat testing or are not seen in fluid suspensions (in some disorders they appear bowl-shaped in suspension). There is no satisfactory unifying molecular explanation for the occurrence of targeting in the variety of disorders listed.

The commonest cause in childhood is obstructive jaundice (usually biliary atresia) or chronic liver disease of mild to moderate degree (severe disease is likely to be associated with crenation, shrinkage and spiculation, p. 90). These target cells have increased surface area due to increase in membrane cholesterol and phospholipid.

The rare familial lecithin: cholesterol acyltransferase (LCAT) deficiency (Norum et al 1989) is characterized by corneal opacities, premature atherosclerosis and sea-blue histiocytes (p. 232) in marrow. Target cells are associated with mild haemolysis. Inheritance is autosomal recessive.

In asplenia target cells are attributed to loss of the splenic function of removing surplus membrane.

PYKNOCYTOSIS (Table 3.15)

Pyknocytes are whole, irregularly contracted erythrocytes, with a few (< 5) irregularly distributed, short, broad-based projections. Some cases of acanthocytosis with an unusual degree of shrinkage may be misidentified as pyknocytosis (Fig. 3.14).

Infantile pyknocytosis (Fig. 3.10, Keimowitz & Desforges 1965)

This is probably an exaggeration of the normal pyknocytosis of the first months of life (p. 4). Normal erythrocytes infused into affected infants become pyknocytic (i.e. extracorpuscular defect). The possible contribution of vitamin E deficiency is obscure (Zipursky et al 1987); in some cases a relation to maternal alcohol ingestion has been suggested.

Haemolytic anaemia and jaundice may be severe enough to require exchange transfusion. Diagnosis requires exclusion of other causes of pyknocytosis (Table 3.21), especially Heinz body haemolysis.

Table 3.14 Target cells in childhood

Artefact (of drying)
Obstructive liver disease
Parenchymal liver damage of mild to moderate degree
Haemoglobinopathy
Thalassaemias
Structural variants — SS,CC,DD,EE
Double heterozygotes of above
Familial LCAT deficiency
Hereditary xerocytosis
Drugs
Phenothiazines
Usually minor component
Normal neonate
Asplenia/splenic hypofunction
Iron deficiency anaemia

Table 3.15 Pyknocytosis in childhood

Normal
First months of life[1]
Infantile pyknocytosis
Vitamin E deficiency (?)
Heinz body/oxidant-induced haemolysis
Fragmentation haemolysis[1]
Chronic renal disease[2]

[1] Minor component only
[2] Some cases only

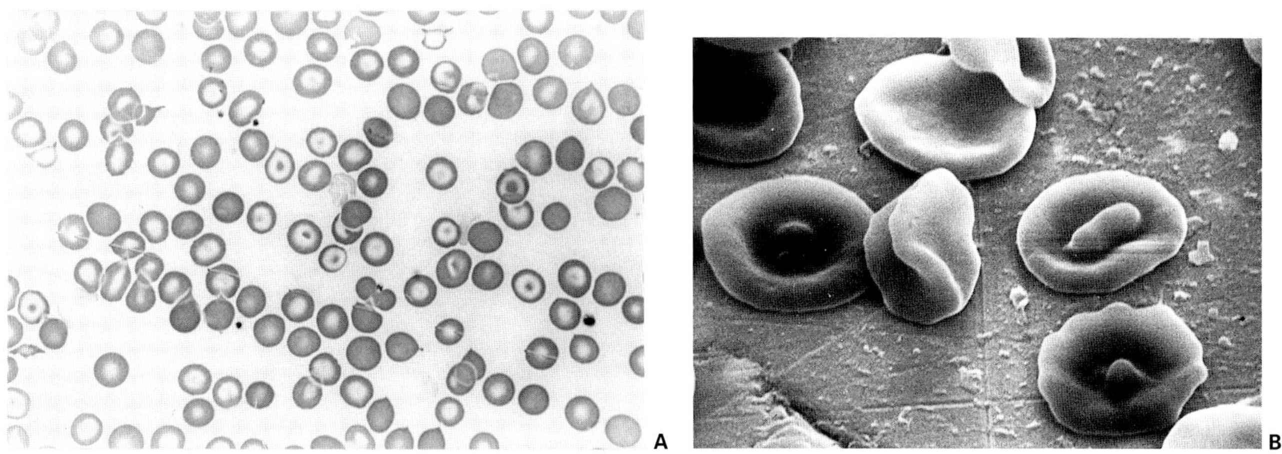

Fig. 3.9 Target cells. **a** Biliary atresia, Hb 9.5 g/dl, MCV 82 fl, serum bilirubin total 342, conjugated 219 μmol/l, liver enzymes 9–13 x upper normal. **b** HbH disease.

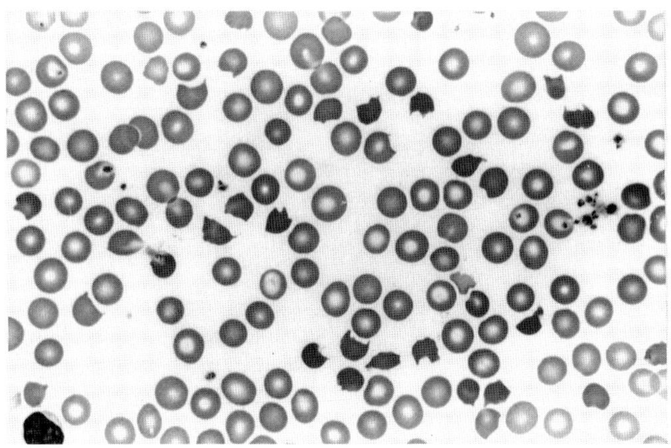

Fig. 3.10 Infantile pyknocytosis, 17-day-old infant with hyperbilirubinaemia (total 256, conjugated 19 μmol/l), Hb 9.5 g/dl.

Neonatal Heinz body haemolysis (Table 3.16, Fig. 3.11)

This diagnosis is appropriate only when the proportion of erythrocytes with Heinz bodies is substantial (> 5%). Lesser increases may be normal (e.g. prematurity) or non-specific.

The Heinz body haemolysis most consistently associated with pyknocytosis is that of oxidant exposure or (the majority) presumed oxidant exposure ('idiopathic'); some spherocytes, fragments and bite cells may be evident. Surprisingly, methaemoglobinaemia is only infrequently associated, and few methaemoglobin producers cause Heinz body formation (Table 2.16).

This haemolysis occurs most commonly in the first weeks of life. Recurrence after recovery is exceptional, which suggests a transient neonatal deficiency of a protective substance (? glutathione reductase, catalase, vitamin E). The greater susceptibility of prematures may be due to more pronounced splenic hypofunction or deficiency of protective components.

Table 3.16 Neonatal Heinz body haemolysis

Neonatal Heinz body haemolysis
Slight increase (5–10% of cells)
Hyposplenism: prematurity
asplenia
Substantial increase
Oxidant drugs, toxins[1,2]
Sulphonamides
Primaquine
Fava beans
Vitamin K, water-soluble analogues
Aminophyllin[3]
Inhalation or skin absorption
Naphthalene
Aniline derivatives
Nitrobenzene derivatives
Resorcin lotions
Insecticides[3]
Methylene blue[4]
Hexose monophosphate shunt defect
G6PD
Glutathione peroxidase
Glutathione synthetase
Unstable Hb[2]
Idiopathic[2]

[1] Infant exposed directly or via breast milk, or fetus via placenta
[2] Likely to be associated with pyknocytosis
[3] Relation to haemolysis uncertain
[4] Instilled into amniotic sac to detect possible leak

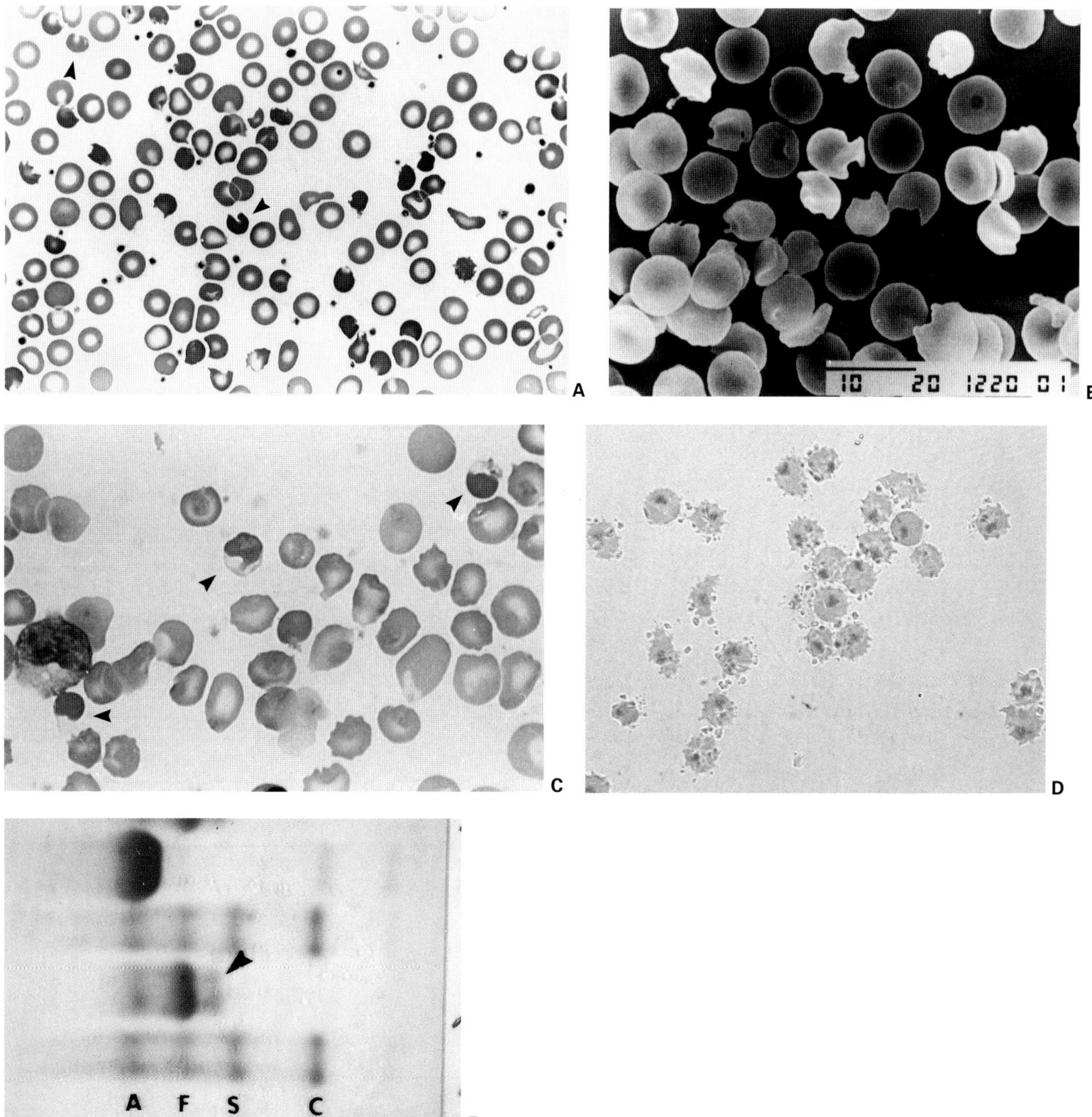

Fig. 3.11 Heinz body haemolysis (idiopathic) in the neonate. **a,b** Irregularly contracted and (arrows) bitten-out cells. **a** 15-day-old, **b** 11-day-old infant. **c,d** 11-day-old infant; arrows show blister cells; Heinz bodies in approximately 90% of cells (**d**, methyl violet). **e** 1-day-old infant, 12% metHb (arrow); this and cell abnormalities had disappeared by 8 weeks. **b** $\times$ 2000; **c,d** $\times$ 750. **e** Courtesy of Dr I D Perel

BITE CELLS (Fig. 3.12)

Bite cells are suggestive of oxidant exposure and/or unstable haemoglobinopathy (e.g. Hb Köln). Naphthalene and sulphasalazine (for inflammatory bowel disease) are common exposures in childhood. Affected cells may or may not show pyknocytosis and Heinz bodies may or may not be demonstrable. Haemolysis is accentuated if G6PD is deficient, but cell damage can occur with (as is usual) normal levels of enzyme.

ACANTHOCYTOSIS (Figs 3.13, 3.14)

Acanthocytes are whole erythrocytes with 5–10 irregularly distributed, elongated, slender projections. There is variable shrinkage. In some cases acanthocytosis coexists with crenation.

The membrane defect may be intrinsic or extracorpuscular (Table 3.17). Although acanthocytes might be expected, because of rigidity, to have shortened survival, significant haemolysis is seen in few disorders (see below).

- Woronets trait

A not uncommon, dominantly inherited, asymptomatic acanthocytosis of minor degree (< 5% of cells, Beutler et al 1980b). A combination of minor acanthocytosis and elliptocytosis (Fig. 3.6) may be a variant.

- Asplenia

There is great variation in degree and morphology of acanthocytosis in asplenic states, e.g. even after splenectomy for the one disorder, such as HS. Acanthocytosis is usually minor (< 10% of cells), and projections usually blunt and few. For other erythrocyte changes, see page 108 and Table 3.29.

- Hallervorden-Spatz disease (Elejalde et al 1979, Fig. 3.13)

Acanthocytosis occurs in most cases. There is no anaemia. The main clinical features are increasing and distressing muscle rigidity and involuntary choreic or athetoid movements, beginning in the first or second decade. Deposition of iron in the globus pallidus and substantia nigra is characteristic. Inheritance is autosomal recessive.

Table 3.17 Acanthocytosis in childhood

Corpuscular
Woronets trait
Hallervordern-Spatz disease[1]
Normolipaemic chorea-acanthocytosis syndrome[2]
McLeod phenotype[1]
Other
Extracorpuscular
Asplenia
Anorexia nervosa
Hypothyroidism[2]
Abetalipoproteinaemia[1]
Hypo-β-lipoproteinaemia
Obstructive jaundice/liver disease[2]
Artefact
Nature unknown

[1] In the majority of cases and likely to be profuse (> 10% of cells)
[2] May be profuse in rare cases

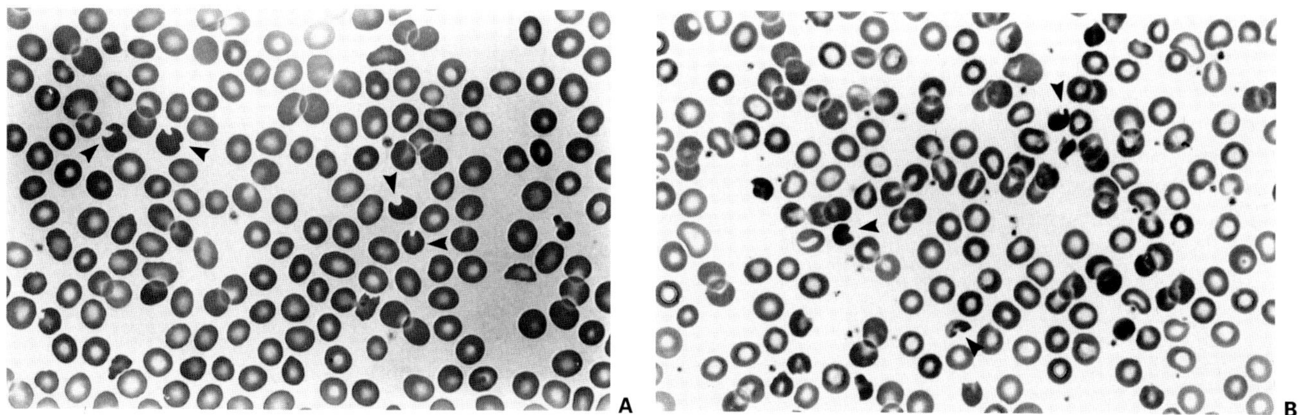

Fig. 3.12 Cell damage from sulpha drugs. **a** Bite cells (arrows), sulphamethoxazole for prophylaxis against pneumocystis infection post-marrow transplant. **b** Contracted and bitten-out cells (arrows), sulphasalazine for ulcerative colitis.

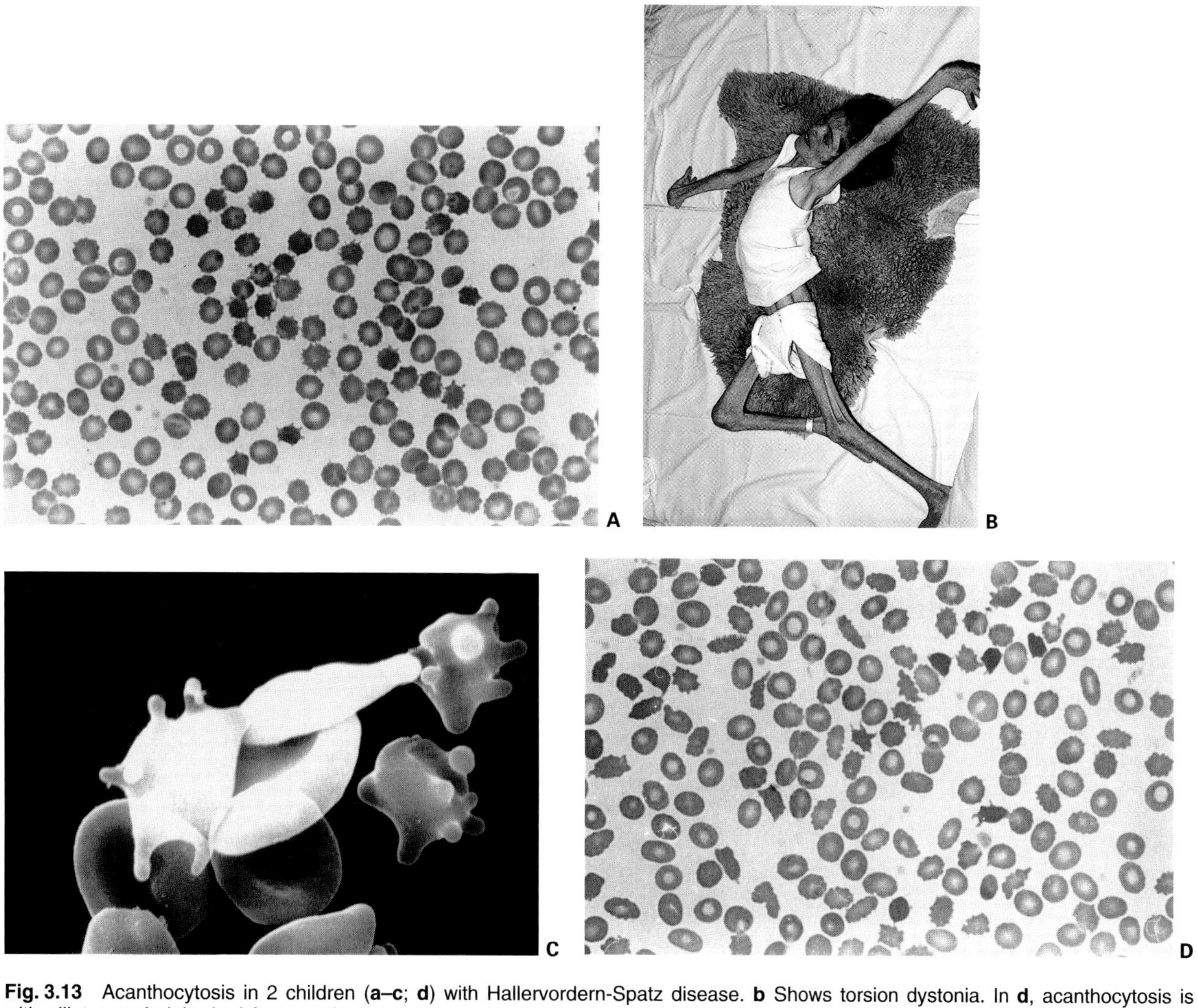

Fig. 3.13 Acanthocytosis in 2 children (**a–c**; **d**) with Hallervordern-Spatz disease. **b** Shows torsion dystonia. In **d**, acanthocytosis is combined with elliptocytosis inherited from mother.

- Normolipaemic chorea-acanthocytosis syndrome (Levine-Critchley syndrome) (Vance et al 1987)
Neurologic disorder manifests in adult life, with choreo-athetoid movements, orofacial dyskinesia, muscle atrophy and variable deterioration of mental function. Atrophy of the caudate nucleus is consistent. It appears to be rare outside Japan. Most cases are sporadic or have autosomal dominant inheritance. A deficiency of erythrocyte membrane monosialogangliosides is described (Gross et al 1982).

- McLeod phenotype (Issitt 1985)
Absence of the Kx antigen is associated with acanthocytosis and haemolysis which is usually mild but occasionally severe (or fatal) and tends to become more severe after 40. Neuromuscular disorder is common, especially after 40, with involuntary choreiform movements, muscle wasting and cardiac enlargement. Inheritance is X-linked recessive; carrier females show, as a result of lyonization, varying degrees of acanthocytosis.

Absence of Kx antigen on granulocytes is a cause of chronic granulomatous disease (normal phagocytosis but defective bactericidal capacity of granulocytes); this may occur independently of, or coexist with, the erythrocyte anomaly.

- Other corpuscular defects
Acanthocytosis is associated with a familial syndrome of motor neurone disease, tics and progressive parkinsonism (Spitz et al 1985) and with a mutant band 3 of the membrane skeleton (Kay et al 1988).

- Anorexia nervosa (Mant & Faragher 1972)
Acanthocytosis is common, affecting usually $< 10\%$ of cells, often with some elliptocytosis. Anaemia is absent or mild (erythrocyte survival normal or slightly shortened). The cause is not known — serum lipoprotein levels are normal; nor is it clear why it affects only some cases. Acanthocytosis disappears slowly (months) as nutrition improves. Other manifestations include marrow hypoplasia (p. 52) and hypofibrinogenaemia (p. 288).

- Hypothyroidism (Wardrop & Hutchison 1969)
Acanthocytosis is notable in some cases (Fig. 3.14), disappearing slowly (months) with treatment. For other haematologic manifestations see page 40.

- Abetalipoproteinaemia (Kane & Havel 1989)
A rare disorder. Prominent acanthocytosis (50–90% of cells) is secondary to absence of low and very low density transporter lipoproteins. Acanthocytosis is attributed to sphingomyelin excess locating preferentially to the outer leaflet of the membrane bilayer to increase the surface area. Hb, reticulocyte count and cell survival are normal or only mildly abnormal. Severe anaemia, if present, suggests deficiency of iron, folate or vitamin E (malabsorption). Molecules carried by β lipoprotein, e.g. triglyceride, cholesterol, are grossly deficient in plasma. Serious clinical manifestations are due to malabsorption of fat and tocopherol and include visual impairment (retinitis pigmentosa) and ataxia and intention tremor (demyelination). Inheritance is autosomal recessive with no sign detectable in parents.

- hypo-β-lipoproteinaemia
The homozygous inherited state (Kane & Havel 1989) is similar to abetalipoproteinaemia. However, neurologic damage is usually milder, and heterozygotes usually show some clinical manifestations, subnormal β lipoprotein and cholesterol and some acanthocytes. In the child shown in Figure 2.2, acanthocytosis was associated with iron deficiency (malabsorption) and t(14;18).

Malabsorption-induced hypo-β-lipoproteinaemia with acanthocytosis may be an epiphenomenon in genetic disorders such as cystic fibrosis and Wolman's disease (Fig. 3.14, Eto & Kitagawa 1970) or may result from acquired bowel disorder.

- Artefact
Bizarre appearances may be noted following transfusion of damaged cells (Fig. 3.14b). Damage may occur before or during transfusion and in subtle ways, e.g. heat of phototherapy lights (Opitz et al 1988).

- Acanthocytosis of obscure origin
A congenital but impermanent acanthocytosis of obscure nature is shown in Figure 3.14e,f. Maxwell et al (1983) reported a similar sibship: the first sib died from intravascular coagulation hours after birth before exchange transfusion could be completed; an extracorpuscular influence could not be demonstrated.

In a personally observed family, acanthocytosis was noted in a child with failure to thrive, unilateral malformations and partial trisomy of 18q, inherited from a pericentric inversion of maternal 18. The clinically normal mother had milder acanthocytosis.

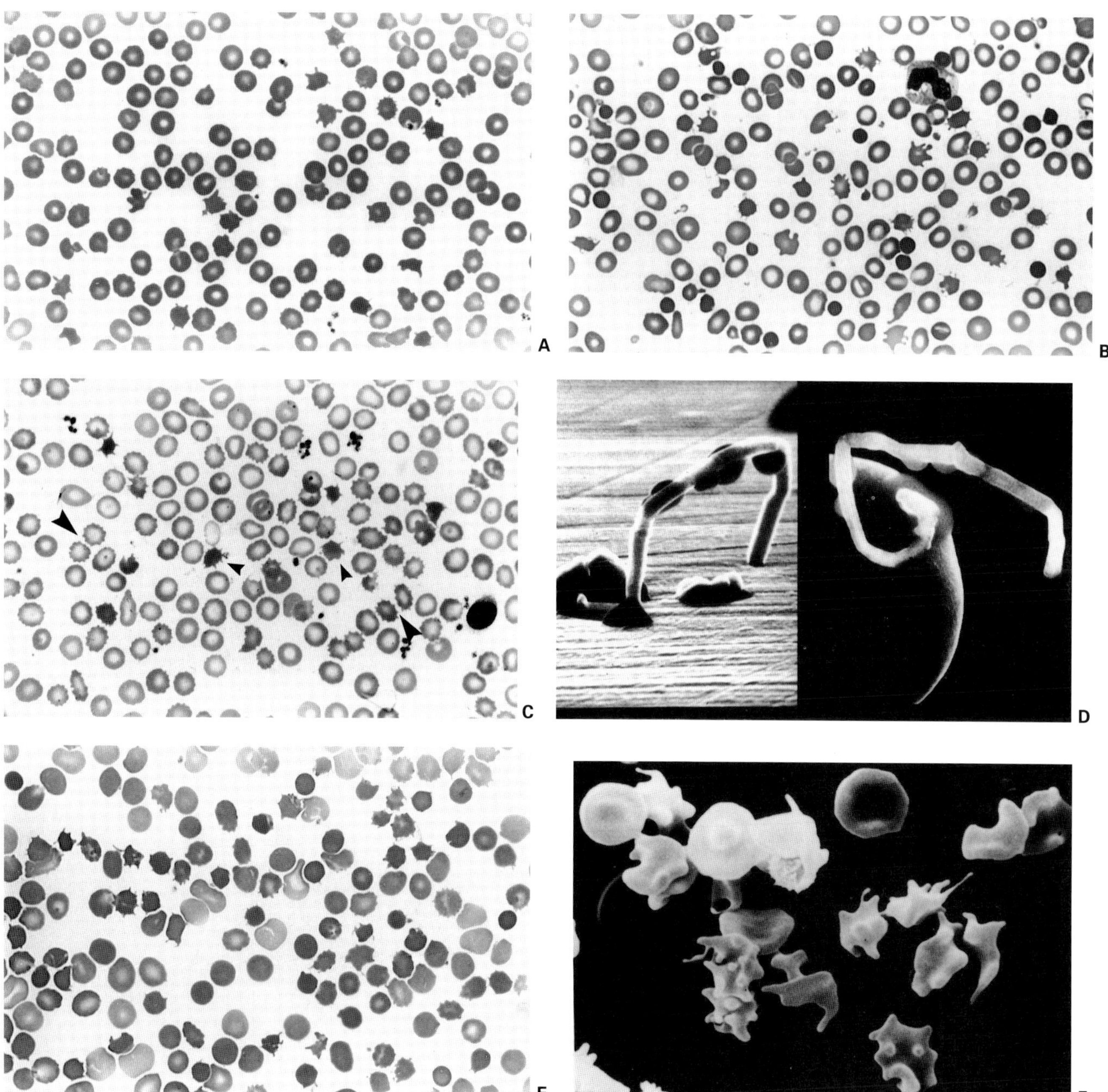

Fig. 3.14 Acanthocytosis. **a** 11-month-old girl with hypothyroidism. **b** With spherocytosis, due to cell damage in transfused blood, cause not determined. **c,d** Acanthocytosis (small arrows) and crenation (large arrows) in a 2-month-old infant with cystic fibrosis; scanning micrograph shows blow-outs; abnormalities were attributed to hypo-β-lipoproteinaemia and hypoalbuminaemia. **e,f** Cord blood, showing dense shrunken acanthocytes and some spherocytes, cause not determined; this was associated with severe unconjugated hyperbilirubinaemia, affected 2 sibs and disappeared at about 8 months. **b** Courtesy of Dr R Rodwell

CRENATION

In crenation (echinocytosis), the membrane is gathered into a continuum of low, usually blunt projections. There is no or minimal shrinkage (Figs 3.8d, 3.14c, 3.15a,b). Crenation is not necessarily associated with significant haemolysis.

Crenation is most commonly an artefact of delay in making films. Genuine crenation (present on repeat examinations, and in wet preps) may be noted in a variety of serious illnesses (electrolyte disturbance, gastroenteritis, infection, burns, renal and liver disease) and may be an early sign of liver transplant rejection. In transfused patients, crenated cells may be derived from stored blood.

SPICULATED (SPUR) CELLS

Contracted, dense cells, bristled with short, fine processes ('whiskered spherocytes', Fig. 3.15); may be accompanied by true spherocytes, into which they may evolve by a process of membrane loss. Haemolysis is usually severe.

Spur cells appear to be intensely shrunken crenated cells — they occur together and an evolution (over about a week) may be discerned from crenation to spur cell formation. This is a (reversible) phenomenon of extracorpuscular origin — accumulation of free cholesterol in the membrane is secondary to decrease in serum lecithin: cholesterol acyltransferase activity and increase in bile salts (Cooper 1969).

Spur cells are prominent in severe obstructive jaundice/liver disease; they may be a presenting manifestation of Wilson's disease. In small numbers they may be noted in renal disease (Fig. 3.22) and in some enzyme deficiencies, especially after splenectomy (Fig. 3.26).

For other erythrocyte changes in obstructive jaundice/liver disease see Table 3.18 and Figure 3.15.

Table 3.18 Red cell morphology in obstructive jaundice/liver disease

	Significance
Macrocytosis	unknown: folate and B_{12} normal marrow aplasia: rare late effect of viral hepatitis
Target cells	mild to moderate disease
Spherocytosis[1]	viral infection: DAT usually pos (C3d)[2] evolution from spur cells ABO mismatch of liver transplant incompatible blood transfusion, e.g. Kell, Kidd
Microcytosis	bleeding — oesophageal varices, hypoprothrombinaemia + thrombocytopenia (hypersplenism)
Crenation	may be early sign of serious disease
Spur cells[1]	serious disease; usually preceded by crenation
Fragmentation[1]	associated: renal disease (hepato-renal syndrome) hypoalbuminaemia intravascular coagulation
Acanthocytosis	rare
'Water-logged' cells	rare; normalize after diuresis

[1] Associated with haemolysis
[2] Often with autoagglutination

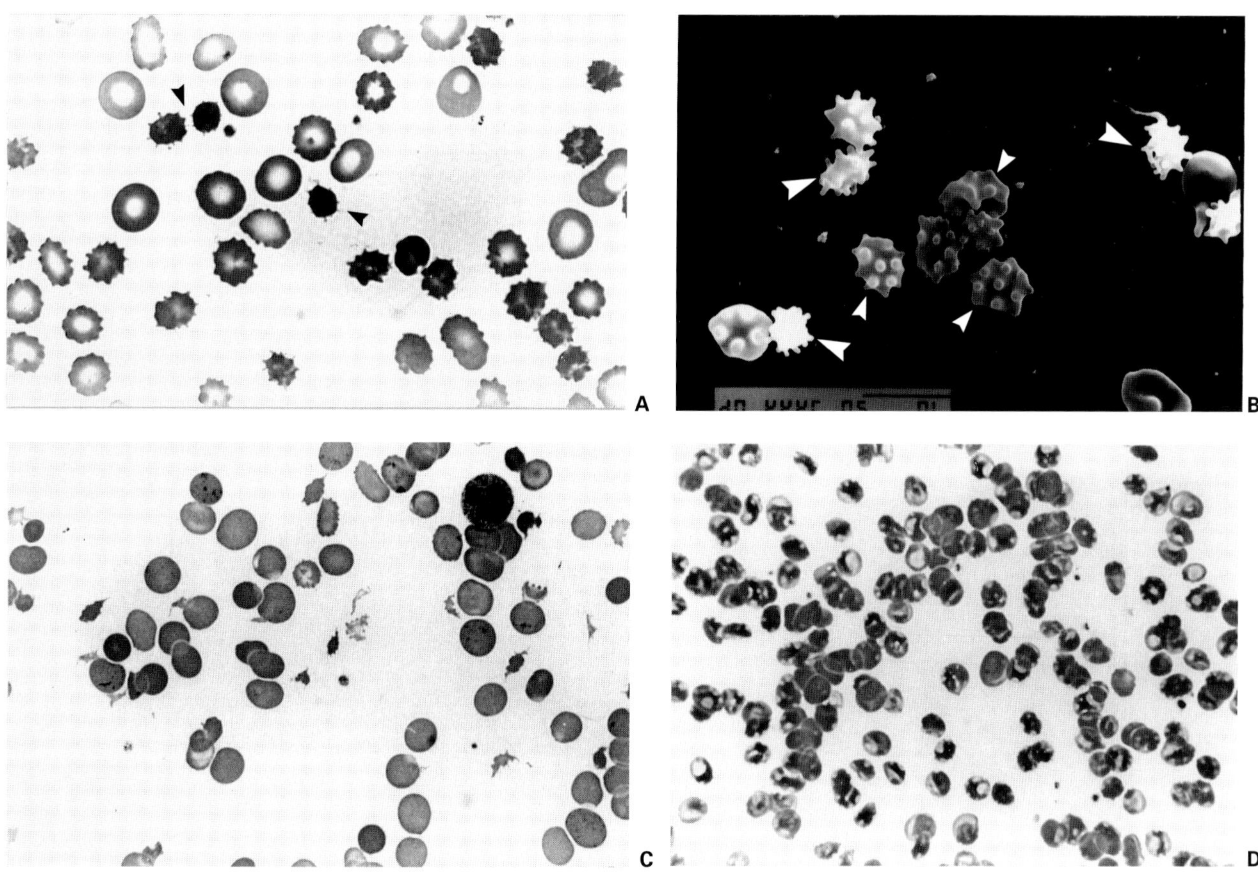

Fig. 3.15 Erythrocyte changes in jaundice/liver failure due to biliary atresia. **a** Crenation and (arrows) dense shrunken spiculated cells. **b** Scanning micrograph, crenation (small arrows) and spiculated cells (large arrows). **c** Component of fragmentation, due to associated renal damage (hepato-renal syndrome). **d** 'Water-logged' cells, a genuine change in an oedematous child, which persisted for 3 weeks until a diuresis occurred. **a,c** × 750; **b** × 2400; **d** × 480

BLISTER CELLS (HEMIGHOSTS, ECCENTROCYTES) (Figs 3.11c, 3.16, Chan et al 1982)

The Hb is concentrated into a dense mass, with empty, crumpled and ragged membrane remaining attached or lost (cf puddling of Hb, Fig. 3.16, in which cell shape is usually maintained). Hb-free ghosts may be noted.

These cells are an indication of severe oxidative injury. Heinz bodies are usually demonstrable, and sometimes methaemoglobinaemia. Small numbers occur in a variety of haemolytic anaemias; large numbers are characteristic in favism and neonatal Heinz body haemolysis.

PUDDLING OF HAEMOGLOBIN

The Hb is condensed into one or two masses or a band at the periphery of the cell (Fig. 3.17). Cell shape is for the most part maintained (cf blister cells, above).

These cells occur in small numbers as an incidental finding in a variety of anaemias, e.g. thalassaemias and severe obstructive jaundice/liver disease. They are an important but usually not prominent feature of hereditary xerocytosis, often with target cells.

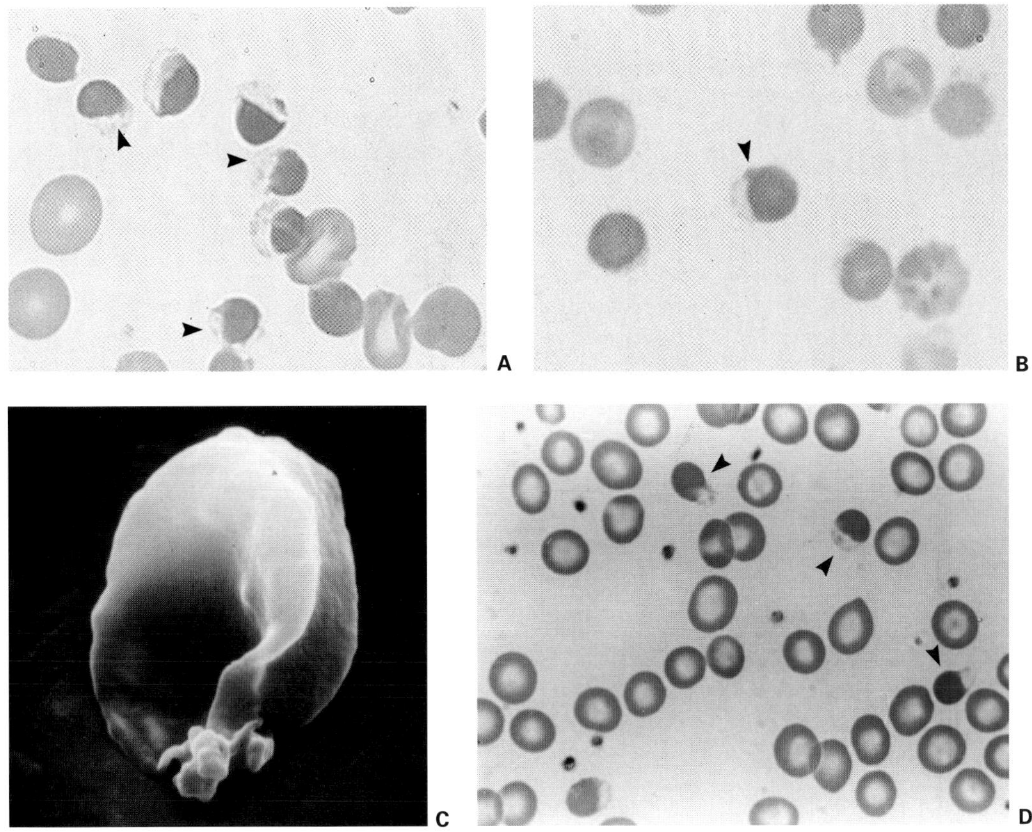

Fig. 3.16 Blister cells (arrows) in 2 children with favism (**a–c**; **d**). In **b**, a Heinz body lies in the Hb-free portion (methyl violet). Associated microcytosis (MCV 67 fl) in **d** was due to β thal trait (courtesy of Dr D Gill). **a,b** × 1200; **c** × 6000; **d** × 750

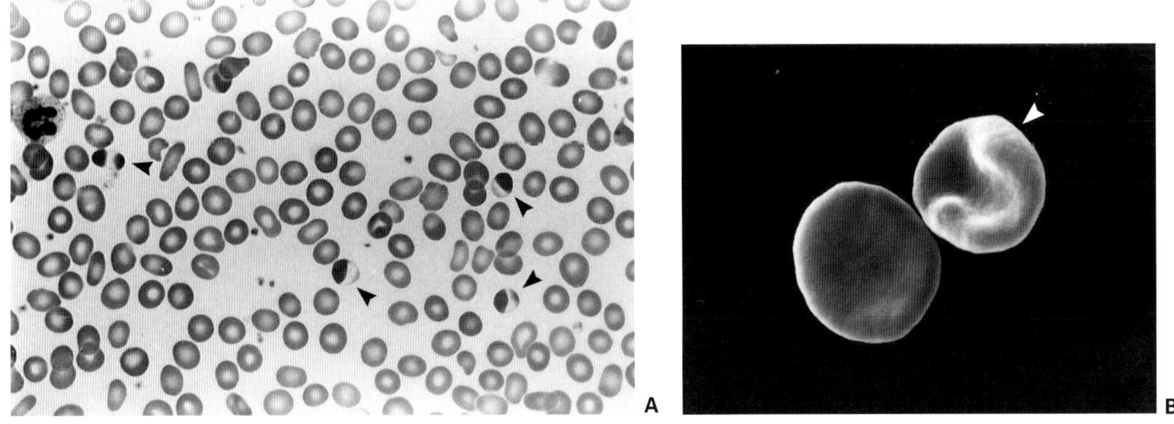

Fig. 3.17 Cells with puddled Hb (arrows), hereditary xerocytosis. **b** × 4500

Hereditary xerocytosis

This is one of a group of uncommon membrane disorders characterized by increased cation flux (Wiley 1984, Table 3.19).

K^+ is lost in excess of Na^+ gain — depletion of total cell cations, with accompanying water loss, leads to cell dehydration. The probable basis is uncontrolled hyperactivity of the K^++Cl^- co-transport system, which shifts K^+ and Cl^- (with water) out of cells in response to swelling in hypotonic states. The molecular basis is not known. There is an unexplained increase in membrane phosphatidylcholine.

The increase in Na influx is not specific but a normal result excludes the diagnosis. Lesser increases in flux occur in a variety of haemolytic disorders, e.g. HS.

Diminution in 2,3 DPG (Fig. 3.18) causes an increase in O_2 affinity, reduced capacity to deliver O_2 to tissues and compensatory increase in Hb. However, though Hb level is often normal, there is persistent haemolysis, with reticulocytosis, low haptoglobin and mild jaundice. Variable numbers of target cells (dehydration) may be noted; in suspension these cells have a bowl shape (compare target cells in thalassaemia, Fig. 3.9). The MCHC is increased because of dehydration.

Exercise often increases haemolysis (Platt et al 1981; abdominal pain may result from splenic distension), due to increase in plasma and erythrocyte acidity which encourages egress of K^+ and water with further cell dehydration.

Inheritance, when demonstrable, is autosomal dominant. Splenectomy is not beneficial for haemolysis, presumably because intravascular haemolysis is more important than sequestration in the spleen, but may be required for reasons of size or exercise-induced discomfort.

STOMATOCYTOSIS (Table 3.20)

Stomatocytes (Fig. 3.19) have a slit-like area of central pallor in blood films and are bowl-shaped in suspensions, which should be used to help exclude artefact (patchy distribution in film, inconstant occurrence). Target cells in certain conditions, e.g. hereditary xerocytosis, also have a bowl shape in suspension.

Table 3.19 Hereditary xerocytosis vs hereditary hydrocytosis

	Hereditary xerocytosis	Hereditary hydrocytosis
Cell cations		
Total	↓	↑↑
Na^+	↑	↑↑
K^+	↓	↓↓
Na^+ influx	>2 × n	>2 × n
MCHC	↑	↓
MCV[1]	n to slight ↑	↑
Blood film	puddling of Hb, targets	stomatocytes
Wet prep	bowl shapes	bowl shapes
Osmotic fragility (fresh)	↓	↑
Haemolysis	mild to moderate	may be severe
Cellular 2,3 DPG	↓	↓
Splenectomy for haemolysis	usually no benefit	beneficial

[1] Determined by size of mature cells + degree of reticulocytosis
n = normal

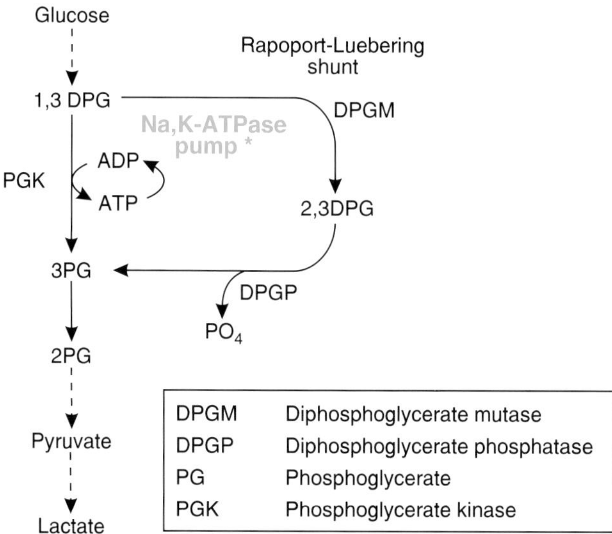

Fig. 3.18 Glycolysis: in states of hyperactivity of the cation pump*, formation of 2,3 DPG via the Rapoport-Luebering shunt (normally about 20% of glycolysis) is curtailed in favour of the direct path from 1,3 DPG to 3 PG.

Table 3.20 Stomatocytosis in childhood

Artefact
Genetic
Melanesian ovalocytosis
'Mediterranean' stomatocytosis[1]
Hereditary hydrocytosis
Rh null, mod
Tangier disease
Stewart's syndrome
Other rare defects
Acquired
Cytotoxics
Phenothiazines
Marathon running
Zinc deficiency (?)
Unexplained, transitory (days)

[1] Unclear if genetic or environmental

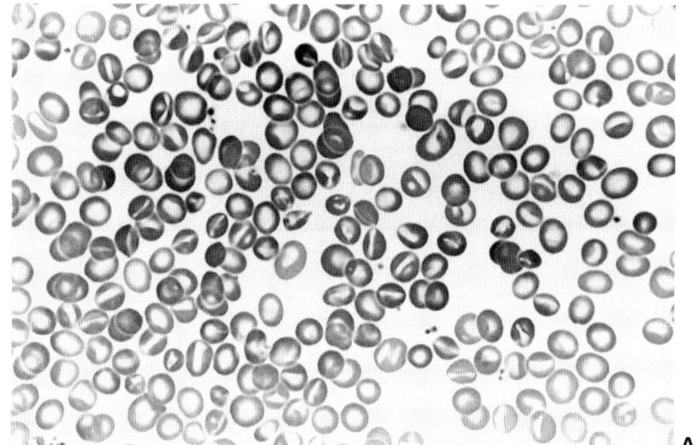

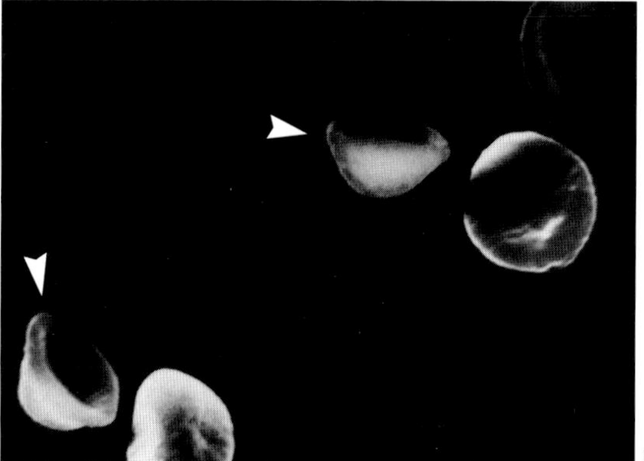

Fig. 3.19 Stomatocytosis. **a** Temporary (weeks) in a child receiving the usual regime of asparaginase, methotrexate and 6MP for ALL. **b** Rh null — scanning electron microscopy; note bowl shapes. **b** × 1800

Melanesian ovalocytosis

See page 78 and Figure 3.6.

Mediterranean stomatocytosis (Ducrou & Kimber 1969)

Stomatocytosis unassociated with recognized disease is not uncommon in adult Mediterranean immigrants into Australia, but is not apparently common in their country of origin, or in their children or in immigrants into other countries. Its development varies from one subject to another (10–40% of cells) and at different times in the same person. Mild haemolytic anaemia and splenomegaly are common (in splenectomized patients Hb and reticulocytes return to normal), as well as macrothrombocytopenia (Table 8.29).

Hereditary hydrocytosis (Becker & Lux 1993, Table 3.19)

A rare disorder of cell volume regulation. Excessive inward flow of Na^+ with lesser K^+ egress leads to increase in total intracellular cations (and water, high Na^+/low K^+ cells). The bloated, inflexible cells are trapped and destroyed in the spleen. Absence of a 28 kD component of membrane protein 7 appears to be the basic defect (Eber et al 1989).

Anaemia and jaundice in the neonate may require exchange transfusion. Anaemia may however be unexpectedly mild because of increase in oxygen affinity from diminution in 2,3 DPG caused by hyperactive cation pumping (Fig. 3.18, Wiley et al 1979).

Macrocytosis results from cell swelling and reticulocytosis (usually > 15%), and MCHC is decreased because of overhydration. Inheritance, when demonstrable, is autosomal dominant.

Diagnosis requires demonstration of an increase in total cell cations (flame photometry) or a substantial (> 2 × normal) increase in inward Na^+ flux (radioisotopes; lesser increases are non-specific). Splenectomy usually gives only partial relief of haemolysis.

Cryohydrocytosis is a rare variant in which autohaemolysis is greater at 4°C than 37°C, and the cold effect is demonstrable with heparin and EDTA but not acid citrate dextrose (Stewart & Ellory 1985).

Other rare genetic defects

- Rh null, Rh mod (Ballas et al 1984, Saji & Hosoi 1979, Fig. 3.19)

Absence (null) or marked reduction (mod) of Rh antigen expression is associated, by unknown mechanisms, with stomatocytosis and moderate haemolysis; small numbers of spherocytes may be noted. In contrast to the stomatocytes of hereditary hydrocytosis, the cells may be dehydrated due to K^+ and net cation loss. Inheritance in most cases appears to be autosomal recessive. Splenectomy results in marked improvement in haemolysis.

- Tangier disease

Virtual absence of high density lipoprotein, which transports cholesteryl esters to the liver, is associated with stomatocytosis and haemolysis (decreased cholesterol, increased phosphatidylcholine in membrane, Reinhart et al 1989), and effects due to accumulation of cholesteryl ester-laden macrophages — orange coloration of a variety of tissues (tonsils, rectal mucosa), peripheral neuropathy, splenomegaly, mild corneal clouding and foam cells in marrow. Inheritance is autosomal recessive.

- Stewart's syndrome (Stewart et al 1987)

Stomatocytosis and mild haemolytic anaemia with severe pseudohomozygous hypercholesterolaemia, tendon sheath xanthomas and macrothrombocytopenia. No abnormality of erythrocyte membrane lipids or proteins or cation transport was found. Stomatocytosis and platelet abnormality persisted despite cure of hypercholesterolaemia and xanthomas with cholestyramine.

- Combined deficiency of proteins 3, 6, 4.1 and 7

Attributed to defective post-translational modification rather than multiple defects, dominantly inherited and associated with congenital stomatocytosis and haemolysis requiring exchange transfusion (Huppi et al 1991).

- Protein 3 mutation (Wada et al 1990)

Mild stomatocytosis associated.

- Protein 4.2 mutation (Inoue et al 1990)

Conspicuous stomatocytosis, autosomal dominant. Other mutations are associated with recessive HS.

- ADA overproduction (Miwa et al 1978)

Haemolysis is attributed to deficiency of ATP (adenosine depleted by conversion to inosine, Fig. 3.20); autosomal dominant. Lesser increases in ADA (about 4 × normal, compared to the 45–85 increase in ADA overproduction) occur in Diamond-

Blackfan anaemia and arthrogryposis, but without significant haemolysis (Mentzer 1993).

Cytotoxics and other drugs

Stomatocytosis is infrequent in children treated with cytotoxics (Fig. 3.19). Cytotoxics and chlorpromazine induce stomatocytosis in vitro (Neville et al 1984).

Marathon running

Stomatocytosis of unknown mechanism may be noted in suspensions (rather than films), reverting to normal within 18 hours (Reinhart & Chien 1985).

SICKLE CELLS

See page 26.

CRYSTALS

See page 28.

PROMINENT BASOPHILIC STIPPLING

Fine stippling, with or without occasional coarsely stippled cells, is common in red cell regeneration of any origin. Coarse stippling in more than occasional cells is notable in:

- thalassaemias
- lead poisoning (Fig. 2.3).

Stippling is probably due to inhibition of pyrimidine-5'-nucleotidase (see below).

- Unstable haemoglobinopathies, e.g. Hammersmith, Bristol

- Genetic pyrimidine-5'-nucleotidase deficiency

The stipples are aggregates of undegraded ribosomal nucleoprotein, derived by ribonuclease digestion of ribosomal RNA surplus to requirements in maturation of the reticulocyte (Fig. 3.20). Stippling occurs in up to 5% of cells and is associated with haemolysis, usually not severe. Mental retardation in some patients is attributed to deficiency of the enzyme in the brain (Beutler et al 1980a). UV spectroscopic examination for pyrimidine nucleotides in perchloric acid extracts may be used as a screening procedure. Inheritance is autosomal recessive.

BIZARRE POIKILOCYTOSIS

A listing is given in Table 3.21.

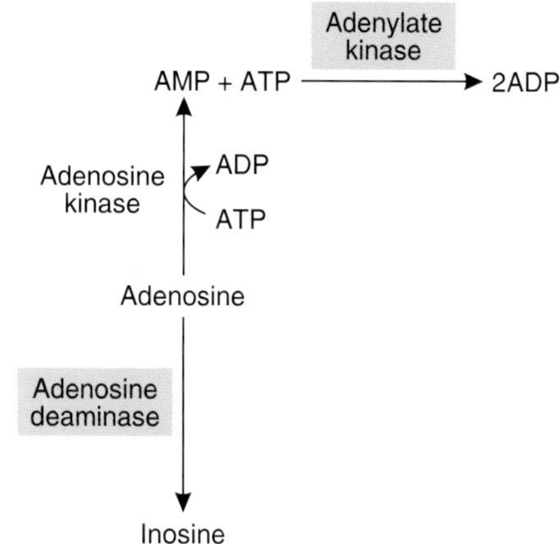

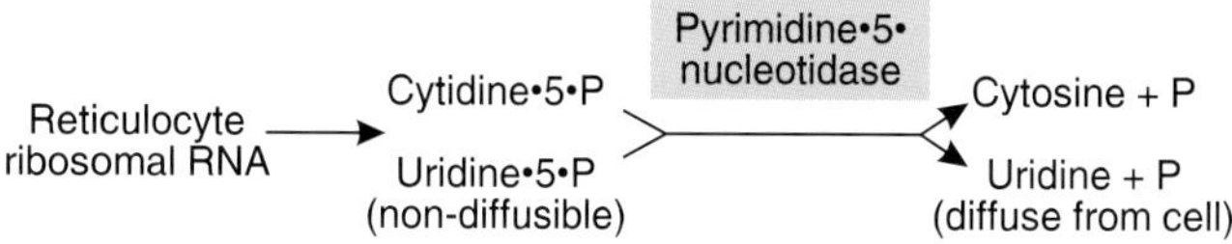

Fig. 3.20 Some aspects of nucleotide metabolism. Enzymes defective in genetic haemolytic anaemias are shown against a blue background.

Table 3.21 Bizarre poikilocytosis in childhood

Fragmentation haemolysis
Neonatal Heinz body haemolysis
Obstructive jaundice/liver failure, ± renal damage intravascular coagulation hypoalbuminaemia
Infantile pyknocytosis (first months of life)
HE + pyknocytosis (first months of life)
HS, variant with poikilocytosis and acanthocytosis
Homozygous mild HE
Haemolytic HE with spherocytosis
Hereditary pyropoikilocytosis
Neonatal iron deficiency + (normal or abnormal degree of) pyknocytosis
Double heterozygosity, e.g. HS + HE
Congenital dyserythropoiesis (some types)
Pyruvate kinase deficiency (some cases)
Transfusion of damaged red cells

Haemolytic anaemias without distinctive erythrocyte morphology

Normal or nondescript morphology is noted in a wide variety of haemolytic disorders (Table 3.22). Disorders not already considered in Chapters 2 and 3 are considered here.

INFECTION

The commonest cause of anaemia in childhood. In a proportion of cases a mechanism is identified (Table 3.23), e.g:

- T activation (p. 74)
- in haemophilus infection, binding to erythrocytes of bacterial capsular polysaccharide and, subsequently, antibody to polysaccharide, with complement (Shurin et al 1986)
- haemolysins may be significant in bacterial infections in particular, and occasionally produce visible effect (Fig. 3.4)
- more than one mechanism for haemolysis may be operating in a patient, e.g. prolonged anaemia after bacterial meningitis may be due to autoimmune effect from superadded viral infection; see also Figure 3.8e.

Table 3.22 Haemolytic anaemias with normal or nondescript red cell morphology[1]

Membrane
Inherited
Congenital dyserythropoietic anaemias
Disorders of cation flux[2]
Congenital erythropoietic porphyria
Acquired
Infection
Alloimmune
Fetomaternal other than ABO
Autoimmune[2]
Neonatal Heinz body haemolysis[2]
Renal disease
Wilson's disease[2]
PNH
Vitamin E deficiency (?)
Selenium deficiency
Hypervitaminosis
Enzyme
Glycolytic pathway
Hexose monophosphate shunt
Adenosine deaminase hyperactivity
Haemoglobin
Unstable haemoglobinopathy

[1] The placement of some disorders in the various categories is tentative
[2] Normal or nondescript morphology in a minority only

In the generality of acute infections, however, a mechanism for the anaemia is not detected; the rapidity of fall in Hb (days) suggests haemolysis, although usual indications of haemolysis are normal: reticulocytes are not increased, and bilirubin and LDH are normal, as well as haptoglobin (whose reduction however would be masked by increase due to acute inflammatory response).

It is not clear why a variety of organisms (e.g. CMV, herpes simplex, rubella, toxoplasma, *Treponema pallidum*, listeria) cause severe anaemia more often in the fetus and neonate than at other ages; anaemia may be severe enough to be associated with hydrops.

ALLOIMMUNE HAEMOLYSIS

Spherocytosis is consistent in ABO, does not occur in Rh (Fig. 3.21) and is rare in other fetomaternal incompatibilities (p. 72). In contrast to fetomaternal incompatibility, incompatible transfusion due to anti-D may be associated with spherocytosis (Mollison et al 1993).

RENAL DISEASE

Anaemia is due to a variety of mechanisms (Table 3.24) and is usually severe (mild in acute nephritis). The commonest change is contraction into various shapes (Fig. 3.22). The component/s in uraemic serum responsible for this change are obscure. In dialysed patients haemolysis may be due to contaminants in dialysis fluid (Carlson & Shapiro 1970, Eaton et al 1973).

Table 3.23 Anaemia in infection

- Haemolysis
  - Autoimmune
    - Virus, mycoplasma (DAT positive, Table 3.10)
    - Cryptantigen exposure (pneumococcus, clostridium)
  - Fragmentation haemolysis, endothelial damage
    - Neuraminidase (pneumococcus-associated HUS)
    - Exotoxin (*E. coli*-, shigella-associated HUS)
  - Binding of bacterial capsular polysaccharide + antipolysaccharide antibody
  - Haemolysins (?)
  - Infection-associated haemophagocytic syndrome
  - Oxidative injury — G6PD deficiency
  - Parasitization — malaria, babesia, bartonella
  - Undefined mechanisms
- Marrow production
  - Erythroblastopenia
    - Parvovirus
    - TEC
  - Marrow aplasia
    - Viral infection
  - Anaemia of chronic disease
- Blood loss
  - Hookworm

Table 3.24 Anaemia in renal disease

Mechanisms/morphology	Disease or other association
Haemodilution	acute glomerulonephritis
Erythropoietin lack	renal destruction of any cause
Haemolysis	
Fragmentation	haemolytic-uraemic syndrome thrombotic thrombocytopenic purpura SLE (some cases)
Nondescript shrinkage	chronic damage of any cause contaminants in dialysis fluid (copper, chloramine, nitrates[1])
Spur cells	chronic damage of any cause
Folate deficiency	anorexia haemodialysis, peritoneal dialysis immunosuppressants
Iron deficiency	bleeding into/from tumour iron loss in nephrosis (rare)

[1] Often with Heinz body haemolysis

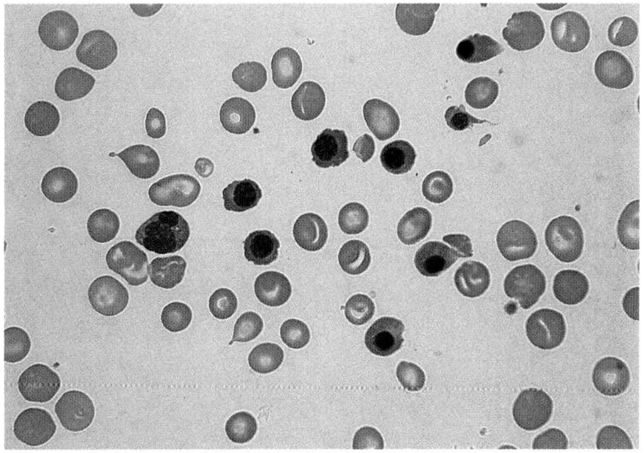

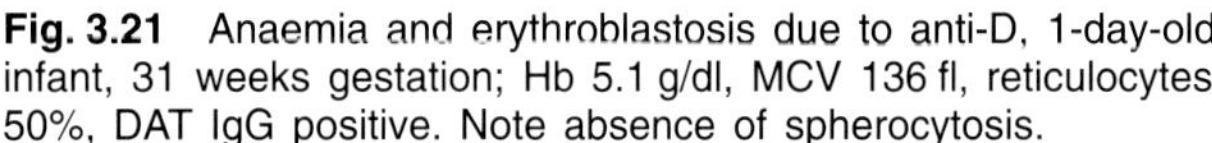

Fig. 3.21 Anaemia and erythroblastosis due to anti-D, 1-day-old infant, 31 weeks gestation; Hb 5.1 g/dl, MCV 136 fl, reticulocytes 50%, DAT IgG positive. Note absence of spherocytosis.

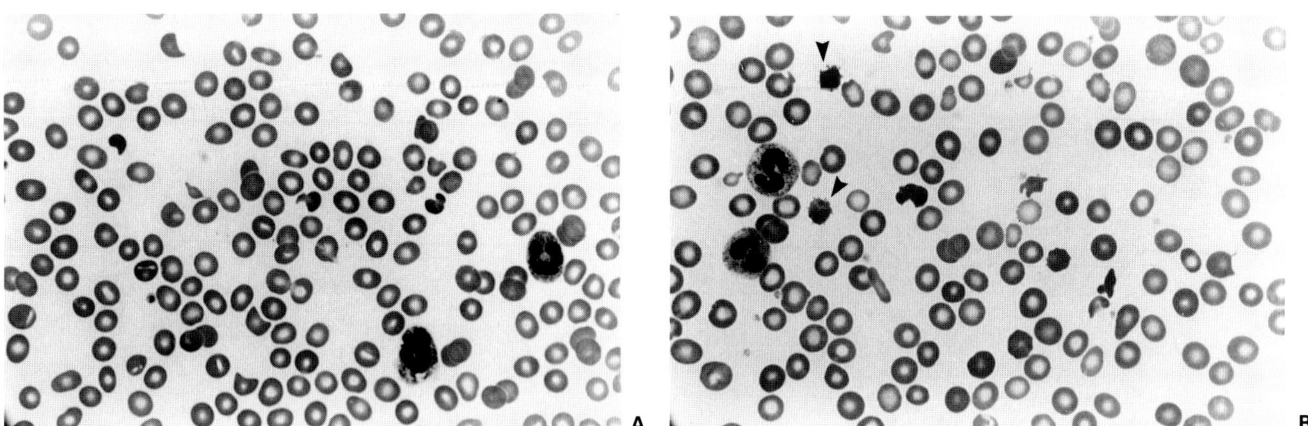

Fig. 3.22 Anaemia in chronic renal disease. **a** Nondescript cell shrinkage, lupus nephritis. **b** Shrunken and (arrows) dense spiculated cells, Wegener's granulomatosis.

VITAMIN DEFICIENCY/EXCESS, TRACE ELEMENT DEFICIENCY, HYPERLIPIDAEMIA (Fig. 3.23)

Deficiency of vitamin E (α tocopherol) has been implicated in pyknocytic haemolysis and thrombocytosis in the neonate; however, the evidence is tenuous (Zipursky et al 1987). Vitamin E deficiency is common in cystic fibrosis, in which it may cause a shortening of red cell life span, but without anaemia (Farrell et al 1977).

High dosage vitamin C has a potential for causing haemolysis with Heinz bodies (Ballin et al 1988).

Selenium deficiency may cause a distinctive brittleness of erythrocytes.

Fragile erythrocytes may be noted in gross hyperchylomicronaemia.

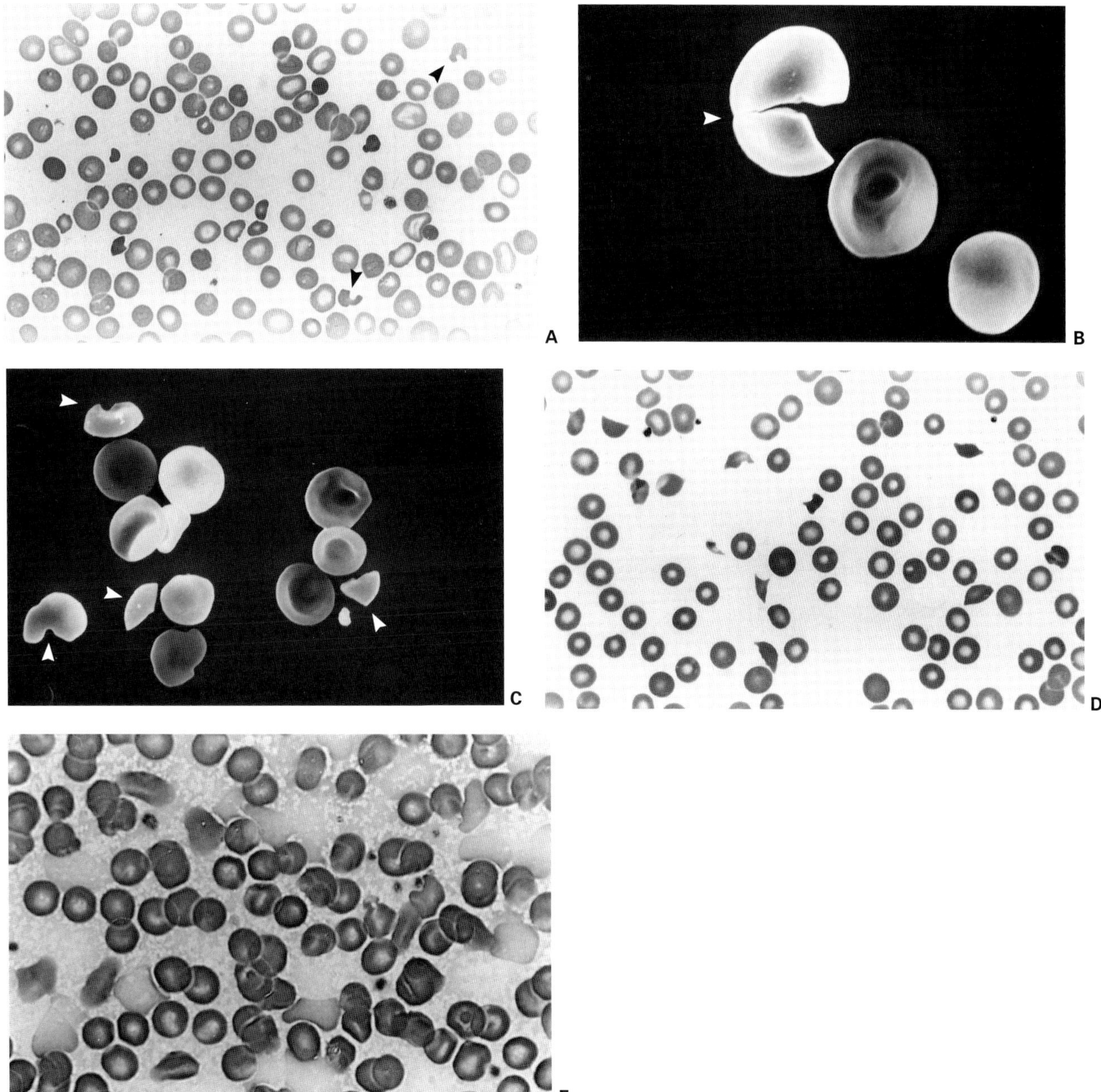

Fig. 3.23 Rare haemolytic disorders. **a–c** Selenium deficiency, 3-year-old girl with cyclosporine-responsive autoimmune enteropathy, Hb 7.9 g/dl. **a** Contracted and (arrows) bite cells. **b** Brittle cell on verge of fragmentation (arrow). **c** Fragments and bite cells (arrows). **d** Nondescript shrinkage in a 2-year-old given toxic doses of a variety of vitamins (for Down's syndrome) by a nutritionist, Hb 8.9 g/dl; haemolysis was probably due to excess of vitamin C. Examination for Heinz bodies was not made. **e** Fragile, decolorized cells in gross hyperchylomicronaemia; note 'moth-eaten' background; courtesy of P Stallybrass.

ENZYME DEFECTS (Lestas & Bellingham 1990, Beutler 1991, Mentzer 1993)

Haemolysis is due to 3 mechanisms (Figs 3.24, 3.25):

- ATP depletion

ATP is essential for the function of the cation pump, synthesis of glutathione and salvage of adenine nucleotides. Depletion occurs in glycolytic enzyme deficiency and in ADA overproduction.

- Depletion of reduced glutathione

An adequate supply of glutathione is essential for detoxication of peroxides and free radical oxidants, which have the capacity to seriously damage Hb and the cell membrane. Deficiency occurs in defects of pentose phosphate pathway enzymes.

- Toxic increase in pyrimidine nucleotides

Toxic amounts accumulate in pyrimidine-5'-nucleotidase deficiency.

With the exception of G6PD and PK deficiency, enzyme defects are rare.

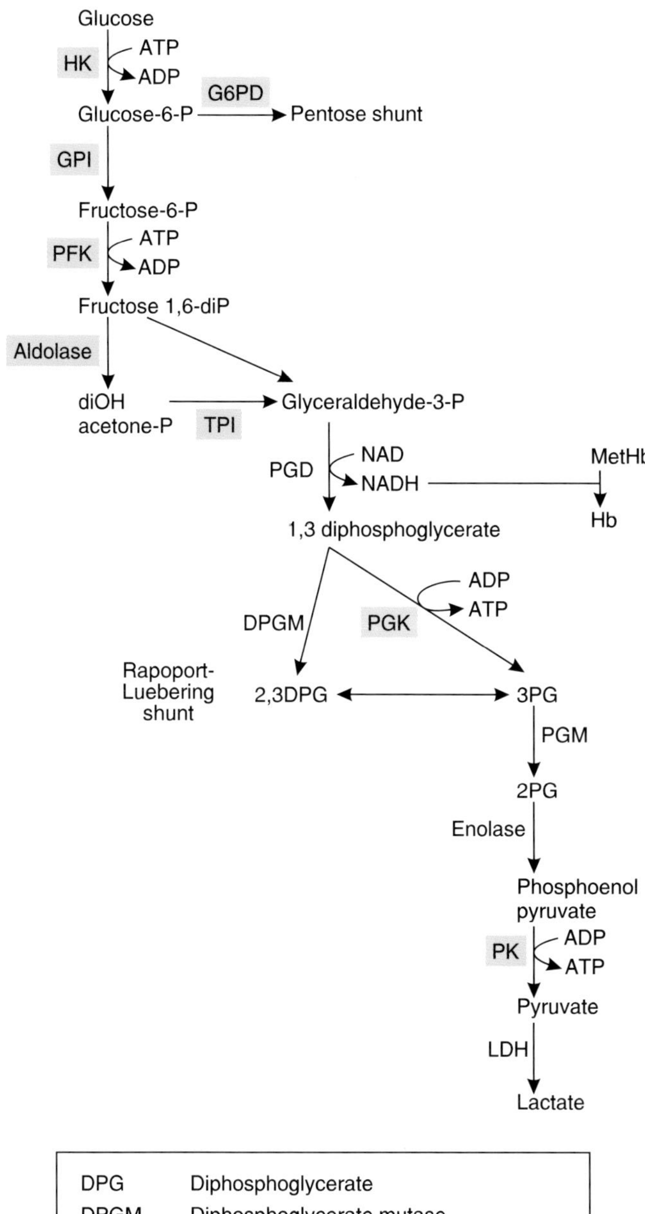

DPG	Diphosphoglycerate
DPGM	Diphosphoglycerate mutase
GPI	Glucose phosphate isomerase
G6PD	Glucose-6-phosphate dehydrogenase
HK	Hexokinase
NAD	Nicotinamide adenine dinucleotide
PGD	Phosphoglyceraldehyde dehydrogenase
PFK	Phosphofructokinase
PGK	Phosphoglycerate kinase
PK	Pyruvate kinase
TPI	Triosephosphate isomerase

Fig. 3.24 The glycolytic pathway, simplified. Enzymes defective in genetic haemolytic disorders are shown against a blue background.

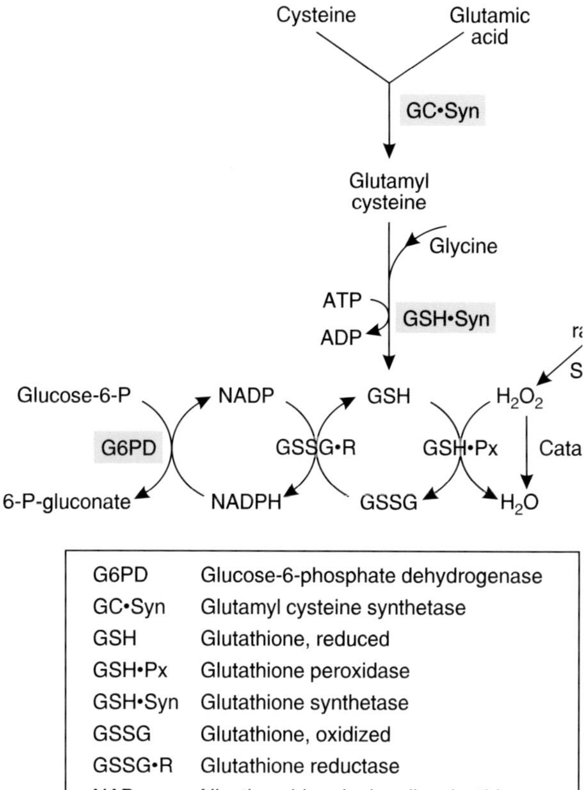

G6PD	Glucose-6-phosphate dehydrogenase
GC•Syn	Glutamyl cysteine synthetase
GSH	Glutathione, reduced
GSH•Px	Glutathione peroxidase
GSH•Syn	Glutathione synthetase
GSSG	Glutathione, oxidized
GSSG•R	Glutathione reductase
NAD	Nicotinamide adenine dinucleotide
SOD	Superoxide dismutase

Fig. 3.25 The hexose monophosphate shunt, simplified. Enzymes defective in genetic haemolytic disorders are shown against a blue background.

Blood morphology and values

- With some rare exceptions (Table 3.6), spherocytosis is a minor component (non-spherocytic haemolytic anaemias).
- Dense spiculated spherocytes occur in some deficiencies, especially after splenectomy (Fig. 3.26, Table 3.25, Nathan et al 1966).
- Blister cells (hemighosts) are common in crises of favism (p. 92, Fig. 3.16).
- Notable poikilocytosis occurs in some patients with PK deficiency (Fig. 3.26).
- Heinz bodies are a feature of the episodic haemolysis of G6PD deficiency (Fig. 3.16) and the rare glutathione deficiency.

Methaemoglobinaemia is (surprisingly) a rare occurrence in G6PD deficiency (Hibbard et al 1978).

Anaemia may be episodic (haemolytic crises of G6PD deficiency) or chronic. In the fetus/neonate anaemia may be severe enough in some deficiencies to cause hydrops. Macrocytosis is usually in proportion to reticulocytosis, but in some cases is inexplicably excessive. As in other anaemias with hyperplasia of the erythron, severe anaemia with reticulocytopenia may result from parvovirus infection (p. 54).

Drug exacerbation of haemolysis

Except for oxidant drugs in G6PD and glutathione deficiencies, and a possible effect of salicylate in PK deficiency, drugs are not known to influence the degree of haemolysis.

Non-erythrocytic manifestations

Enzyme deficiency in non-erythroid tissues may cause clinical disturbance (Table 3.25). Neuromuscular dysfunction occurs in a few rare deficiencies. See also G6PD deficiency, below.

Inheritance

Inheritance is X-linked in G6PD and phosphoglycerate kinase deficiencies, and autosomal dominant in ADA overproduction. Other defects have autosomal recessive transmission. Where the enzyme has numerous variants (e.g. PK), severe deficiency may be due to homozygosity or compound heterozygosity.

Effect of splenectomy

In general splenectomy gives little or only partial benefit (compare HS). Splenectomy is most commonly done for PK deficiency, in which it is often followed by striking reticulocytosis (to 90% of cells).

Table 3.25 Features of some glycolytic enzyme deficiencies[1]

	Morphology	Non-haematologic disease	Inheritance[2]
Hexokinase	dense spiculated cells in some cases post-splenectomy		AR; rare ?AD are probably manifesting heterozygotes
Glucose phosphate isomerase	spherocytes or dense spiculated spherocytes in some cases, esp after splenectomy. Stomatocytosis in rare cases	neuromuscular dysfunction in occasional cases	AR
Phosphofructokinase	prominent stippling in some cases	fatigue, myopathy and exertional myoglobinuria in some cases	AR
Triosephosphate isomerase	dense spiculated cells in small numbers in some cases	severe neurologic dysfunction, onset usually at 6–12 months: spasticity, psychomotor retardation, muscle weakness; death (cardiac failure) often before 5 yr	AR
Phosphoglycerate kinase	dense spiculated cells in some cases	psychomotor retardation, seizures, aphasia, tetraplegia in severe deficiency. Rhabdomyolysis in some variants	XLR
Pyruvate kinase	anaemia 0 to severe; dense spiculated cells in some cases, esp after splenectomy	chronic leg ulcers in rare families	AR

[1] Listed in order of appearance in glycolytic pathway
[2] AD = autosomal dominant; AR = autosomal recessive or compound heterozygosity; XLR = X-linked recessive

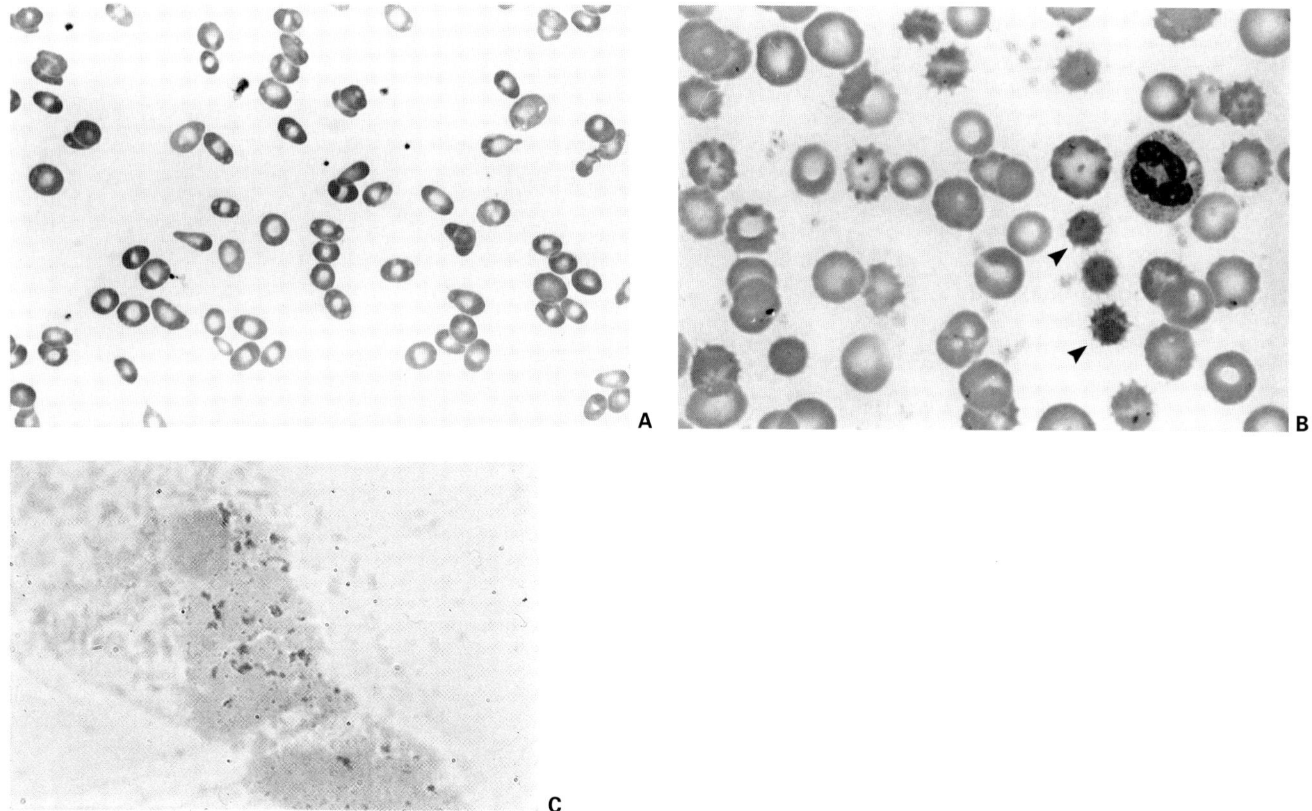

Fig. 3.26 Pyruvate kinase deficiency. **a** Unsplenectomized patient, showing poikilocytosis. **b** Post-splenectomy (different child), crenated and dense spiculated cells (whiskered spherocytes, arrows). **c** Intracellular haemosiderin, spun deposit of urine, Perls stain. **b** $\times$ 750; **c** $\times$ 1000. **b** Courtesy of Dr G Tauro

Diagnosis
Autohaemolysis and osmotic fragility are non-specific and have been replaced by assay of enzymes or intermediates and gene analysis. Procedures for G6PD and PK at the least (Dacie & Lewis 1991) should be routine in work-up for haemolysis. See also G6PD deficiency, diagnosis, below.

Assays of enzymes other than G6PD and PK and identification of variants are best done in a specialist laboratory.

G6PD deficiency

Worldwide, this is the commonest genetic defect. Identification of deficiency, therefore, does not necessarily mean that this is the cause of haemolysis.

Clinical manifestations
Deficiency is often asymptomatic. Manifestations fall into 3 major groups:

1. Neonatal jaundice
Jaundice is evident at 2–3 days, rarely at birth, and may be severe enough to require exchange transfusion. Anaemia by contrast is rarely a problem, suggesting that hepatic dysfunction (? G6PD deficiency) is the major component in jaundice. The incidence of jaundice varies, even among apparently homogeneous populations, suggesting that environmental factors (e.g. naphthalene, camphor) may be significant. Temporary deficiency of protective enzymes such as glutathione peroxidase, glutathione reductase and superoxide dismutase (Fig. 3.25) may explain the greater frequency of jaundice in the neonate.

2. Episodic haemolysis
Agents with accepted potential for precipitating haemolysis are listed in Table 3.26. Omitted are drugs (e.g. aspirin) which were once incriminated for haemolysis which was in fact due to accompanying infection (Beutler 1991). During infection, some physicians would advise restraint in use of drugs additional to those listed, e.g. aspirin, additional sulphonamides and antimalarials, chloramphenicol, vitamin C and aqueous vitamin K. The ingredient/s of the fava bean active in haemolysis are not clear. The haemolytic potential of infections is attributed to peroxide production in cells.

Because of the multitude of enzyme variants, there is considerable individual variation in susceptibility to these agents. For example, all persons with favism are deficient, but most G6PD deficient subjects are not susceptible to favism. Favism is more likely in Mediterraneans (G6PD Med, virtually absent activity) than Africans (G6PD A-, about 10% activity, mostly in reticulocytes).

Irregularly contracted cells, blister cells (Fig. 3.16) and occasional bites and spherocytes may be noted in films. Heinz bodies (Fig. 3.16) may be transient because of splenic pitting and removal of affected cells by macrophages. Haemoglobinuria is common (Table 3.27). Parvovirus infection (Fig. 2.20) will aggravate anaemia, with erythroblastopenia and reticulocytopenia (Fig. 2.20).

Between haemolytic episodes, Hb and reticulocytes are normal, though there may be some shortening of erythrocyte survival.

3. Chronic haemolysis
This is less common than episodic haemolysis. Haemolysis is obvious, manifested by anaemia, reticulocytosis, splenomegaly, (mild) jaundice and high incidence of gallstones; though chronic, it may be exacerbated by exposures which precipitate episodic haemolysis (Table 3.26). The distinctiveness of the group may be due not so much to degree of deficiency as to impairment in binding to ligands such as glucose-6-phosphate, NADP and NADPH (Fig. 3.25).

Deficiency in non-erythroid tissues
These manifestations are rare, and include:
(i) defective bactericidal capacity (especially for *S. aureus*) of granulocytes, attributed to restriction in oxidative burst due to NADPH deficiency; (ii) early onset of cataracts in juveniles.

Diagnosis (Dacie & Lewis 1991)
Because deficiency is severe, diagnosis of affected males is not difficult. Screening procedures, e.g. fluorescent spot test, will detect levels < 30% normal (clinically significant illness is unlikely above this; most carriers will not be identified).

Spuriously normal or low normal results may be obtained (for PK as well) if reticulocytes are increased or there is contamination with granulocytes and platelets, which contain significant amounts of enzyme when mature erythrocytes are deficient.

If testing cannot wait until a quiescent phase 2–3 weeks after the acute episode, the following approaches may be used:

- use of reticulocyte-poor lower fractions of centrifuged samples
- simultaneous assay of other age-dependent enzymes, e.g. PK
- use of controls with comparable reticulocytosis
- cytochemical identification of deficiency in individual cells.

Because of their double population of normal and deficient cells, female carriers may be difficult to identify. Low percentages are best identified cytochemically or by gene analysis. Carrier mothers are less frequently identified if the child has chronic rather than episodic haemolysis.

Identification of variants (best done by DNA analysis) can assist in identifying the cause of haemolysis in G6PD patients, for example G6PD A- and G6PD Med are not associated with chronic haemolysis.

CONGENITAL ERYTHROPOIETIC PORPHYRIA (GÜNTHER'S DISEASE)

Very rare. Deficiency of uroporphyrinogen III cosynthase results in curtailment of synthesis of (normal) type III and excess of damaging type I porphyrins. These accumulate in skin (severe photosensitivity, bullous eruptions, scarring), teeth (red-brown discoloration, red fluorescence in UV light), erythrocytes (fluorescence in UV, mainly nuclei, Schmid et al 1955), erythrocytes (haemolysis) and urine (pink to brown discoloration). Inheritance is autosomal recessive. Diagnosis requires identification of the type I porphyrins or the enzyme defect.

Table 3.26 Drugs and other agents which may cause haemolysis in G6PD deficiency[1]

Food
Fava beans[2]
Drugs
Sulphonamides, sulphones
Sulphamethoxazole
Sulphacetamide
Sulphasalazine
Dapsone
Antimalarials
Primaquine
Pamaquine
Antihelminth
Niridazole
Nitrofurans
Nitrofurantoin
Furazolidone
Other
Phenazopyridine
Doxorubicin
Nalidixic acid
Methylene blue
Dimercaprol (BAL)
Chemicals
Naphthalene
Infection
Pneumococcus
Salmonella
Viral hepatitis

[1] Secretion in milk by nursing mother will affect G6PD-deficient infant
[2] Harmful if eaten raw rather than cooked, frozen or tinned

Table 3.27 Haemoglobinuria in childhood

Autoimmune haemolysis
Cold rather than warm types
G6PD deficiency
Blackwater fever
Incompatible blood transfusion
PNH

Asplenia, splenic atrophy/hypofunction
(Table 3.28, Corrigan et al 1983)

Recognition is important because of the associated risk of serious infection.

Erythrocyte changes (Fig. 3.27, Table 3.29) are variable, even for the same degree of hypofunction, e.g. asplenia. The most consistent is the presence of Howell-Jolly bodies (as an isolated finding this may be normal in the neonate, Fig. 1.1). The pitted ('pocked') cell count (Table 1.7), using differential interference phase-contrast, is a valuable aid to diagnosis, except in HS (p. 66). Confirmation may be made by [^{99m}Tc] sulphur colloid uptake (liver and spleen) or the more sensitive uptake of technetium-labelled heat-damaged patient erythrocytes (spleen only).

- In Ivemark syndrome the most common anomalies are dextrocardia, transposition of viscera, transposition of great arteries, anomalous pulmonary venous return and pulmonary hypertension, with resultant cyanosis and polycythaemia (McKusick 1988, Fig. 3.27). Most cases are sporadic but familial occurrence is not rare.
- Stormorken et al (1985) described a syndrome of asplenia with platelet dysfunction, muscle fatigue, contracted pupils, migraine, dyslexia and ichthyosis.
- In sickle cell disorders, hypofunction is earlier (6 months–3 years) and more severe in sickle cell anaemia (SS) and Sβ° thal (Fig. 2.8) than in SC and Sβ^{+} thal. Anatomic enlargement is followed by infarction and fibrosis (Pearson et al 1985).

- For Pearson's syndrome, see page 216.
- Atrophy may be familial (Kevy et al 1968).
- Atrophy is a late (1–2 years) effect of graft vs host disease following marrow transplantation (Kalhs et al 1988).
- Hypofunction in cyanotic heart disease may result from congestion (Pearson et al 1971).
- Hypofunction is a rare effect of cytotoxics, malnutrition and acute haemolysis (? reticuloendothelial blockade).

Table 3.28 Asplenia, splenic atrophy/hypofunction in childhood

Asplenia
Surgical removal
Ivemark syndrome
Rarer syndromes
Stormorken
Atrophy: anatomic presence but destruction sufficient to impair function
HbS disorders
Pearson's syndrome
Familial
Graft vs host disease
Splenic artery/vein thrombosis
Hypofunction: variable anatomic change (including enlargement) and decrease in function
Temporary or potentially reversible
Prematurity
Cyanotic congenital heart disease
Cytotoxics
Malnutrition
Acute haemolysis
May proceed to atrophy but rarely before adulthood
Coeliac disease
Connective tissue disease
SLE
Rheumatoid arthritis
Inflammatory bowel disease
Dermatitis herpetiformis

Table 3.29 Red cell morphology in asplenia/splenic atrophy

Howell-Jolly bodies
Target cells
Acanthocytes
'Holes' in cells
Siderocytes[1]
Spherocytes, small numbers
Heinz bodies (usually > 5% of cells)
Increase in pitted (pocked) cells (interference-phase contrast)

[1] Unlikely to be prominent unless spleen has been removed for conditions such as hereditary sideroblastic anaemia, thalassaemia major, histiocytosis

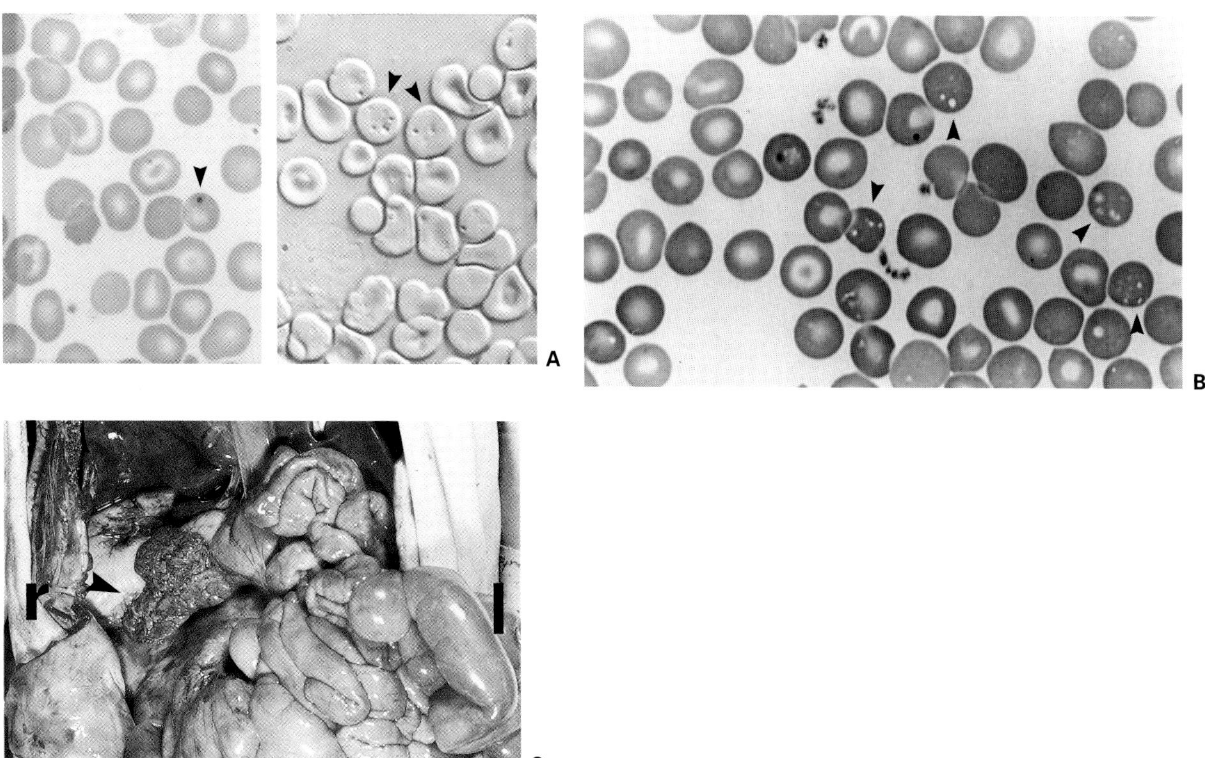

Fig. 3.27 Asplenia/splenic atrophy. **a** Routine morphology (left) shows target cells and Howell-Jolly body (arrow); differential interference phase-contrast (right) shows target cells and pocked cells (some arrowed); 11-year-old girl with unidentified collagen disease and splenic atrophy. **b** Ivemark syndrome, routine film showing holes corresponding to pits visible by differential interference phase. **c** Ivemark syndrome, pancreas in right abdomen (r) and pointing to right, as part of transposition of viscera.
a × 800; **b** × 750

REFERENCES

Abdalla S, Weatherall D J 1982 The direct antiglobulin test in P. falciparum malaria. British Journal of Haematology 51: 415–425

Balari A S, Espinosa J V, Fuertes I F 1989 A new modification of the "Pink test" for the diagnosis of hereditary spherocytosis. Acta Haematologica 82: 213–214

Ballas S K, Clark M R, Mohandas N et al 1984 Red cell membrane and cation deficiency in Rh null syndrome. Blood 63: 1046–1055

Ballin A, Brown E J, Koren G, Zipursky A 1988 Vitamin C-induced erythrocyte damage in premature infants. Journal of Pediatrics 113: 114–120

Becker P S, Lux S E 1993 Disorders of the red cell membrane. In: Nathan D G, Oski F A (eds) Hematology of infancy and childhood, 4th edn. W B Saunders, Philadelphia, ch 17

Becton D L, Kinney T R 1986 An infant girl with severe autoimmune hemolytic anemia: apparent anti-Vel specificity. Vox Sanguinis 51: 108–111

Beutler E 1991 Glucose-6-phosphate dehydrogenase deficiency. New England Journal of Medicine 324: 169–174

Beutler E, Baranko P V, Feagler J et al 1980a Hemolytic anemia due to pyrimidine-5'-nucleotidase deficiency: report of eight cases in six families. Blood 56: 251–255

Beutler E, West C, Tavassoli M, Grahn E 1980b The Woronets trait: a new familial erythrocyte anomaly. Blood Cells 6: 281–287

Bird G W G, Wingham J, Martin A J et al 1976 Idiopathic non-syphilitic paroxysmal cold haemoglobinuria in children. Journal of Clinical Pathology 29: 215–218

Booth P B, Serjeantson S, Woodfield D G, Amato D 1977 Selective depression of blood group antigens associated with hereditary ovalocytosis among Melanesians. Vox Sanguinis 32: 99–110

Bucx M J L, Breed W P M, Hoffmann J J M L 1988 Comparison of acidified glycerol lysis test, Pink test and osmotic fragility test in hereditary spherocytosis: effect of incubation. European Journal of Haematology 40: 227–231

Carlson D J, Shapiro F L 1970 Methemoglobinemia from well water nitrates: a complication of home dialysis. Annals of Internal Medicine 73: 757–759

Carpentieri U, Gustavson L P, Haggard M E 1977 Pyknocytosis in a neonate: an unusual presentation of hereditary elliptocytosis. Clinical Pediatrics 16: 76–78

Chan T K, Chan W C, Weed R I 1982 Erythrocyte hemighosts: a hallmark of severe oxidative injury in vivo. British Journal of Haematology 50: 575–582

Chilcote R R, Le Beau M M, Dampier C et al 1987 Association of red cell spherocytosis with deletion of the short arm of chromosome 8. Blood 69: 156–159

Cooper R A 1969 Anemia with spur cells: a red cell defect acquired in serum and modified in the circulation. Journal of Clinical Investigation 48: 1820–1831

Corrigan J J, Van Wyck D B, Crosby W H 1983 Clinical disorders of splenic function: the spectrum from asplenism to hypersplenism. Lymphology 16: 101–106

Curtis B R, Lamon J, Roelcke D, Chaplin H 1990 Life-threatening, antiglobulin test-negative, acute autoimmune hemolytic anemia due to a non-complement-activating IgG1 k cold antibody with Pr_a specificity. Transfusion 30: 838–843

Dacie J V, Lewis S M 1991 Practical haematology, 7th edn. Churchill Livingstone, Edinburgh

Dean H M, Decker C L, Baker L D 1967 Temporary survival in clostridial hemolysis with absence of circulating red cells. New England Journal of Medicine 277: 700–701

Ducrou W, Kimber R J 1969 Stomatocytes, haemolytic anaemia and abdominal pain in Mediterranean migrants. Some examples of a new syndrome? Medical Journal of Australia 2: 1087–1091

Duru F, Gürgey A, Öztürk G et al 1992 Homozygosity for dominant form of hereditary spherocytosis. British Journal of Haematology 82: 596–600

Eaton J W, Kolpin C F, Swofford H S et al 1973 Chlorinated urban water: a cause of dialysis-induced hemolytic anemia. Science 181: 463–464

Eber S W, Lande W M, Iarocci T A et al 1989 Hereditary stomatocytosis: consistent association with an integral membrane protein deficiency. British Journal of Haematology 72: 452–455

Eichner E R 1984 Spider bite hemolytic anemia: positive Coombs' test, erythrophagocytosis, and leukoerythroblastic smear. American Journal of Clinical Pathology 81: 683–687

Elejalde B R, De Elejalde M M J, Lopez F 1979 Hallervorden-Spatz disease. Clinical Genetics 16: 1–18

Eto Y, Kitagawa T 1970 Wolman's disease with hypolipoproteinemia and acanthocytosis: clinical and biochemical observations. Journal of Pediatrics 77: 862–867

Farrell P M, Bieri J G, Fratantoni J F et al 1977 The occurrence and effects of human vitamin E deficiency. A study in patients with cystic fibrosis. Journal of Clinical Investigation 60: 233–241

Fraga J R, Reichelderfer T E, Scott R B, Said D M 1968 Giant cell hepatitis associated with hereditary spherocytosis. Clinical Pediatrics 7: 364–372

Giblett E R, Varela J E, Finch C A 1956 Damage of the bone marrow due to Rh antibody. Pediatrics 17: 37–44

Greenberg J, Curtis-Cohen M, Gill F M, Cohen A 1980 Prolonged reticulocytopenia in autoimmune hemolytic anemia of childhood. Journal of Pediatrics 97: 784–786

Gross K B, Skrivanek J A, Emeson E E 1982 Ganglioside abnormality in amyotrophic chorea with acanthocytosis. Lancet 2: 772

Harrison C R, Hayes T C, Trow L L, Benedetto A R 1986 Intravascular hemolytic transfusion reaction without detectable antibodies: a case report and review of literature. Vox Sanguinis 51: 96–101

Hernandez J A, Steane S M 1984 Erythrophagocytosis by segmented neutrophils in paroxysmal cold hemoglobinuria. American Journal of Clinical Pathology 81: 787–789

Hibbard B Z, Koenig H M, Lightsey A L et al 1978 Severe methemoglobinemia in an infant with glucose-6-phosphate dehydrogenase deficiency. Journal of Pediatrics 93: 816–818

Holtzman N A, Elliott D A, Heller R H 1966 Copper intoxication. Report of a case with observations on ceruloplasmin. New England Journal of Medicine 275: 347–351

Hughes D W O'G, Lovric V A 1962 Multiple red-cell population in association with cyanotic congenital heart-disease. Lancet 1: 726–727

Huppi P S, Ott P, Amato M, Schneider H 1991 Congenital haemolytic anaemia in a low birth weight infant due to congenital stomatocytosis. European Journal of Haematology 47: 1–9

Inoue T, Kanzaki A, Ata K et al 1990 An unique duplet band 4.2 (72 kD/74 kD) disease of autosomal dominantly inherited stomatocytosis. Blood 76 (suppl 1): 9a

Issitt P D 1985 Applied blood group serology, 3rd edn. Montgomery Scientific Publications, Miami

Jones G L, Edmundson H M, Wesche D, Saul A 1990 Human erythrocyte band-3 has an altered N terminus in malaria-resistant Melanesian ovalocytosis. Biochimica et Biophysica Acta 1096: 33–40

Kalhs P, Panzer S, Kletter K et al 1988 Functional asplenia after bone marrow transplantation. A late complication related to extensive chronic graft-versus-host disease. Annals of Internal Medicine 109: 461–464

Kane J P, Havel R J 1989 Disorders of the biogenesis and secretion of lipoproteins containing the B apolipoproteins. In: Scriver C R, Beaudet A L, Sly W S, Valle D (eds) The metabolic basis of inherited disease, 6th edn. McGraw-Hill, New York, ch 44

Kaplan B S, Levin M, De Chadarevian J-P 1992 The hemolytic-uremic syndrome. In: Edelman C M (ed) Pediatric kidney disease, 2nd edn. Little Brown, Boston, ch 60

Kay M M B, Bosman G J C, Lawrence C 1988 Functional topography of band 3: specific structural alteration linked to functional aberrations in human erythrocytes. Proceedings of National Academy of Sciences USA 85: 492–496

Keimowitz R, Desforges J F 1965 Infantile pyknocytosis. New England Journal of Medicine 273: 1152–1155

Kempin J 1993 Personal communication

Kevy S V, Tefft M, Vawter G F, Rosen F S 1968 Hereditary splenic hypoplasia. Pediatrics 42: 752–757

Klock J C, Williams H E, Mentzer W C 1974 Hemolytic anemia and somatic cell dysfunction in severe hypophosphatemia. Archives of Internal Medicine 134: 360–364

Krueger H C, Burgert E O 1966 Hereditary spherocytosis in 100 children. Mayo Clinic Proceedings 41: 821–830

Lestas A N, Bellingham A J 1990 A logical approach to the investigation of red cell enzymopathies. Blood Reviews 4: 148–157

Letsky E A 1991 Haemolytic disease of the newborn. In: Hann I M, Gibson B E S, Letsky E A (eds) Fetal and neonatal haematology. Baillière Tindall, London, ch 5

McCann S R, Jacob H S 1976 Spinal cord disease in hereditary spherocytosis: report of two cases with a hypothesized common mechanism for neurologic and red cell abnormalities. Blood 48: 259–263

McGrath K M, Zalcberg J R, Slonim J, Wiley J S 1982 Intralipid induced haemolysis. British Journal of Haematology 50: 376–378

McKusick V A 1988 Mendelian inheritance in man, 8th edn. Johns Hopkins University Press, Baltimore

Malorni W, Iosi F, Donelli G et al 1993 A new, striking morphologic feature for the human erythrocyte in hereditary spherocytosis: the blebbing pattern. Blood 81: 2821–2822

Mant M J, Faragher B S 1972 The haematology of anorexia nervosa. British Journal of Haematology 23: 737–749

Maxwell D J, Seshadri R, Rumpf D J, Miller J M 1983 Infantile pyknocytosis: a cause of intrauterine haemolysis in 2 siblings. Australian and New Zealand Journal of Obstetrics and Gynaecology 23: 182–185

Mentzer W C 1993 Pyruvate kinase deficiency and disorders of glycolysis. In: Nathan D G, Oski F A (eds) Hematology of infancy and childhood, 4th edn. Saunders, Philadelphia, ch 18

Miwa S, Fujii H, Matsumoto N et al 1978 A case of red-cell adenosine deaminase overproduction associated with hereditary hemolytic anemia found in Japan. American Journal of Hematology 5: 107–115

Moake J L 1994 Haemolytic-uraemic syndrome: basic science. Lancet 343: 393–397

Moiseyev V S, Korovina E A, Polotskaya E L et al 1987 Hypertrophic cardiomyopathy associated with hereditary spherocytosis in three generations of one family. Lancet 2: 853–854

Mollison P L, Engelfriet C P, Contreras M 1993 Blood transfusion in clinical medicine, 9th edn. Blackwell Scientific Publications, London

Murphy W G, Moore J C, Barr R D et al 1987a Relationship between platelet aggregating factor and von Willebrand factor in thrombotic thrombocytopenic purpura. British Journal of Haematology 66: 509–513

Murphy W G, Moore J C, Kelton J G 1987b Calcium dependent cysteineprotease activity in the sera of patients with thrombotic thrombocytopenic purpura. Blood 70: 1683–1687

Nathan D G, Oski F A, Sidel V W et al 1966 Studies of erythrocyte spicule formation in haemolytic anaemia. British Journal of Haematology 12: 385–395

Neville A J, Rand C A, Barr R D, Mohan Pai K R 1984 Drug-induced stomatocytosis and anemia during consolidation chemotherapy of childhood acute leukemia. American Journal of the Medical Sciences 287: 3–7

Norum K R, Gjone E, Glomset J A 1989 Familial lecithin:cholesterol acyltransferase deficiency, including fish eye disease. In: Scriver C R, Beaudet A L, Sly W S, Valle D (eds) The metabolic basis of inherited disease, 6th edn. McGraw-Hill, New York, ch 46

Novak R W 1990 The pathobiology of red cell cryptantigen exposure. Pediatric Pathology 10: 867–875

O'Grady J G, Harding B, Egan E L et al 1984 'Pitted' erythrocytes: impaired formation in splenectomized subjects with congenital spherocytosis. British Journal of Haematology 57: 441–446

Opitz J C, Baldauf M C, Kessler D L, Meyer J A 1988 Hemolysis of blood in intravenous tubing caused by heat. Journal of Pediatrics 112: 111–113

Pati A R, Patton W N, Harris R I 1989 The use of the Technicon H1 in the diagnosis of hereditary spherocytosis. Clinical and Laboratory Haematology 11: 27–30

Pearson H A, Schiebler G L, Spencer R P 1971 Functional hyposplenia in cyanotic congenital heart disease. Pediatrics 48: 277–280

Pearson H A, Gallagher D, Chilcote R et al 1985 Developmental pattern of splenic dysfunction in sickle cell disorders. Paediatrics 76: 392–397

Pegels J G, Helmerhorst F M, van Leeuwen E F et al 1982 The Evans syndrome: characterization of the responsible autoantibodies. British Journal of Haematology 51: 445–450

Platt O S, Lux S E, Nathan D G 1981 Exercise induced hemolysis in xerocytosis. Erythrocyte dehydration and shear sensitivity. Journal of Clinical Investigation 68: 631–638

Popat N, Weatherall D J, Wood W G, Turnbull A C 1977 Pattern of maternal F-cell production during pregnancy. Lancet 2: 377–378

Ramsey G, Nusbacher J, Starzl T E, Lindsay G D 1984 Isohemagglutinins of graft origin after ABO-unmatched liver transplantation. New England Journal of Medicine 311: 1167–1170

Ravenel S D, Johnson J D, Sigler A T 1969 Intravascular hemolysis associated with coarctation of the aorta. Journal of Pediatrics 75: 67–73

Reeve J D 1971 Haemorrhage mimicking intravascular haemolysis. British Medical Journal 1: 654

Reinhart W H, Chien S 1985 Stomatocytic transformation of red blood cells after marathon running. American Journal of Hematology 19: 201–204

Reinhart W H, Gössi U, Bütikofer P et al 1989 Haemolytic anaemia in analpha-lipoproteinaemia (Tangier disease): morphological, biochemical, and biophysical properties of the red blood cell. British Journal of Haematology 72: 272–277

Saji H, Hosoi T 1979 A Japanese Rh_{mod} family: serological and haematological observations. Vox Sanguinis 37: 296–304

Schmid R, Schwartz S, Sundberg R D 1955 Erythropoietic (congenital) porphyria: a rare abnormality of the normoblasts. Blood 10: 416–428

Schröter W, Kahsnitz E 1983 Diagnosis of hereditary spherocytosis in newborn infants. Journal of Pediatrics 103: 460–463

Seger R, Joller P, Baerlocher K et al 1980 Hemolytic-uremic syndrome associated with neuraminidase-producing microorganisms: treatment by exchange transfusion. Helvetica Paediatrica Acta 35: 359–367

Shurin S B, Anderson P, Zollinger J, Rathbun R K 1986 Pathophysiology of hemolysis in infections with Hemophilus influenzae type b. Journal of Clinical Investigation 77: 1340–1348

Simpkins H, Kahlenberg A, Rosenberg A et al 1971 Structural and compositional changes in the red cell membrane during Clostridium welchii infection. British Journal of Haematology 21: 173–182

Sivan Y, Merlob P, Nutman J, Reisner S H 1983 Direct hyperbilirubinemia complicating ABO hemolytic disease of the newborn. Clinical Pediatrics 22: 537–538

Sokol R J, Hewitt S, Stamps B K 1982 Erythrocyte autoantibodies, autoimmune haemolysis and pregnancy. Vox Sanguinis 43: 169–176

Sokol R J, Hewitt S, Stamps B K, Hitchen P A 1984 Autoimmune haemolysis in childhood and adolescence. Acta Haematologica 72: 245–257

Spitz M, Jankovic J, Killian J M 1985 Familial tic disorder, parkinsonism, motor neurone disease, and acanthocytosis: a new syndrome. Neurology 35: 366–370

Stewart G W, Ellory J C 1985 A family with mild hereditary xerocytosis showing high membrane cation permeability at low temperatures. Clinical Science 69: 309–319

Stewart G W, O'Brien H, Morris S A et al 1987 Stomatocytosis, abnormal platelets and pseudo-homozygous hypercholesterolaemia. European Journal of Haematology 38: 376–380

Stormorken H, Sjaastad O, Langslet A et al 1985 A new syndrome:

thrombocytopathia, muscle fatigue, asplenia, miosis, migraine, dyslexia and ichthyosis. Clinical Genetics 28: 367–374
Streichman S, Gesheidt Y, Tatarsky I 1990 Hypertonic cryohemolysis: a diagnostic test for hereditary spherocytosis. American Journal of Hematology 35: 104–109
Torlontano G, Fioritoni G, Salvati A M 1979 Hereditary haemolytic ovalocytosis with defective erythropoiesis. British Journal of Haematology 43: 435–441
Upshaw J D 1978 Congenital deficiency of a factor in normal plasma that reverses microangiopathic hemolysis and thrombocytopenia. New England Journal of Medicine 298: 1350–1352
Vance J M, Pericak-Vance M A, Bowman M H et al 1987 Chorea-acanthocytosis: a report of three new families and implications for genetic counselling. American Journal of Medical Genetics 28: 403–410
Wada H, Kanzaki A, Ata K et al 1990 A new band 3 variant with increased hemolysis, decreased anion transport, glycophorin A anomaly and abnormal rheology. Blood 76 (suppl I): 20a
Wardrop C, Hutchison H E 1969 Red-cell shape in hypothyroidism. Lancet 2: 1243
Wheeler D E, Pettigrew B 1986 A simplified approach to the detection and assessment of intravascular haemolysis following prosthetic cardiac valve implantation. Australian Journal of Medical Laboratory Science 7: 48–50
Wiley J S 1970 Red cell survival studies in hereditary spherocytosis.Journal of Clinical Investigation 49: 666–672
Wiley J S 1984 Inherited red cell dehydration: a hemolytic syndrome in search of a name. Pathology 16: 115 116
Wiley J S, Cooper R A, Adachi K, Asakura T 1979 Hereditary stomatocytosis: association of low 2,3-diphosphoglycerate with increased cation pumping by the red cell. British Journal of Haematology 41: 133–141
Willis C, Foreman C S 1988 Chronic massive fetomaternal haemorrhage: a case report. Obstetrics and Gynecology 71: 459–461
Zipursky A, Brown E J, Watts J et al 1987 Oral vitamin E supplementation for the prevention of anemia in premature infants: a controlled trial. Pediatrics 79: 61–68

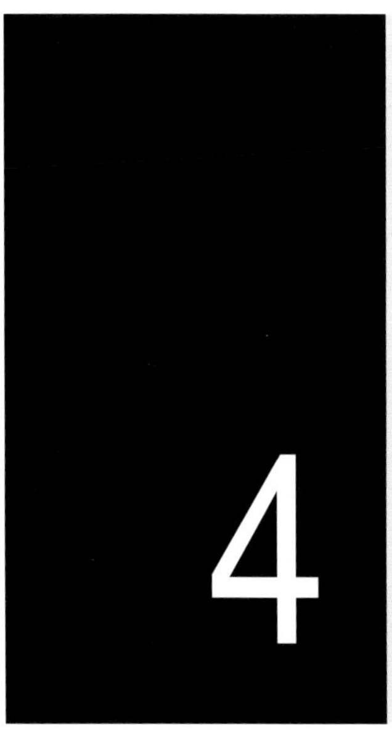

4 Lymphocytic leukaemias

ALL is the commonest malignancy of childhood. An expanding variety of procedures is revealing an increasing heterogeneity, to the point of individuality.

Abbreviations and notes

AcPh: acid phosphatase; ALL: acute lymphoblastic leukaemia; AML: acute myeloid leukaemia; ANAE: α naphthyl acetate esterase; ANBE: α naphthyl butyrate esterase; c: cytoplasmic; CAE: chloroacetate esterase; CSF: cerebrospinal fluid; H: heavy chain; Ig: immunoglobulin; H & E: haematoxylin and eosin; MPO: myeloperoxidase; ORO: oil red O; PAS: periodic acid-Schiff; SBB: sudan black B; TCR: T-cell antigen receptor; TdT: terminal deoxynucleotidyl transferase.

Magnifications: × 750 unless otherwise stated.
Karyotypes: for complex karyotypes, only the alteration deemed the most significant is given.

Acute lymphoblastic leukaemia 114
Essential for diagnosis 114
Marrow infiltration 114
Cell morphology 114
Myeloperoxidase 114
Immunophenotype 116
Other characteristics of the leukaemic cells 118
Morphology 118
Cytochemistry 124
Cytogenetics 126
Gene rearrangements 128
Morphology of infiltrated marrows 128
Necrosis 128
Myelofibrosis 130
Apoptosis 130
Abnormal macrophages 132
Necrobiotic multinucleate cells 132
Blood 132
Lymphoblastosis 132
Eosinophilia 132
Erythrocytes 132
Haemostasis 132
Prodromes for ALL 134
Cytopenias 134
Other 134
Relapse, residual disease 134
Differential diagnosis of leukaemic lymphoblastosis 136
Benign lymphoblastosis 136
Non-lymphocytic leukaemias 136
Non-haemopoietic malignancies 138
Non-Hodgkin lymphoma 138
Hodgkin's disease 140
Chronic lymphocytic leukaemia 140

Acute lymphoblastic leukaemia

ESSENTIAL FOR DIAGNOSIS

Marrow infiltration

At diagnosis, infiltration with lymphoblasts is gross (Fig. 4.1), usually ≥ 60% (up to 100%, normal < 3%). Lesser infiltration should raise suspicion of other conditions (see differential diagnosis, p. 136). Sampling from one site is sufficient because the disease is diffuse at this stage. At relapse, lesser degrees of infiltration are common and sampling from at least 2 sites may be needed.

Cell morphology

Important characteristics (Fig. 4.1) are immaturity, lymphoid appearance, small to medium size and absence of evidence of myeloid differentiation (myeloid granulation, Auer rods).

In cytospin preparations (Fig. 4.2) nuclear distortion (clover-leaf shapes, budding) is common. On occasion, assessment by morphology alone is inconclusive, confident diagnosis requiring cytochemistry, monoclonal antibodies and, if the count is high, immunophenotyping (Fig. 4.2). Meningeal disease may be asymptomatic and leukaemic cells may be evident in CSF whose cell count is normal.

Myeloperoxidase

MPO activity in < 3% of blast cells is essential. This figure is accepted as the upper limit for immature myeloid cells which might survive in ALL marrows, and which might be confused with leukaemic lymphoblasts. Ultrastructural methods and monoclonal antibodies are more sensitive for detection of MPO than standard cytochemistry.

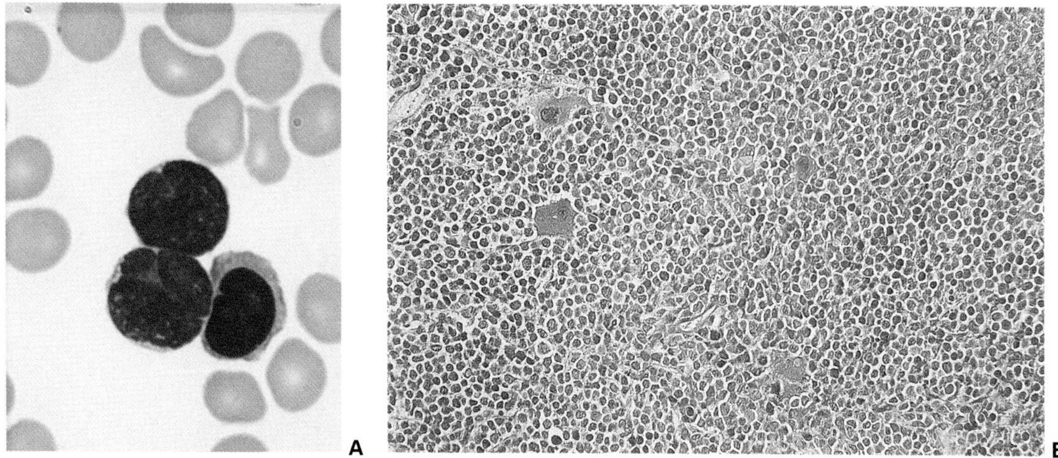

Fig. 4.1 ALL. **a** 2 leukaemic lymphoblasts vs normal lymphocyte. **b** Trephine biopsy, showing almost complete replacement by lymphoblasts; residual megakaryocytes. **a** × 1200; **b** × 200

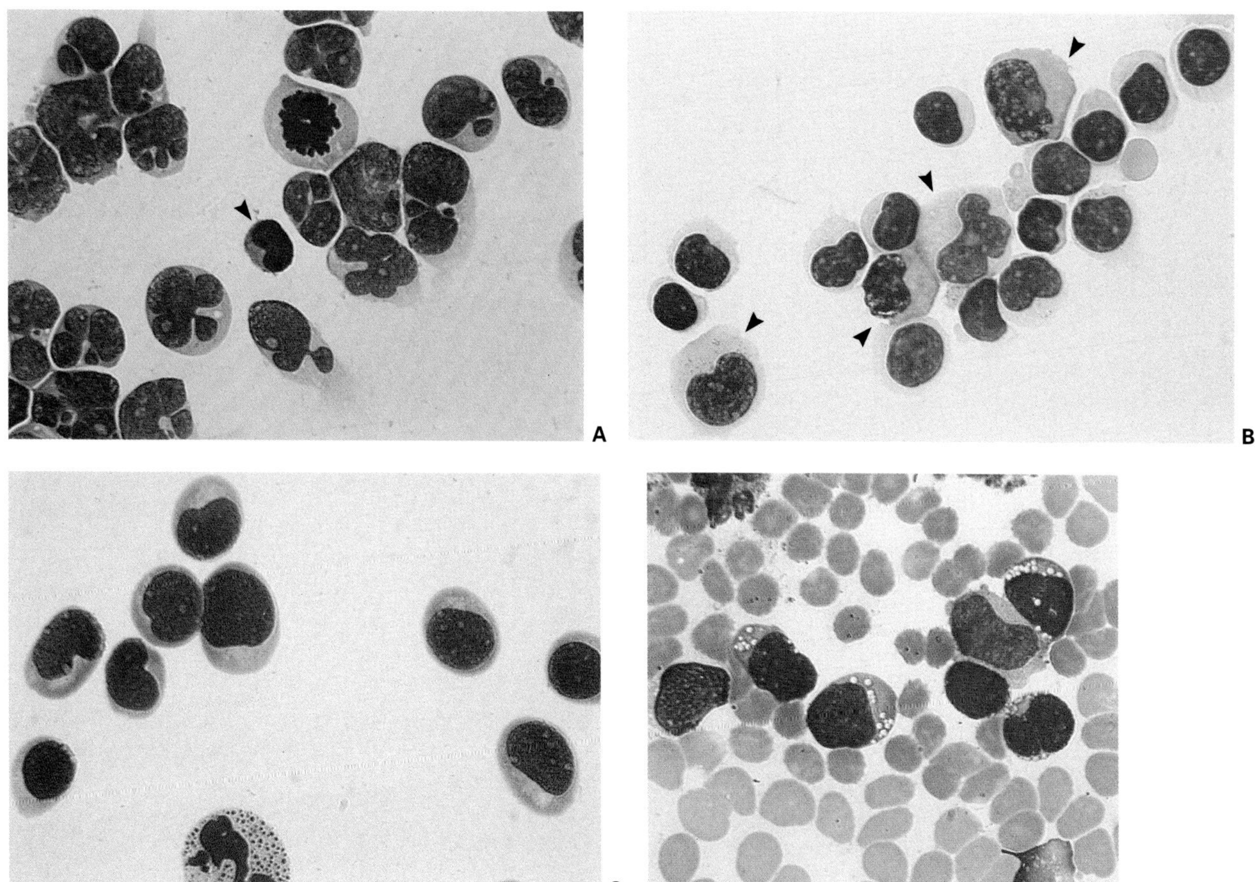

Fig. 4.2 Cytospins of CSF in ALL. **a** Lymphoblasts and (arrow) normal lymphocyte. **b** In remission, showing normal and (arrows) reactive lymphocytes. **c** A 'problem' CSF in treated T lymphoma. Interpretation was uncertain because of differences from the (L3-like) marrow lymphoblasts (**d**) in morphology and cytochemistry (CSF cells AcPh negative, marrow cells positive). Immunophenotyping of CSF was possible because of high count (370/mm^3) and showed T markers.

Table 4.1 Major immunologic types of childhood ALL

	CD34	CD19	CD10	CD20	cμ[1]	sIg	T markers[2]	Approx frequency %
Early precursor B	+	+/–	–	–	–	–	–	5
Common	+	+	+	+	–	–	–	55–60
Pre-B	–	+	+/–	+	+	–	–	10–15
B	–	+	+/–	+	–	+	–	<5
T	+/–	–	–	–	–	–	+	15

[1] c = cytoplasmic
[2] e.g. CD1,2,3,4,5,8

Immunophenotype (Ludwig et al 1994)

This is essential for:

- Excluding lineages which may have lymphoid appearance, e.g. AML M0, blastic M6 AML, AML M7.

ALL is an expansion of a population corresponding, in most cases at least, to a discrete point in normal cell maturation (Fig. 4.3). Major types of ALL are summarized in Table 4.1. However, additional heterogeneity occurs; early and late antigens may, for example, be expressed together (asynchrony), e.g. in B lineage ALL, CD34 (early) with CD20 (late).

Immunophenotype per se is not diagnostic of ALL, as substantial expansions of populations with, for example, common markers may occur in marrow from children with no evidence of malignancy (Sandhaus et al 1993).

- Recognition of mixtures of populations of more than one lineage (Fig. 4.4). Only rarely can this be suspected from morphology.

Identification of mixed lineage is acceptable if, for each lineage, a score of ≥ 2 points is obtained in a scale which weights characteristics according to their value for specific lineage recognition (Table 4.2). A lower score in possible lineage admixture may even be a normal phenomenon.

Co-occurrence of features of two lineages occurs most commonly within the same cell (biphenotypic leukaemia). Co-occurrence of two different populations (bilineage leukaemia) appears to be rare. Lineages which may manifest together are lymphoid (B or T) with myeloid (Fig. 4.4), less often B with T lymphoid. On the criteria in Table 4.2 the incidence of ALL with myeloid admixture is approximately 3% (Catovsky et al 1991). Some karyotypes such as t(11;19) may be over-represented in these cases.

Table 4.2 Scoring system for lineage specificity in diagnosis of biphenotypic/bilineage ALL[1]

Points	B lineage	T lineage	Myeloid lineage
2	cyto CD22 cyto μ chain	cyto CD3	MPO (any method) Auer rods
1	CD10 CD19 CD24	CD2 CD5 TCR gene rearrangement, β or δ chain	CD33 CD13, surface or cyto CD14, surface or cyto other AML type cytochemistry[2]
0.5	TdT IgH gene rearrangement	TdT CD7	CD11b CD11c CD15

[1] Adapted from Catovsky et al 1991. A score at ≥ 2 points is taken as evidence of lineage specificity
[2] Myeloid type ANAE, fluoride sensitive, and/or positive SBB

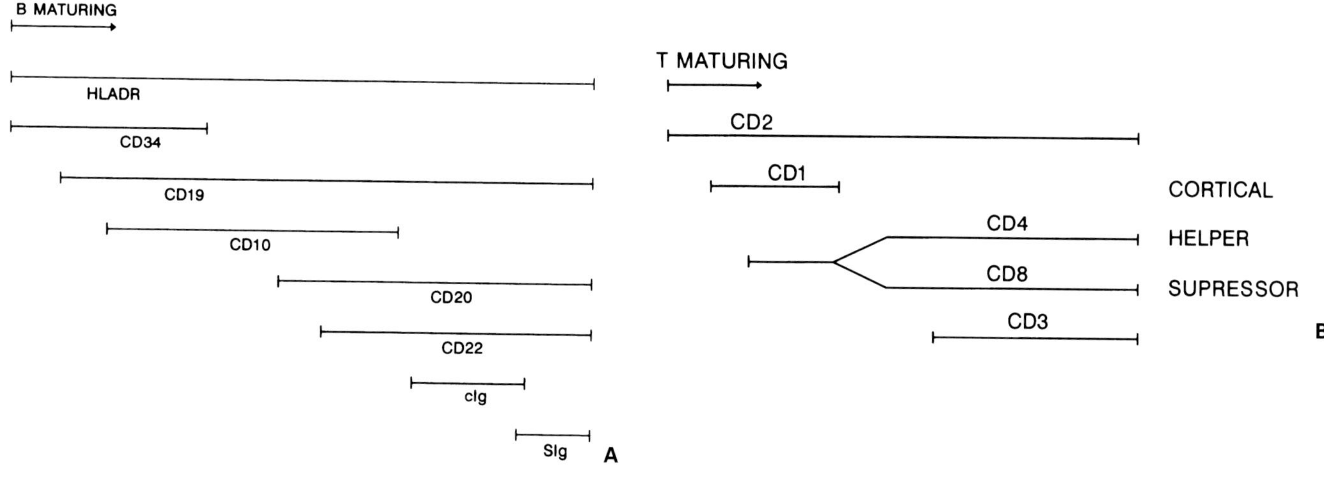

Fig. 4.3 Sequence of antigen expression during maturation of **a**, B cells and **b**, T cells.

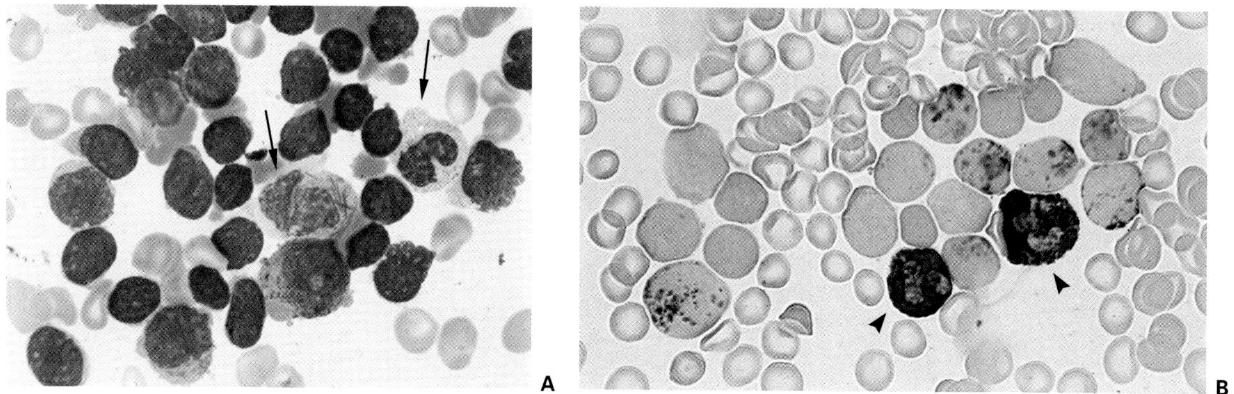

Fig. 4.4 Bilineage ALL. **a** Pelgerized neutrophil and neutrophil containing Auer rods (arrows) lie among lymphoblasts; the presence of a minor granulocyte population was not revealed by immunophenotyping. Disseminated intravascular coagulation was associated (rare in pure ALL). The child, aged 11 at diagnosis, remains in continuous remission 6 years later. **b** SBB-positive ALL; arrows show granulocytes. Positive SBB and CD13 were taken as evidence of myeloid presence. This was a relapse 28 months after first presentation, when CD13 was negative (i.e. lineage switch at relapse); karyotype del 9p on both occasions.

OTHER CHARACTERISTICS OF THE LEUKAEMIC CELLS

Morphology

FAB types (Bain 1990)

The three FAB categories (Fig. 4.5) for Romanowsky-stained films of marrow aspirates are:

- L1: fairly uniform population of small cells; nuclei of regular outline, nucleoli inconspicuous; cytoplasm scanty and moderately basophilic; vacuolation variable.
- L2: population not as homogeneous as L1 or L3; cell size variable with preponderance of large cells; majority have irregular nuclei, conspicuous nucleoli and moderate amount of cytoplasm; cytoplasmic basophilia variable but less intense than in L3; vacuolation variable.
- L3 (Burkitt-like): homogeneous population of medium-sized to large cells, cytoplasm strongly basophilic, usually vacuolated; nuclei regular in outline, nucleoli usually prominent (1 or more); cytoplasm moderate in amount, often completely surrounding nucleus; mitoses usually frequent.

L3 is the most consistently identifiable. The distinction between L1 and L2 has evolved from the semiquantitative assessment of whole populations to identification of individual cells as L1 or L2 (Table 4.3), with a marrow identified as L2 if it contains ≥ 10% L2 cells and L1 if this figure is < 10%. L1 morphology has traditionally been associated with better prognosis than L2, nucleolar frequency and nuclear/cytoplasmic ratio determining the association rather than nuclear contour and cell size (Lilleyman et al 1986). The distinction between L1 and L2 is tending to diminish in importance as more intensive treatments improve survival.

There are no specific associations between FAB type and immunophenotype except between L3 and B phenotype. However, L3 or L3-like morphology may on occasion be associated with common or T markers (Fig. 4.2), while L1 and L2 ALL may occasionally have B markers.

The 'hand-mirror' variant (Schumacher et al 1989) is an uncommon curiosity in which most of the leukaemic cells are elongated into a 'uropod' (Fig. 4.5). The direction of elongation is random (artefactual elongation tends to point in the same direction). There are no specific associations with other characteristics such as FAB morphology and immunophenotype.

Atypical morphology may be a predictor of unsatisfactory response to treatment (Fig. 4.5).

Table 4.3 Identification of L1 and L2 ALL cells on Children's Cancer Study Group criteria[1]

L1 features	Score	L2 features	Score
High N/C ratio[2]	+1	Low N/C ratio[2]	–1
Small inconspicuous nucleoli	+1	Conspicuous nucleoli	–1
Regular nuclear outline	0	Convoluted/clefted nuclear contour	–1
Small size[3]	0	Large size[3]	–1

Total score: 0 to 2+ = L1 cell
–1 to –4 = L2 cell

[1] Miller et al 1985

[2] High N/C (nuclear/cytoplasmic) ratio = cytoplasm < 20% of cell area; low ratio = cytoplasm > 20% of area

[3] Small = < 2 × diameter of small lymphocyte; large = > 2 × diameter

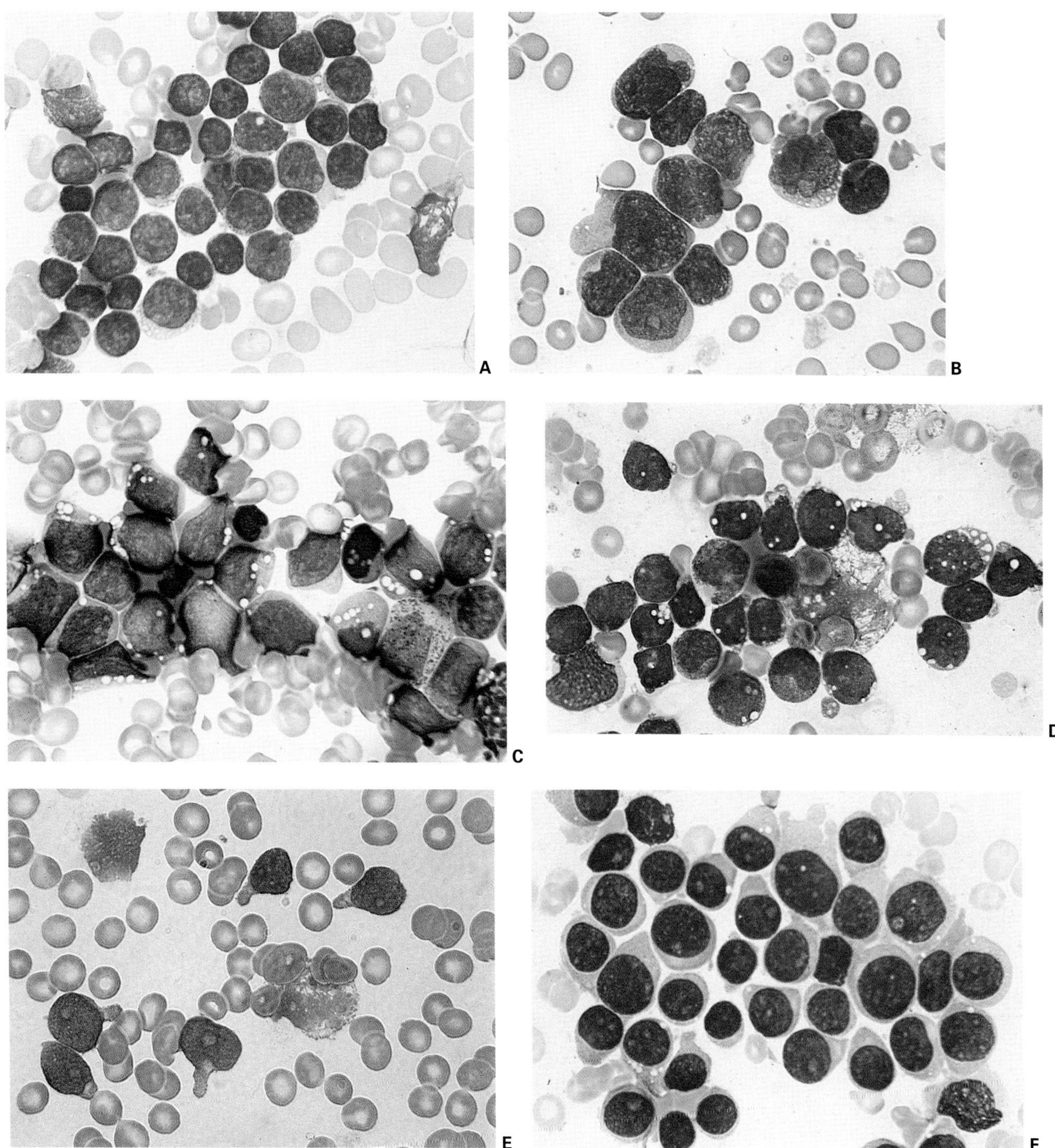

Fig. 4.5 Morphologic types of ALL. **a** L1. **b** L2. **c** L3. **d** Vacuolated L1. **e** 'Hand-mirror', markers common. **f** Atypical morphology (pre-B), poorly responsive to treatment. **b** Courtesy of Dr G Tauro

Cytoplasmic inclusions

- Azurophil granules

The presence of some azurophil granules in the cytoplasm of blast cells is not uncommon, but as an easily discernible feature is infrequent — 7% of cases had > 5% granular blast cells in one series (Darbyshire & Lilleyman 1987). Some of these cases show strong punctate AcPh, ANAE and PAS reactions. Electron microscopy in a personal case showed only granules of unremarkable structure (Fig. 4.6). There is no known relation to prognosis.

An unusual azurophil-like granulation of distinctive ultrastructure is shown in Figure 4.6.

- Vacuoles

Vacuoles in leukaemic lymphoblasts are deposits of neutral fat (Fig. 4.11) or of glycogen (Fig. 4.10) or lysosomes. They occur most consistently in L3 B ALL. In ALL, excluding the SIg positive, vacuolation (> 10% of cells) is associated with PAS positivity, a leucocyte count at diagnosis of $< 50 \times 10^9/l$, common (CD10 positive) phenotype and a favourable prognosis (Lilleyman et al 1988).

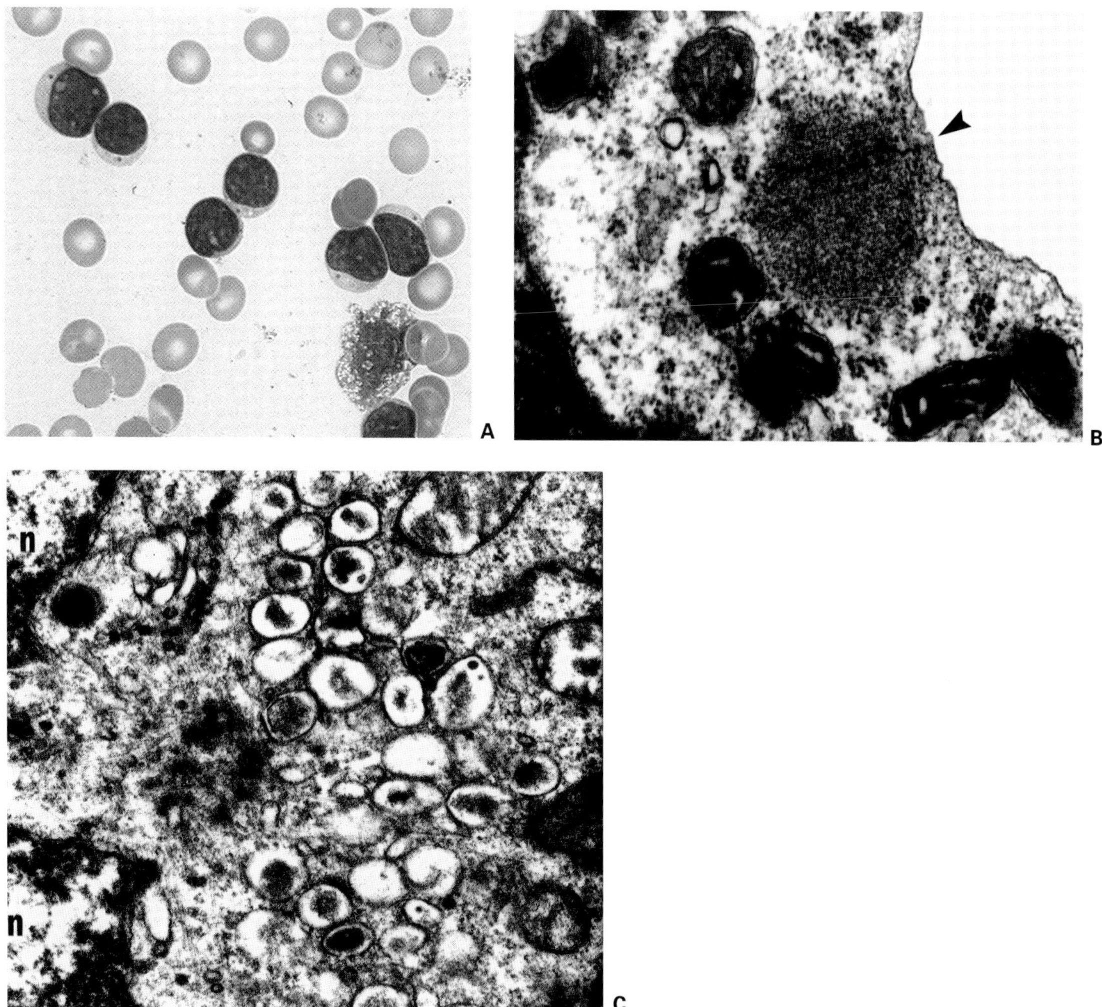

Fig. 4.6 Granulated ALL. **a,b** T ALL. 28% of lymphoblasts contained a single granule (shown in 5 cells in **a**). The granules (**b**, arrow) were of coarse amorphous structure and not membrane-bound. **c** Common markers. Unremarkable membrane-bound granulation. Fine azurophil granulation in 27% of lymphoblasts by light microscopy. n = nucleus. **b** × 45 000; **c** ×30 000. **b** Reproduced with permission from: Smith H, Collins R J 1990 Acute lymphoblastic leukaemia with cytoplasmic granules or inclusions. British Journal of Haematology 75: 440. Copyright, Blackwell Scientific Publications

• Altered chromatin

Altered heterochromatin can be identified in cytoplasm by electron microscopy and is derived from degenerate areas in the cell nucleus (Smith et al 1986, Fig. 4.7). Altered chromatin may be an indication of gene deletion.

• Collections of virus-like particles

Collections of virus-like particles may be seen by light microscopy in lymphoblasts of about 40% of children with ALL (usually rare, in some cases up to about 10% of cells). They have distinctive morphology and staining and appear to be specific for ALL. A proportion stain with PAS. The particles are 40–100 nm in size and show eccentric thickening (vesicles in normal structures such as multivesicular bodies do not show thickening). There is some evidence that the particles are viral (Fig. 4.8, Smith 1978, Smith et al 1986, 1991).

• Other

Cells or cellular material may occasionally be phagocytosed (Fig. 4.8). Other types of inclusion may be noted (Brunning et al 1974).

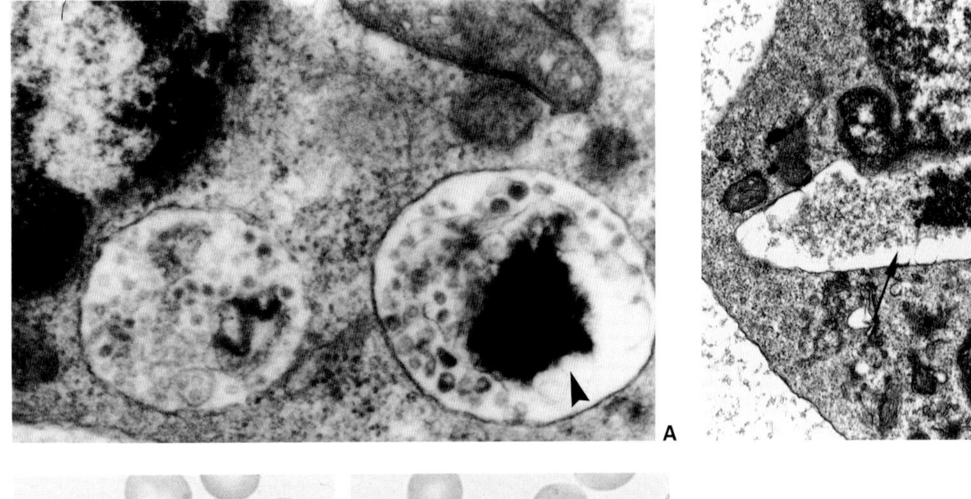

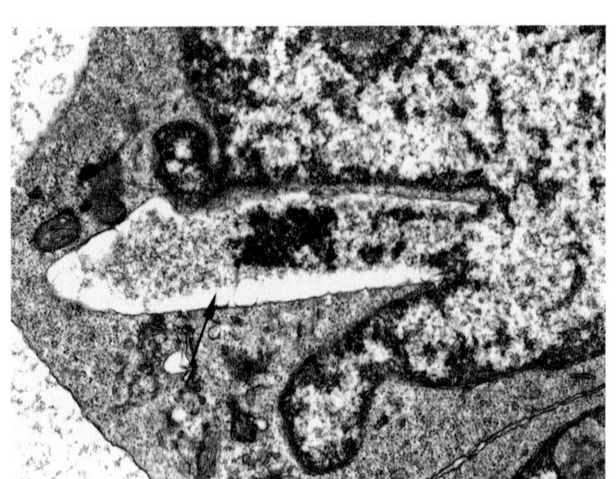

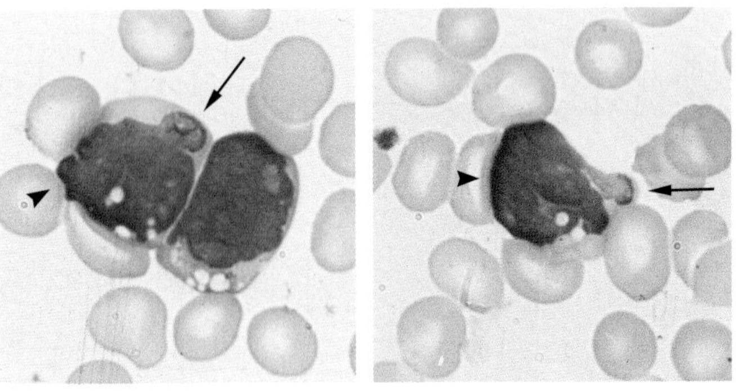

Fig. 4.7 Altered chromatin in leukaemic lymphoblasts. **a** Altered chromatin (arrow) with virus-like particles in membrane enclosure. **b** In situ degeneration of part of nucleus (arrow). **c** Cap at rim of nucleus (arrows) interpreted as damaged chromatin; cf artefactual thickening from compression by neighbouring cells (arrowheads). **a** × 48 000; **b** × 15 000; **c** × 1200. **a** Reproduced with permission from British Journal of Experimental Pathology 1986, 67: 551. Copyright, Blackwell Scientific Publications

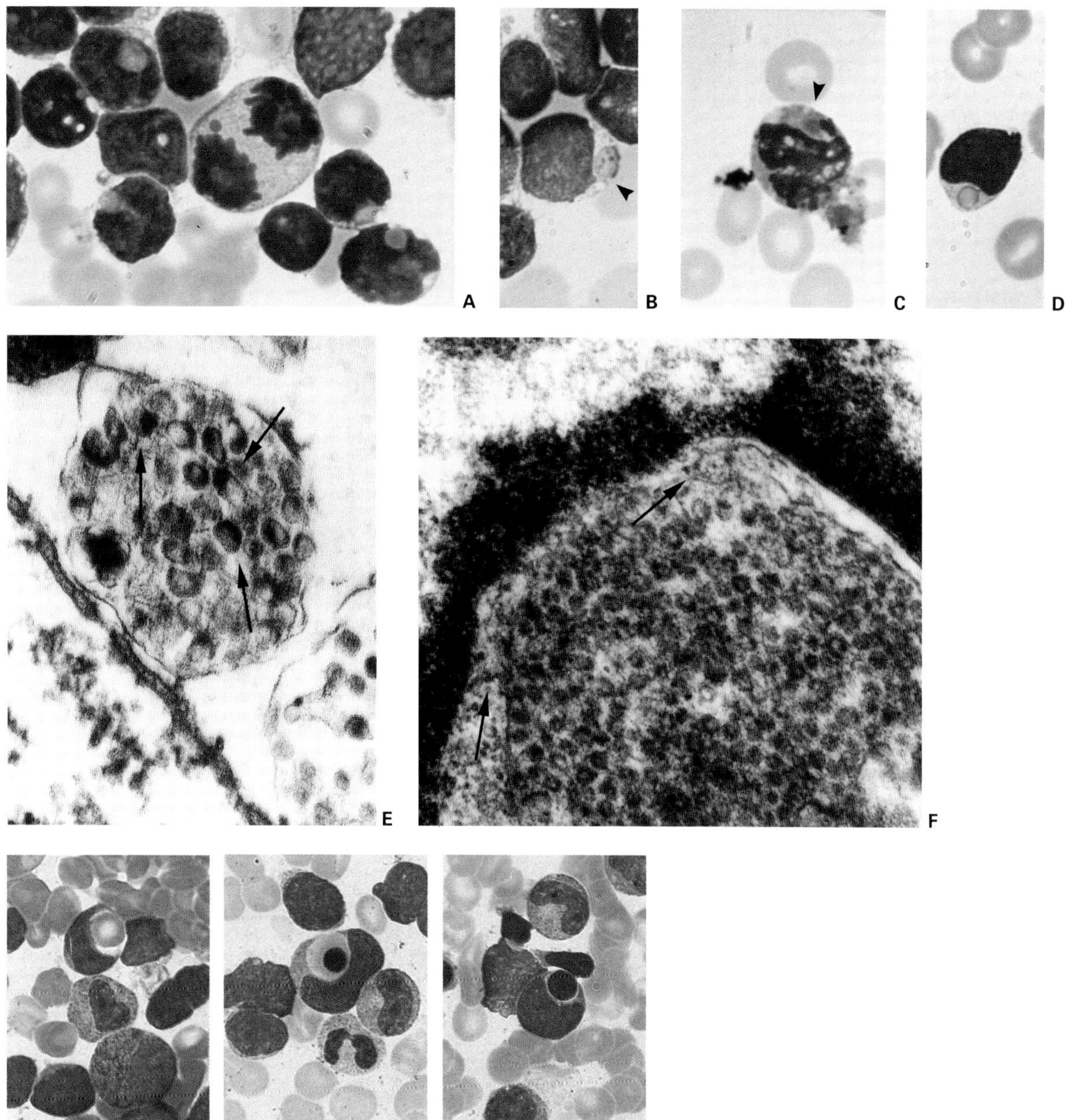

Fig. 4.8 Inclusions in leukaemic lymphoblasts. **a–f** Collections of virus-like particles, **g** corpuscular elements. **a** Inclusions in 5 lymphoblasts, in the cell in mitosis attached by a stalk to one nucleus. Inclusion in dead cell in **c** (arrow), and attached to nucleus by stalk in **d**. **e** Particles, showing eccentric thickening (arrows). **f** Confluence of particle collection with nucleus; arrows show continuity of outer nuclear membrane with membrane enclosing particle collection. **g** Inclusions of erythrocyte, erythroblast, unidentified nucleated cell (from same child with T ALL). **a–d** × 1200; **e** × 80 000; **f** × 48 000; **g** × 750. **e** Reproduced with permission from Pathology 1990, 23: 207. Copyright, Modern Medicine. **f** Reproduced with permission from Leukemia Research 1978, 2: 135. Copyright, Pergamon Press Ltd

Intranuclear demarcations

These are visible only by electron microscopy (Fig. 4.9) and, as a fetal characteristic (Smith et al 1982), suggest that childhood ALL has fetal origins.

Other evidence for fetal origins of childhood malignancy includes the following:

- the fact that malignancies may be clinically manifest at birth
- associations between malignancies in childhood and fetal exposures (radiation, chemicals/drugs, viruses) in amounts which suggest that the fetus is unusually sensitive (Rice 1988, Preston-Martin 1989)
- the kinetics of ALL, which suggest an origin from a single cell at or before birth (Mauer et al 1973)
- the apparent identity of leukaemias in identical twins (cytology, karyotype, gene rearrangements), which, together with a high rate of concordance, suggest, as one explanation, origin in one fetus and metastasis to the other via the common placenta (Chaganti et al 1979, Pombo de Oliveira et al 1986).

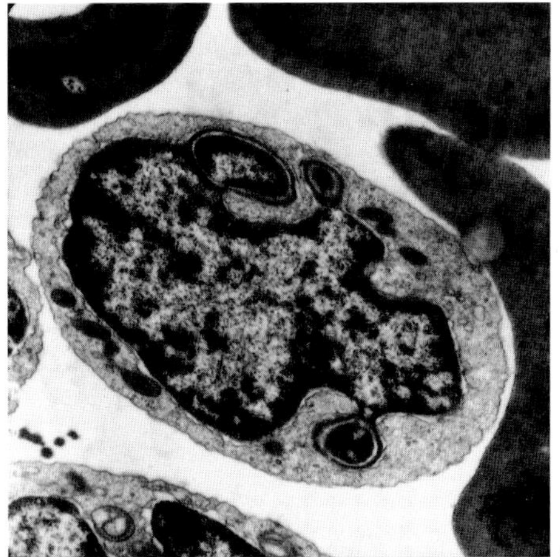

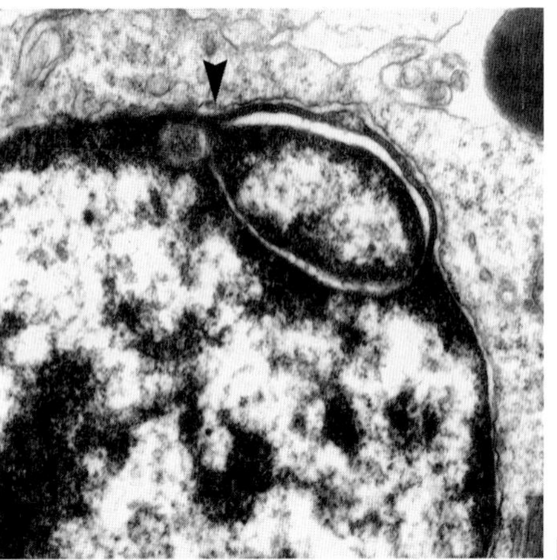

Fig. 4.9 Intranuclear demarcations in leukaemic lymphoblasts (T ALL). **a** 3 demarcations at periphery of nucleus. **b** Demarcated portion connected to main nucleus by stalk (arrow, probably all demarcated areas are so connected). **a** × 8000; **b** × 20 000. **b** Reproduced with permission from Leukemia Research 1982, 6: 677. Copyright, Pergamon Press Ltd

Cytochemistry

Though not specific, cytochemistry is an important support for diagnosis.

- MPO

See above.

- SBB

Positivity in < 3% of blasts is, like MPO, compatible with a diagnosis of ALL. However, occasional cases of genuine ALL or biphenotypic ALL show positive reaction in > 3% of cells (Fig. 4.4). SBB positivity is regarded as evidence of myeloid differentiation (Table 4.2). In most if not all of these cases the lymphocyte markers are early precursor B or common. In some cases azurophil granulation is obvious in Romanowsky-stained films ('granulated' ALL, p. 120).

- PAS

Glycogen stains as granules, blocks, or occasionally 'lakes' against a clear background (Fig. 4.10). Reaction is positive in about 80% of B-lineage ALL (excluding SIg-positive), though the proportion of positive cells varies from patient to patient. Reaction is of lower intensity in T ALL but the difference from B lineage is of limited value as a guide to phenotype. Reaction is absent in most cases of SIg-positive B ALL. Glycogen is to be distinguished from the less intensely staining, larger, rounded inclusions of virus-like particles (p. 122).

- ANAE

In most cases the reaction is negative. In some cases of B-lineage ALL a proportion of cells contain scattered granules or patches (Fig. 4.10, compare the more intense, diffuse and granular pattern in monocytes, Fig. 5.11). Strong scattered granulation may be noted in granular ALL. Occasional cases of T ALL show strong dot positivity (Fig. 4.10) or focal aggregates like the AcPh. ANAE reaction in ALL is variably inhibited by fluoride (inhibited in monocytes).

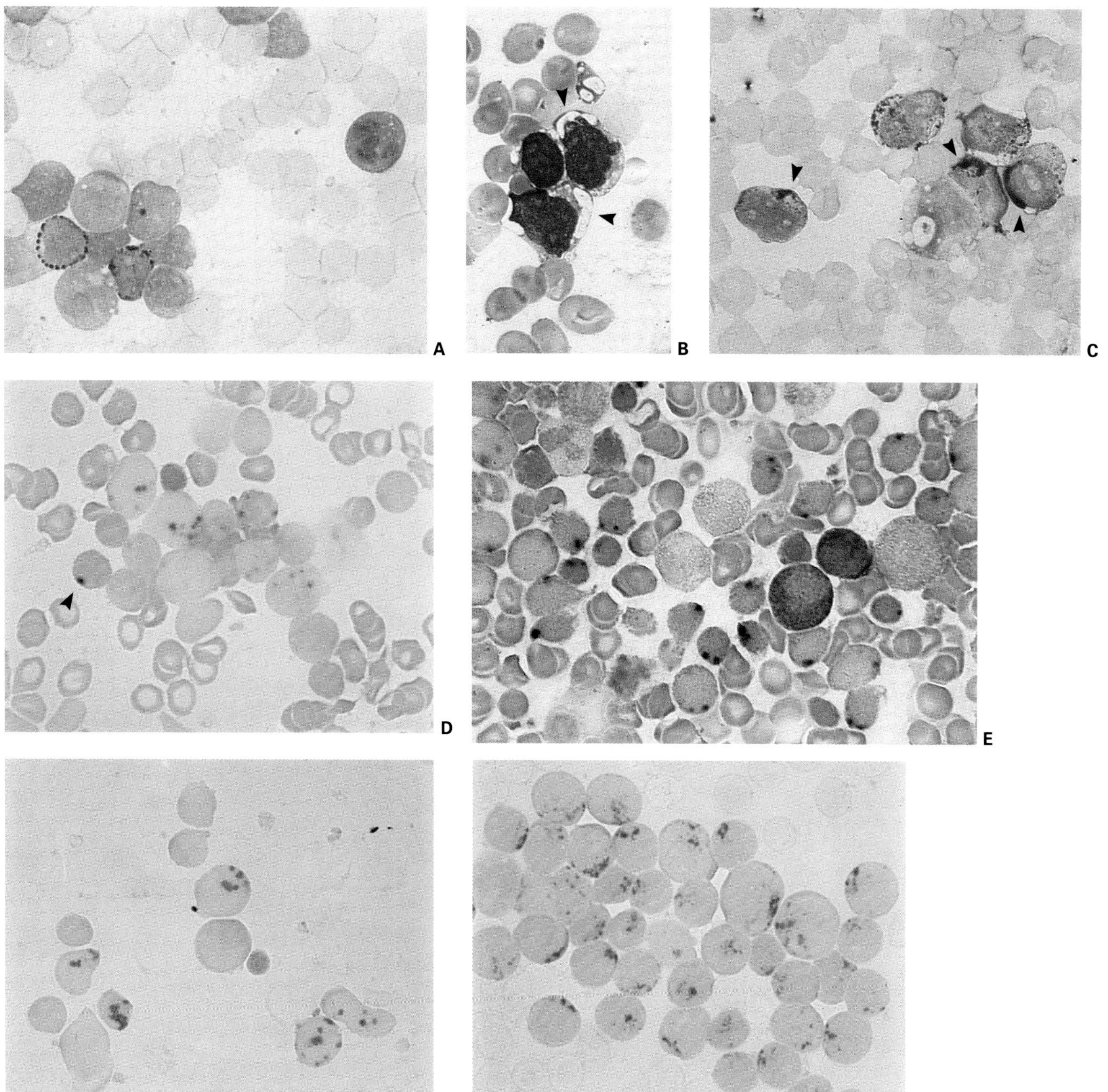

Fig. 4.10 Cytochemistry in ALL. **a** PAS, showing typical spotty pattern (cf neutrophil). **b,c** Romanowsky and PAS, showing lakes (arrows), 11-day-old infant, deletion 6q. **d** ANAE, common ALL, showing scattered granulation; arrow shows normal lymphocyte with strong, single dot. **e** ANAE, T ALL, strong dot positivity in lymphoblasts (fluoride resistant); cf diffuse reaction in 2 granulocytes (fluoride sensitive). **f** AcPh, common ALL, showing scattered granulation. **g** AcPh, T ALL, more focal aggregation.

- ANBE

Reactions tend to be stronger than for ANAE. Typical reactions are: single dense dot in T ALL, negative in SIg-positive ALL and scattered granulation in other types. Activity is not inhibited by fluoride.

- AcPh

Most cases of T ALL are positive, with activity in the majority of cells, and strong and predominantly paranuclear (Golgi zone, Fig. 4.10). In about 20%, activity is scattered granular or negative. Most cases of non-T ALL are negative; if positive, activity appears as scattered granules or patches (Fig. 4.10), or occasionally as 'T' type pattern. Activity is inhibited by tartrate.

- β glucuronidase

Most cases of non-T ALL show a spotty pattern (Fig. 4.11); a minority are negative. In T ALL the reaction is negative or (in a minority) tends to paranuclear location, like the AcPh.

- ORO

Though most consistent in ALL L3, ORO-positive vacuoles (neutral fat) are not infrequent in vacuolated ALL of other types.

- CAE

A positive CAE is rare in ALL (Keifer et al 1985).

Cytogenetics (Raimondi 1993)

Acquired abnormalities of karyotype are a confirmation of malignancy as well as an indication of heterogeneity. Associations are established of karyotype with immunophenotype (Tables 4.4, 4.5) and with prognosis; for example: hyperdiploidy and good prognosis; translocations, especially (9;22), (4;11), (8;14), and poor prognosis.

Abnormalities which appear by conventional cytogenetics to be positioned at the same band can often be shown by PCR to be heterogeneous, for example in up to half of cases of Ph-positive ALL the t(9;22) is that of adult CML.

Table 4.4 ALL cytogenetics: change in number[1]

	% of ALL overall	Structural abnormalities	Associations
Hyperdiploid 51–65	25–30	62%	early pre-B, age 2–10 yr
Hyperdiploid 47–50	10–15	76%	precursor B
Pseudodiploid	40	all[2]	see Table 4.5
Diploid	10–15	0[2]	diploidy in up to 30% T ALL
Hypodiploid	7–8	most	

[1] Adapted from Raimondi 1993
[2] By definition

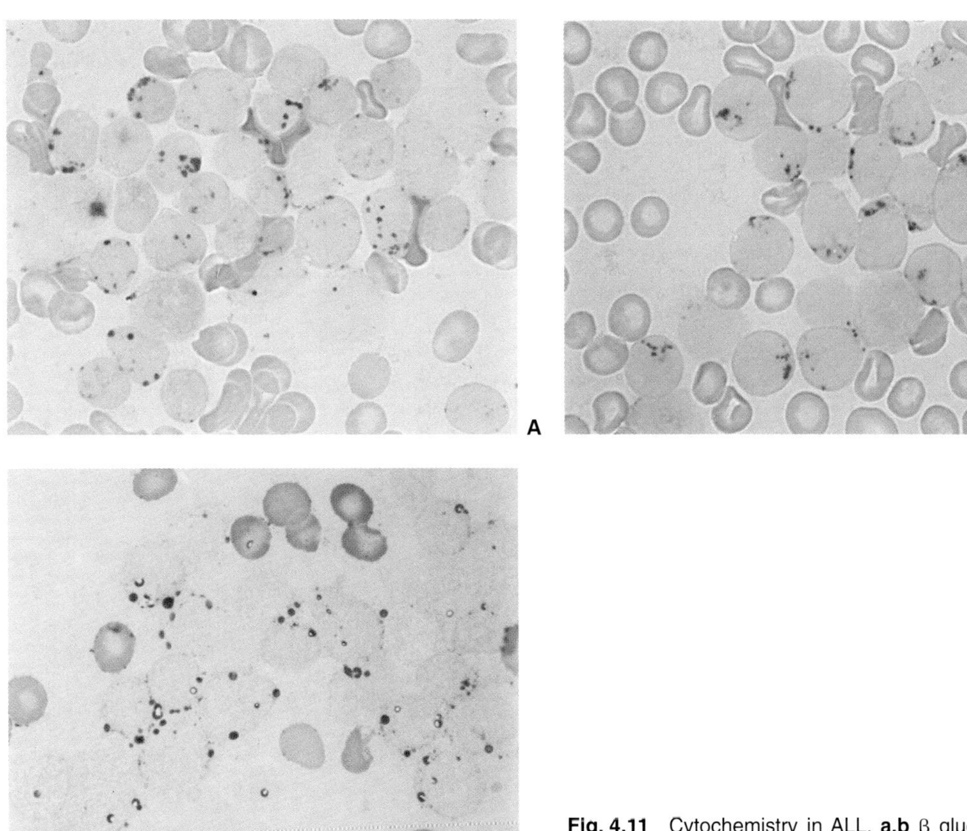

Fig. 4.11 Cytochemistry in ALL. **a,b** β glucuronidase. **a** Common ALL, scattered granulation. **b** T ALL, more focal aggregation. **c** ORO-positive deposits, vacuolated L1 ALL.

Table 4.5 ALL karyotype: more common structural alterations[1]

	% of ALL overall	Predominant immunophenotype associated	Gene loci involved
t(8;14)(q24;q32)	3	B	8q24 CMYC proto-oncogene; 14q32 Igμ
t(2;8)(p12;q24)	< 1	B	2p12 Igκ
t(8;22)(q24;q11)	< 1	B	22q11 Igλ
t(1;19)(q23;p13)	5–6	pre-B	1q23 PBX 1; 19p13 E2A Ig-binding enhancer
t(9;22)(q34;q11) (Ph)[2]	2–5	early pre-B	9q34 ABL proto-oncogene; 22q11 BCR
t(4;11)(q21;q23)	2	early pre-B, infantile (< 1 yr), mixed lymphoid/myeloid/monocytic, hyperleucocytosis	11q23 THY1, NCAM, parts of TCR; ETS 1 and CBL 2 proto-oncogenes; MLL gene
Abnormal 11q23	4.5–6	1. early pre-B 2. secondary myeloid leukaemia post treated ALL	above
t(5;14)(q31;q32)	rare	eosinophilia	5q31 interleukin-3; 14q32 Igμ
t(11;14)(p13;q11)	1	T (7% of T)	14q11 TCR α/δ
t(10;14)(q24;q11)	1	T (5–10% of T)	
t(8;14)(q24;q11)	< 1	T (2% of T)	8q24 CMYC proto-oncogene
Abnormality of: 14q11, 7q34–36, 7p15	5	T (30–40% of T)	7q34–36 TCRβ; 7p15 TCRγ
del(6q)	4–13	non-specific	
t/del(9p)	7–12	non-specific	interferon α and β genes
t/del(12p)	10–12	non-specific	

MLL = mixed lineage leukaemia; TCR = T cell receptor
[1] Adapted from Raimondi 1993
[2] The ALL-type Ph disappears in remission (but is detectable by PCR); the adult CML-type Ph persists

A normal karyotype may be due to failure to induct leukaemic cells into mitosis or (less often) to true normality. Excess or deficit of DNA may be demonstrated (if ≥ 5%) by cell sorting, using propidium iodide as DNA binder (Fig. 4.12). Fluorescent in situ hybridization also may detect cytogenetic abnormality not revealed by conventional analysis (Le Beau 1993). Karyotype abnormalities disappear in morphologic remission, except for adult CML-type Ph.

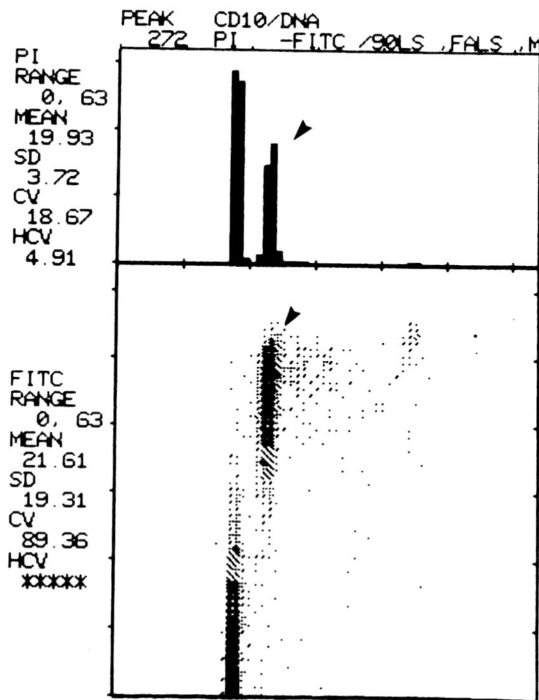

Fig. 4.12 Abnormal DNA content by cell sorting (propidium iodide) in ALL with normal conventional cytogenetics. **a** Population with DNA content 1.3 × normal (arrow). **b** (Immunophenotyped for CD10): the hyperdiploid but not the normal population CD10 positive.

Gene rearrangements (Hurwitz & Mirro 1990)

Examination for gene rearrangements is not routine in the diagnostic work-up for ALL and does not at present add significantly to the diagnostic information obtained from other investigations. Ig gene rearrangements are not specific for B-lineage ALL — about 20% of T-cell malignancies contain rearranged IgH genes (more frequent in leukaemia than lymphoma). These rearrangements occur also in about 11% of cases of AML.

TCR β chain rearrangements occur in 29%, and γ chain rearrangements in 56% of B-lineage ALL (again, more frequent in leukaemia than lymphoma). TCR rearrangements are infrequent (about 5%) in AML.

MORPHOLOGY OF LYMPHOBLAST-INFILTRATED MARROWS

Marrow necrosis (Fig. 4.13)

Necrosis is uncommon (about 1%) in ALL, and may be seen in marrow from only one site, or from all of several sites. It may occur at presentation, or precede overt blastosis by several months, or occur during chemotherapy.

In gross appearance the marrow resembles red soup or pus, and consists of amorphous, pink- or grey-staining material containing cell ghosts and pyknotic nuclei and, often, free-lying Charcot-Leyden crystals (Fig. 4.13). In some cases attempts at aspiration result in a dry tap. Necrosis may be patchy within one trephine biopsy. If well-preserved marrow cannot be obtained, diagnosis and assessment of treatment have to depend on blood findings alone. Necrosis is usually associated with pancytopenia or neutropenia, but not necessarily with poor prognosis.

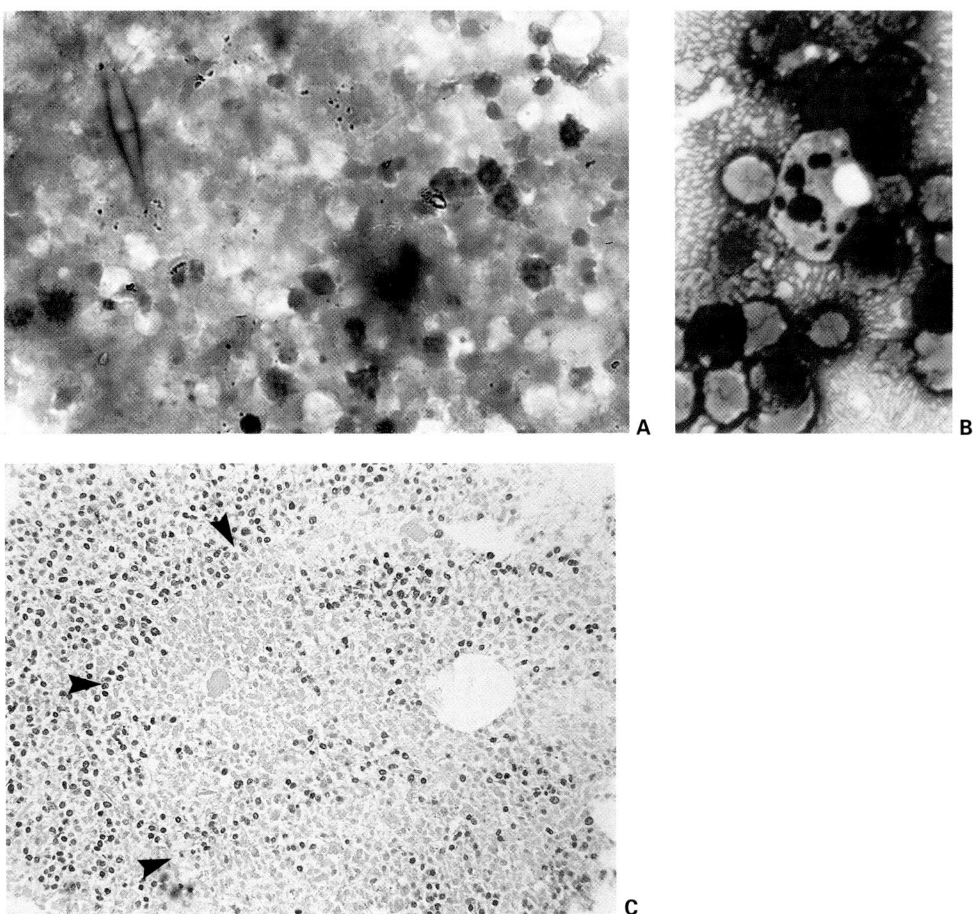

Fig. 4.13 Bone marrow necrosis in 3 cases of ALL at presentation. **a** Charcot-Leyden crystal also in field. **b** Leucocyte outlines more discernible than in **a**. **c** Trephine biopsy; arrows outline necrotic area. **a** × 600; **b** × 1000; **c** H & E × 200

A variety of explanations has been proposed (e.g. vessel obstruction, high O_2 demand, Habboush & Hann 1987), though other mechanisms such as viral destruction are possible.

Excessive numbers of smudge cells may on occasion be an indication of incipient necrosis. They are a common artefact in ALL, but occurrence in large numbers, together with tumour lysis syndrome (main features being irritability, decreased responsiveness, opisthotonos, hypocalcaemia, hyperphosphataemia, hyperuricaemia), suggests genuine cell degeneration (Fig. 4.14).

Myelofibrosis

Fibrosis is not uncommon in ALL (Hann et al 1978). Leucoerythroblastosis may be associated. Rarely, fibrosis is severe enough to cause problems in diagnosis (Fig. 4.15).

Apoptosis

Dead lymphoblasts are common in pre- (and post-) treatment marrow (genuine only in unanticoagulated films; anticoagulants induce apoptosis).

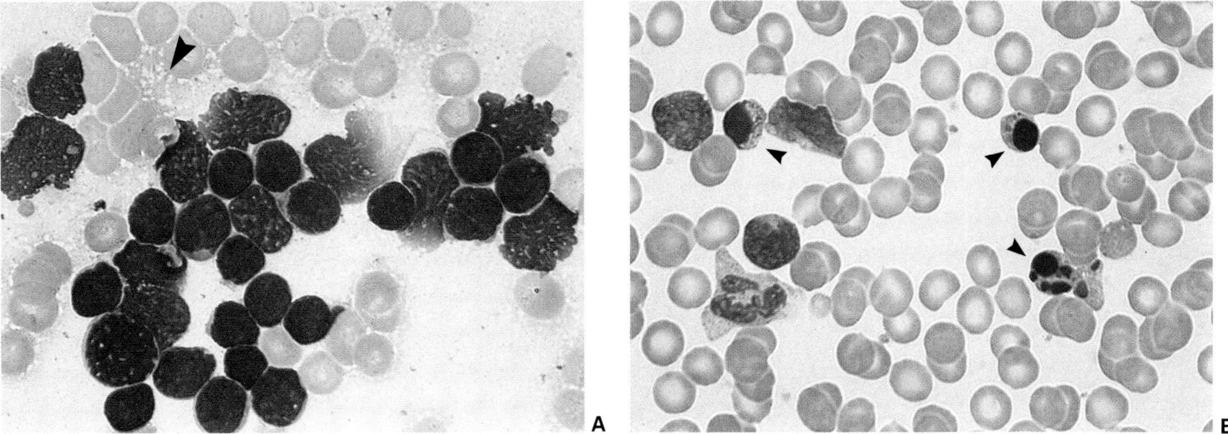

Fig. 4.14 Tumour lysis syndrome. **a** Marrow, preserved lymphoblasts together with smudge cells regarded as genuinely degenerate because of profuse numbers and association with tumour lysis; 'moth-eaten' background (arrow) due to hyperchylomicronaemia; pre-B ALL, t(11;19). **b** Blood, T lymphoma, pre-treatment, spontaneous death of lymphoblasts (arrows); leucocyte count rose from 22 to 109 × 10^9/l in 3 days.

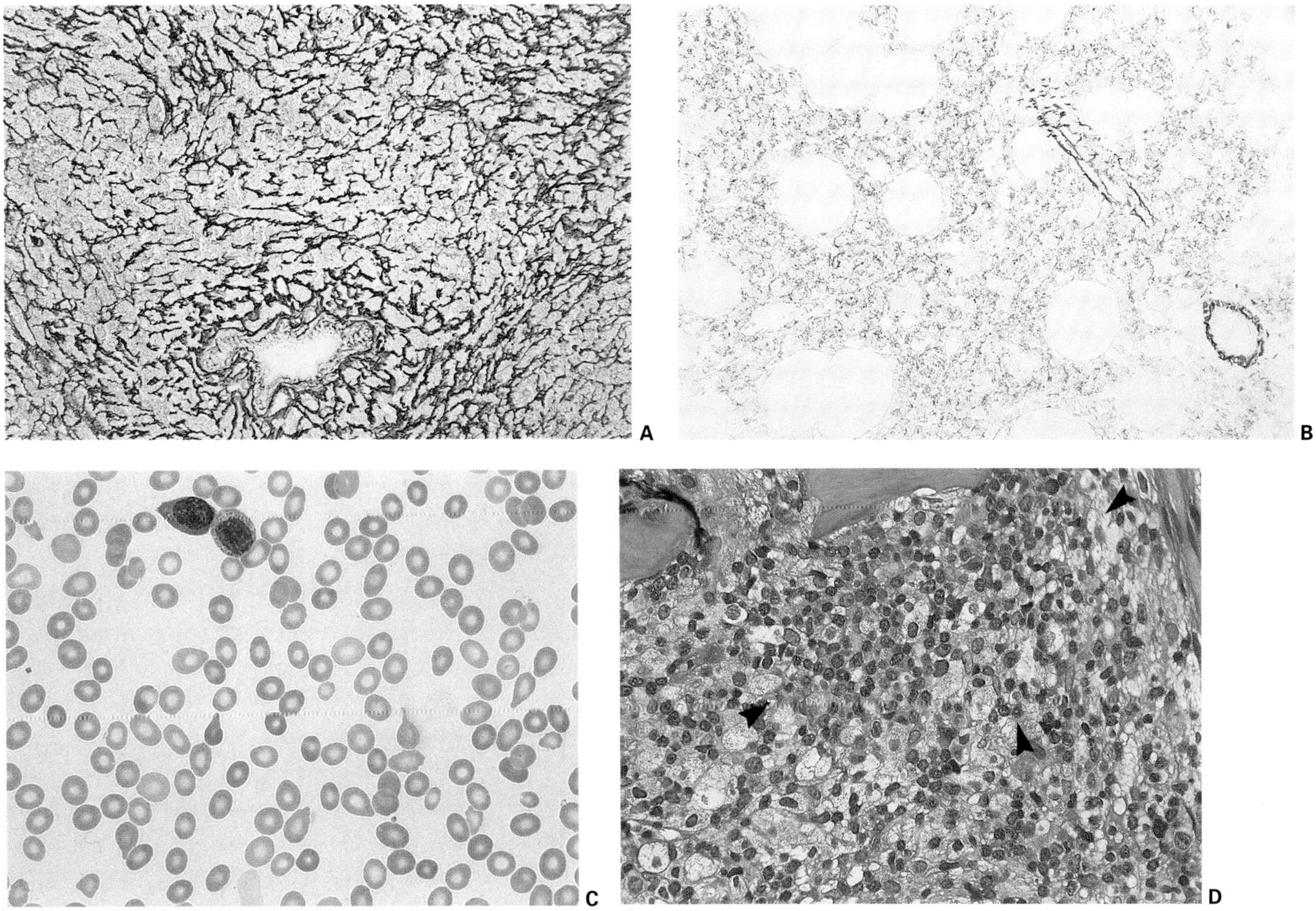

Fig. 4.15 Marrow fibrosis in ALL (common markers). Reticulin **(a)** compared with normal of same age **(b)**. Blood film (**c**, same child as **a**) shows leucoerythroblastosis — pear-shaped erythrocytes, myelocyte and erythroblast. **d** Another child, showing loose aggregate of lymphoid cells (arrows) among macrophage-type and connective tissue cells (reticulin increased); an aspirate, obtained with difficulty, contained 22% lymphoblasts. **a,b** × 200; **c** × 500; **d** H & E × 330

Abnormal macrophages

Foamy macrophages and Gaucher-like cells are seen rarely (Carrington et al 1992, Fig. 4.16), and are attributed to cell turnover which is excessive for available degradation mechanisms. They are more prominent in treated children (Figs 6.37, 6.42) and in T lymphoma (whether marrow is infiltrated or not). Intracellular opportunistic organisms such as histoplasma and candida are more likely after treatment than at presentation. Sea-blue histiocytes occur in rare cases (Fig. 6.43). Intracellular Charcot-Leyden crystals occur in myeloid leukaemias (Fig. 5.6) but not in ALL.

Eosinophilia

See blood, below.

Necrobiotic multinucleate cells of unknown nature

A phenomenon of necrobiosis in multinucleate cells of unknown nature is shown in Figure 4.16. The marrow was infiltrated (96%) by lymphoblasts. Necrobiotic cells were no longer present in remission. These cells could be macrophages damaged by lymphoid cells which had been phagocytosed or wandered inside (emperipolesis), or they could be formations of fused and degenerating lymphoblasts; the clear surround might be an effect of a cytotoxin.

BLOOD CHANGES

Although normal values for one or other of the formed elements are not unusual, complete normality of values and morphology is seen in < 0.5% of cases at diagnosis.

Lymphoblastosis

Lymphoblasts are noted at presentation in almost all cases (in relapse the proportion is lower). There is no clear relation between abundance of lymphoblasts in blood and degree of marrow infiltration.

High lymphoblast counts suggest T rather than non-T ALL (medians for total count 63.3 vs $12.5 \times 10^9/l$); high counts are also common in the first year of life and with certain karyotypes, e.g. t(11;19). A leucocyte count of $< 10 \times 10^9/l$ is found in about half of cases.

Blood transfusion may diminish lymphoblasts to a greater degree than can be explained by simple dilution, and severe infection may induce temporary clearing of leukaemic cells from blood and marrow. Large numbers of dead lymphoblasts may accompany tumour lysis syndrome (Fig. 4.14).

Although the presence of one or two lymphoblasts in an otherwise normal blood film is not necessarily abnormal (p. 8), ALL should be considered in appropriate clinical circumstances, e.g. arthropathy which is poorly responsive to conventional treatment (antinuclear antibody may be present in serum in these cases).

Eosinophilia

Eosinophilia in blood and marrow is uncommon in ALL. It may precede (up to 9 months), or coincide with or follow by some months overt lymphoblastosis. Eosinophilia may occur in common-marker ALL, T ALL and T lymphoblastic lymphoma and may be accompanied by increase in basophils. In CSF, increase in eosinophils may accompany or precede lymphoblastosis and may not be accompanied by eosinophilia in blood and marrow.

Extreme eosinophilia (to $110 \times 10^9/l$) if chronic may be accompanied by the hypereosinophilic syndrome (p. 256). A distinctive translocation (5;14) has been noted in some of these cases (Hogan et al 1987).

Although the eosinophils may show some abnormality (e.g. hypogranularity, Pelgerization, Fig. 4.16), it would appear that, in most cases at least, eosinophilia is a reaction to an eosinopoietin produced by lymphoblasts (Catovsky et al 1980); the eosinopoietin is most likely interleukin-3, which, in t(5;14) cases, is activated (gene at 5q31) by juxtaposition of the IgH gene (from 14q32, Meeker et al 1990).

In remission the eosinophil count diminishes but may not become normal. Eosinophilia (or neutrophilia) may herald relapse.

Erythrocyte changes

See Table 4.6.

Haemostatic changes

See Table 4.7.

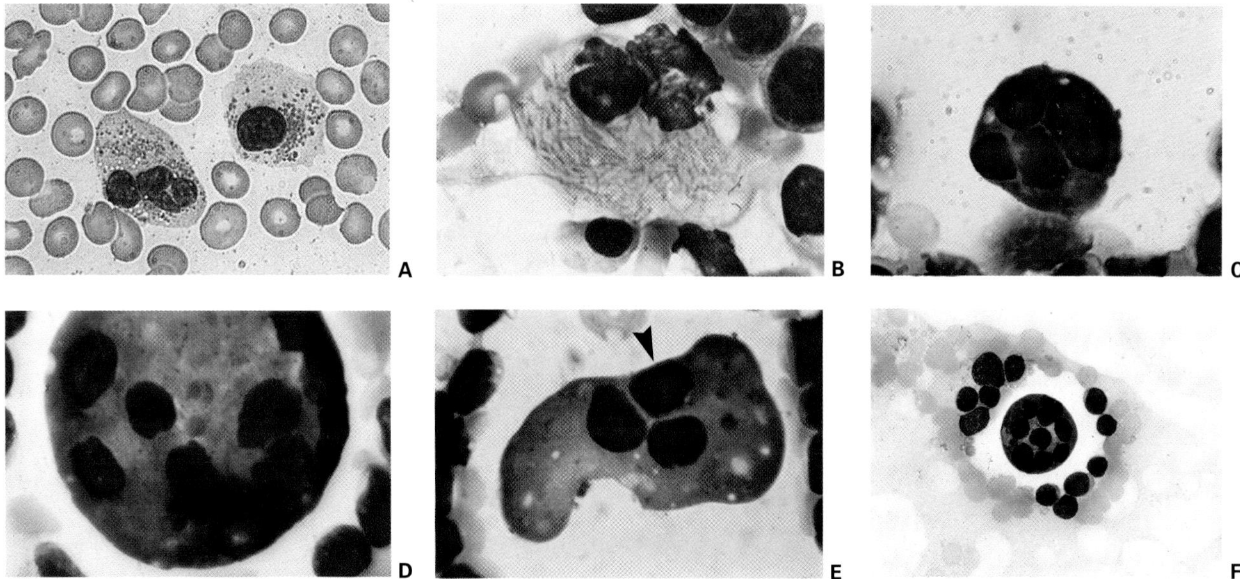

Fig. 4.16 Unusual manifestations in 3 cases of (untreated) ALL. **a** Eosinophilia (13.2×10^9/l) with Pelgerized and hypogranular eosinophils; karyotype normal. **b** Gaucher-like cell in marrow. **c–f** Multinucleate necrobiotic cells of unknown nature in marrow. **c** Early phase — conglutination of lymphoid nuclei. **d,e** Older cells; arrow shows lymphoid cell with cytoplasm retained. **f** Characteristic clearing around cell. All × 1000, except **a** (× 750) and **f** (× 380)

Table 4.6 ALL: erythrocyte changes in blood

At diagnosis
- Anaemia (about 85% of cases), usually normocytic, normochromic
- Macrocytosis rare — folate deficiency (dietary, malabsorption)
- Microcytosis rare, most likely B lymphoma/ALL (bleeding, malabsorption from bowel infiltration) or unrelated, e.g. thalassaemia
- Erythroblasts usually sparse; together with minimal polychromasia suggests marrow infiltration (important if no or few convincing lymphoblasts)
- Myeloid leucoerythroblastosis + tear-drop poikilocytes (myelophthisis) may suggest marrow fibrosis (Fig. 4.15)
- Fragmentation haemolysis rare (tumour or infection)
- HbF > 10% rare

After treatment
- Macrocytosis (cytotoxics, especially methotrexate, cytosine arabinoside)
- Target cells (liver damage from cytotoxics, especially methotrexate)
- Elliptocytosis (cytotoxics)
- Changes of asplenia (in some cases, for a few weeks during induction)
- Fragmentation haemolysis, rare (infection)
- Autoagglutination, uncommon (infection)
- HbF > 10%, in some cases, temporarily after marrow transplantation
- Pancytopenia from marrow destruction by graft vs host disease in transplanted or transfused children

Table 4.7 ALL: haemostatic abnormalities

At diagnosis
- Thrombocytopenia (about 80%), due to ↓ production
- Hypoprothrombinaemia, uncommon — vitamin K deficiency from anorexia, antibiotics, malabsorption (bowel infiltration), liver disease (infection, tumour)
- Intravascular coagulation, rare (tumour, infection); characteristic of the rare t(17;19) (Inaba et al 1992); fragmentation haemolysis inconstant
- Hypofibrinogenaemia, uncommon — intravascular coagulation, liver damage (infection, tumour, L-aspariginase)
- Platelet dysfunction and vessel fragility (infection)

After treatment
- Haemostatic problems may worsen — cytotoxic effects on marrow and liver, infection, graft vs host disease in those transfused or transplanted; immune thrombocytopenia rare (Rao & Pang 1979)

PRODROMES FOR CHILDHOOD ALL

Cytopenias

Transient cytopenias precede overt blastosis in about 2% of cases (Wegelius 1986), manifesting usually as anaemia with neutropenia or as pancytopenia (Fig. 4.17).

The marrow is depleted, usually with some fibrosis. Depletion may be noted in only some or in all of several sites sampled. Rarely, cellularity is normal or increased. Evidence of viral infection includes:

- atypical lymphocytosis preceding or during episodes (Fig. 4.17)
- serologic evidence of herpes simplex or non-A non-B hepatitis (Ireland et al 1988)
- increased chromatid breaks on karyotype.

Transient fragmentation haemolysis may occur.

Cytopenias last for up to one month, improvement occurring spontaneously or following, often within days, blood transfusion or corticosteroid or androgen treatment. Rapid improvement, being uncharacteristic of true aplasia, should suggest the possibility of pre-leukaemia. In some cases only the neutropenia and thrombocytopenia of a pancytopenia remit, to expose an erythroblastopenia which may be steroid/androgen responsive (de Alarcon et al 1978). More than one episode may occur. Overt blastosis appears within 5 weeks to 10 months, usually within 4 months, of first presentation of cytopenia.

This phenomenon occurs in common-marker (including Ph-positive) rather than other types of ALL and is rare or does not occur in non-lymphocytic leukaemias. It is more common in girls than boys (about 3/1; childhood ALL has a male preponderance).

In some cases leukaemia can be demonstrated in the depleted marrow (Fig. 4.17). The relation between the leukaemia and the hypoplasia is unknown.

Eosinophilia

See page 132.

RELAPSE, RESIDUAL DISEASE

Detection may be important for timing of cessation of treatment and of marrow transplantation.

- Morphology

Blast cell counts of < 5% are evidence of disease if the leukaemic cells are of distinctive morphology (e.g. large size, cytoplasmic basophilia). Detection of marrow infiltration may require sampling from more than one site.

- Cytogenetics

Cytogenetics is useful if karyotype at diagnosis was abnormal. Cytogenetics may be abnormal in morphologically normal marrow. A donor karyotype does not necessarily indicate that a relapse post-transplant is of donor origin (see below).

Fluorescent in situ hybridization of interphase cells may detect abnormality in marrows which are normal by conventional cytogenetics (Anastasi et al 1991).

- Immunophenotype

Significant changes in phenotype may occur in relapse (see below). Immunophenotyping alone, however, may overdiagnose relapse (p. 136).

- Gene rearrangements

Gene rearrangements unique for the leukaemia may be amplified at diagnosis by PCR, sequenced and a homologous probe constructed for hybridization to PCR-amplified sequences in subsequent samples. This technique detects leukaemic cells down to about 1 in 10^5 cells (Potter 1992). In some cases of recipient-origin relapse post-transplant, gene rearrangements show that a donor karyotype was obtained because recipient cells failed to enter mitosis (Naoe et al 1989).

Relapse in ALL usually shows minor change, if any, from the original in morphology and phenotype. In some cases the relapse is myeloid, e.g. to AML M5 (Fig. 5.12) or to CML (Fig. 5.17). The change in phenotype may however be more subtle (Fig. 4.4).

A change to myeloid lineage (Bain & Catovsky 1990) may be due to:

- True lineage switch — treatment has selected an originally minor, myeloid subclone; the two leukaemias have the same karyotype (Figs 4.4, 5.17) and gene rearrangements.
- Secondary leukaemia — treatment has been leukaemogenic to residual normal stem cells; the two leukaemias differ in karyotype and gene rearrangements. There is preferential aberration of 11q23 in myeloid leukaemias post-chemotherapy for ALL (especially T ALL) and Hodgkin's disease (Pedersen-Bjergaard & Philip 1991).

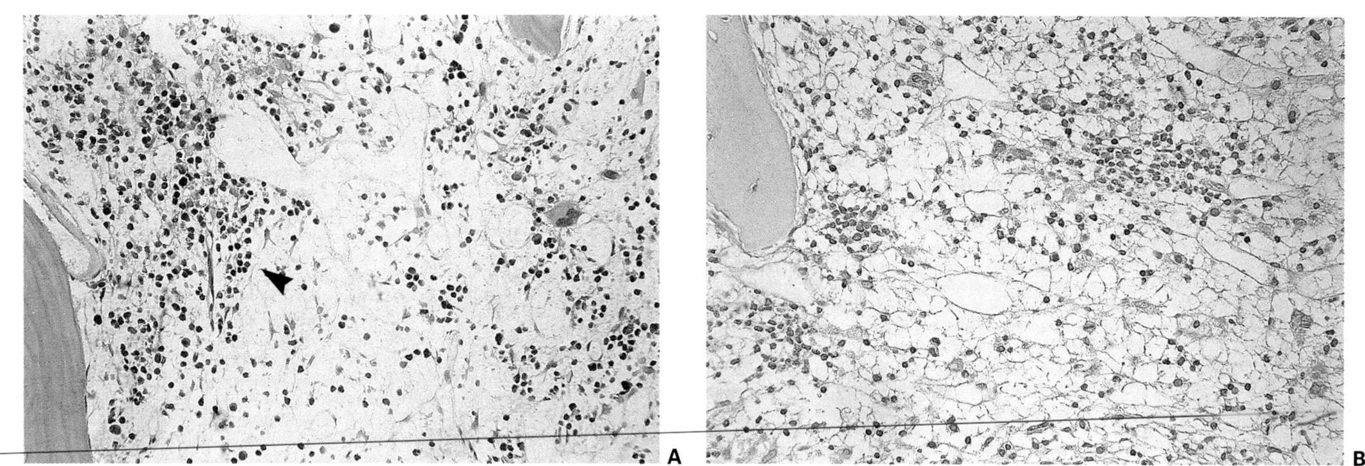

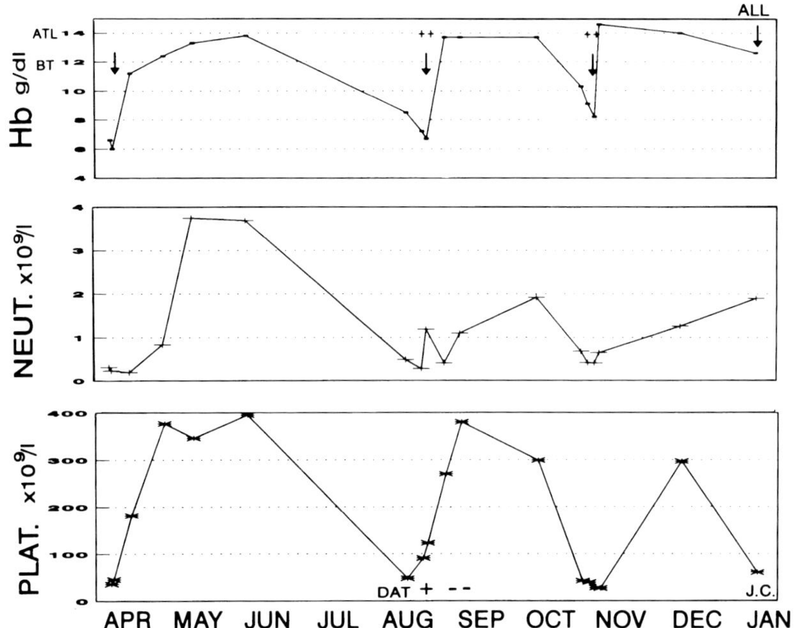

Fig. 4.17 Marrow hypoplasia preceding/accompanying ALL. **a** 17-month-old girl, small focus of normal cells (arrow) in depleted marrow. ALL (common markers) manifested 5 months later. **b** 4-year-old boy with pancytopenia and depleted marrow containing a sprinkling of lymphoid cells; an aspirate obtained with difficulty contained 45% hyperdiploid lymphoblasts (DNA index 1.1). **c** 4-year-old girl with Down's syndrome and ALL (common) 9 months after first episode of pancytopenia; atypical lymphocytes (ATL) were notable in blood before at least 2 episodes; direct antiglobulin test (DAT) positive (IgG) in second episode; BT = blood transfusion. **a** H & E $\times$ 200; **b** PAS $\times$ 200

DIFFERENTIAL DIAGNOSIS OF LEUKAEMIC LYMPHOBLASTOSIS

Benign lymphoblastosis

Marrow in normal children often contains blastic cells resembling leukaemic lymphoblasts, as well as other immature cells (haematogones) which may be confused with these (Fig. 1.4). The recognition of leukaemia rests on morphology. Immunophenotyping alone is insufficient, as substantial expansions of populations with common, early precursor B or B phenotype may occur in children with no evidence of leukaemia (Sandhaus et al 1993).

Benign lymphoblastosis may occur in marrow of children with vague ill-health (Fig 4.18). CMV, EBV or other virus can be demonstrated in some cases. With the exception of treated ALL, in which marrow blastosis of even minor degree is suspicious of relapse, lymphoblastosis in marrow might be considered benign in the following circumstances:

- blastosis < 60%
- clinical features atypical for ALL
- karyotype atypical for ALL, e.g. chromatid breaks (suggesting viral infection)
- serologic evidence of viral infection (but viral infection may coexist with ALL or be introduced by transfusion)
- disappearance of blastosis within 6 weeks. ALL and lymphoma show progression, usually rapid, in this period.

Benign lymphoblastosis of marrow is sometimes persistent. Woessner et al (1985) described 5 children with 5–10% blasts in marrow, thought to be pre-B, and persisting for up to 6 years (in one adult to 21 years).

Benign lymphoblastosis appears to be rare. The cure rate for treated ALL is unlikely to be unduly high as a result of unwitting inclusion of these cases.

Blastic, reactive (atypical) lymphocytes may occur in such numbers in (rare cases of) viral infection as to raise a suspicion of leukaemia (Fig. 4.18).

Non-lymphocytic leukaemias

MPO-negative non-lymphocytic leukaemias may have lymphoid morphology, e.g. AML M0, M6, M7. Immunophenotyping is essential for diagnosis. See Chapter 5.

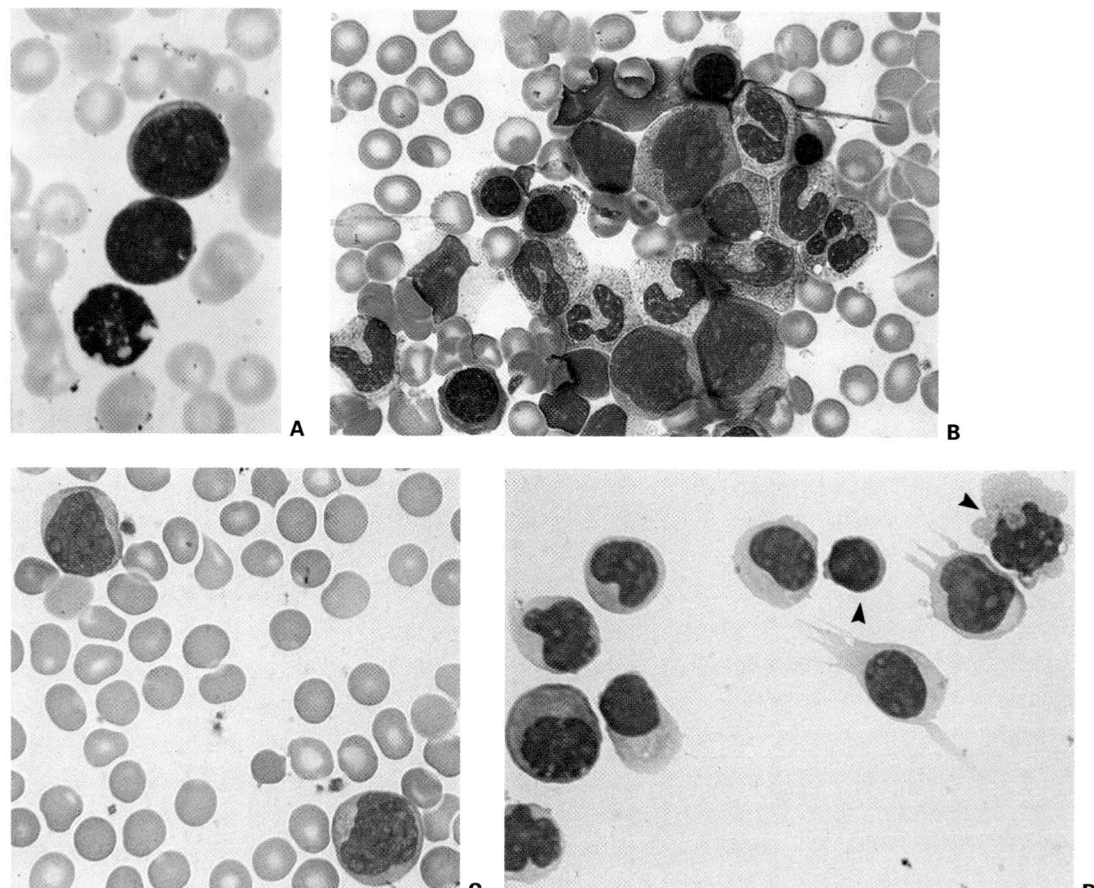

Fig. 4.18 Benign lymphoblastosis. **a** 4-month-old infant with 55% MPO-negative blast cells in marrow (2 in this field), regarded as ALL (immunophenotype and cytogenetics not available in those times); after 3 doses of 6MP was lost to follow-up until reappearance 19 years later for unrelated minor symptoms. **b** Marrow containing 10% lymphoblasts 2 months after cessation of (effective) treatment for abdominal B lymphoma. Marrow not involved at diagnosis. Immunophenotype and cytogenetics of marrow normal. Blast cells had disappeared spontaneously 3 weeks later. **c** Blastic reactive lymphocytes in blood, 10-week-old infant with fever and splenomegaly; the frequency of these cells (15% of lymphocytes) led to suspicion of leukaemia; however, marrow contained only 5% blast cells and CSF cytology was viral (**d**, arrows show normal lymphocyte and macrophage); adenovirus isolated from CSF. **a** × 1000. **c,d** Courtesy of Dr P O'Regan

Non-haemopoietic malignancies

Non-haemopoietic malignant cells, e.g. neuroblastoma, may resemble leukaemic lymphoblasts. However, other cytologic features such as cell grouping, cytochemistry, immunophenotype and cytogenetics enable identification (see Ch. 5).

Non-Hodgkin lymphoma

As a generalization, marrow involvement in lymphoma is metastatic from an extramedullary source (lymph nodes, mediastinum) and therefore usually light (< 25%) and/or spotty; sampling from more than one site may be needed. Lymphoma is usually biologically different to ALL — lymphoma cells may differ in morphology and karyotype from ALL cells (Fig. 4.19), and tend to be more mature in phenotype.

The combination of gross marrow involvement with extramedullary mass disease is appropriately regarded as lymphoma if cellular characteristics are unusual for ALL (Fig. 4.19), and as leukaemia if characteristics are typical.

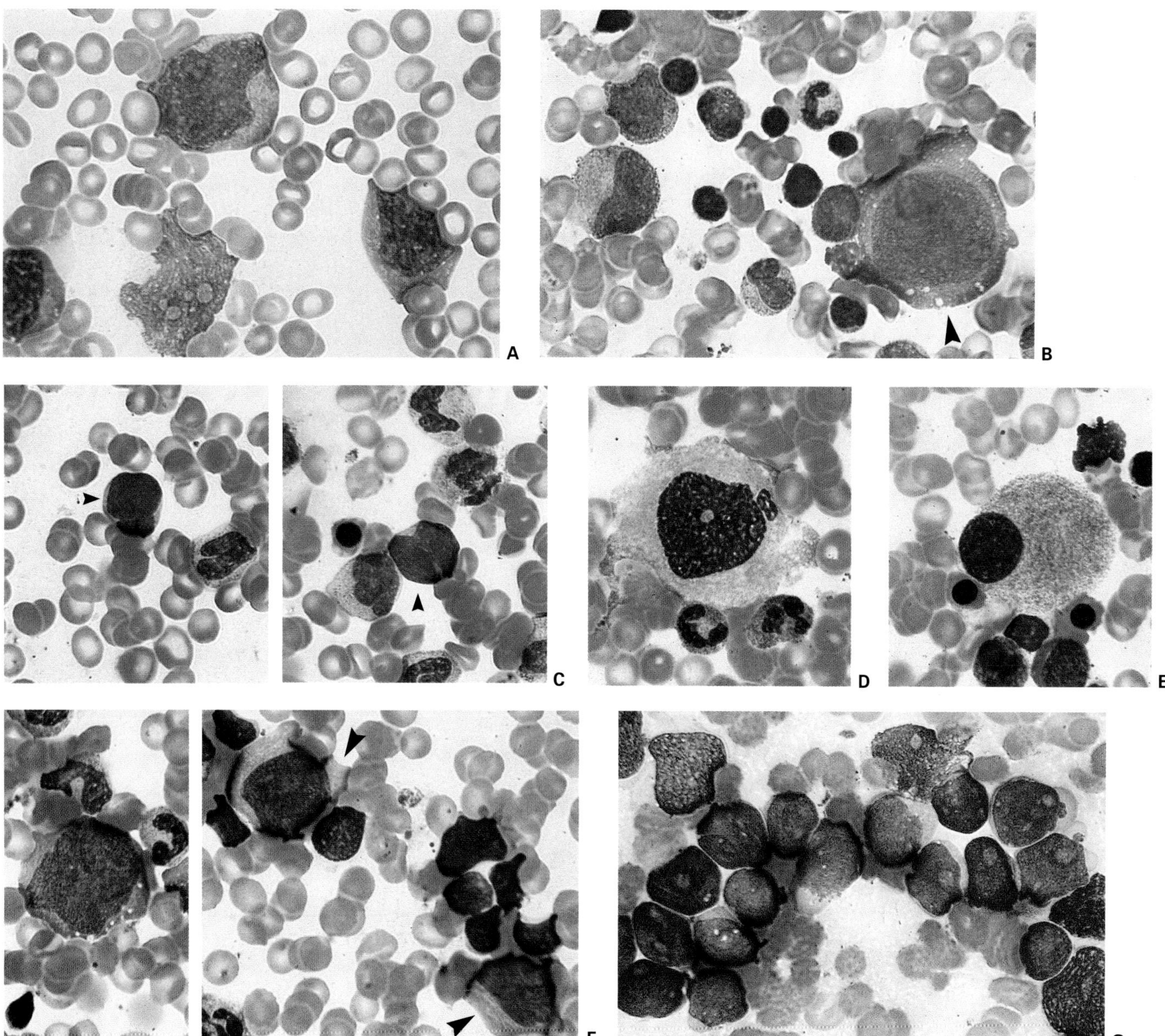

Fig. 4.19 Non-Hodgkin lymphoma. **a** Blood, 9-year-old boy with B lymphoma due to cyclosporin treatment post-liver transplant; these cells contained EBV antigen. **b** Marrow, 3-year-old girl with abdominal B lymphoma (cell arrowed). **c** Marrow (lymphoma cells arrowed), 6-year-old boy with T lymphoma clinically confined to a cervical lymph node. **d** Marrow, 9-year-old boy with T lymphoma clinically localized to skin (cf immature megakaryocyte, **e**). **f** Marrow, 15-month-old child with unilateral retinoblastoma (no morphologic evidence in marrow); lymphoma cells in right frame arrowed; deletion 4p in 5% of metaphases, skin karyotype normal. There has been no increase in abnormality (3.5% of marrow cells) over a follow-up of 11 months. **g** Heavy (74%) lymphoblastic infiltration in marrow, 13-year-old boy, early precursor B ALL. An unusual karyotype (62–89 hyperdiploid) and association with a retroperitoneal mass suggested lymphoma rather than ALL.

Hodgkin's disease.

This is a rare occurrence in marrow (Fig. 4.20).

Chronic lymphocytic leukaemia

Diagnosis of this exceedingly rare leukaemia might be considered if an increase of normal-appearing lymphocytes persists or becomes more pronounced over at least 3 months. In most cases the proliferated cells have B markers (evidence of clonal restriction, e.g. κ or λ chains required). The karyotype may be abnormal, e.g. t(12;14) (Sonnier et al 1983). Normal serum immunoglobulins may be diminished, but paraproteins have not been demonstrated in the few cases reported.

For the differential diagnosis of lymphocytosis of normal-appearing lymphocytes see Table 7.11.

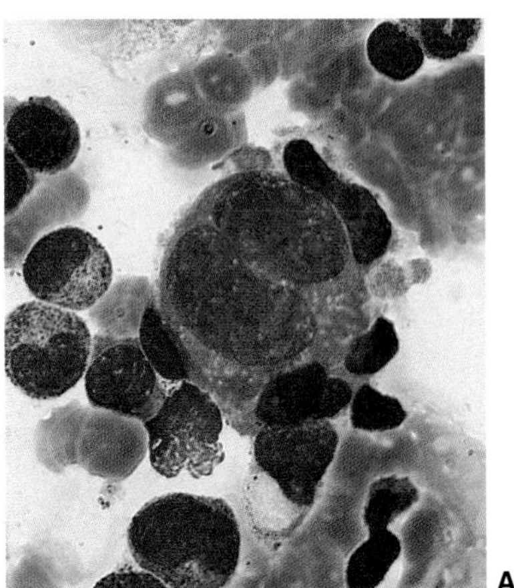

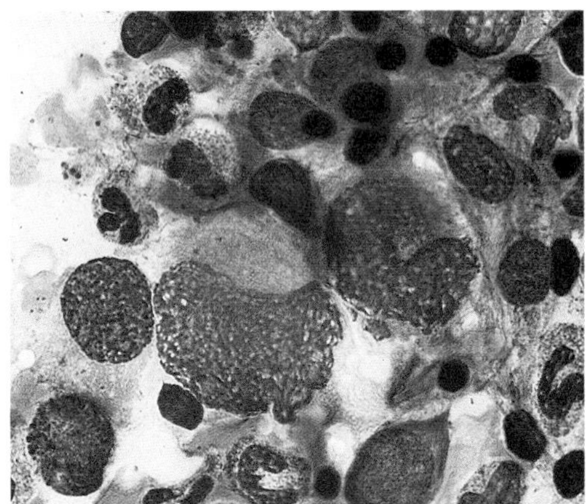

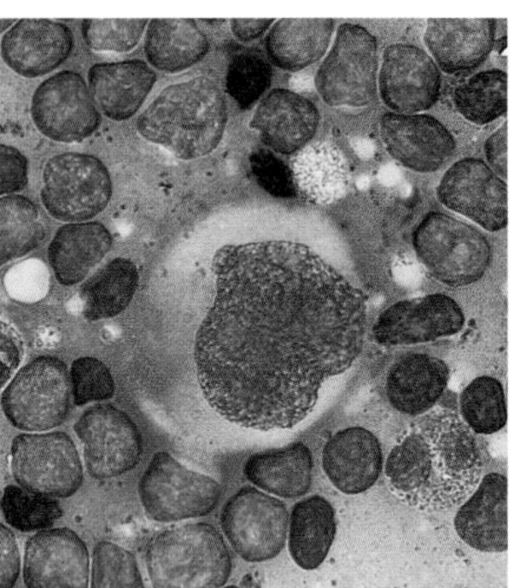

Fig. 4.20 Hodgkin's disease in marrow aspirates. Reed-Sternberg **(a)** and uninucleate cells **(b)**. Compare with lymph node imprint (**c**, same child as **b**).

REFERENCES

Anastasi J, Thangavelu M, Vardiman J W et al 1991 Interphase cytogenetic analysis detects minimal residual disease in a case of acute lymphoblastic leukemia and resolves the question of origin of relapse after allogeneic bone marrow transplantation. Blood 77: 1087–1091

Bain B 1990 Leukaemia diagnosis. A guide to the FAB classification. Gower Medical Publishing, London

Bain B, Catovsky D 1990 Current concerns in haematology 2: classification of acute leukaemias. Journal of Clinical Pathology 43: 882–887

Brunning R D, Parkin J, Dick F, Nesbit M 1974 Unusual inclusions occurring in the blasts of four patients with acute leukemia and Down's syndrome. Blood 44: 735–741

Carrington P A, Stevens R F, Lendon M 1992 Pseudo-Gaucher cells. Journal of Clinical Pathology 45: 360

Catovsky D, Bernasconi C, Verdonck P J et al 1980 The association of eosinophilia with lymphoblastic leukaemia or lymphoma: a study of seven patients. British Journal of Haematology 45: 523–534

Catovsky D, Matutes E, Buccheri V et al 1991 A classification of acute leukaemia for the 1990s. Annals of Haematology 62: 16–21

Chaganti R S K, Miller D R, Meyers P A, German J 1979 Cytogenetic evidence of the intrauterine origin of acute leukemia in monozygotic twins. New England Journal of Medicine 300: 1032–1034

Darbyshire P J, Lilleyman J S 1987 Granular acute lymphoblastic leukaemia of childhood: a morphological phenomenon. Journal of Clinical Pathology 40: 251–253

de Alarcon P A, Miller M L, Stuart M J 1978 Erythroid hypoplasia: an unusual presentation of childhood acute lymphocytic leukemia. American Journal of Diseases of Children 132: 763–764

Habboush H W, Hann I M 1987 Bone marrow necrosis in acute lymphoblastic leukaemia. Scottish Medical Journal 32: 177–180

Hann I M, Evans D I K, Marsden H B et al 1978 Bone marrow fibrosis in acute lymphoblastic leukaemia of childhood. Journal of Clinical Pathology 31: 313–315

Hogan T F, Koss W, Murgo A J et al 1987 Acute lymphoblastic leukemia with chromosomal 5;14 translocation and hypereosinophilia: case report and literature review. Journal of Clinical Oncology 5: 382–390

Hurwitz C A, Mirro J 1990 Mixed-lineage leukemia and asynchronous antigen expression. Hematology/Oncology Clinics of North America 4: 767–794

Inaba T, Roberts W M, Shapiro L H et al 1992 Fusion of the leucine zipper gene HLF to the E2A gene in human acute B-lineage leukemia. Science 257: 531–534

Ireland R, Gillett D, Mieli-Vergani G, Mufti G 1988 Pre-ALL and non-A, non-B hepatitis infection. Leukemia Research 12: 795–797

Keifer J, Abromowitch M, Stass S A 1985 Chloroacetate esterase positivity in acute lymphoblastic leukemia. American Journal of Clinical Pathology 83: 647–649

Le Beau M M 1993 Detecting genetic changes in human tumor cells: have scientists "gone fishing?". Blood 81: 1979–1983

Lilleyman J S, Hann I M, Stevens R F et al 1986 French American British (FAB) morphological classification of childhood lymphoblastic leukaemia and its clinical importance. Journal of Clinical Pathology 39: 998–1002

Lilleyman J S, Hann I M, Stevens R F et al 1988 Blast cell vacuoles in childhood lymphoblastic leukaemia. British Journal of Haematology 70: 183–186

Ludwig W-D, Raghavachar A, Theil E 1994 Immunophenotypic classification of acute lymphoblastic leukaemia. Baillière's Clinical Haematology 7: 235–262

Mauer A M, Evert C F, Lampkin B C, McWilliams N B 1973 Cell kinetics in human acute lymphoblastic leukemia: computer simulation with discrete modeling techniques. Blood 41: 141–154

Meeker T C, Hardy D, Willman C et al 1990 Activation of the interleukin-3 gene by chromosome translocation in acute lymphocytic leukemia with eosinophilia. Blood 76: 285–289

Miller D R, Krailo M, Bleyer W A et al 1985 Prognostic implications of blast cell morphology in childhood acute lymphoblastic leukemia: a report from the children's cancer study group. Cancer Treatment Reports 69: 1211–1221

Naoe T, Kiyoi H, Yamanaka K et al 1989 A case of cALL relapse after allogeneic BMT: recurrence of recipient cell origin, initially determined as being that of donor cell origin by sex chromosome analysis. British Journal of Haematology 73: 420–422

Pederson-Bjergaard J, Philip P 1991 Balanced translocations involving chromosome bands 11q23 and 21q22 are highly characteristic of myelodysplasia and leukemia following therapy with cytostatic agents targeting at DNA-topoisomerase II. Blood 78: 1147–1148

Pombo de Oliveira M S, Awad el Seed F E K, Foroni L et al 1986 Lymphoblastic leukaemia in Siamese twins: evidence for identity. Lancet 2: 969–970

Potter M N 1992 The detection of minimal residual disease in acute lymphoblastic leukaemia. Blood Reviews 6: 68–82

Preston-Martin S 1989 Epidemiological studies of prenatal carcinogenesis. In: Napalkov N P, Rice J M, Tomatis L, Yamasaki H (eds) Perinatal and multigeneration carcinogenesis. Scientific publications no 96. International Agency for Research on Cancer, Lyon, p 289

Raimondi S C 1993 Current status of cytogenetic research in childhood acute lymphoblastic leukemia. Blood 81: 2237–2251

Rao S, Pang E J-M 1979 Idiopathic thrombocytopenic purpura in acute lymphoblastic leukemia. Journal of Pediatrics 94: 408–409

Rice J M 1988 Fetal susceptibility to viral and chemical carcinogens. Laboratory Investigation 58: 1–4

Sandhaus L M, Chen T L, Ettinger L J et al 1993 Significance of increased proportion of CD 10-positive cells in non-malignant bone marrows of children. American Journal of Pediatric Hematology and Oncology 15: 65–70

Schumacher H R, Desai S N, McClain K L 1989 Acute lymphoblastic leukemia — hand mirror variant. Analysis for endogenous retroviral antibodies in bone marrow plasma. American Journal of Clinical Pathology 91: 410–416

Smith H 1978 Inclusion bodies containing virus-like particles in acute lymphocytic leukaemia of childhood. Leukemia Research 2: 133–140

Smith H, Collins R J, Martin N J, Siskind V 1982 A developmental characteristic of the ultrastructure of childhood leukaemic lymphoblasts. Leukemia Research 6: 675–683

Smith H, Collins R J, Martin N J, Siskind V 1986 Altered chromatin in childhood leukaemic lymphoblasts: association with virus-like particles. British Journal of Experimental Pathology 67: 549–561

Smith H, Collins R J, Curley M G et al 1991 Viral-like characteristics of particle aggregates in a lymphoblastic cell line. Pathology 23: 206–211

Sonnier J A, Buchanan G R, Howard-Peebles P N et al 1983 Chromosomal translocation involving the immunoglobulin kappa-chain and heavy-chain loci in a child with chronic lymphocytic leukemia. New England Journal of Medicine 309: 590–594

Wegelius R 1986 Preleukaemic states in children. Scandinavian Journal of Haematology 36 (suppl 45): 133–139

Woessner S, Sans-Sabrafen J, Lafuente R, Florensa L 1985 Asymptomatic bone marrow infiltration by blast cells. New England Journal of Medicine 312: 1129

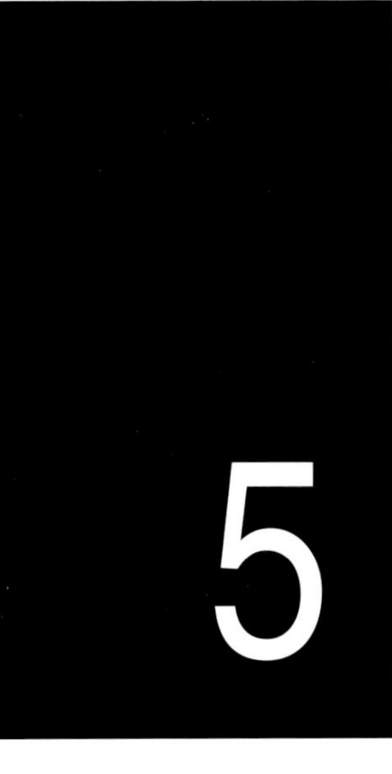

5 Myeloid leukaemias. Non-haemopoietic malignancies in marrow

An account of myeloid leukaemias, non-haemopoietic malignancies of marrow and histiocytoses of childhood. Some of these disorders are confined to childhood. Benign conditions which mimic leukaemia are a significant consideration in differential diagnosis.

Abbreviations and notes

AcPh: acid phosphatase; ALL: acute lymphoblastic leukaemia; AML: acute myeloid leukaemia/s; ANAE: α naphthyl acetate esterase; ANBE: α naphthyl butyrate esterase; c: cytoplasmic; CAE: chloroacetate esterase; CML: chronic myeloid leukaemia; CSF: cerebrospinal fluid; Gp: glycoprotein; H & E: haematoxylin and eosin; JCML: juvenile chronic myeloid leukaemia; MDS: myelodysplastic syndrome; MPD: myeloproliferative disease; MPO: myeloperoxidase; NAP: neutrophil alkaline phosphatase; ORO: oil red O; Ph: Philadelphia; PPO: platelet peroxidase; RAEB: refractory anaemia with excess blasts; SBB: sudan black B; TAM: transient abnormal myelopoiesis; TdT: terminal deoxynucleotidyl transferase.

Magnifications: × 750 unless otherwise stated. Karyotypes: are banded karyotypes of marrow except those done before availability of banding (designated 'pre-banding').

AML 144

FAB classification, general remarks 144
M0 144
M1 144
M2 146
M3 152
M4 156
M5 160
M6 162
M7 166

Chronic myeloid leukaemias, myelodysplasias 170

Juvenile chronic myeloid leukaemia 170
Monosomy 7 MPD 174
Adult type CML 176
Myelodysplastic syndromes 178
Essential thrombocythaemia 180
Rarer myeloproliferative disorders 182

Non-haemopoietic malignancies in marrow 183

Neuroblastoma 184
Retinoblastoma 188
Medulloblastoma 188
Rhabdomyosarcoma 190
Ewing's sarcoma 192
Other 192

Histiocytoses 194

Langerhans cell histiocytosis 194
Non-Langerhans histiocytosis 196
Malignant histiocytosis 198
Sinus histiocytosis with massive lymphadenopathy 198

Acute myeloid leukaemias

AML accounts for about 15% of all childhood leukaemias in the 'developed' countries.

FAB CLASSIFICATION, GENERAL REMARKS

The FAB classification (Bain 1990) is used here, with modifications, including those of Bloomfield & Brunning (1985). Changes we have found useful are:

- Definition of blast cells

The designation of 2 types of blast cell unnecessarily complicates assessments. 'Blast cells' refers here to agranular cells.

- Definition of MDS

Myeloblastoses with < 30% blast cells are not classified as MDS if the appearances are simply a quantitatively muted or early version of classic AML (> 30% blasts). A diagnosis of MDS is appropriate if there is conspicuous dysplasia of at least one cell line as well as a low percentage (< 30%) of blast cells (p. 178).

- Differential counts

To avoid confusion from use of more than one set of figures, differential counts on marrow are for total nucleated cells, except for AML M6 (% of non-erythroid cells).

Table 5.1 Self-limiting or reversible hyperplasias which may mimic leukaemia

Myeloid	
M0	TAM of neonatal trisomy 21
M2	Leukaemoid reactions due to virus or undetermined cause
M3	CMV infection
M4	CMV infection
M7	TAM of neonatal trisomy 21
Juvenile CML	EBV infection
	Self-limiting myelomonocytoses of obscure origin (some familial)
Adult CML	EBV infection
	Thrombocytopenia–absent radius syndrome
Myelodysplastic syndromes	Megaloblastic anaemias
Essential thrombocythaemia	Reactive thrombocytosis
Lymphoblastic	CMV, EBV infection
	Temporary lymphoblastosis of obscure origin
	Lymphocytosis of blastic atypical (reactive) lymphocytes

Descriptions of leukaemias are set out under these headings:

- identifying characteristics
- other characteristics

and, where appropriate:

- morphologic variants
- differential diagnosis (summary in Table 5.1).

The most common types of AML in childhood are M1, 2, 3 and 5.

AML M0 (AML WITH MINIMAL DIFFERENTIATION) (Bennett et al 1991)

About 2–3% of AML.

Identifying characteristics

- Blast cells ≥ 30% of marrow nucleated cells
- < 3% of blast cells positive for MPO (light microscopy) and SBB
- Negative for lymphocyte markers (Tables 4.1, 4.2)
- Positive (≥ 20% of cells) for at least one myeloid-associated marker, e.g. CD13, CD33
- Positive for MPO by either electron microscopy (Matutes et al 1988) or immunocytochemistry
- Serum lysozyme normal or not substantially increased.

Other characteristics

Blast cells in most cases appear 'myeloid' (Fig. 5.1), with open chromatin, one or more prominent, widely spaced nucleoli, and usually a low nuclear/cytoplasmic ratio; less commonly cells resemble L2 or L1 ALL. Auer rods do not occur. Markers additional to CD13 and CD33, e.g. CD11b, CD11c, CD14 and CD15, may be positive. TdT is positive in a minority.

Differential diagnosis

- Other acute leukaemias negative for MPO by light microscopy: ALL, erythroblastic 'ALL' (p. 164), AML M7 (p. 166).
- TAM of neonatal trisomy 21. In most cases the proliferated population is of megakaryocytic lineage (p. 168).

AML M1 (AML WITHOUT MATURATION) (Fig. 5.1)

Up to 10% of AML.

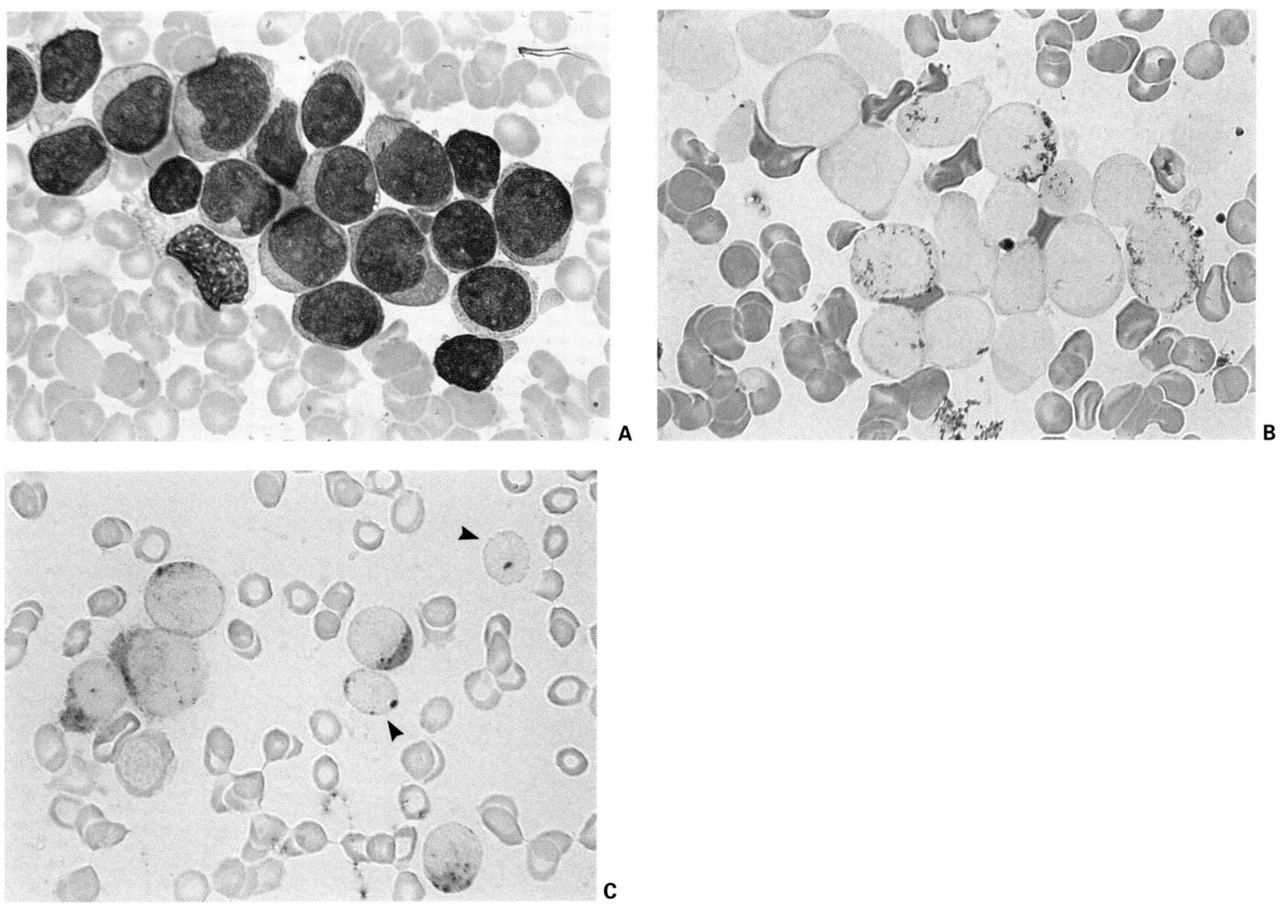

Fig. 5.1 AML M1. **a** Romanowsky, **b** MPO, **c** β glucuronidase. In **c**, 5 blast cells show granular and diffuse staining; 2 lymphocytes (arrows) show spotty staining.

Identifying characteristics

- Blast cells 'myeloid', ≥ 30% of marrow nucleated cells (down to 5% if Auer rods present, Bloomfield & Brunning 1985)
- ≥ 3% of blast cells positive for MPO (Fig. 5.2) or SBB (may be the more sensitive)
- Minimal maturation — promyelocytes and more mature forms < 30% of cells
- Erythroblasts < 50% of cells
- Monocytic forms < 30% of marrow cells or of blood leucocytes.

Other characteristics

Auer rods are often present, usually single and in only a minority of cells. They are positive for MPO and SBB and may be weakly positive with PAS. Occasional blasts may contain erythrocytes. Trilineage dysplasia occurs in a minority (6% in an adult series, Brito-Babapulle et al 1987).

Table 5.2 Cytogenetic abnormalities (at diagnosis) in childhood AML

M0	various	
M1	common:	5q–,–5,7q–,–7,+8,+21,–17, t(9;22)(q34;q11)[1]
	other:	t(8;21), inv(3)(q21q26)[2]
M2	common:	t(8;21)(q22;q22) and variants of this, often with –X in females, –Y in males, +8, partial deletion of 7q,9q
	other:	t(6;9)(p23;q34), +8,+4, t(9;22), inv(3)
M3		t(15;17)(q22;q12–21) probably specific; in about 1/3, additional trisomy 8, isochromosome of derived 17
M4		t/del(11)(q23), t(6;9)(p23;q34), +4
M4Eo		inv(16)(p13q22)
M5	common:	t(9;11)(p22;q23)[3], t/del(11)(q23)
	other:	t(8;16)(p11;p13)[4]
M6 blastic		various
di Guglielmo		hyperdiploidy, marker chromosomes, rings, double minutes, deletions (20q,–5,5q–,–7,7q–)
M7		abnormalities of 21 (translocation, deletion, multiple copies, isochromosome and ring formation), inv 3, ring 7 and other chromosomes

[1] Disappears in remission, unlike the t(9;22) of adult CML
[2] Associated with only mild thrombocytopenia (or thrombocytosis) and megakaryocyte or trilineage dysplasia
[3] Breakpoint at 11q not the same as in t(11;19) ALL (Cherif et al 1992)
[4] Associated with haemophagocytic variant

PAS negative or mild diffuse, sometimes with superimposed fine granulation. In some cases a proportion of cells is ANAE positive, fluoride sensitive. β glucuronidase is usually positive, in a 'myeloid' pattern (Figs 5.1, 5.12). CAE may be positive, AcPh is usually positive (diffuse). A substantial increase (> 10%) in HbF may occur.

Cytogenetics
See Table 5.2.

AML M2 (AML WITH MATURATION) (Fig. 5.3)

About one fifth to one quarter of AML.

Identifying characteristics

- Blast cells ≥ 30% of marrow nucleated cells (down to 5% if Auer rods are present)
- ≥ 3% of blast cells positive for MPO or SBB
- Evidence of maturation: promyelocytes and beyond > 30%
- Erythroblasts < 50% of nucleated cells
- Monocytic forms < 30% of marrow cells or blood leucocytes.

Other characteristics

Auer rods are common, usually single in blast cells and later forms; occasional cases are positive for ANAE, fluoride sensitive (Fig. 5.3, normal neutrophil precursors sometimes are positive). Blast cells or maturing cells may be CAE positive.

Cytogenetics
See Table 5.2.

Variants

M2 is the most heterogeneous of the myeloid leukaemias. Perverted development may be noted in one or more types of granulocyte. Cases in which aberrant development is confined to, or most evident in eosinophils or basophils are designated M2Eo or M2Baso. Even in small numbers, aberrant cells are an important indication of active disease.

Neutrophils (Fig. 5.3)

- In occasional cases maturing neutrophils appear agranular, with basophilia restricted to the periphery. Electron microscopy shows appearances of granule degeneration. This change may occasionally be seen also in MDS and reactive marrows.

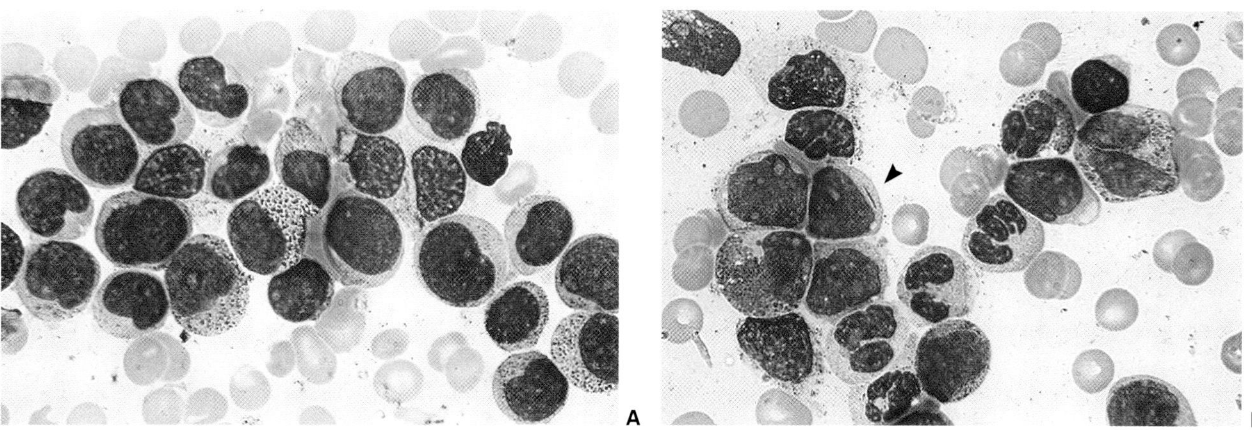

Fig. 5.2 Marrow, AML M2. **a** Typical appearance; blast cells 34%, neutrophil promyelocytes 60%, more mature neutrophils 1%, eosinophils < 1%, monocytic forms < 1%, karyotype normal. **b** Marrow with 12% myeloblasts, diagnosed as AML M2 rather than MDS because of absence of conspicuous myelodysplasia, presence of Auer rods (arrow) and characteristic karyotype, t(8;21).

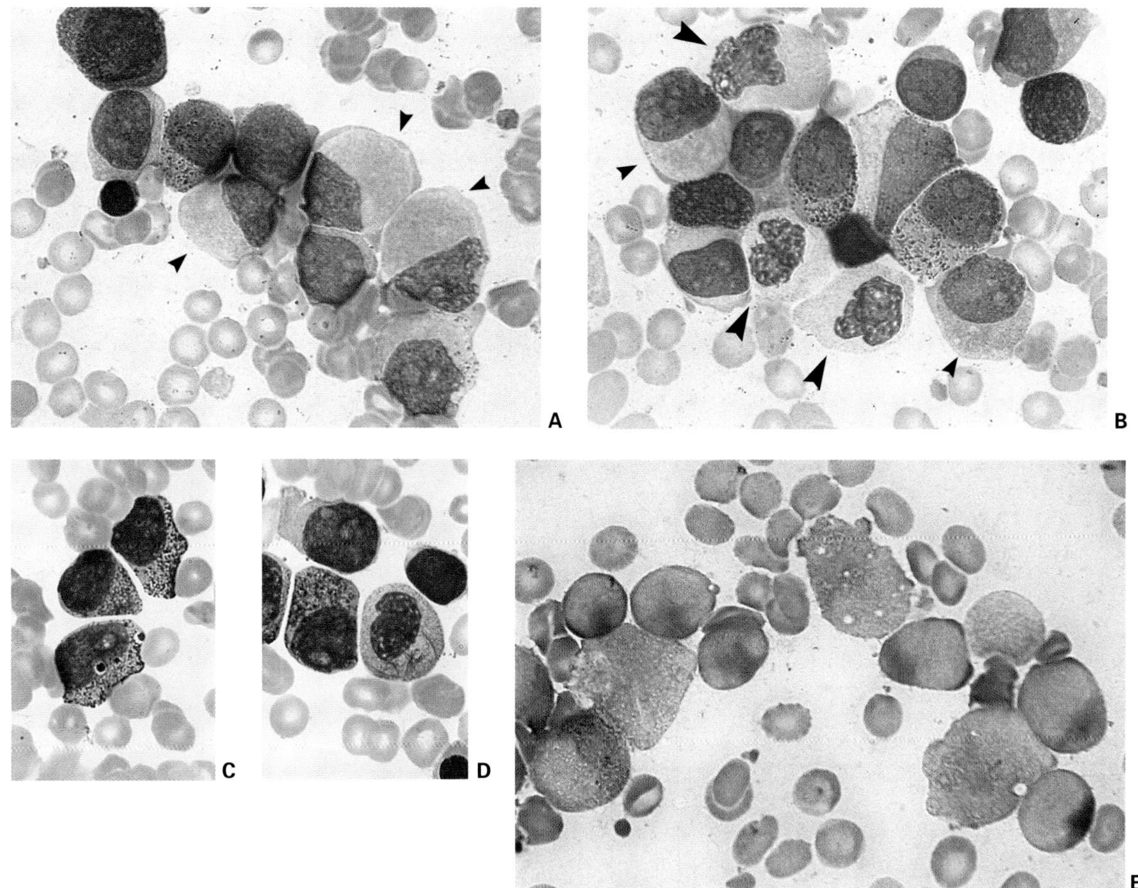

Fig. 5.3 AML M2 with abnormal neutrophils. **a**,**b** 5-year-old boy, karyotype normal. **c**,**d** 2-year-old boy with prominent lymph node enlargement, karyotype not done. **e** 9-year-old girl, monosomy X the only cytogenetic abnormality. In **a**, 3 promyelocytes contain agranular, orange-grey cytoplasm (arrows, compare with normal promyelocyte in field). **b** shows 2 granulated promyelocytes, 2 agranular promyelocytes (small arrows) and 3 Pelgerized, agranular, segmented neutrophils (large arrows). In **c**, a promyelocyte contains large, densely-staining granules. **d** The segmented neutrophil contains fine Auer rods. **e** ANAE positive myeloid cells (fluoride inhibited).

- In a rare variant, a few precursor cells contain sparse, large, densely-staining granules, with Auer rods most frequent in or confined to mature cells (Fig. 5.3, more readily detectable in blood than in marrow). The occurrence of Auer rods in mature neutrophils may be specific to AML M2 (Stass et al 1984).
- Intracellular Charcot-Leyden crystals in leukaemia are a sign of dyspoiesis (Fig. 5.6). These differ from Auer rods in Romanowsky staining (colourless or grey), size (larger), shape (needle, boat, compass-needle), cytochemistry (negative with routine stains) and ultrastructure (no discernible ordered structure).
- Giant, Chediak-Higashi-like granules are noted in rare cases (Tulliez et al 1979).
- Other kinds of aberration may be noted (Figs 5.4, 5.5).

Eosinophils (Fig. 5.4)
- Atypical cytochemistry, e.g. CAE positivity.
- Abnormality in structure, with or without increase in number. In mature cells, specific granules are large and crowd the cytoplasm giving the cell a cobbled outline ('sago grain' appearance). The granule rim is prominent and grey-coloured granules may be conspicuous. Primary granules may be unusually coarse in myelocytes and persist into mature stages. Electron microscopy shows asynchrony in maturation of nucleus and granules. The granules may be PAS positive (normally negative or mildly positive). The abnormality differs from that in M4Eo (p. 158).
- Hypogranulation (Fig. 5.5).
- Auer rods.
- Intracellular Charcot-Leyden crystals. These may occur in normal eosinophils and macrophages in gross, benign eosinophilias (Fig. 6.49). In the absence of gross eosinophilia (Fig. 5.4), they are an indication of dyspoiesis (gross eosinophilia is rare in myeloid leukaemias). They are not seen in ALL (but free-lying crystals may be seen in marrow necrosis, Fig. 4.13).

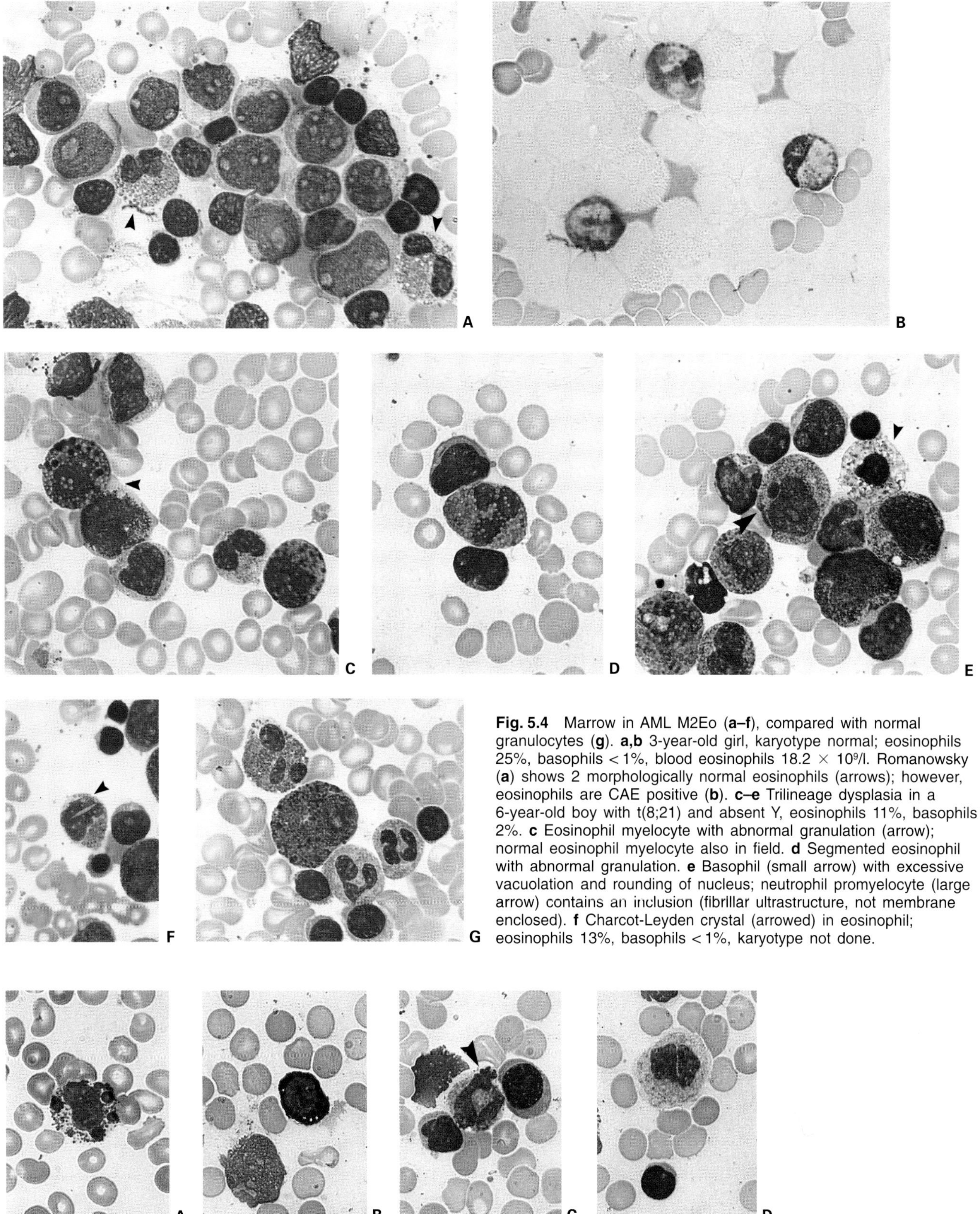

Fig. 5.4 Marrow in AML M2Eo (**a–f**), compared with normal granulocytes (**g**). **a,b** 3-year-old girl, karyotype normal; eosinophils 25%, basophils < 1%, blood eosinophils 18.2 × 10^9/l. Romanowsky (**a**) shows 2 morphologically normal eosinophils (arrows); however, eosinophils are CAE positive (**b**). **c–e** Trilineage dysplasia in a 6-year-old boy with t(8;21) and absent Y, eosinophils 11%, basophils 2%. **c** Eosinophil myelocyte with abnormal granulation (arrow); normal eosinophil myelocyte also in field. **d** Segmented eosinophil with abnormal granulation. **e** Basophil (small arrow) with excessive vacuolation and rounding of nucleus; neutrophil promyelocyte (large arrow) contains an inclusion (fibrillar ultrastructure, not membrane enclosed). **f** Charcot-Leyden crystal (arrowed) in eosinophil; eosinophils 13%, basophils < 1%, karyotype not done.

Fig. 5.5 Trilineage dysplasia, marrow AML M2, del 7q and monosomy 7. **a** Basophil with giant granulation. **b** Micro mast cell. **c** Pyknosis in extrusion of neutrophil nucleus. **d** Large, hypogranular eosinophil. Differential included basophils 6%, eosinophils 4%.

Basophils (Fig. 5.6)

- Intracellular Charcot-Leyden crystals in the absence of gross increase in cell number.
- Coarse densely-staining granules, usually metachromatic with toluidine blue or astra blue (Fig. 5.6). Karyotypes which may be preferentially associated with this variant are t/del(12)(p11–13) and t(6;9)(p23;q34).
- Giant, Chediak-Higashi-like granulation (Fig. 5.5).

Mast cells

Aberrant mast cells occur in rare cases (Fig. 5.5).

Differential diagnosis

Myeloid leukaemoid reactions with a small percentage of myeloblasts may occur in viral infections, often with anaemia and thrombocytopenia, and may persist for weeks to months. Marrow myeloblasts however are not, or are only slightly, increased (< 5%).

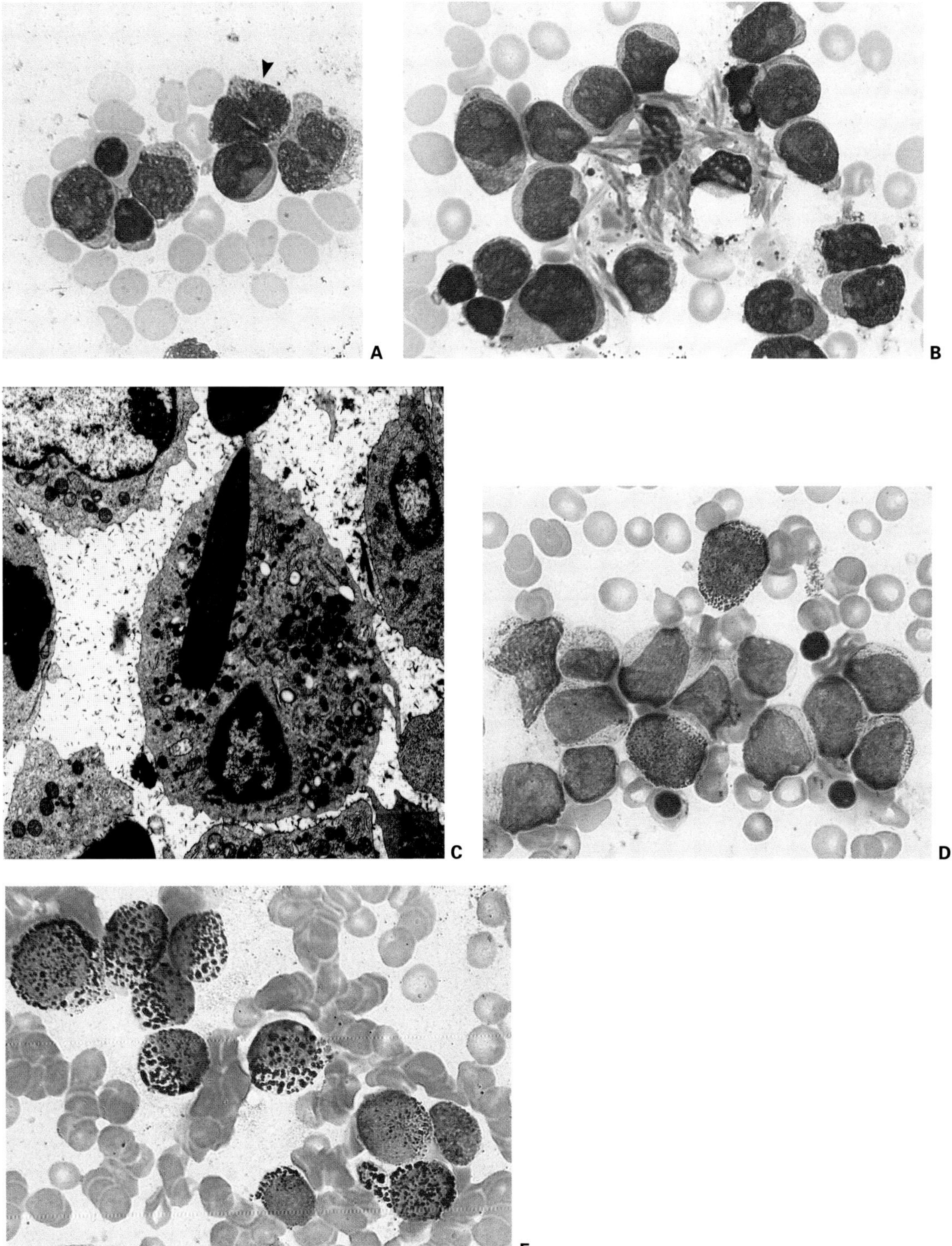

Fig. 5.6 Marrow, AML M2Baso. **a–c** Charcot-Leyden crystals in an 8-year-old with trisomy 8, eosinophils 0.5%, basophils 5.5%. **a** Crystal in basophil (arrow). **b** Crystals in macrophage. **c** Crystal in neutrophil; absence of containing vacuole suggests in situ formation rather than phagocytosis. × 6000. **d** M2 in a 2-year-old relapsing 2 ½ years later as M2Baso (**e**); granulation only weakly metachromatic with toluidine blue. Karyotype of **e** showed clonal evolution only.

AML M3 (ACUTE PROMYELOCYTIC LEUKAEMIA, APML) (Fig. 5.7)

About 10% of AML.

Identifying characteristics

1. A dominant population (> 50%) in marrow of promyelocytes with specific abnormality:

- azurophilic granulation usually profuse and obscuring the Golgi area and often nucleus. Overspill of granules outside cells is characteristic.
- contortion of nuclei into folds, reniform or bilobed shapes; these cells may be sparse, but should be carefully sought because of their importance for diagnosis.

2. MPO, SBB and CAE positive.
3. Blast cell numbers variable, usually less than the 30% required for diagnosis of acute leukaemia.
4. Erythroblasts < 50% of nucleated cells.
5. Monocytic forms < 30% of marrow cells or blood leucocytes.

Other characteristics

In occasional cases granulation is sparse or apparently absent (Fig. 5.7). Auer rods occur in about half of patients, usually with some grouping into faggots; they are MPO, SBB and CAE positive and weakly PAS positive. Auer rods may occur, by phagocytosis, in marrow macrophages.

A diffuse pink flush with PAS is characteristic; occasional cases are ANAE positive, fluoride inhibited; AcPh is strongly positive. Trilineage dysplasia is rare (compare with other types of AML).

Cytogenetics
See Table 5.2.

Depletion of coagulation factors is common and may become more pronounced or manifest first after chemotherapy. Although release of thromboplastic and fibrinolytic substances in the granules is a possible explanation, hyperfibrinolysis and proteolysis from hyperplasminaemia due to α_2 antiplasmin deficiency appear to be important (Kahle et al 1985).

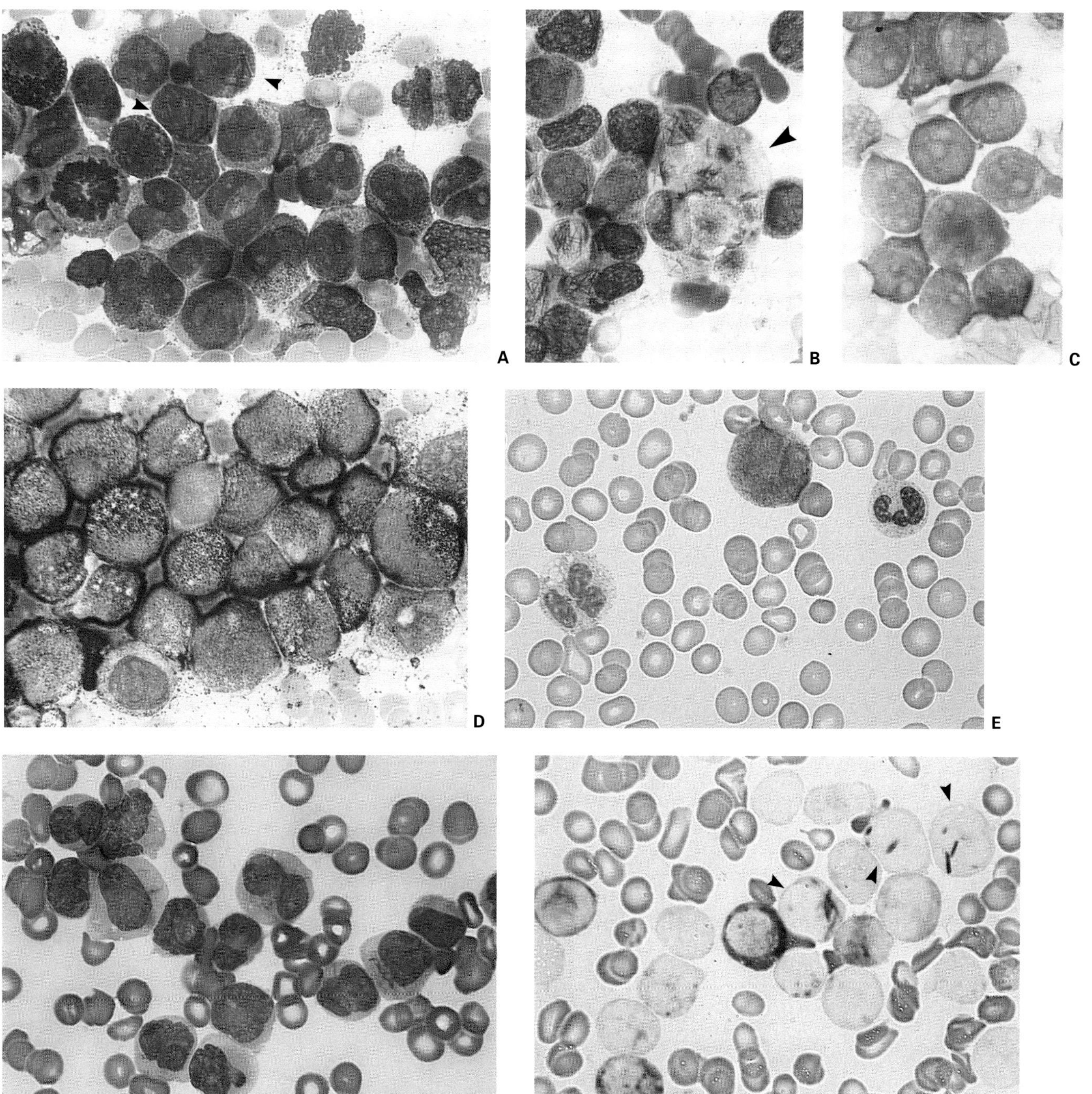

Fig. 5.7 AML M3. **a–c** Typical disease, karyotype t(15;17); arrows show Auer rods in leukaemic cells (**a**) and in marrow macrophage (**b**). Blush with PAS (**c**). **d,e** Atypical M3 in a 14-month-old with trisomy 6 and pericentric inversion of 3, no t(15;17). **d** Marrow, there are no Auer rods. **e** Blood, promyelocyte with contorted nucleus, a normal and a large neutrophil. **f,g** Blood, atypical M3 in an 11-year-old, karyotype not done. The profusion (leucocyte count 162 × 10^9/l) of monocytoid, agranular leukaemic cells was strongly positive with CAE (**g**) as well as with MPO. Arrows show CAE-positive Auer rods. Marrow was typical M3.

Variants (Fig. 5.8)

- Microgranular

This is less common than the hypergranular form. Granules are finer or not discernible (electron microscopy shows numerous granules), and Auer rods less profuse. Some hypergranular cells or cells with contorted nucleus are usually present, however, and should be carefully sought because of their importance for diagnosis. Blood leucocyte count is usually higher than in standard M3. In other aspects — cytochemistry, karyotype and association with coagulopathy — microgranular and standard M3 are similar.

- Other

An unusual promyelocytic leukaemia is shown in Figure 5.8. Marrow differential included blast cells 4% and neutrophil promyelocytes 68%. The occurrence of granule 'balls' and their ultrastructure suggest that the inclusions are granule agglutinates formed as a perverted development of the normal evolution/ discharge of granules in immature neutrophils. A slight increase in fibrin degradation products was the only coagulation abnormality.

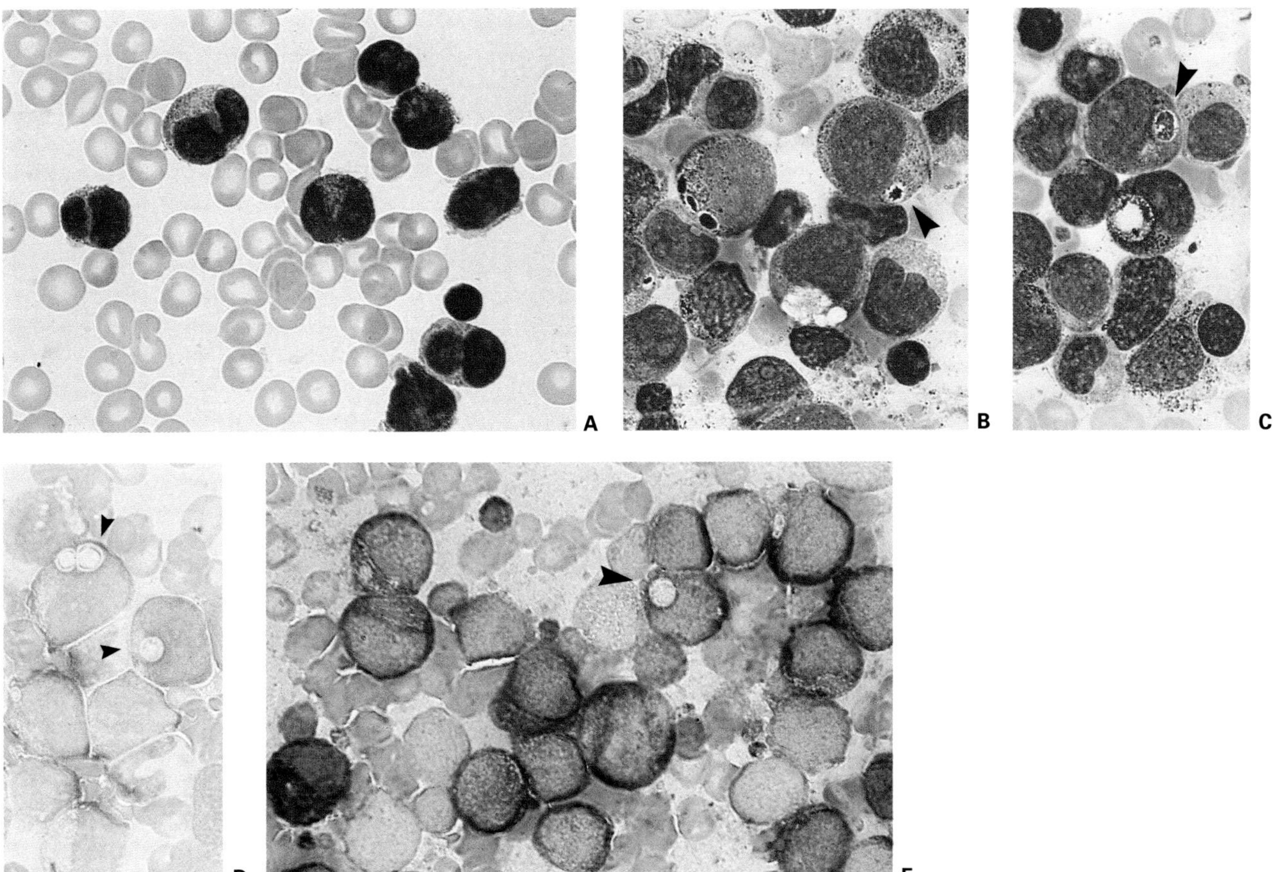

Fig. 5.8 AML M3 variants. **a** Microgranular, normal karyotype (pre-banding). **b–e** 18-month-old girl, t(11;19). **b,c** Promyelocytes contain granulated and smooth bodies within vacuoles; arrows show granule balls interpreted as an early stage in formation of inclusions. **d** Metachromatic rings (toluidine blue). **e** ANAE, strong staining of myeloid cells (fluoride sensitive); arrow shows positive ring in vacuole.

Differential diagnosis

Promyelocytic hyperplasia in marrow may occur in infection and drug induced marrow damage (Innes et al 1987). The promyelocytes show only minor changes; obscuration of the Golgi zone by granules, nuclear contortion and Auer rods do not occur. In CMV infection, the marrow may contain small numbers of multinucleate cells with intranuclear inclusions, which appear to be specific for CMV (Fig. 5.9, Chesney et al 1978).

AML M4 (ACUTE MYELOMONOCYTIC LEUKAEMIA, AMML)

Less than 5% of AML. A leukaemia with simultaneous participation of granulocytes and monocytes.

Identifying characteristics

- Granulocytic component:
1. undifferentiated blast cells > 5% of marrow cells
2. evidence of maturation — blast cells + more mature forms ≥ 20%.
- Monocytic component:
1. marrow monoblasts, promonocytes + monocytes ≥ 20%, and/or
2. blood monocytes ≥ $5.0 \times 10^9/l$
3. lysozyme in serum or urine significantly increased (> 3 × upper normal).
- Erythroblasts < 20% of marrow cells.

Other characteristics

Auer rods are usually sparse (granulocytes, monocytes or both). In most cases the monocytic cells are ANAE positive, fluoride sensitive. Trilineage dysplasia occurs in about 15%.

Cytogenetics
See Table 5.2.

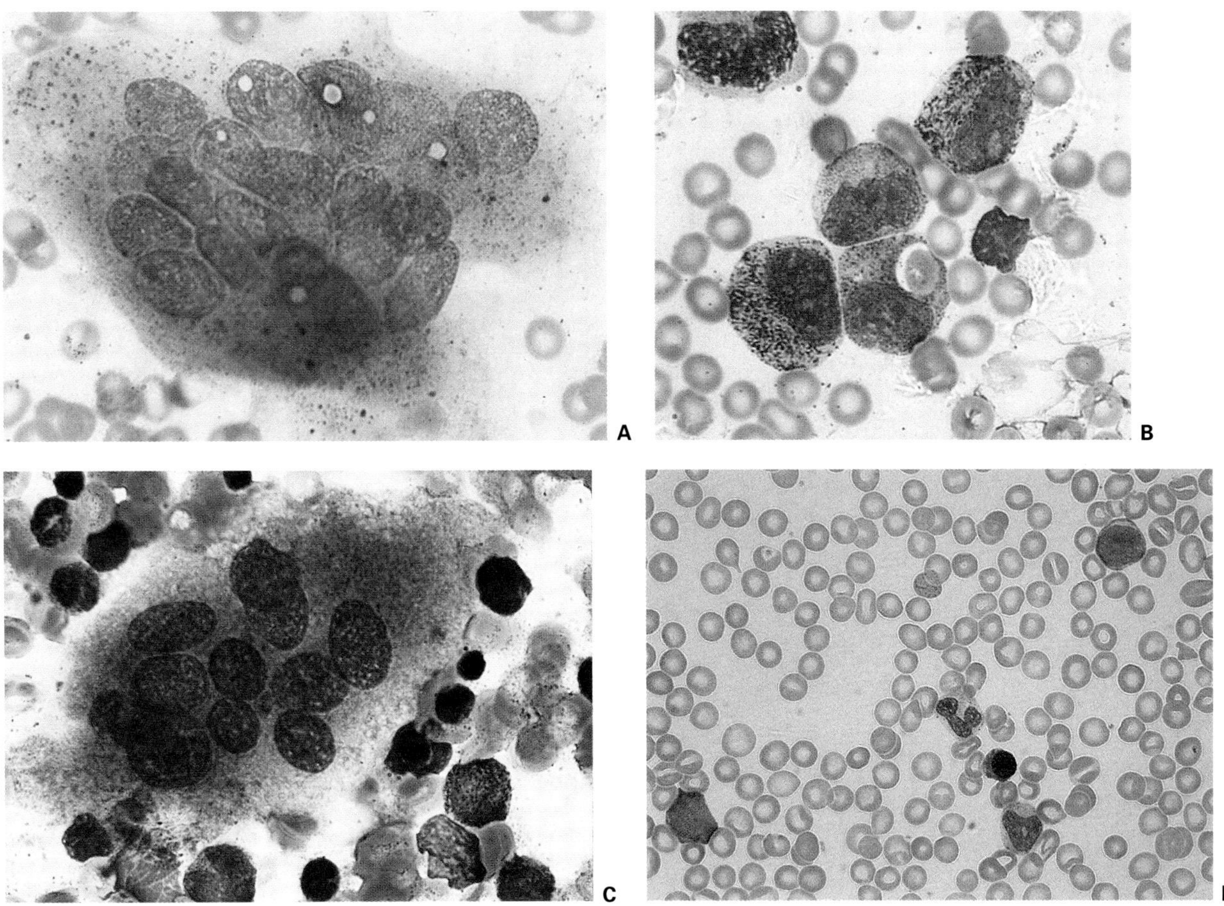

Fig. 5.9 Myeloid leukaemoid reactions. **a,b** CMV infection mimicking AML M3. Marrow of 19-month-old child with pancytopenia and promyelocytic hyperplasia (51% of cells), fibrinogen 95 mg/100 ml and serum paraprotein band (?CMV antibody) which disappeared over several months. **a** Multinucleate cell of unknown nature with intranuclear inclusions; cf osteoclast (**c**). **b** Promyelocytes, one containing an erythrocyte, no Auer rods. **d** Blood, M4-like myelomonocytosis in a 2-month-old with CMV infection; field includes 2 leucoblasts and an erythroblast; monocytes 5.4, platelets 117 $\times$ 10^9/l; marrow blasts $<$ 1%. **d** $\times$ 500

Variants

M4Eo (Fig. 5.10)
In childhood, most M4 cases are M4Eo. In marrow, coarse densely-staining primary granules are prominent in precursor eosinophils; segmented forms may show persistence of azurophil granules and deficiency of specific granules, vacuolation may be prominent and unusually large forms are frequent. Eosinophil cytochemistry may be atypical, e.g. PAS and CAE (Fig. 5.4). Charcot-Leyden crystals may be evident in macrophages. Marrow eosinophils may be increased. In contrast to marrow, eosinophils in blood are usually normal in structure and numbers.

Cytogenetics
See Table 5.2.

M4Baso
Perverted development of basophils or of both eosinophils and basophils is rarer than M4Eo.

Differential diagnosis

Viruses such as CMV may produce a myelomonocytosis (Fig. 5.9).

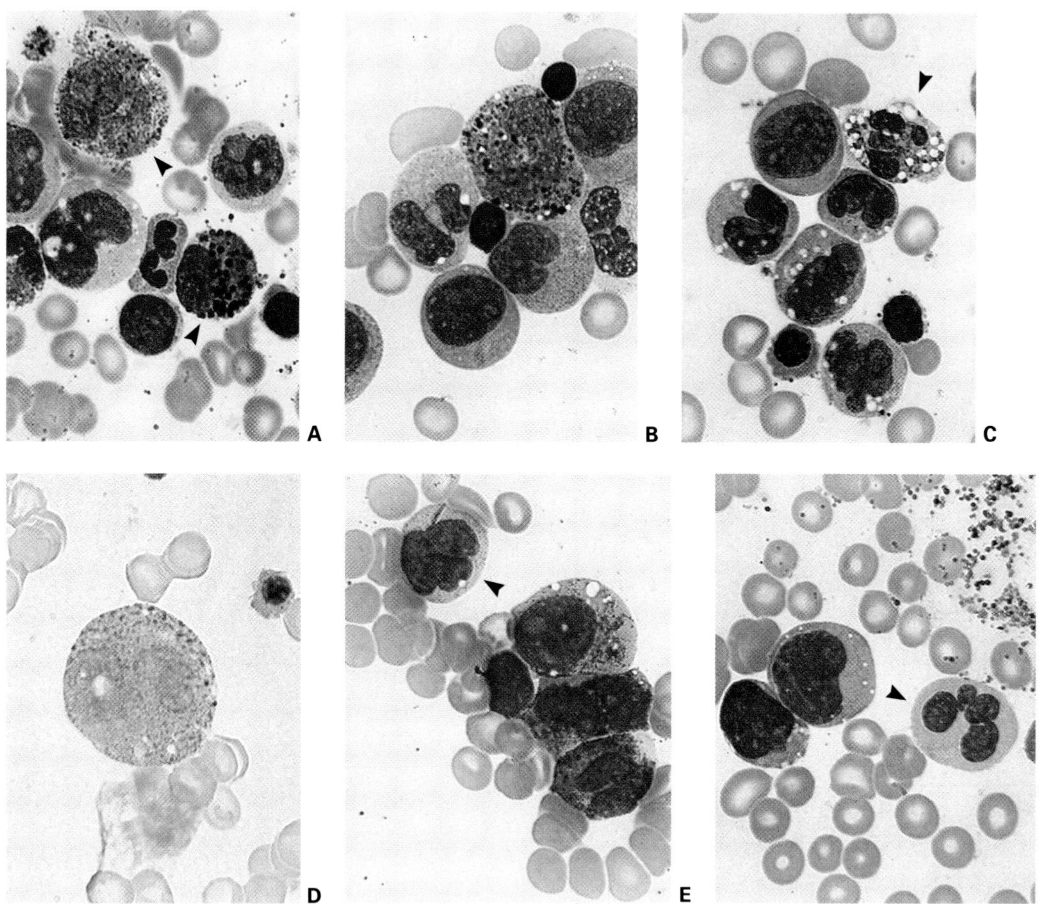

Fig. 5.10 AML M4Eo. **a** 12-year-old, karyotype (pre-banding) normal; coarse azurophil granulation in myelocyte and persisting azurophil granulation in mature form (arrows). **b–d** 15-year-old, pericentric inversion of 16 and terminal deletion 9q. Large stab eosinophil with persisting azurophil granulation, large neutrophil adjacent in **b**. Vacuolation and persisting azurophil granulation in segmented eosinophil (arrow) in **c**. Large eosinophil with diffuse and granular PAS staining in **d**. **e,f** 10-month-old with pericentric inversion of 16 and del 11q; monoblast containing Auer rod, and an agranular monocyte (arrows).

AML M5 (ACUTE MONOCYTIC)

(Figs 5.11, 5.12)

About 15% of AML. 5a is more common than 5b.

Identifying characteristics

Monocytoid cells ≥ 80% of marrow cells:

- 5a (monoblastic): ≥ 80% of monocytoid cells are monoblasts, the remainder promonocytes and monocytes
- 5b (monocytic): < 80% of monocytoid cells are monoblasts.

Other characteristics

Auer rods are rare. Occasional cells may contain erythrocytes or nucleated cells.

Usually a majority of cells is positive for ANAE and ANBE, with fluoride inhibition; rarely, reaction is negative (Fig. 5.12). MPO and SBB are rarely strong and occasionally negative. AcPh is diffusely positive, with tartrate inhibition. CAE is negative to weak; rare cases show an aberrant strong reaction. PAS is negative, or if positive, in a diffuse pattern with or without superimposed granulation or rarely blocks. β glucuronidase is usually strong (myeloid pattern).

An increase in lysozyme in serum or urine occurs in most cases (≥ 3 × upper normal to be considered significant). Depletion of coagulation factors is noted in about one fifth of cases, usually not as severe as in AML M3. Adenovirus particles were noted in one of our cases (Fig. 5.11); although this was most likely a secondary infection, adenovirus has oncogenic potential for animal cells (Benjamin & Vogt 1991). Monoblasts often mark for the T cell marker CD4 (receptor for HIV).

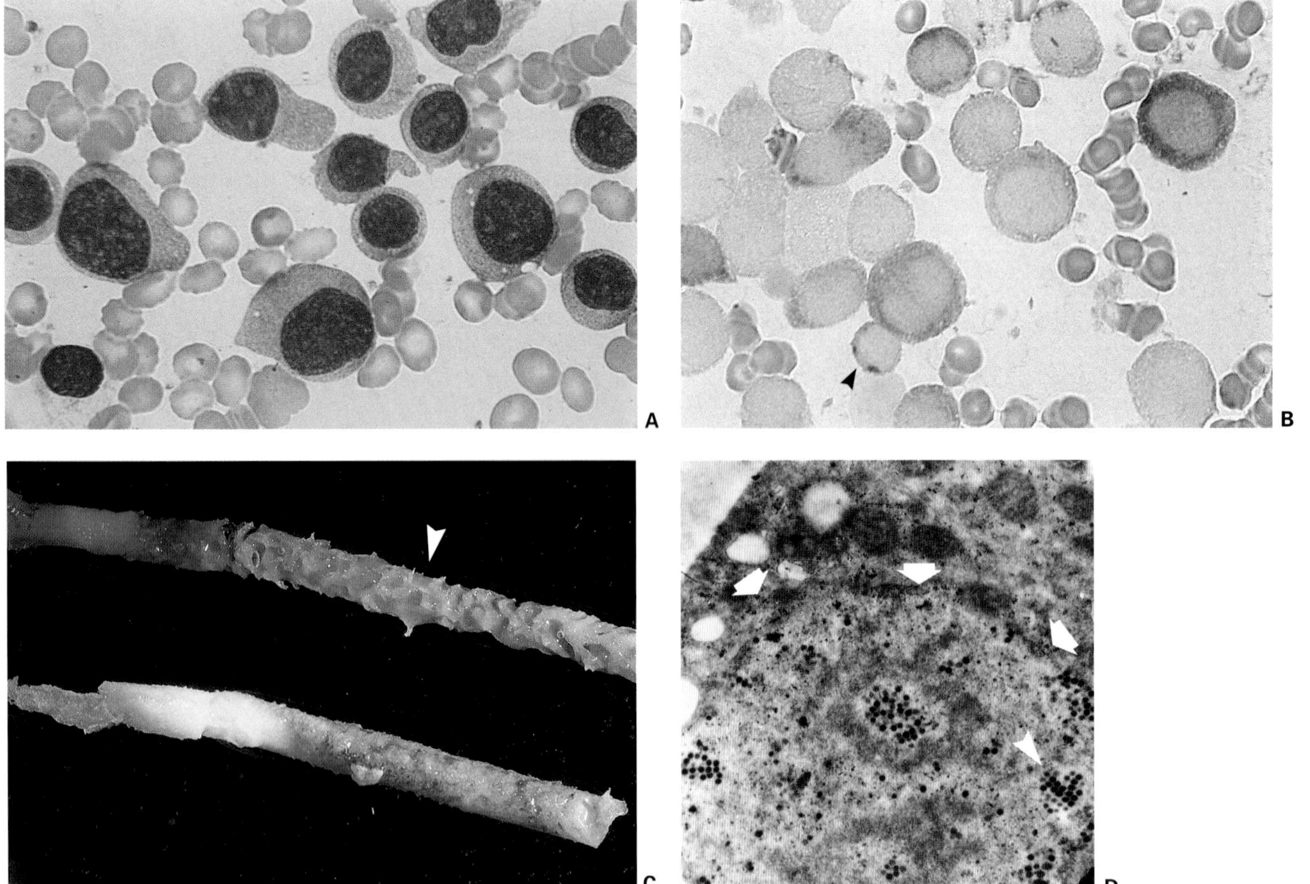

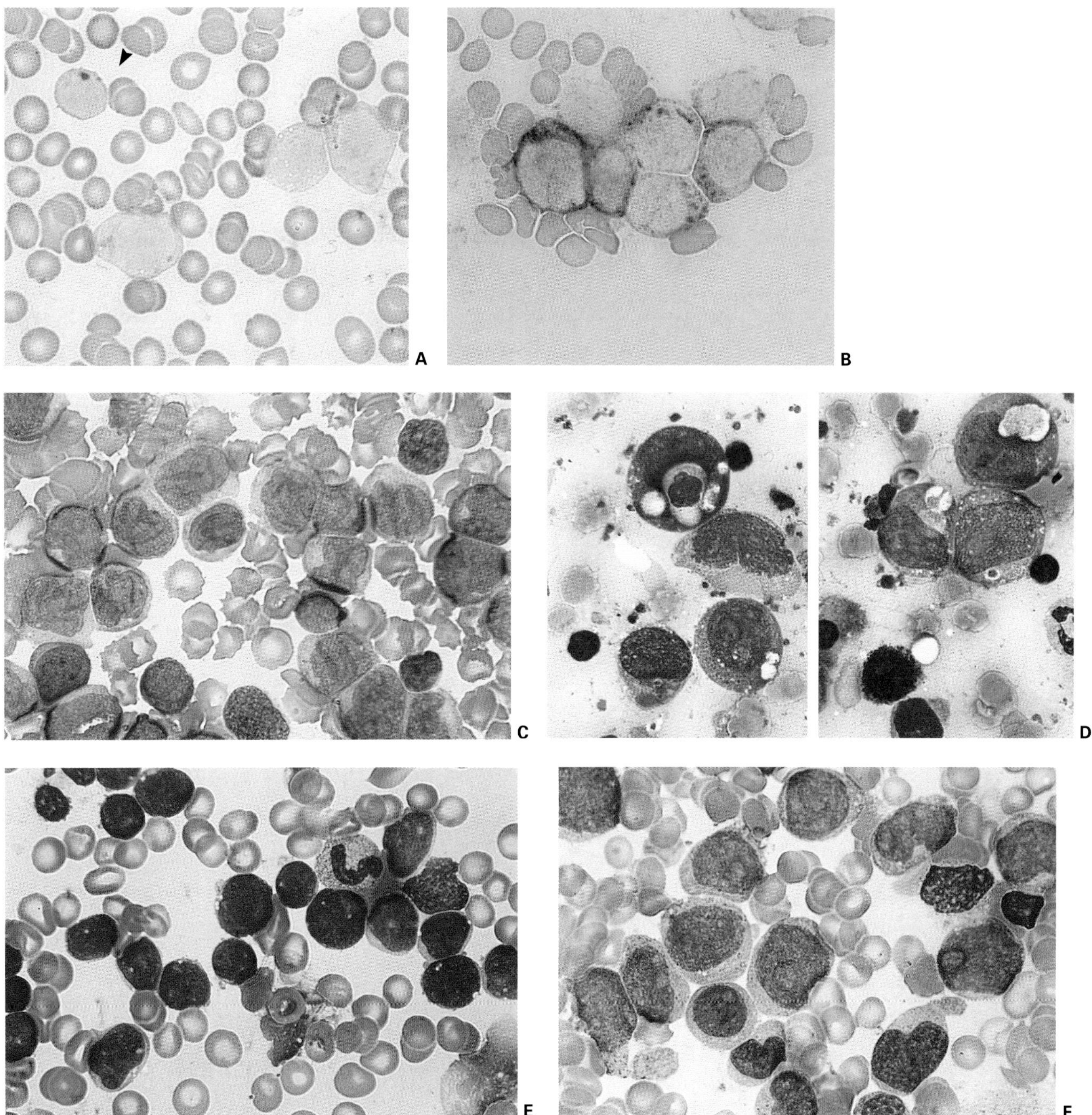

Fig. 5.12 AML M5a, unusual types. **a–c** ANAE negative. **a,b** Marrow, 18-month-old, serum muramidase only slightly raised, deletion 11q. **a** ANAE, showing 3 monoblasts (negative) and lymphocyte (arrow). **b** β glucuronidase, showing granular + diffuse myeloid pattern. **c** Blood, 1-day-old infant, leucocytes 632 × 10⁹/l, serum muramidase 4.3 × upper normal. **d** Haemophagocytic variant, 7-month-old girl, karyotype hyperdiploidy only; inclusions of erythrocytes and unidentified cellular material. **e,f** As a relapse (**f**) 15 months after ALL 'common' markers (**e**). Karyotype of **e** unobtainable because of insufficient metaphases; karyotype of **f** normal. **d** Courtesy of Dr B Williams

Fig. 5.11 (facing page) AML M5a. **a,b** Some cells are elongated. ANAE (**b**) shows diffuse and granular reaction; cf spotty reaction in lymphocyte (arrow). **c** Trephine biopsies, patient (arrow) vs normal (× 7). **d** Adenovirus particles, approx 50 nm, in nucleus of degenerate eukaemic cell; arrows show outline of nucleus; arrowhead shows crystalline array. × 12 000. These particles were not seen in 8 other cases examined by electron microscopy.

A proportion of cases is congenital (Fig. 5.12). In these cases clinical evidence of leukaemia (e.g. subcutaneous infiltrates) may disappear spontaneously to be followed, however, by aggressive disease, usually within 18 months. The marrow may be morphologically normal early in the disease. The karyotype, however, may be abnormal when the marrow is of normal morphology.

Monocytic leukaemia may rarely present as a relapse after ALL (Fig. 5.12).

Cytogenetics
See Table 5.2.

Variant

A variant (Fig. 5.12) is characterized by prominent haemophagocytosis (especially erythrophagocytosis), and often t(8;16).

AML M6 (AML WITH PREDOMINANTLY ERYTHROID DIFFERENTIATION)

This is rare in childhood (< 5% of AML). Two varieties occur — classic M6 (di Guglielmo disease) and blastosis of morphologically undifferentiated cells.

Classic AML M6 (di Guglielmo disease)
(Fig. 5.13)

Identifying characteristics

- Erythroblasts ≥ 50% of marrow cells
- Blast cells ≥ 30% of non-erythroid cells (lower if Auer rods present).

Other characteristics

Dyserythropoiesis is usual, with megaloblastosis, giant forms and phagocytosis, especially of erythroblasts. Erythroblasts often are PAS positive, in a diffuse or granular pattern. Some erythrocytes may be diffusely PAS positive. Erythroblasts may be positive for ANAE, ANBE and AcPh (which may be focal). In a minority ringed sideroblasts are prominent.

Macrocytic megaloblastic anaemia, usually as part of a pancytopenia, and resistant to treatment with folate and B_{12}, is common and may precede overt myeloblastosis (Fig. 5.13).

The non-erythroid component resembles AML except M3. Auer rods are usual.

Cytogenetics
See Table 5.2.

The natural history is of progression to blastic AML M1, 2 or 4.

Differential diagnosis

Dyserythropoiesis occurs in:

- megaloblastic anaemias; erythroblasts may be positive for AcPh, ANAE and rarely PAS
- congenital dyserythropoietic anaemias
- patients receiving cytotoxics, especially cytosine arabinoside or methotrexate
- thalassaemia major; erythroblasts may be PAS positive; thalassaemic blood changes (p. 24)
- iron deficiency anaemia, severe haemolysis — minor dysplasia only; associated blood changes.

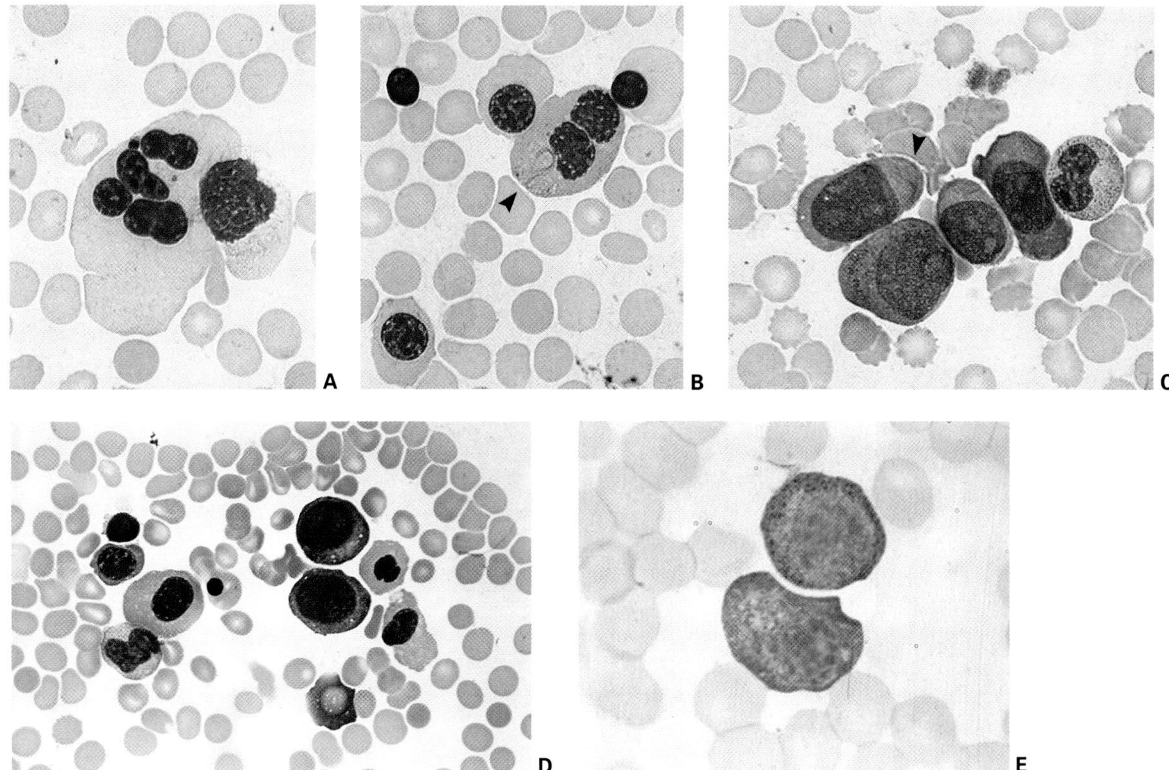

Fig. 5.13 Marrow, AML M6. **a–c** 13-year-old boy. **a** Giant erythroblast. **b** Cabot ring (arrow) in erythroblast in mitosis. **c** Field containing 2 myeloblasts (one with Auer rods, arrow), neutrophil promyelocyte, megaloblastoid erythroblast, Pelgerized neutrophil.
d,e 9-month-old boy presenting as refractory megaloblastic anaemia. PAS (**e**) shows diffuse and granular staining in erythroblasts. Myeloblastosis was not evident till 3 months later. **d** × 500; **e** × 1000

AML M6 with morphologically undifferentiated blast cells (blastic AML M6) (Fig. 5.14)

Identifying characteristics

- Blast cells ≥ 30% of marrow cells
- Evidence of erythroblastic differentiation:

1. Demonstration by monoclonal or polyclonal antibodies of specifically erythroblastic components, e.g. MN antigens. Monoclonals for glycophorins A and C are suitable for marrow films and trephine biopsies, the A giving a stronger reaction and in a greater proportion of erythroblasts than C.
2. Lymphoid markers negative.

Other characteristics

Cells in some cases are ALL-like in morphology, and in others appear myeloid. Siderotic granules may be demonstrable. Ultrastructural cytochemistry is negative for MPO.

Differential diagnosis

From other blastic leukaemias, by immunophenotyping.

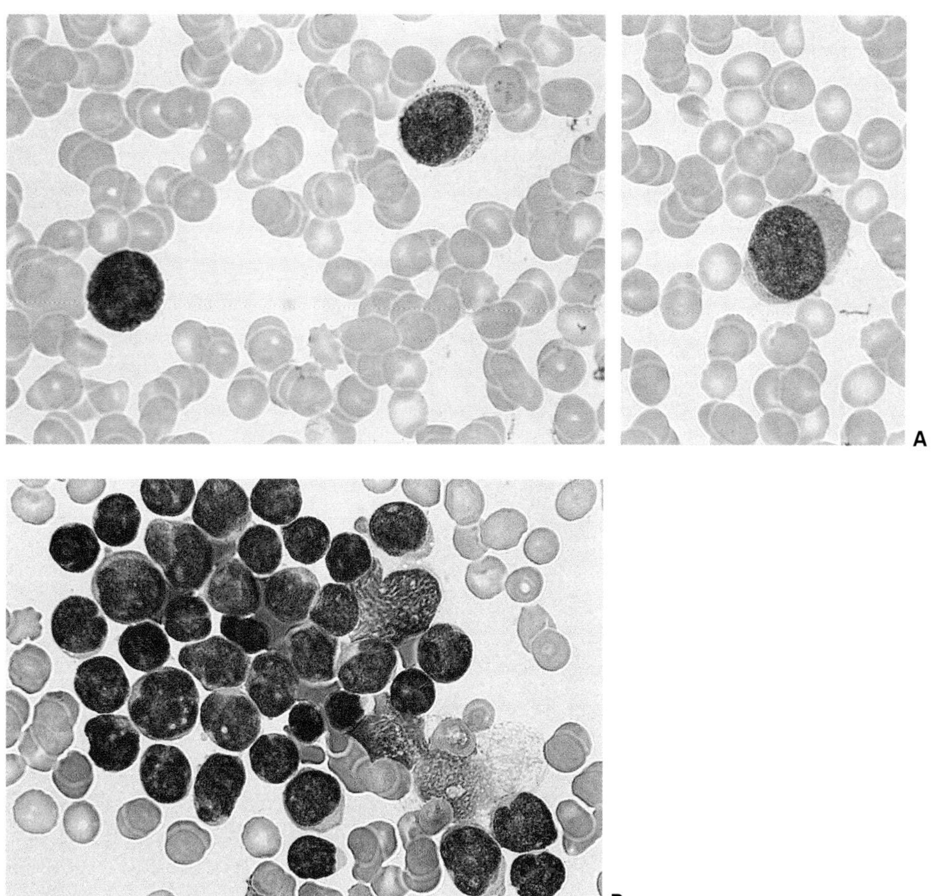

Fig. 5.14 Blastic AML M6. **a** Blastic and granulated leukaemic cells in a 2-year-old with Down's syndrome; MPO (light microscopy) equivocal. **b** ALL-like morphology in a 5-year-old boy, MPO negative.

AML M7 (ACUTE MEGAKARYOBLASTIC LEUKAEMIA) (Fig. 5.15)

Less than 5% of AML. Fetal leukaemia is described (Swirsky D M 1993, personal communication).

Identifying characteristics

- Blast cells ≥ 30% of marrow cells
- Evidence of megakaryocytic differentiation:

1. Cytology

Features suggestive of megakaryocytic differentiation include: oval, elongated or tailed forms, blebs, paranuclear clustering of vacuoles, micro and mononuclear megakaryocytes and large or bizarre platelets.

2. Cytochemistry

Leukaemic cells may be ANAE positive (stronger in more mature cells), fluoride sensitivity variable; cells are negative for MPO, SBB and CAE.

3. Immunophenotype

The most specific and useful monoclonal antibodies for films and trephine biopsies are:

a. CD61 (GpIIIa on megakaryocytes, platelets, endothelium). GpIIIa is expressed early in megakaryocyte development and CD61 identifies > 90% of cases.
b. CD42a,b (Gp Ib–IX on megakaryocytes, platelets) is positive in about 75% of cases.
c. Antibodies to FVIII Rag are less useful as FVIII is not expressed till late in maturation.

4. Ultrastructural cytochemistry

PPO is glutaraldehyde and formaldehyde sensitive and localized to the perinuclear space and endoplasmic reticulum.

Other characteristics

In some cases the leukaemic cells resemble lymphoblasts or myeloblasts.

PAS is positive in more mature cells, as granules or coarse deposits, with or without a diffuse background. Granules may be clustered within blebs; AcPh is usually positive, tartrate sensitive. ANBE is weak to negative.

Myelofibrosis is common and attributed to excessive production of platelet-derived growth factor. Difficulty in aspiration may necessitate use of collagenase-treated trephine samples to obtain satisfactory cell suspensions.

Cytogenetics

See Table 5.2. Patients with Down's syndrome are at risk for AML M7 (Zipursky et al 1992). About 20% of leukaemias in Down's syndrome are M7, compared with approximately 1% in non-Down's children.

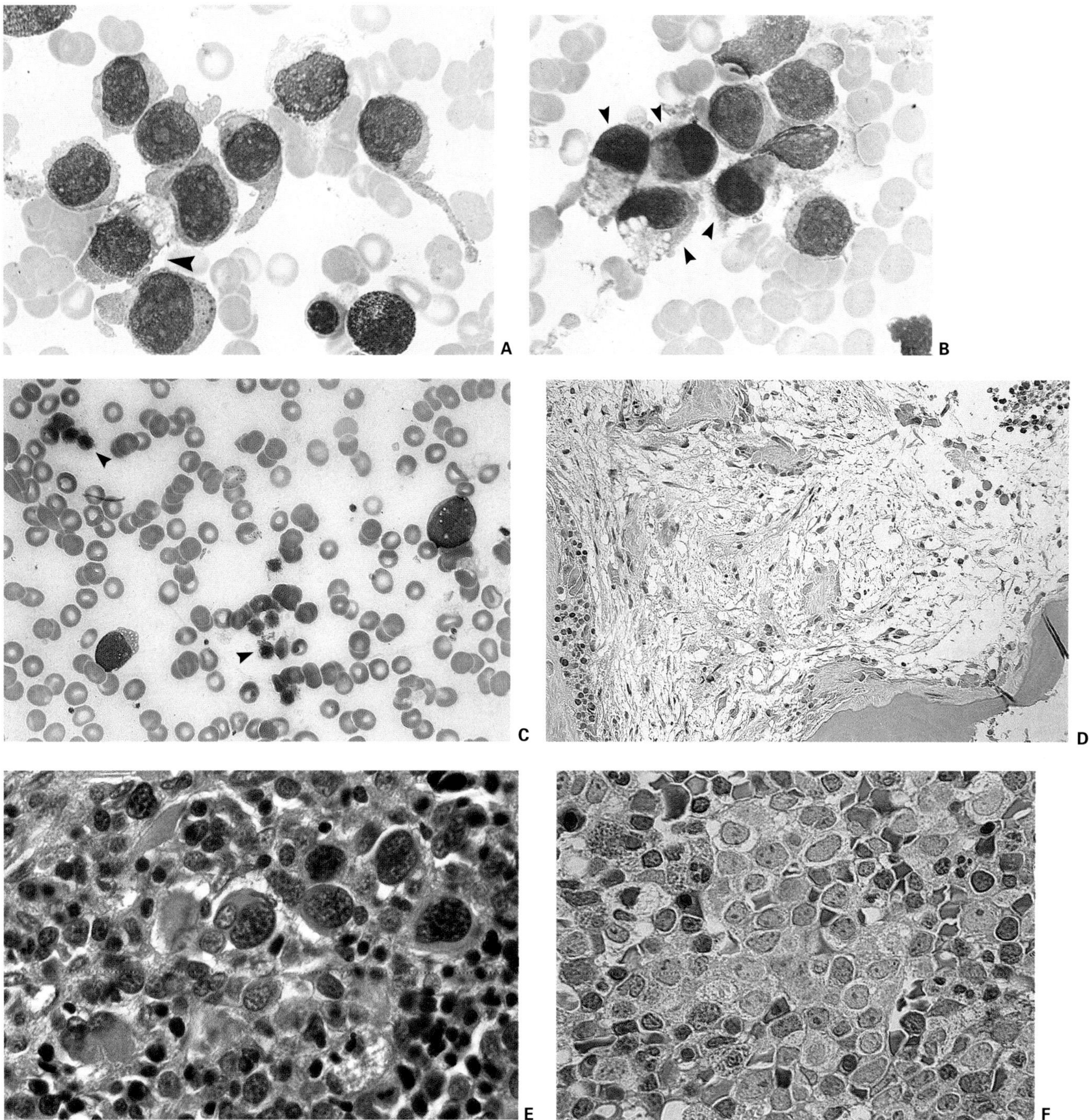

Fig. 5.15 Marrow, AML M7. **a,b** 22-month-old girl, isochromosome 21q. **a** Cells with tails and pseudopodia, and a micromegakaryoblast (arrow). **b** 4 micromegakaryocytes (arrows) and 3 blast cells. **c,d** 5-year-old girl, insufficient metaphases for karyotype. **c** Hypocellular aspirate, 2 undistinguished blast cells (29% of total), groups of large platelets (arrows) which had normal surface Gp. **d** Hypocellular, fibrotic trephine biopsy. **e** 7-year-old girl, abnormal megakaryocytes in trephine biopsy; reticulin stain showed increase in fibrous tissue.
f 18-month-old boy, complex karyotype including ring 7. Infiltrate of undistinguished blast cells in cellular marrow, no fibrosis. **a,b** × 750; **c** × 500; **d** H & E × 200; **e** H & E × 600; **f** H & E × 750. **e** Courtesy of Dr J Bell

Differential diagnosis

Transient abnormal myelopoiesis (TAM) of neonatal trisomy 21 (Bain 1991, Fig. 5.16, Table 5.3)
The TAM of neonatal trisomy 21 is to be considered as a cause of blastosis in infants under the age of 3 months. It is rare in older children.

The blast cells are negative for MPO and SBB, and in most cases ANAE is negative and PAS is negative to mild diffuse. A majority of blast cells are of megakaryocytic lineage on morphology (hypolobulated and micromegakaryocytes, giant and bizarre platelets), immunophenotype and ultrastructural evidence of PPO. A proportion of blast cells are undifferentiated myeloblasts or primitive erythroblasts.

Blood leucocyte counts of up to $470 \times 10^9/l$ are described (Nakagawa et al 1988). The percentage of blast cells in marrow is usually lower than in blood, and occasionally there is no blastosis in marrow when the blood is grossly affected. There is no or only mild anaemia, the neutrophil count is usually normal to high, and the platelet count variable — thrombocytopenia is common, but the count may exceed $1000 \times 10^9/l$. Eosinophils and basophils are increased in some cases. NAP is normal to high. Intravascular coagulation may occur, whilst hypoxia due to cardiac anomalies or hyperviscosity (from high leucocytosis) may produce coagulation factor deficiencies. Hepatosplenomegaly is usual. Transient subcutaneous masses, probably infiltrations, were noted in a personal case.

The trisomy may take one of 3 forms:

- constitutional, regular, clinically evident Down's syndrome
- constitutional mosaicism for trisomy 21, with the partial clinical appearances of Down's syndrome
- trisomy 21 confined to the abnormal cell population; these infants do not have the phenotype of Down's syndrome, the trisomy being demonstrable only in unstimulated blood and marrow and disappearing with the abnormal population.

An additional, cytogenetically abnormal clone of variable type occurs in a minority, and double minutes, characteristic of malignancy, occur in some cases. Analysis of chromosomal and DNA polymorphisms suggests that TAM is a result of disomic homozygosity, in most cases of maternal origin, for a mutant gene in the region 21q11.2 (Niikawa et al 1991).

Table 5.3 TAM vs AML in infants and children with trisomy 21

	TAM	AML
Age at onset	almost all < 3 months; likelihood of MPD in Down's neonate being TAM about 47%	any age; likelihood of MPD in Down's child > 3 months old being TAM about 2%
Subcutaneous infiltrates	occasionally	common in neonatal leukaemias
General health	usually not ill, unless has heart anomaly	usually ill, failure to thrive
Anaemia, neutropenia, thrombocytopenia	none or mild	common
Auer rods	very rare	often
Cytogenetics		
Marrow	trisomy 21; additional clonal abnormality in some	trisomy 21; additional clonal abnormality common[1]
Constitutional	trisomy 21 (regular or mosaic) or normal (trisomy confined to abnormal cells in phenotypically normal infant)	trisomy 21
Natural history	spontaneous resolution in < 3 months; true leukaemia later in up to 20%	remission rare and temporary, as in other neonatal leukaemias

[1] Hyperdiploidy, trisomy 8,19, quadrisomy or pentasomy 21 commonest

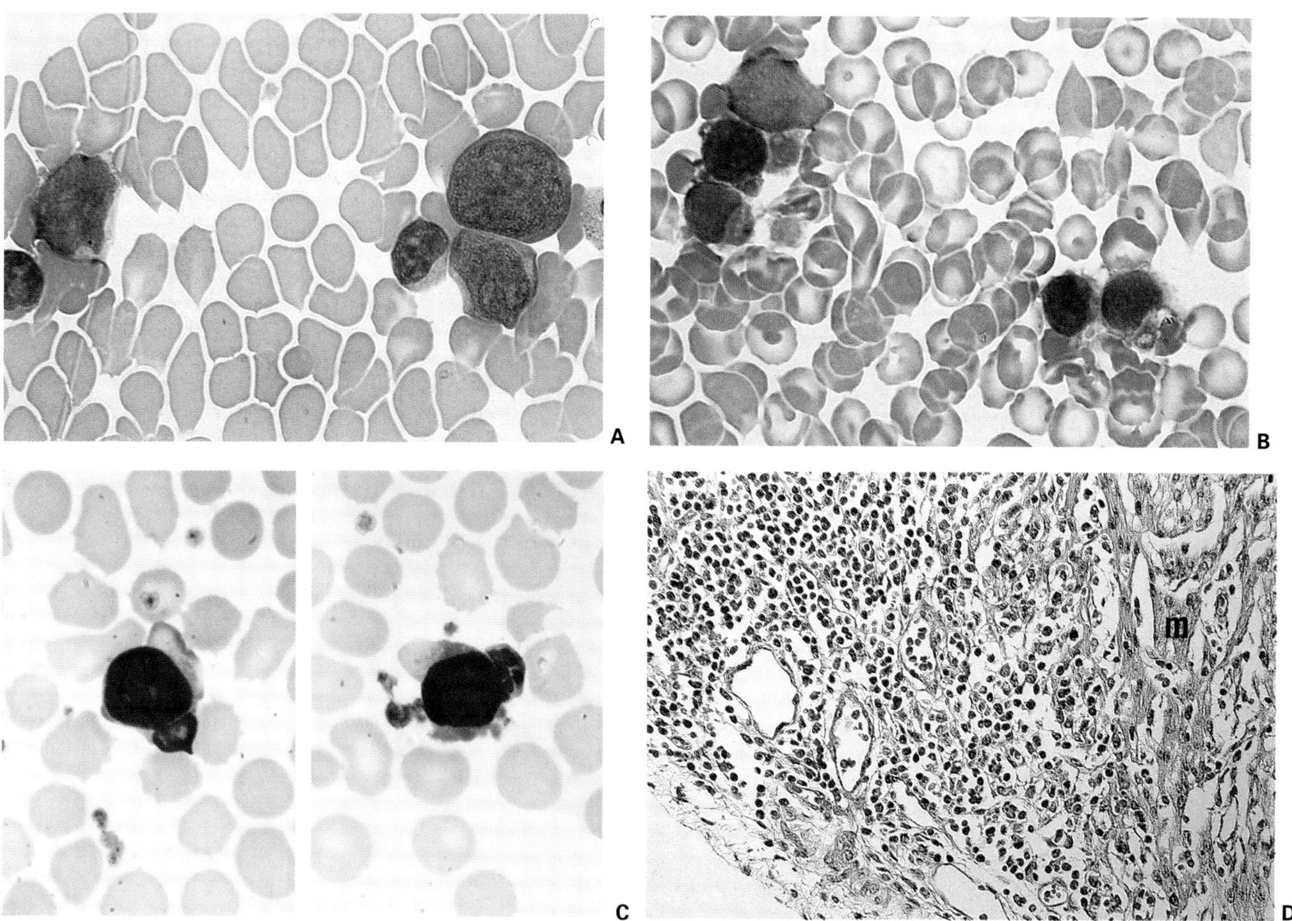

Fig. 5.16 TAM in neonatal/fetal trisomy 21. **a,b,d** Constitutional; **c** phenotypically normal infant. **a** Day 3, field with 3 blast cells. **b** Same infant, day 8, one blast cell and 4 megakaryoblasts (returned at 18 months with AML M7). **c** Another infant, day 13, degenerate blast cells, × 1000 (unanticoagulated blood film). **d** Nodule of myeloid cells at epicardial surface of heart (m = myocardial fibres) in 19-week-old Down's syndrome fetus, H & E × 200.

The blast cells disappear within 3 months. In infants who have died after disappearance of the blast cells, no morphologic evidence of blastic infiltration has been found. Death of blast cells (Fig. 5.16) may be noted as they disappear.

In up to 20% of cases a true leukaemia arises within 6 months to 3 years after the blast cells have disappeared. In most, the leukaemia is AML and, in a significant proportion, M7. It is not possible to predict with certainty which infants will develop leukaemia later. The occurrence of cytogenetic abnormality additional to trisomy 21 does not necessarily mean that true leukaemia will follow.

The reasons for the infrequency of TAM (of the order of 1% suggested) in, and its apparent specificity for trisomy 21 are unknown. We have noted the phenomenon as an apparently incidental histologic finding in one Down's syndrome fetus (of 5 whose blood or tissues were examined, Fig. 5.16).

Transient megakaryocytic dyspoiesis

A syndrome of transient (months) myelodysplasia, with megakaryoblasts and micromegakaryocytes in blood and an unusual haemoglobin (?embryonic, 11% of total) is described in a newborn (Smith et al 1979). Clinical phenotype and cytogenetics were normal. The relationship of this syndrome to TAM is uncertain.

Other causes of myelofibrosis

See Table 5.40.

Table 5.4 Myelofibrosis in childhood

AML M7
Non-haemopoietic malignancy, e.g.
neuroblastoma
rhabdomyosarcoma
Hodgkin's disease
Monosomy 7 MPD
ALL (some cases)
Histiocytosis
Grey platelet syndrome
Idiopathic

Chronic myeloid leukaemias. Myelodysplasias

These are uncommon (< 5% of total, Table 5.5). Some are peculiar to childhood. As with AML, the possibility of mimicry is important in diagnosis.

JUVENILE CHRONIC MYELOID (MYELOMONOCYTIC) LEUKAEMIA (JCML)

(Castro-Malaspina et al 1984, Fig. 5.17, Table 5.6)

The commonest (about 14%) of this group.

Identifying characteristics

- Myelomonocytosis (more easily recognized in blood than in marrow). The total leucocyte count does not exceed 200 × 10^9/l. The granulocytosis is entirely or almost entirely neutrophilic. Monocytes exceed 5 × 10^9/l in 80% of cases (up to 50 × 10^9/l). Lysozyme may be increased in concert with the monocytosis.

In some cases the granulocytic component is inconspicuous in a prolonged (months) lead-in period before manifestations become typical. Misinterpretation as idiopathic monocytosis or atypical histiocytosis may be made in this period.

- Marrow karyotype normal (in about 80%) or showing only non-specific changes, e.g. C group trisomy or abnormalities at 11p15; 7 is normal, no Ph chromosome.
- Exclusion of viral infection, especially EBV.

Table 5.5 Chronic myeloid leukaemias and myelodysplasias of childhood

Uncommon
Juvenile CML
Monosomy 7 MPD
Adult type CML
Myelodysplasias (FAB criteria)
— primary
— secondary to chemotherapy
Essential thrombocythaemia
Rare
Familial MPD
t(1;5) MPD with eosinophilia
5q– syndrome
Polycythaemia vera
Eosinophilic leukaemia

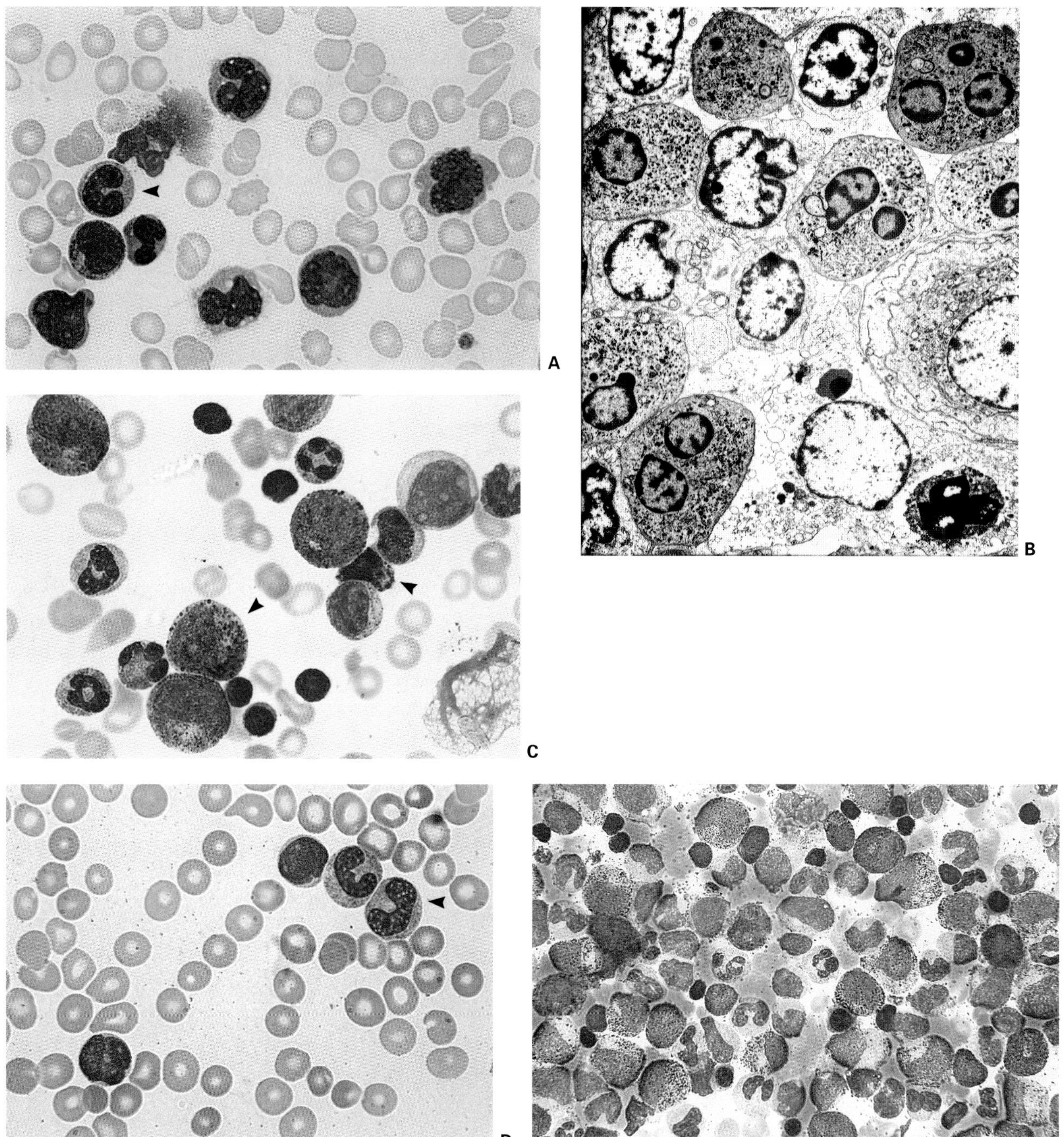

Fig. 5.17 Chronic myeloid leukaemias. **a** JCML, blood, 16-month-old boy, showing, from left, a myeloblast, 3 neutrophils (one Pelgerized, arrow), 2 atypical monocytes and 2 monoblasts. Leucocyte count 52.4 × 10^9/l, including neutrophils 21.5, lymphocytes 14.7, monocytes 6.8 and blast cells 7.9 × 10^9/l; HbF 45% of total. **b** Axillary lymph node in a 19-week fetus, showing neutrophils and lymphocytes, × 2500. (Lymphadenopathy in JCML may be due to reactivation of fetal granulopoiesis.) **c** Blood, 9-month-old girl with adult CML, Ph positive. Field includes 2 basophils (arrows) and blast cell. Leucocytes 291 × 10^9/l, including neutrophils 166, eosinophils 12, basophils 12, monocytes 18 and lymphoid cells 76 × 10^9/l. **d** Ph positive common ALL in a 2-year-old boy (blood × 750) relapsing as Ph positive adult type CML 24 months later (**e**, marrow × 500). Lymphoblasts and neutrophils (one Pelgerized, arrow) in **d**, granulocytic hyperplasia in **e**.

Other characteristics (see also Table 5.6)

Cells indistinguishable from lymphocytes may be abundant. Pelgerization and hypogranularity of neutrophils are common. Auer rods are not described.

In marrow, myeloid hyperplasia, megakaryocyte deficiency and a degree of dyspoiesis are usually the only abnormalities. Myeloblasts do not exceed 30% (usually < 20%); monocytes are usually < 10%.

Reversion to or persistence of fetal haemopoiesis is a significant component. Evidence of this includes:

- Increase in HbF (heterogeneous distribution). HbA_2 is normal or decreased. High levels of HbF diminish in remission and may become normal in long survivors.
- Increase in i antigen.
- Fetal enzyme pattern in erythrocytes.
- Persistence (at low level) of embryonic globin chains.
- Lymph node enlargement as a possible reactivation of the granulopoiesis which may be noted in fetal lymph nodes (Fig. 5.17).

A skin eruption occurs in about 40% of cases (on the face this is often of butterfly distribution). Usually this is a non-diagnostic infiltration with lymphocytes and histiocytes, or is xanthogranulomatous (Cooper et al 1984). It may precede overt leukaemia by many months.

JCML in most cases appears to originate as such. In some, however, the disorder evolves from an aplastic anaemia or RAEB (Inaba et al 1988). Deceptively encouraging spontaneous improvement in leucocyte count and organ size may occur over time. With deterioration, blast cells increase in blood but a blast crisis, as in Ph positive CML, does not occur. About 15% survive for > 10 years. Although leucocyte abnormalities may disappear, some abnormality, especially monocytosis, usually persists, as well as organomegaly. A possibly distinctive feature of this group is absence of thrombocytopenia. The condition in long survivors may differ from the usual (see also spontaneously resolving myelomonocytoses, below).

Differential diagnosis

- Monosomy 7 MPD

The platelet count is usually higher and increase in HbF less frequent and less substantial than in JCML. However, confident distinction requires karyotype.

- Adult type CML (Table 5.6)

- Viral infection

JCML, including fetal characteristics, can be mimicked by persisting EBV infection. However, skin infiltrations are not described, blastosis is usually minimal and reactive lymphocytes may be seen at some stage in blood films to suggest viral infection. In 2 children described by Herrod et al (1983) there was improvement within one year.

- Spontaneously resolving myelomonocytosis of obscure origin

A disorder resembling JCML, with hepatosplenomegaly, may occur without obvious cause and resolve spontaneously over periods of up to 12 years. Karyotype is normal or aneuploid. Some cases are familial.

Randall et al (1965) described a kindred of 9 children (7 first cousins), with anaemia, leucocytosis (to 129 $\times$ 10^9/l, monocytes to 10.5), thrombocytopenia (to 30 $\times$ 10^9/l) and blastosis in blood (to 24%) and marrow (to 45%). Histologic examination of liver and spleen showed extramedullary haemopoiesis and multinucleate giant cells, but no leukaemic infiltration. Three children died within periods of 4 days to 6 months from diagnosis (no necropsies).

- Other

Misinterpretation as idiopathic monocytosis or atypical histiocytosis may be made in (rare) cases of JMCL in which granulocytosis has not yet become conspicuous (see above).

Table 5.6 Juvenile vs adult CML at presentation

	Juvenile	Adult
Age	usually < 2 yr	usually > 2 yr
Lymph node enlargement	about 1/5, tendency to suppurate	occasional only
Skin rash	about 40%, predominantly facial	no
Splenomegaly	variable	marked
Anaemia	about 80%	uncommon
Normoblastosis	about 80%	uncommon
HbF	↑ in about 1/2, usually > 15%, to 80% of total Hb[1]	no or slight ↑, to 10% of total Hb
i antigen	increased	normal
Leucocyte count	usually $< 100 \times 10^9/l$	usually $> 100 \times 10^9/l$
Monocytosis	by definition	no
Eosinophilia	uncommon	common
Basophil increase	rare	common
Myeloblasts (blood)	to 30%, most < 10%	to about 5%
NAP decrease	in about 1/3	usual
Thrombocytopenia	in about 80%	rare
Serum immunoglobulins	↑ in about 1/2; antinuclear antibodies, anti-IgG antibodies in about 1/2	normal
Marrow karyotype	normal or non-specific	almost all Ph positive

[1] In some cases increase does not occur till late in the disease

MONOSOMY 7 MPD (Chessells 1991, Figs 5.18, 5.19)

Monosomy 7 may occur in AML (Table 5.2), but the term monosomy 7 MPD is customarily limited to a chronic 'sub-leukaemic' disorder which appears to be peculiar to childhood, presents usually before 5 years of age and often proceeds to frank AML.

Identifying characteristics

- Myeloid or myelomonocytic excess. Muramidase excretion parallels monocyte excess.
- Dysplasia is conspicuous in at least one cell line — often in the megakaryocytic lineage, with abnormality of megakaryocytes and Bernard-Soulier-like abnormality of platelets (impaired ristocetin aggregation, deficiency of Gp Ib–IX, Berndt et al 1988). In marrow, macrophages containing megakaryocytes or platelet aggregates suggest ineffective thrombopoiesis (Fig. 5.18). Charcot-Leyden crystals may be noted in marrow macrophages, derived presumably from abnormal eosinophils or basophils. In the erythron, dysplasia manifests as abnormal erythroblasts, as macrocytosis and as thalassaemia-like impaired synthesis of β chains (Sheffer et al 1988).
- Blast cells in marrow < 30% of cells, usually < 15%.
- Marrow hypoplasia or fibrosis is frequent at some stage in the disease (Fig. 5.19). Fibrosis is attributed to excessive production of platelet-derived growth factor by the abnormal megakaryocyte/platelet clone.
- Marrow karyotype is essential for diagnosis (blood lymphocytes have normal karyotype).

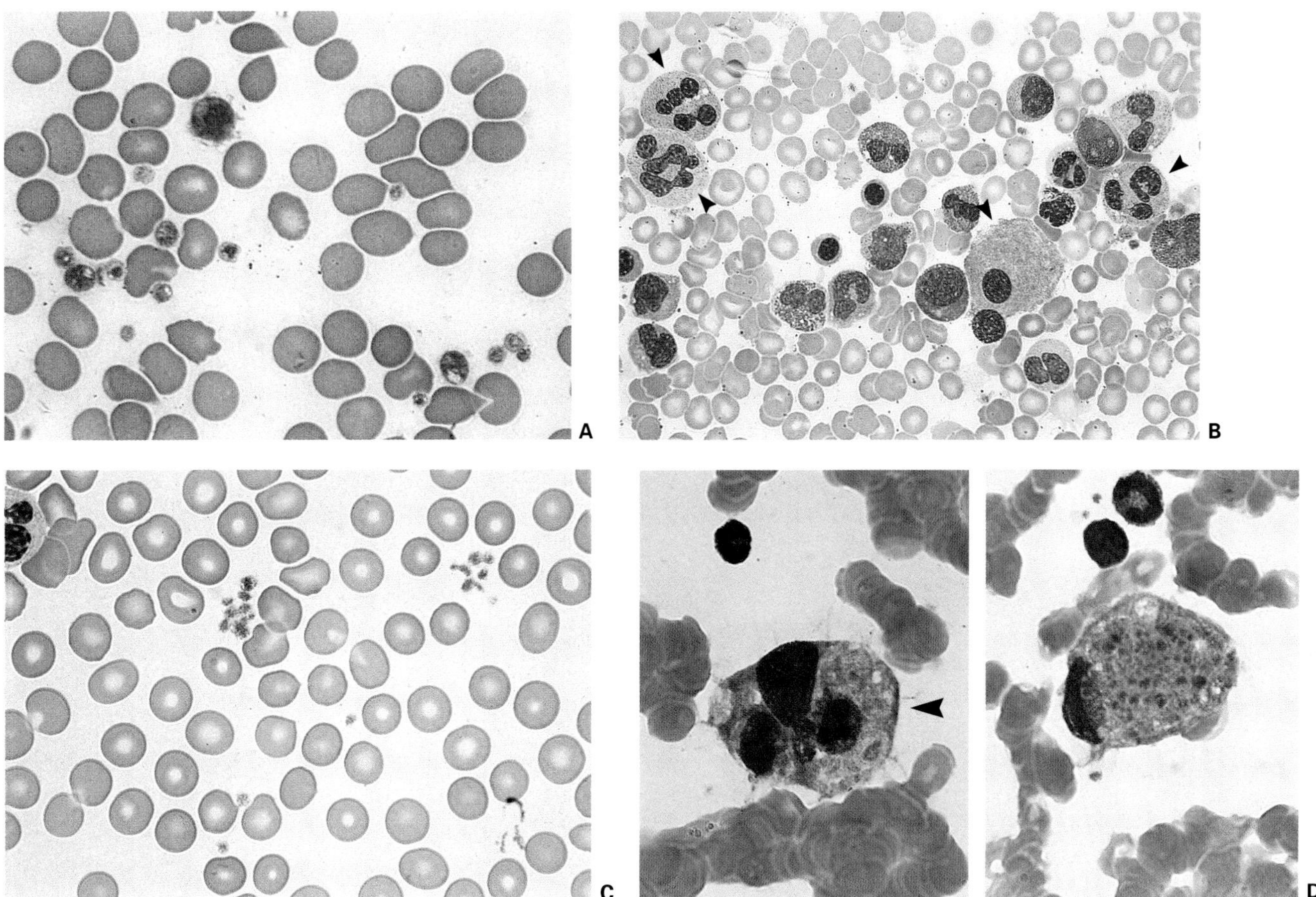

Fig. 5.18 Monosomy 7 MPD. **a–c** 12-year-old boy, **d** 8-year-old girl. **a** Blood, Bernard-Soulier-like platelets (subnormal aggregation with ristocetin). **b** Marrow (× 500), normal cellularity and (arrows) granulocyte and megakaryocyte dysplasia; blast cells 1%. **c** Blood, post-marrow transplant, showing normal platelets. **d** Marrow macrophages containing **left**, a micromegakaryocyte (arrow), and **right**, platelet aggregate (or megakaryocyte fragment).

Other characteristics

Unexplained macrocytosis may be noted within months of birth. HbF is usually normal, and rarely > 15%.

Blood leucocyte counts are usually lower (most < 25, rarely > 50 × 10^9/l) than those characteristic of JMCL or adult CML. Increase affects neutrophils and often monocytes. A percentage of myeloblasts is usual. Eosinophilia occurs in about 1/5. Platelet count is variable (may be increased in early stages).

The majority of patients present before the age of 5 years, often before 2 years, with boys affected more often than girls. Marked hepatosplenomegaly is usual. The skin eruptions common in JCML appear to be rare if they occur at all. Genuine leukaemic infiltration of the skin may occur. Rare cases are familial.

The natural evolution is, in most cases and usually within 2 years, to treatment-resistant AML. Spontaneous remissions after splenectomy may occur. The course can be prolonged. One of our cases (Fig. 5.19) presented at 16 months with palmar space infection, macrocytosis and cyclic neutropenia with 'maturation arrest' at the myelocyte stage in marrow; the neutropenia later became constant. Death occurred at the age of 10 years.

Differential diagnosis

- JCML
In JCML blood leucocyte counts are usually higher, thrombocytopenia is more frequent and more severe, increase in HbF is more frequent and more substantial and there is less propensity to evolve to AML. However, distinction requires karyotype.

- Refractory anaemia, refractory anaemia with excess blasts (RAEB), RAEB in transformation
Distinction requires karyotype.

- Idiopathic myelofibrosis, marrow panhypoplasias
These are not associated with monosomy 7.

- Genetic Bernard-Soulier anomaly (p. 315)

ADULT TYPE CML (Table 5.6, Fig. 5.17)

This is the same disorder as in adults, though features may be atypical in infancy.

Identifying characteristics

- Granulocytic hyperplasia with shift to left — mainly neutrophils, with some basophils and often eosinophils; monocytes increased in some infants (see below).
- Marrow Ph chromosome positive.

Other characteristics

Children under 2 years of age may have anaemia, thrombocytopenia, monocytosis, erythroblastosis and increase in lymphoid cells (Fig. 5.17, Gay et al 1984).

In about 5% of cases conventional karyotype is normal, t(9; 22) being detectable by PCR.

Although most cases appear to originate as such, some originate as Ph positive ALL (Fig. 5.17).

Differential diagnosis

- JCML (Table 5.6).
- Chronic EBV infection may produce Ph negative granulocytic hyperplasia.
- A transient CML-like reaction may occur in thrombocytopenia-absent radius syndrome (p. 300).

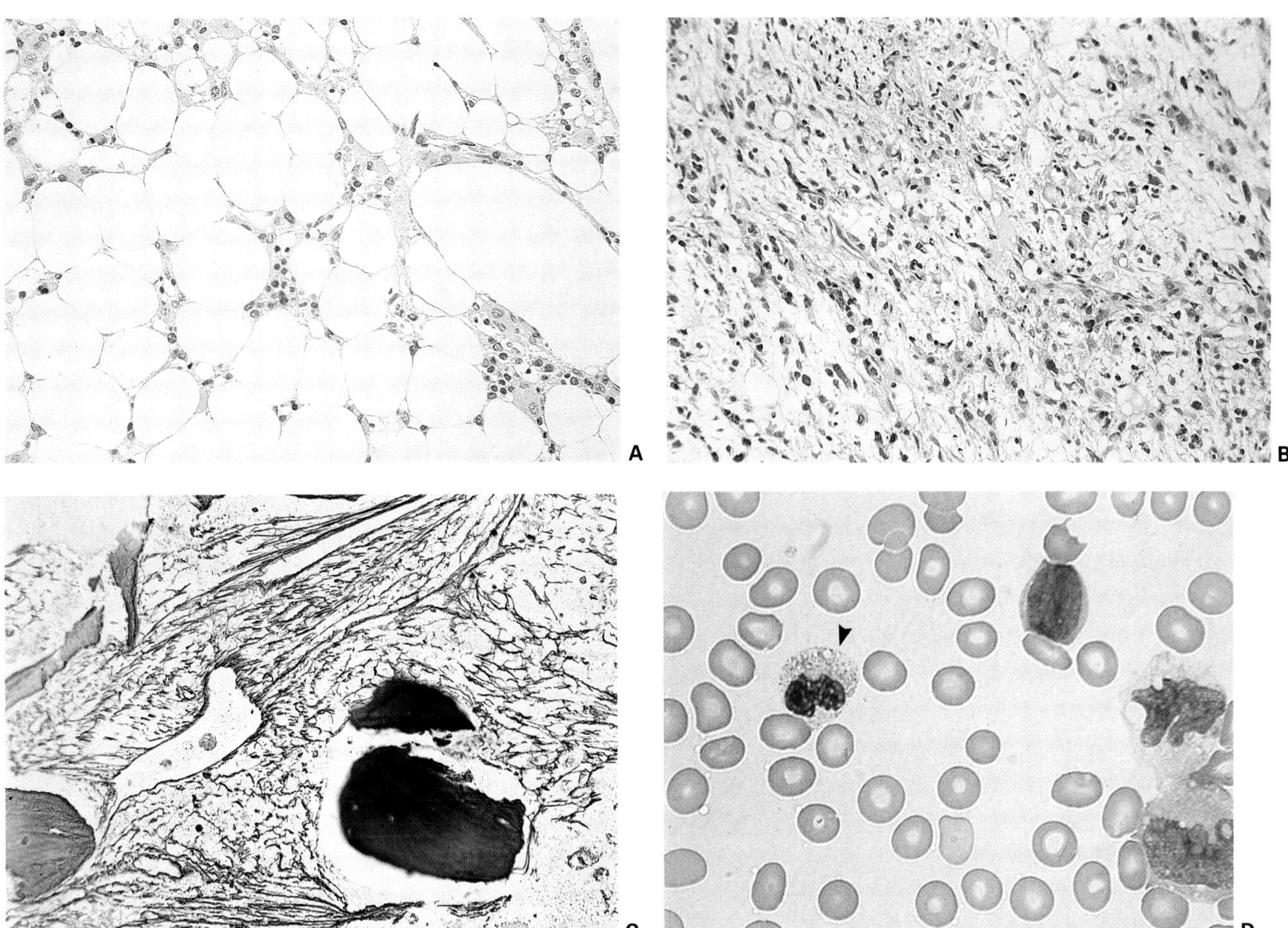

Fig. 5.19 Monosomy 7 MPD in evolution through marrow hypoplasia/fibrosis (**a–c**) to terminal blastic phase (**d**). In **a** and **b** (H & E) haemopoietic elements are predominantly immature myeloid cells. **a** 8-year-old girl at presentation. **b** More fibrotic marrow in a 10-year-old boy, 9 years after presumed onset with cyclic neutropenia. **c** 2-year-old girl with Down's syndrome showing increased reticulin. **d** Blood, 10-year-old boy, hypogranular neutrophil (arrow), blast cell and 2 monocytes (count 5.4×10^9/l). **a–c** $\times$ 200; **d** $\times$ 750

MYELODYSPLASTIC SYNDROMES (MDS)

These are rare in childhood.

Identifying characteristics

Although myelodysplasia is common in a variety of leukaemias, the term MDS is restricted to disorders meeting the FAB criteria (Table 5.7), with the following characteristics common to the group:

- blast cells in marrow < 30% of cells
- conspicuous myelodysplasia in at least one cell line (Fig. 5.20)
- non-specific karyotype (e.g. no Ph).

Other characteristics

MDS may arise de novo (Fig. 5.20) or be secondary to chemotherapy for other malignancy (Fig. 5.21). Karyotype abnormalities occur in about 60% of primary and 90% of secondary MDS. Of the large variety described (Chessells 1991), abnormality of 5 or 7 is especially common in secondary MDS. MDS very rarely is congenital. In an infant described by McMullin et al (1991) dysplasia was most conspicuous in the erythron; karyotype was normal.

Differential diagnosis

- From other chronic myeloid leukaemias, e.g. monosomy 7 MPD

Karyotype is essential for diagnosis.

- Congenital sideroblastic anaemia (p. 20)

There is no dysplasia of other cell lines and the karyotype is normal.

- Megaloblastic anaemia

Myeloblasts are not increased, there are no Auer rods, karyotype is normal and serum folate or B_{12} is subnormal (in the common forms; normal to high in MDS/myeloid leukaemia due to granulocyte hyperplasia).

Table 5.7 Myelodysplastic syndromes[1]

	Blood	Marrow
Refractory anaemia (RA)[2]	blasts < 1%	blasts < 5%
RA with ringed sideroblasts (RARS)	blasts < 1%	blasts < 5%; ringed sideroblasts ≥ 15% of erythroblasts
RA with excess blasts (RAEB)	blasts < 5%	blasts 5–20%
RAEB in transformation (RAEB-t)	blasts usually > 5%	blasts < 20–30% or Auer rods

[1] After Mufti & Galton 1986

[2] It is usual to include those cases (approx 5%) with similar marrow findings but without anaemia

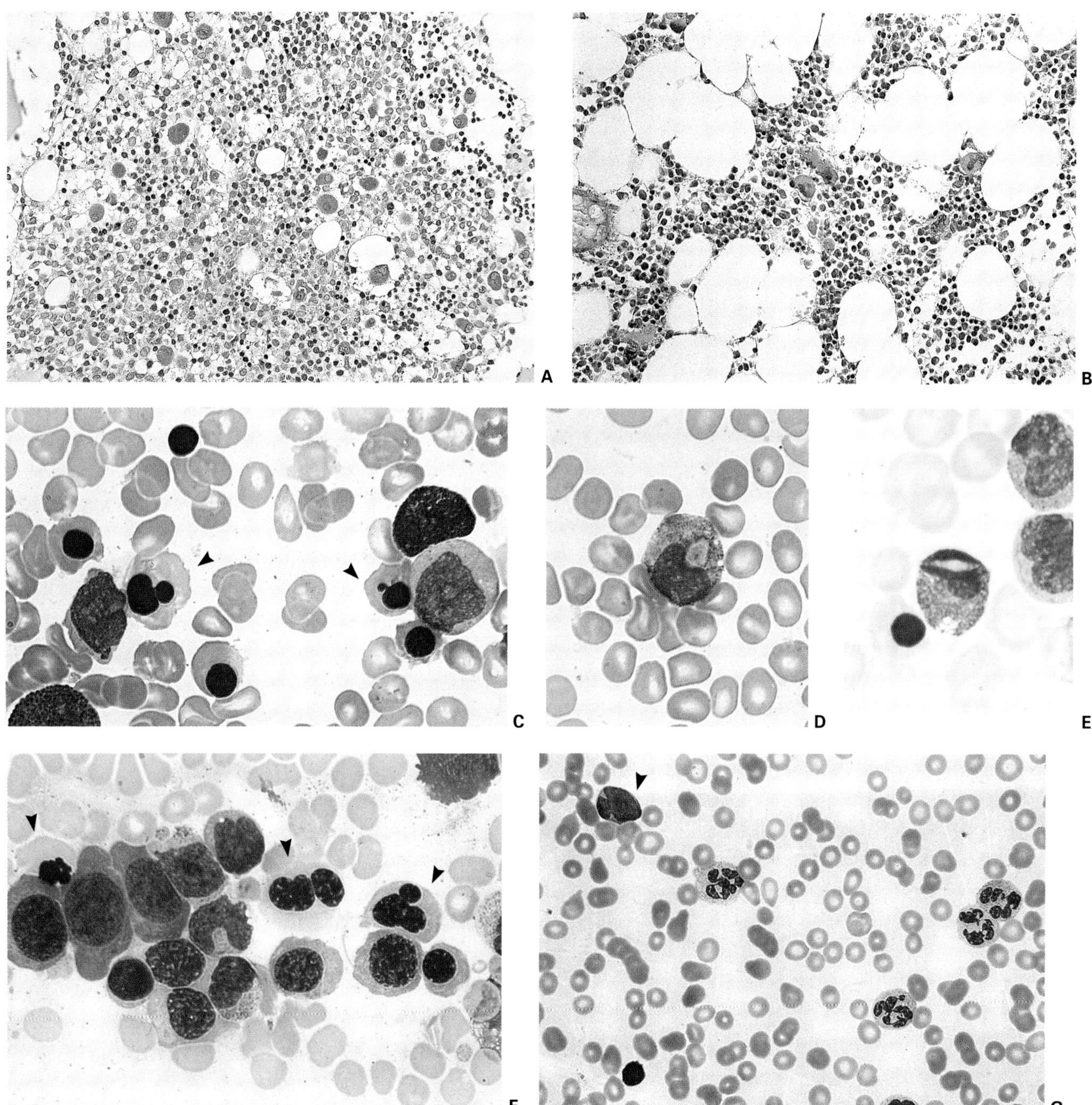

Fig. 5.20 De novo MDS, RAEB-t. **a,c,d** 13-year-old boy, karyotype normal. **a** Abundant small megakaryocytes; cf normal (**b**). **c** Dyserythropoiesis (arrows). **d** Inclusion of unknown nature in neutrophil metamyelocyte. **e** Charcot-Leyden crystal in eosinophil, 3 year old boy, karyotype normal, eosinophil count in blood and marrow normal. **f,g** 3-year-old boy, karyotype normal; marrow (**f**) shows megaloblastosis, distorted nuclei (arrows); blood (**g**) shows hypersegmented neutrophils and blast cell (arrow). **a,b** PAS × 200; **e** × 1000; **g** × 500

Table 5.8 Reactive thrombocytosis vs essential thrombocythaemia

	Reactive thrombocytosis	**Essential thrombocythaemia**
Platelet: count mean volume function	rarely > 1200 × 10^9/l decreased normal	> 600, often > 1200 × 10^9/l increased may be abnormal[1]
Megakaryocyte ploidy[2]	normal or minimal shift to higher ploidy — about 2/3 16n, 1/6 8n, 1/6 32n	shift to higher ploidy, especially ≥ 32n
Marrow trephine large,	normal	↑ cellularity; ↑ megakaryocytes, especially higher ploidy forms; fibrosis common
Karyotype (marrow)	normal	usually normal; Ph rarely
NAP	normal or ↑	↓ in about 1/3
Cause	see Table 5.9	unknown
Natural history	resolution after cause subsides or is removed; duration < 12 weeks	permanent; increasing platelet count; about 10% evolve to AML and 10% to myelosclerosis

[1] e.g. aggregation with ADP
[2] Mazur et al 1988

ESSENTIAL THROMBOCYTHAEMIA

(Schwartz & Cohen 1988, Table 5.8, Fig. 5.21)

This is rare in childhood, and similar to that in adults, but with a more benign course because of greater tolerance of thrombocytosis by children. Diagnosis requires a chronic (> 3 months) thrombocytosis for which a cause cannot be found (Table 5.9). There may be mild leucocytosis (neutrophils, and often basophils and eosinophils). Coagulation factor deficiencies (fibrinogen, V, VIII) of obscure origin (?hypercoagulable state) may occur, as well as thrombocytopathy.

Table 5.9 Reactive thrombocytosis in childhood*

Infection	infection, acute or chronic
Inflammation	burns inflammatory bowel disease collagen disease, e.g. SLE, rheumatoid, sarcoid nephrotic syndrome graft vs host disease Kawasaki disease
Trauma	
Bleeding	
Thrombosis	
Spleen	absence, removal, atrophy
Malignancy	neuroblastoma hepatoblastoma Wilms tumour lymphoma AML M7 adult type CML monosomy 7 MPD
Drugs	steroids adrenalin vinca alkaloids folinic acid
Anaemia	iron deficiency vitamin E deficiency/infantile pyknocytosis other anaemias
Miscellaneous	histiocytosis Caffey's disease (infantile cortical hyperostosis)

*Modified from Schwartz & Cohen 1988

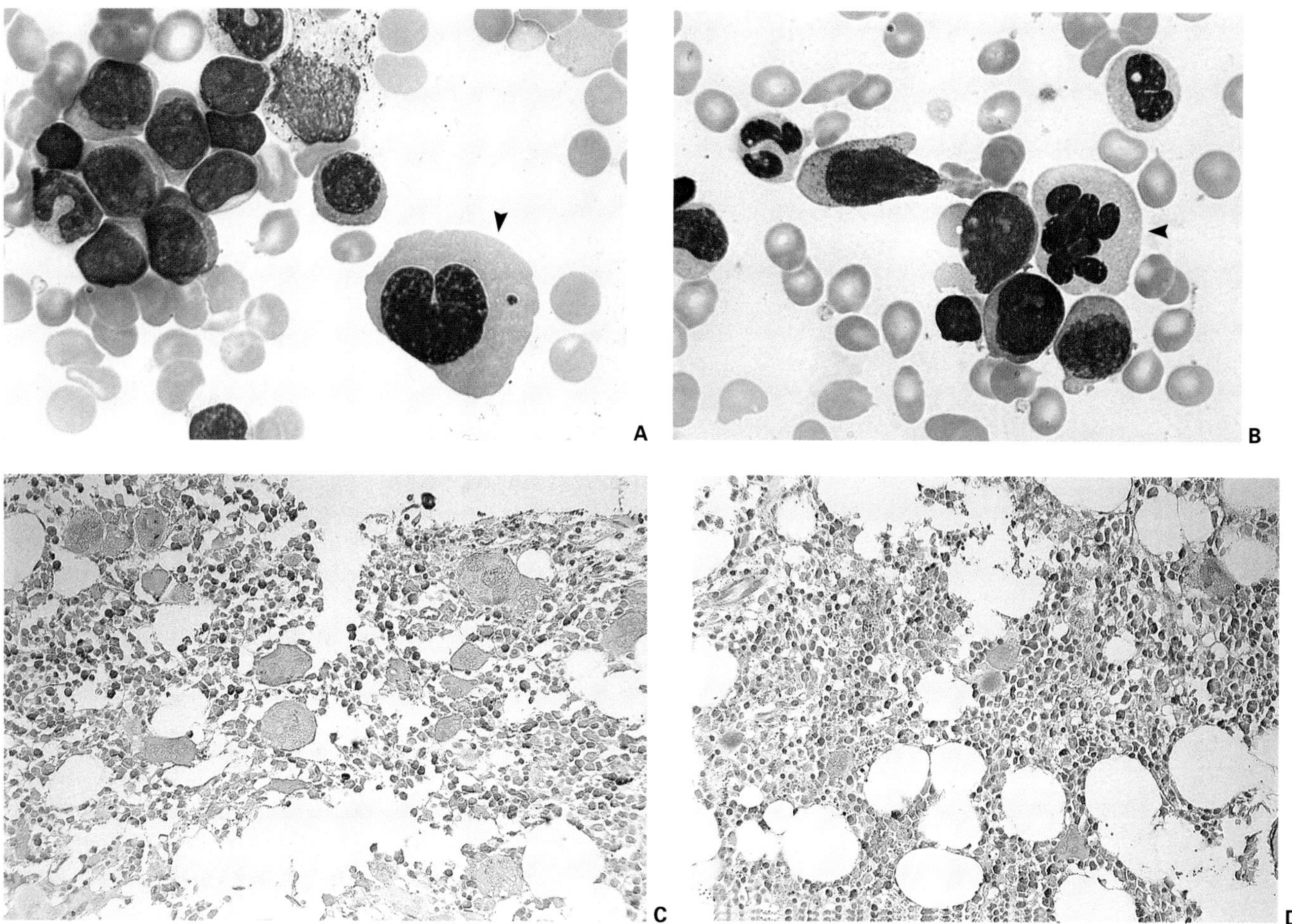

Fig. 5.21 Chronic myeloproliferative disorders. **a,b** RAEB type MDS in a 10-year-old boy, 6 years after chemotherapy and local irradiation for Hodgkin's disease. Arrows show dyspoietic erythroblast and neutrophil. Trisomy 21 and deletion 20q; 5 and 7 normal. **c** Essential thrombocythaemia, 11-year-old boy, platelets 2064 × 10^9/l; trephine biopsy shows profusion of large megakaryocytes; cf normal (**d**). **c,d** PAS × 200

RARER MYELOPROLIFERATIVE DISORDERS

1. t(1;5) MPD with eosinophilia

Darbyshire et al (1987) described two infants presenting before 6 months of age with hepatosplenomegaly, anaemia, eosinophilia (to $40 \times 10^9/l$), thrombocytopenia and t(1;5) confined to myeloid cells. HbF and NAP were normal. The marrow showed hyperplasia, especially of mature and immature eosinophils, and in one case dyspoiesis of neutrophils (hypo-, hyper-granulation); blast cells in marrow were normal or only slightly increased (to 6%). One of the children has died of infection (no blast cell crisis). This MPD may be peculiar to childhood.

2. 5q– syndrome (Bunn 1986)

Deletion of 5q occurs usually in association with other cytogenetic abnormalities (Table 5.2). Isolated 5q– occurs most commonly in elderly women and is very rare in childhood.

Table 5.10 Polycythaemia in childhood[1]

Relative polycythaemia (normal red cell mass, decreased plasma volume)
Dehydration
True polycythaemia
Excess erythropoietin
Appropriate (decreased tissue oxygenation, arterial oxygen saturation < 92%)
Altitude
Cardiac (right to left shunt)
Pulmonary disease
Hypoventilation (Pickwickian syndrome)
Low oxygen-affinity Hb or increased 2,3 DPG
Inappropriate
Tumours
Renal disease
Decreased or normal erythropoietin (primary polycythaemia)
Polycythaemia vera
Adult type CML

[1] After Schwartz & Cohen 1988

3. Polycythaemia vera (Danish et al 1980, Schwartz & Cohen 1988)

Only 0.1% of patients with polycythaemia vera are < 20 years of age at diagnosis. Diagnosis requires exclusion of secondary causes (Table 5.10) and demonstration of myeloproliferative characteristics:

a. increased red cell mass (> 36 ml/kg for males, > 32 for females)
b. splenomegaly, or if absent, two of the following:
   - platelet count $\geq 400 \times 10^9/l$
   - leucocyte count $\geq 12.0 \times 10^9/l$
   - increased serum B_{12} or unbound B_{12}-binding capacity.

The marrow shows trilineage hyperplasia. Deficiencies are described, in separate cases, of factors II, V, VII, X (returning to normal after heparin treatment), and of I, V and VIII with increased fibrin degradation products. Platelet aggregations may be abnormal. There is usually a transition, after an average of about 10 years, to a stable phase of cytopenias due to marrow fibrosis. There is a risk (10–15%), in time, of myeloid leukaemia.

4. Eosinophilic leukaemia

A diagnosis of this exceptionally rare leukaemia might be considered for gross eosinophilia associated with cytogenetic abnormality, especially of 12q (Keene et al 1987). Marrow blast cells are only slightly, if at all, increased. For ALL with eosinophilia, see page 132.

Non-haemopoietic malignancies in marrow

Only a limited number of non-haemopoietic malignancies of childhood (referred to here as 'malignancies') affect marrow with any frequency (Table 5.11). General features will be summarized here before individual malignancies are considered. Emphasis is given to the haematology of aspirates rather than histology of trephine biopsies.

Marrow may be the first (or only) source of tissue for diagnosis. Misdiagnosis as leukaemia may occur if clinical manifestations of the primary tumour are inconspicuous and malignant cells occur in substantial numbers in blood (Fitzmaurice et al 1991).

- Cytology

In few cases is the morphology of malignant cells diagnostic. In contrast to leukaemic cells, malignant cells:
- — are usually larger
- — are more often multinucleate
- — tend to cohere into tighter groups
- — tend to involve marrow in spotty fashion
- — form rosettes in some malignancies.

- Neurofibrils

Occur in some malignancies.

- Cytochemistry

Though not diagnostic, cytochemistry may be of value in suggesting the diagnosis and in distinguishing malignancies from leukaemias, e.g. PAS in neuroblastoma and Ewing's sarcoma.

- Immunophenotype

Only a restricted range of monoclonal antibodies is suitable for use on marrow aspirates (e.g. neuroblastoma, rhabdomyosarcoma); more comprehensive work-up is possible on cell suspensions.

- Cytogenetics

Specific karyotypes occur in some malignancies.

Table 5.11 Non-haemopoietic malignancies in marrow in childhood

Common
Neuroblastoma
Uncommon
Rhabdomyosarcoma
Retinoblastoma
Ewing's sarcoma
Rare
Medulloblastoma
Malignant histiocytosis
Askin tumour
Wilms tumour

Note: common, etc, refers to the proportion which metastasize to marrow, not to the frequency of the condition per se

NEUROBLASTOMA (Figs 5.22–5.24)

Marrow is involved in about one half of cases. A tumour may be found whether X-ray of bone at the site of sampling is abnormal or not.

Identifying characteristics

1. Neuroblastoma cells are usually larger than ALL cells, with rare cells elongated into processes (neuroblasts, specific for diagnosis). Infiltration varies from extensive replacement to the presence of isolated cells or islets or rosettes in otherwise normal marrow, requiring systematic search.
2. Cell grouping:
   - Usually some cells are in tight groups.
   - Rosettes. An important indication of neural malignancy. Because they may be sparse and disrupted during preparation of films, careful search may be needed. In mature malignancies (ganglioneuroblastoma) sparse rosettes may be the only evidence of infiltration. Similar structures occur (rarely) in other malignancies (Fig. 5.27) and rarely rosette-like knots may be discerned in marrow of children with no evidence of malignancy (Fig. 5.23).
3. Neurofibrils. Another important indication of neural malignancy, these occur as oriented bundles of grey or pink fibres (non-birefringent) set in a grey to grey-pink matrix. By contrast, normal supporting fibrils form unordered tangles of naked, red-staining, non-birefringent strands (Fig. 5.24); cotton-wool fibres, which may stray onto slides, are coarse, twisted and birefringent.
4. Immunophenotype. A variety of monoclonal antibodies may give positive staining, e.g. UJ13A (Fig. 5.24), neurone-specific enolase, glial fibrillary acidic protein and S100 protein. Though these react also with other neuro-ectodermal tumours such as retinoblastoma, they are valuable for diagnosis of minor infiltration.

Other characteristics

Marrow
Neuroblastoma cells have no or minimal reaction with PAS and β glucuronidase.

Myelofibrosis is not infrequent and may precede overt tumour by weeks or months.

Karyotype abnormalities (Van Roy et al 1994) include:

- in children under one year, hyperdiploidy to near triploidy
- in older children, markers of chromosome 1, homogeneously staining regions and double minutes
- abnormalities of 17q, e.g. t(1;17), constitutional in some cases.

In children under 2 years of age, hyperploidy and single-copy levels of N-myc are associated with good prognosis, in contrast to diploidy and gene amplification (Look et al 1991).

Blood
A mild anaemia, almost always normocytic, is common. A presence of erythroblasts unexpected for the mildness of the anaemia, and some left shift in granulocytes are suspicious of marrow infiltration. Microcytosis may be due to bleeding into the tumour. Thrombocytosis is common, but thrombocytopenia occurs occasionally. A substantial increase in ESR (> 50 mm in 1 h Westergren) is frequent at onset and relapse. In substantial numbers at least, tumour cells are rare in blood, even in those with advanced disease (compare leukaemia); however occurrence in small numbers may not be rare. A defibrination type coagulopathy may occur in disseminated disease or as part of a tumour lysis syndrome after start of treatment. In rare cases a deposit (? tumour secretion) is evident in stained blood films (Fig. 5.28).

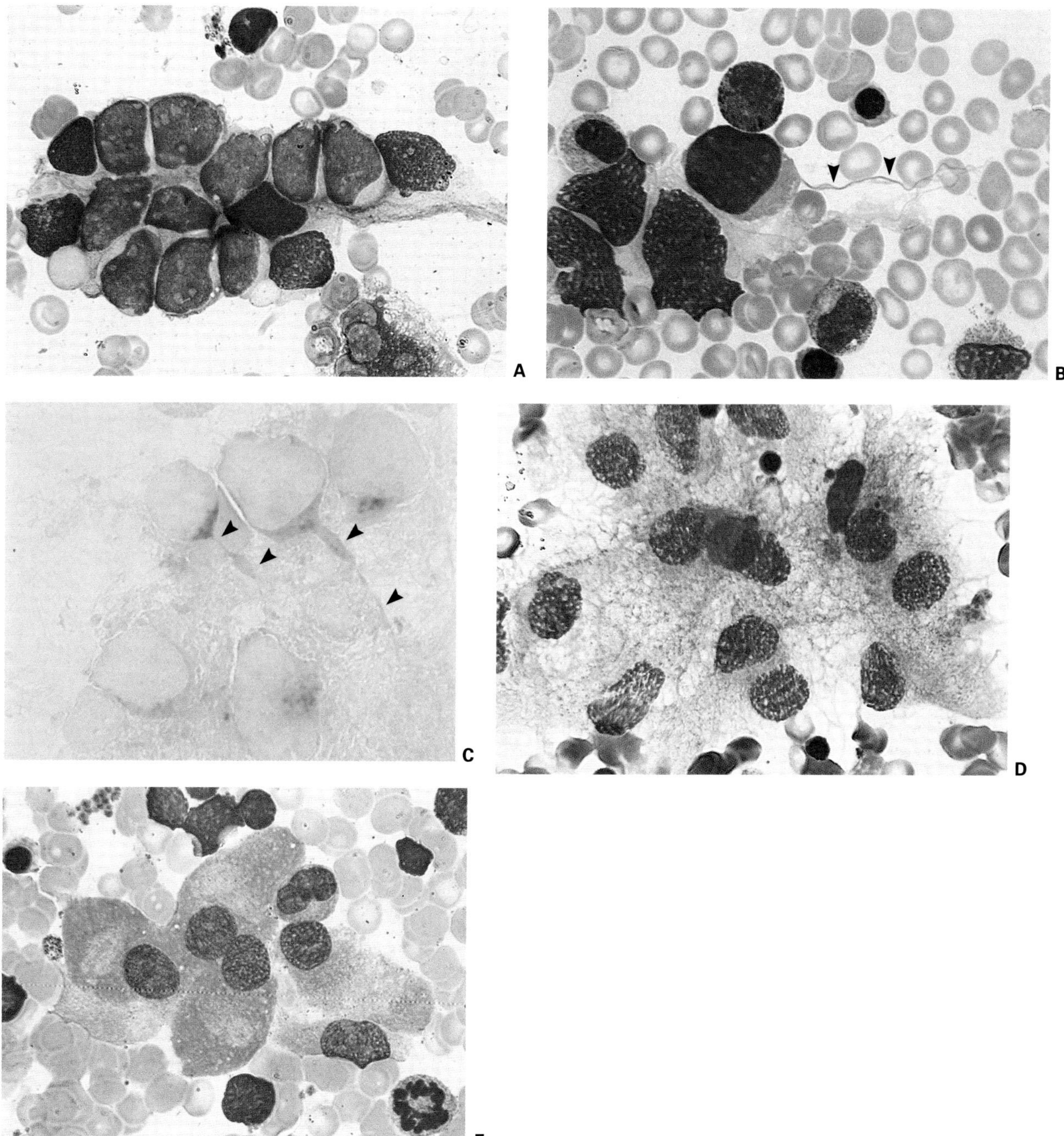

Fig. 5.22 Neuroblastoma vs normal cells in marrow. **a** Group of malignant cells. **b,c** Neuroblasts. Arrows show cell processes (**c**, AcPh). **d** Normal supporting cells. **e** Normal osteoblasts.

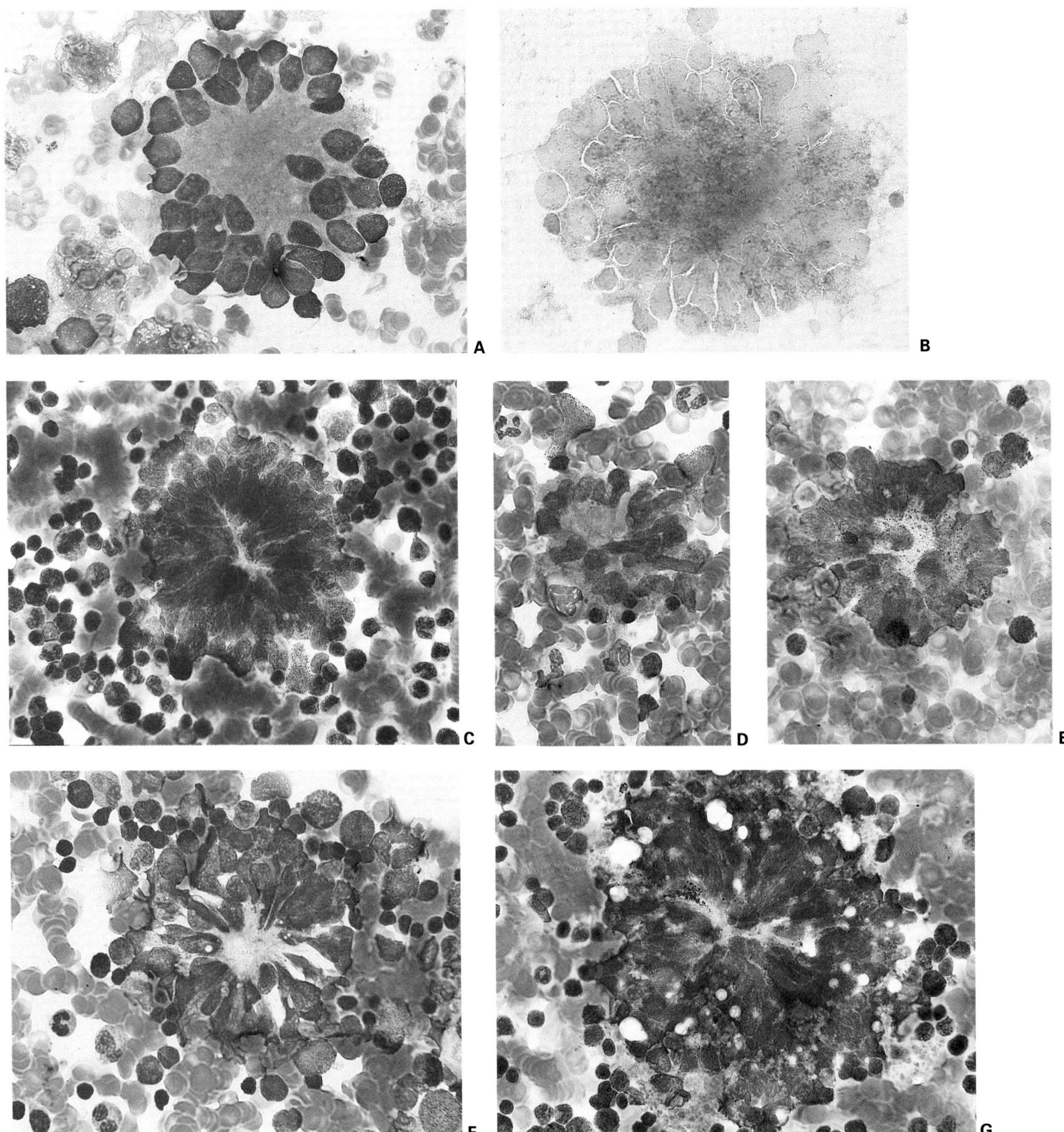

Fig. 5.23 Rosettes in marrow aspirates. **a,b** 2-year-old child, neuroblastoma; AcPh (**b**) in cells and within rosette. **c** More closely palisaded, empty rosette; sparse rosettes were the only evidence of disease in marrow; 6-month-old child with differentiating thoracic neuroblastoma. **d** Rosette-like knot in child with no evidence of malignancy. **e** Rosette-like group of unidentified cells in 5-day-old infant with benign haemangioendothelioma of liver, no rosettes in primary tumour. **f** (Viable) and **g** (degenerate) rosettes in untreated 4-month-old girl with retinoblastoma. All × 500

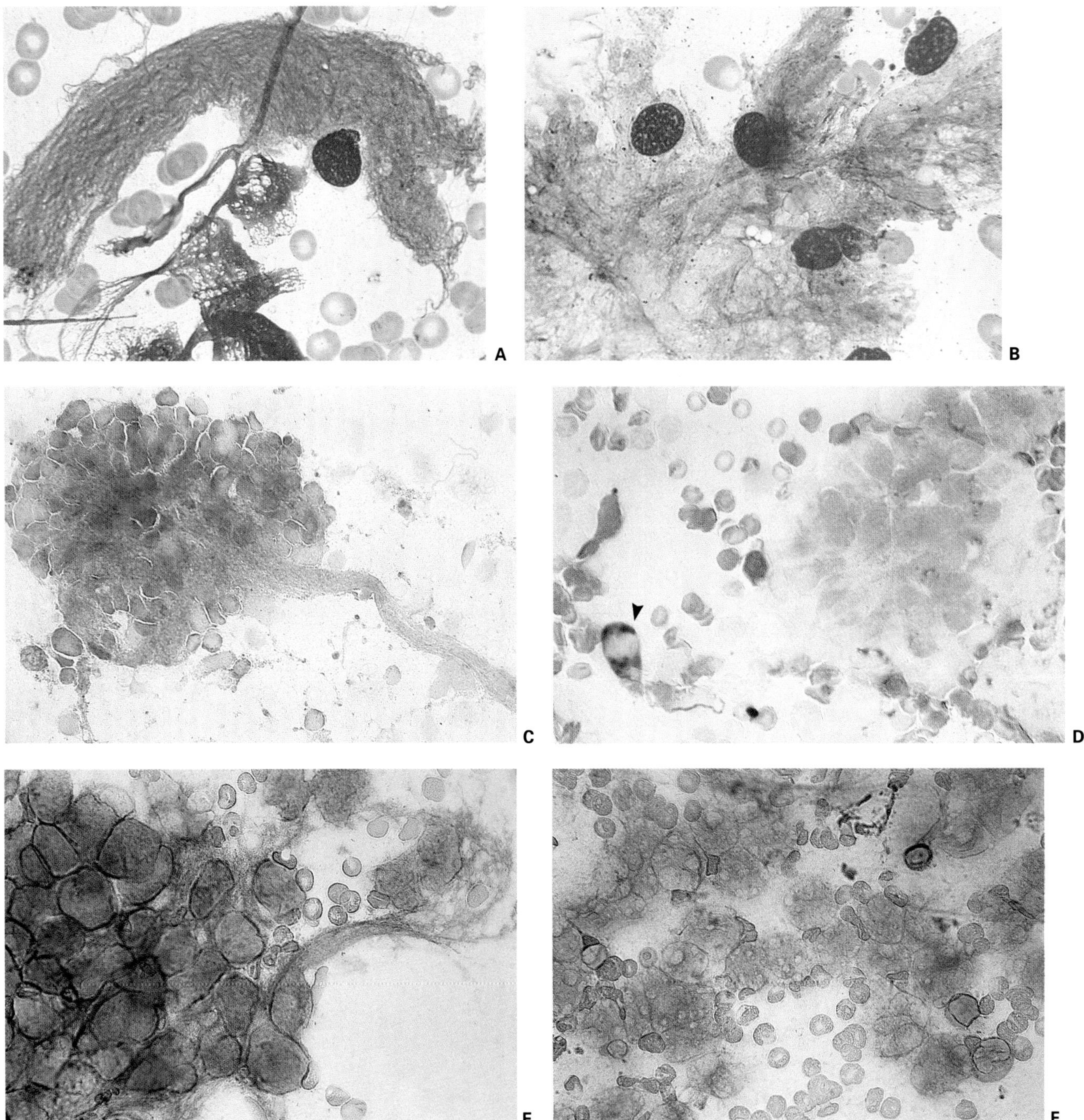

Fig. 5.24 Neuroblastoma in marrow. **a** Neurofibrils vs normal supporting fibrils (**b**). **c** AcPh, neurofibril bundle positive. **d** β glucuronidase, rosette negative, macrophage (arrow) positive. **e** UJ13A monoclonal, cells and neurofibrils positive. **f** CD45, leucocytes positive, tumour cells negative. **a,b** × 750; **c** × 330; **d–f** × 480

Differential diagnosis

- ALL

See Table 5.12. In addition, clinical features (especially presence and location of mass disease) and catecholamine excretion in urine are important.

- Other malignancies

Unless characteristics specific for individual malignancies (qv) are present, a confident distinction cannot be made on cytologic features.

- Normal elements

Normal cells, e.g. osteoblasts and connective tissue cells, should not be confused with malignant cells, and connective tissue fibrils with neurofibrils (Figs 5.22–5.24).

Table 5.12 Neuroblastoma vs ALL

	Neuroblastoma	ALL
Marrow infiltration	spotty in otherwise normal marrow, or diffuse infiltrate	diffuse take-over
Cell size	medium to large	usually small to medium
Cell clumping	usual	uncommon
Rosettes	often	absent
Neurofibrils	often	absent
PAS	rarely if ever pos	often pos
β glucuronidase	rarely if ever pos	often pos
Immunophenotype	neg for leucocyte markers; pos neuro-ectodermal	pos leucocyte and lymphocyte markers; neg neuro-ectodermal
Karyotype	see text	see Tables 4.4, 4.5
Malignant cells in blood	rare	common

pos = positive; neg = negative

RETINOBLASTOMA

This is less frequent than neuroblastoma. Rosette formation may be evident (Fig. 5.23).

The specific karyotype (deletion 13q14) is found also in lymphocytes and fibroblasts in those children (< 5%) with bilateral tumour and a constitutional anomaly of mental and growth retardation, hypotonia, microcephaly, microphthalmia, high arched palate and low-set ears.

Neuro-ectodermal monoclonals such as N-CAM (CD56), though not specific for retinoblastoma, are valuable for detection of minor infiltration.

MEDULLOBLASTOMA

Medulloblastoma rarely metastasizes to marrow. Cytology may resemble that of ALL and misdiagnosis may occur if localizing clinical signs of the primary tumour are inconspicuous. A positive reaction may be obtained with the monoclonal antibody N-CAM (CD56). Medulloblastoma is more likely to be seen in cerebrospinal fluid than in marrow (Fig. 5.25).

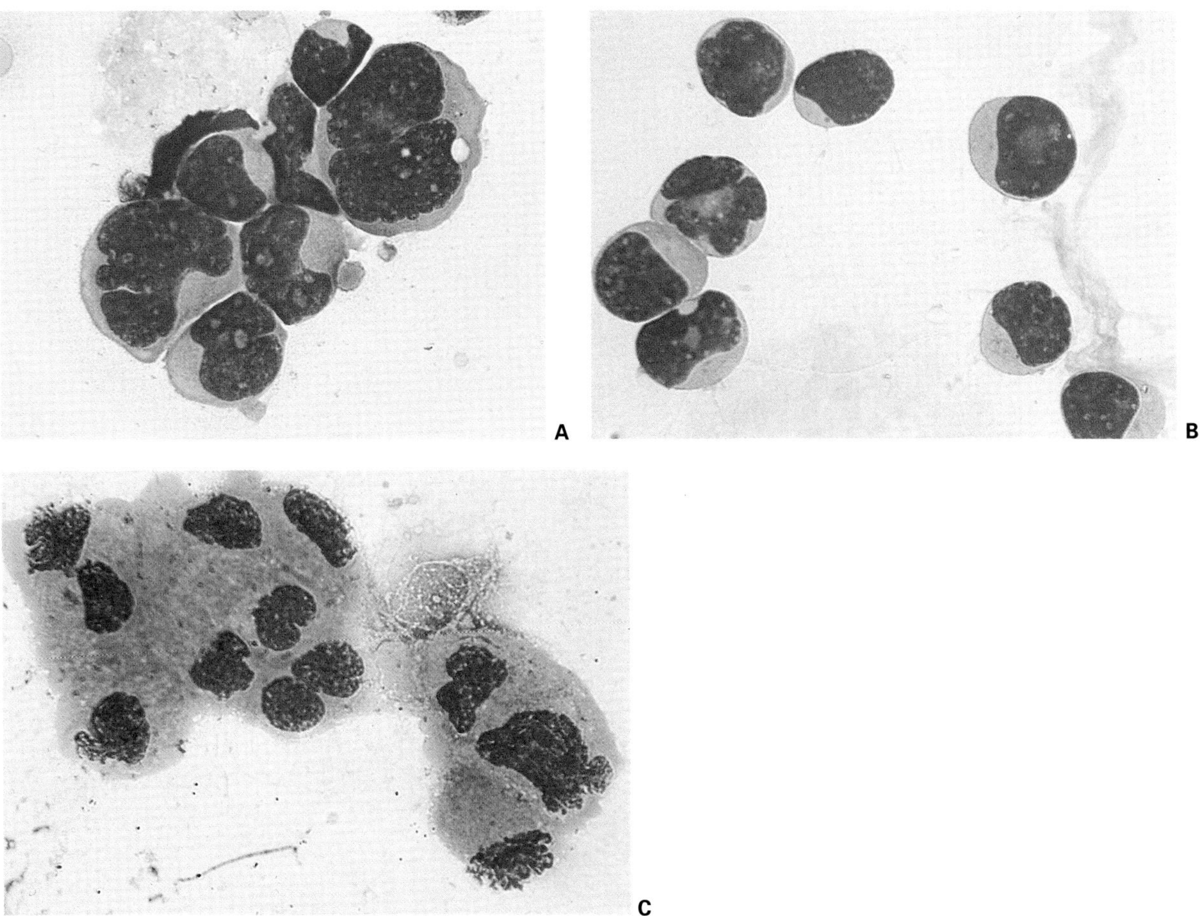

Fig. 5.25 Medulloblastoma in CSF of 2 children (**a,b**), compared with normal mesothelial cells (**c**). In **b**, lack of clumping and lymphoid appearance led to initial suspicion of lymphoma.

RHABDOMYOSARCOMA (Fig. 5.26)

Rhabdomyosarcoma, especially of alveolar histology, may present with marrow infiltration at diagnosis (7/32 patients of Reid et al 1992). Marrow infiltration together with blastic cells in blood and inconspicuous evidence of primary tumour may cause confusion with leukaemia (Fitzmaurice et al 1991).

Infiltration is usually gross and associated with marrow failure. The cells are large and often multinucleated (up to 10). 'Tadpole' cells (tailed, with cross striations) and 'strap' cells (elongated, with blunt end) suggest myoblastic differentiation (Ng et al 1989). Vacuolation is usual, vacuoles often coalescing into lakes. PAS positivity in some or most cells is usual, the reaction corresponding for the most part to the vacuoles and lakes (compare ALL, Fig. 4.10). Some malignant cells contain inclusions of red cells, erythroblasts or other nucleated cells.

In trephine biopsies, the infiltrate is intersected by fibrous septa (compare the uniform infiltration of leukaemia, Fig. 4.1).

Immunophenotyping (usually more satisfactory for aspirates than trephine biopsies) is positive for one or more of: desmin, actin, vimentin, N-CAM (UJ13A) and myoglobin. Desmin gives consistently positive results. Anti-myoglobin is technically less satisfactory and less sensitive because of affinity only for more differentiated cells.

A translocation, t(2;13)(q37;q14), is characteristic of alveolar rhabdomyosarcoma; some cases however show only the 2q+ or other karyotypes (Whang-Peng et al 1992).

In some cases marrow is only sparsely infiltrated and fibrotic, with a prominent macrophage reaction (Fig. 5.26).

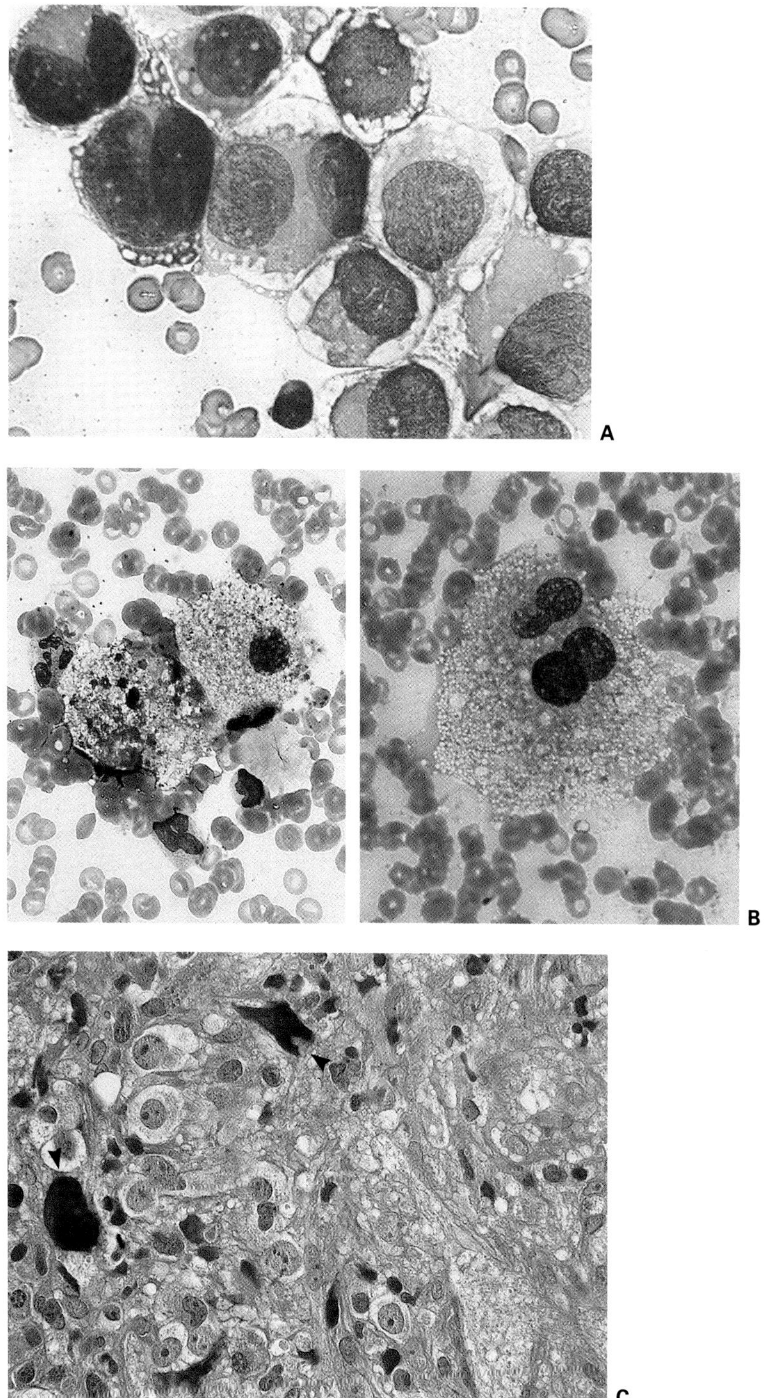

Fig. 5.26 Rhabdomyosarcoma in marrow. **a** Large cells, some binucleate, with cytoplasmic vacuoles and lakes (which were PAS positive). **b,c** Another child. Aspirate (**b**) was difficult to obtain and contained prominent macrophages but no convincing malignant cells. Trephine biopsy (**c**, H & E) contained sparse malignant cells (arrows) in fibrous stroma. **b,c** × 500. **a** Courtesy of Dr G Tauro

EWING'S SARCOMA

This rarely metastasizes to marrow. Malignant cells may be found in marrow taken (inadvertently) from the site of the primary, e.g. in the pelvis (Fig. 5.27). Usually some cells contain vacuoles or lakes of glycogen. Rosettes may rarely be seen. MIC2 is a specific marker (Ambros et al 1992); t(11;22)(q24;q12) appears to be specific; variant translocations may be found, together with markers derived from 11 and 22.

Askin tumour, which may be related to Ewing's sarcoma, occasionally metastasizes to marrow (Fig. 5.27).

OTHER MALIGNANCIES

Blood changes in other malignancies are shown in Figure 5.28.

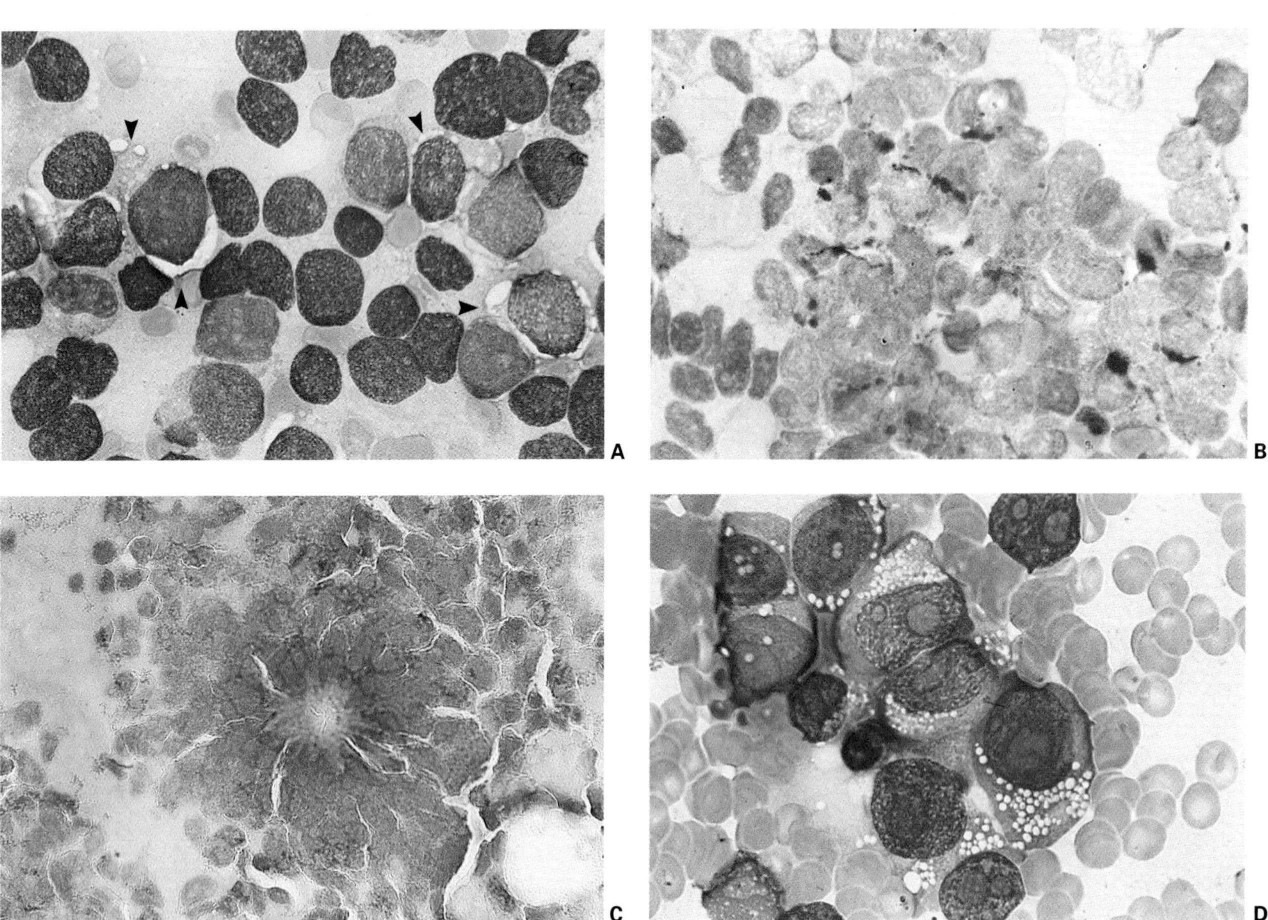

Fig. 5.27 Sarcoma in (iliac) marrow. **a–c** Ewing's sarcoma, site of primary. **a** Clear vacuoles and lakes (arrows), some of which were PAS positive (**b**). **c** Rosette (β glucuronidase × 500). **d** Askin tumour metastasis (primary in chest wall 6 years previously). Cells PAS negative, some vacuoles ORO positive.

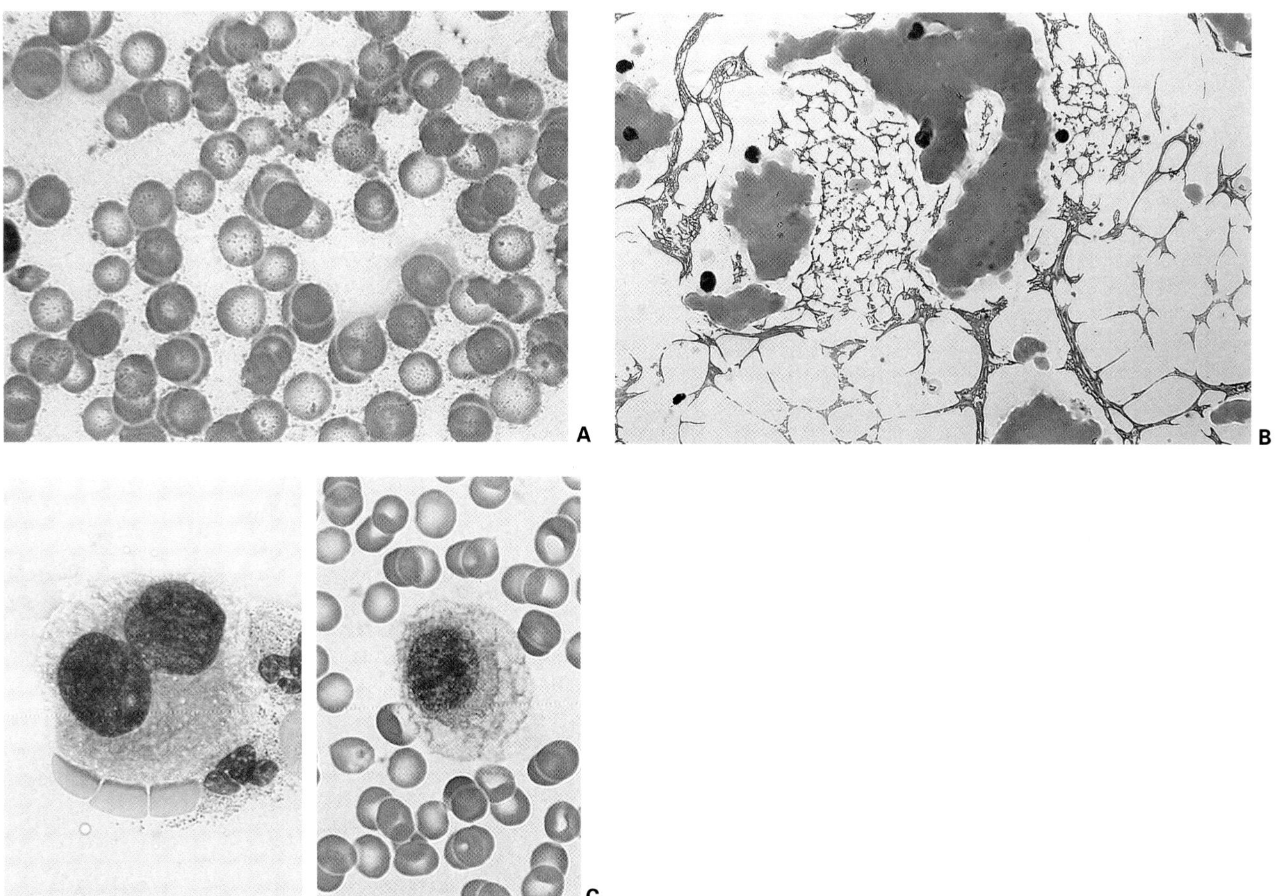

Fig. 5.28 Blood in non-haemopoietic malignancy. **a** Deposit, ?tumour secretion, treated neuroblastoma; deposit not evident at diagnosis 2 weeks earlier. **b** Mucoid deposit, Wilms tumour (× 330). **c** Malignant cells in routine blood film of 9-year-old girl with disseminated melanoma.

Histiocytoses of childhood (Malone 1991)

The designation of histiocytosis is appropriately restricted to proliferations of unknown cause (Table 5.13), to exclude infection-associated haemophagocytosis (p. 267) and reactive histiocytosis in immunodeficiency syndromes such as chronic granulomatous disease and Omenn's syndrome.

The important distinction between Langerhans and non-Langerhans histiocytosis is usually not difficult (Table 5.14).

LANGERHANS CELL HISTIOCYTOSIS

Though it is likely that Langerhans cell histiocytosis is a fairly homogeneous disorder ('histiocytosis X'), cases may be classified according to degree of dissemination. Localized disease (skin, bone) has a good prognosis, organ dysfunction (e.g. liver) a poor prognosis, while multifocal disease without organ dysfunction has an intermediate prognosis.

Letterer-Siwe disease is the multisystem disease of infancy, affecting skin, bone (lytic lesions, especially of skull), liver, spleen, lymph nodes, gingiva and lung. Hand-Schüller-Christian disease is the combination of diabetes insipidus (pituitary disease) and bone lesions in the orbit (exophthalmos) and elsewhere.

Langerhans cell histiocytosis manifests between birth and 20 years, with peak incidence at 2–4 years.

Blood changes are summarized in Table 5.15. Microcytosis is due to diversion of iron to the expanded histiocyte system and may be misdiagnosed as true iron deficiency in children with as yet unmanifest mass disease. Rarely, crystals may be noted in blood monocytes (Fig. 5.30). Rare cases evolve to AML M5a (Fontana et al 1987).

Marrow changes are summarized in Table 5.16. In aspirates the commonest abnormality is the presence, in small numbers, of hypertrophied, basophilic macrophages (Fig. 5.29). The chromatin is ropey and phagocytosis is usual; stainable iron is common (normal marrow macrophages are iron negative in the first years of life). After treatment (cytotoxics, steroids, transfusions) these cells become larger and foamy, with more nuclei and more inclusions. In a minority the aspirate contains sparse non-phagocytic cells resembling Langerhans cells (Fig. 5.29).

Table 5.13 Histiocytoses of childhood

- Langerhans cell
  - Single lesion or system
    - Bone, skin
    - Congenital or later onset
    - Self-healing or persistent
  - Multisystem
- Non-Langerhans
  - Disseminated histiocytosis
  - Malignant histiocytosis[1]
  - Sinus histiocytosis with massive lymphadenopathy

[1] True malignancy of Langerhans cells is exceptionally rare

Table 5.14 Monocytes/macrophages vs Langerhans cells

	Mononuclear/ macrophage	Langerhans
Phagocytosis	+	–
ANAE[1]	+	–
AcPh[1]	+	–
CD68[2]	+	–
CD1[1]	–	+
S100 protein[3]	–	+
Birbeck granules (electron microscopy)	–	+

[1] Marrow aspirate or frozen section of tissue
[2] Frozen section
[3] Applicable to formalin-fixed, paraffin-embedded material. KP-1 and Mac 387 (for macrophages) may also be used on this material

Table 5.15 Histiocytoses: blood changes

	Occurrence
Microcytic anaemia	disseminated/multifocal disease: eosinophilic granuloma of bone or soft tissue disease
Pancytopenia	disseminated histiocytosis
Isolated thrombocytopenia	disseminated disease
Neutrophilia	uncommon
Eosinophilia	rare: eosinophilic granuloma
Malignant mononuclear cells	malignant histiocytosis, histiocytosis terminating as AML M5

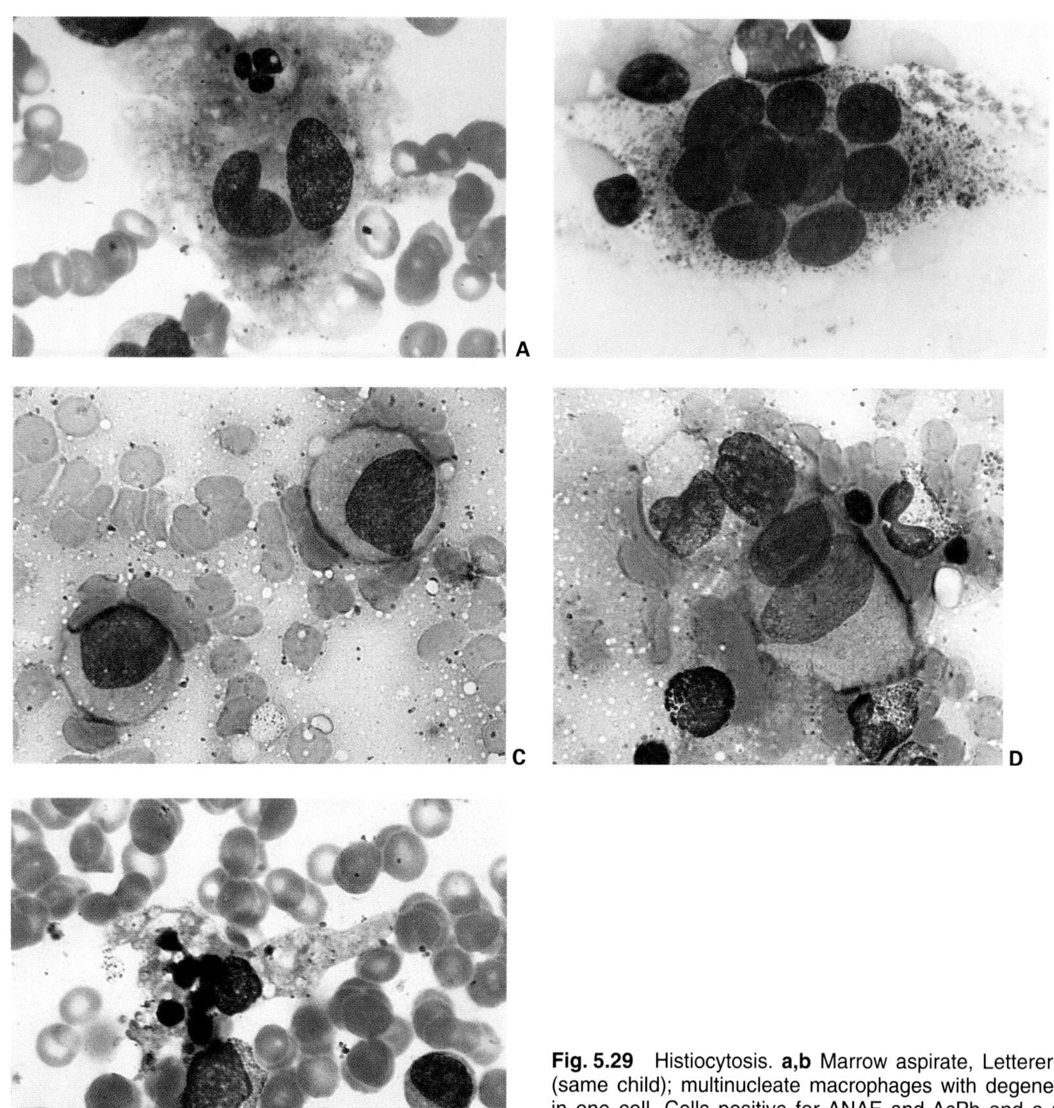

Fig. 5.29 Histiocytosis. **a,b** Marrow aspirate, Letterer-Siwe disease (same child); multinucleate macrophages with degenerate neutrophil in one cell. Cells positive for ANAE and AcPh and a proportion for iron also; cf Langerhans cells (**c,d** imprint of eosinophilic granuloma of bone) and normal marrow macrophage (**e**).

Table 5.16 Histiocytoses: marrow changes

	Occurrence		Occurrence
Aspirate[1]		Trephine biopsy	
Hypertrophied macrophages	disseminated/multifocal disease: eosinophilic granuloma of bone or soft tissue disease	Focus of eosinophilic granuloma	disseminated/multifocal disease — focus at site of biopsy
Langerhans cells[2]	unusual, even in disseminated disease	Diffuse histiocytic infiltration, Langerhans or non-Langerhans; variable eosinophils, lymphocytes, macrophages, fibrosis	disseminated histiocytosis
No abnormality	single focus eosinophilic granuloma of bone; often also in disseminated disease		
Malignant monocytoid/ histiocytoid cells	malignant histiocytosis	Infiltrate of malignant histiocytoid cells	malignant histiocytosis

[1] Aspirates alone may be unrepresentative of marrow disease

[2] Monoclonal antibody to CD1a applied to marrow aspirates (APAAP technique) may reveal Langerhans type cells not identifiable by routine haematologic staining

Trephine biopsies (Fig. 5.30) are more likely to show involvement than aspirates, with variable numbers of eosinophils, lymphocytes, macrophages and multinucleate giant cells (the last 2 may contain inclusions). Necrosis may be discernible, often with numerous eosinophils (eosinophilic 'abscesses'). In the later stages cellularity diminishes, with an increase in fibrosis.

NON-LANGERHANS HISTIOCYTOSIS

(Fig. 5.30)

In disseminated non-Langerhans histiocytosis (Fig. 5.30), the infiltrating cells are non-phagocytic and CD68 positive, but do not have the immunophenotype or ultrastructure of Langerhans cells. Skin involvement may occur, gross hepatosplenomegaly is usual, lymph node enlargement is variable and bone involvement is diffuse instead of occurring as focal lytic lesions. Anaemia, thrombocytopenia or pancytopenia is usual, but general health, at least initially, is good. A case without marrow involvement is described by Russo & Seidman (1990).

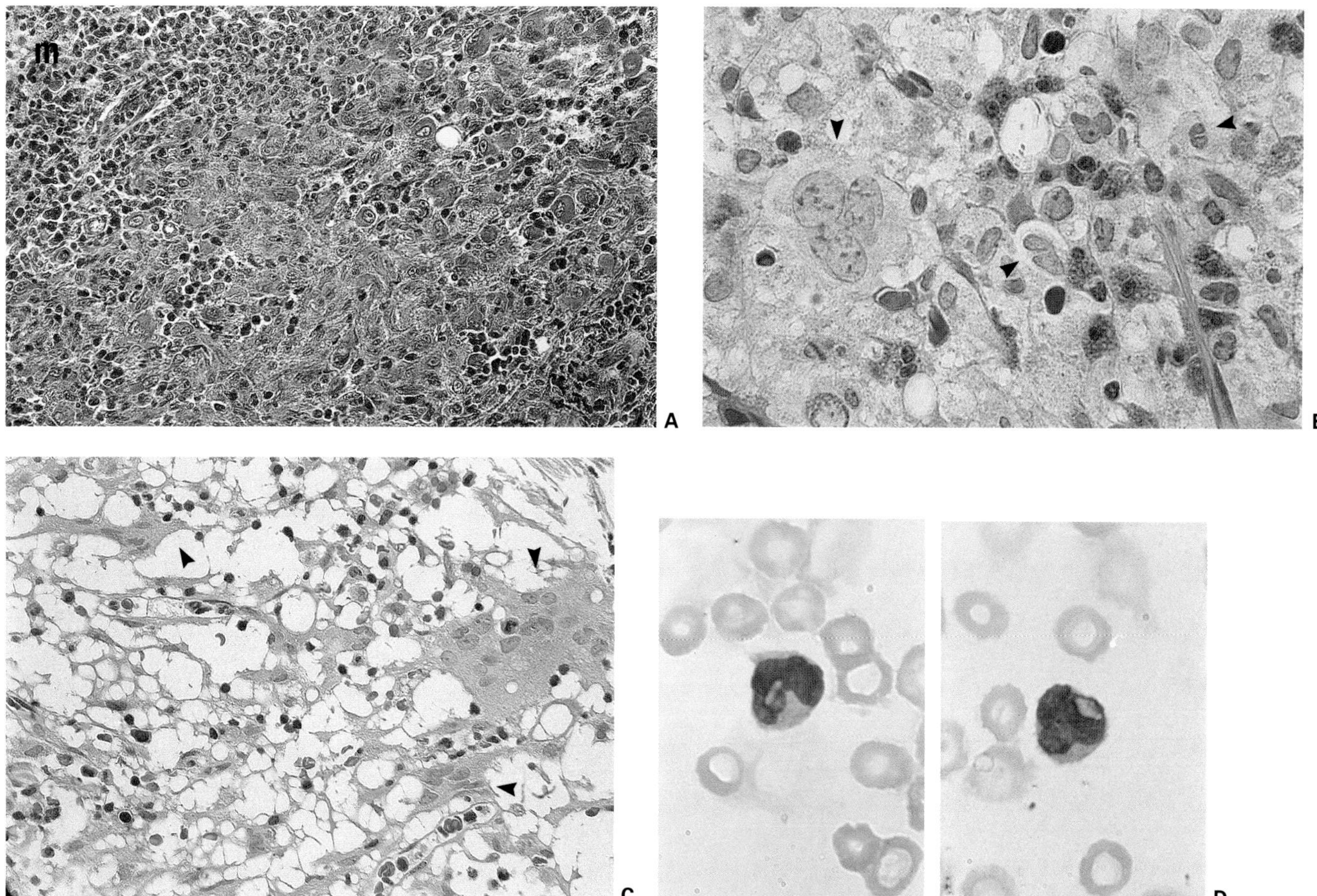

Fig. 5.30 Histiocytosis. **a** Discrete eosinophilic granuloma adjacent to normal marrow (m), 11-year-old girl. **b** Marrow, diffuse infiltration with histiocytes and eosinophils, 10-year-old girl; large arrow shows giant cell, small arrows histiocytes with grooved nuclei. Birbeck body negative, blood eosinophils 1.6 × 10^9/l. **c** 12-month-old child with systemic non-Langerhans histiocytosis (main features pancytopenia and gross hepatosplenomegaly); arrows show giant cells. **d** Unidentified crystals in blood monocytes, treated Letterer-Siwe disease. **a** H & E × 200; **b** H & E × 750; **c** H & E × 330; **d** × 1000. **a** Courtesy of Dr J Bell. **d** Courtesy of R Tracey

MALIGNANT HISTIOCYTOSIS (Fig. 5.31)

In contrast to the histiocytoses above, this is a true malignancy, with the clinical characteristics of lymphoma or leukaemia (Di Sant'Agnese et al 1983). The malignant cells are (often) vacuolated, negative for MPO (unless containing phagocytosed granulocytes) and variably positive for ANAE (fluoride sensitive) and AcPh. Immunophenotype is that of mononuclear phagocytes (Table 5.14), though there is variation from case to case (Hibi et al 1988). A translocation, t(2;5)(p23,q35), is described (Benz-Lemoine et al 1988), though a similar karyotype has been observed in 'phagocytic T cell' lymphoma (Kaneko et al 1989).

SINUS HISTIOCYTOSIS WITH MASSIVE LYMPHADENOPATHY (ROSAI-DORFMAN DISEASE)

This rare histiocytosis (of lymph nodes mainly) is associated with systemic effects (fever, neutrophilia, normocytic anaemia, polyclonal hyperimmunoglobulinaemia, increase in ESR). Histiocytosis of marrow and osteolytic lesions occur in some cases (Foucar et al 1990).

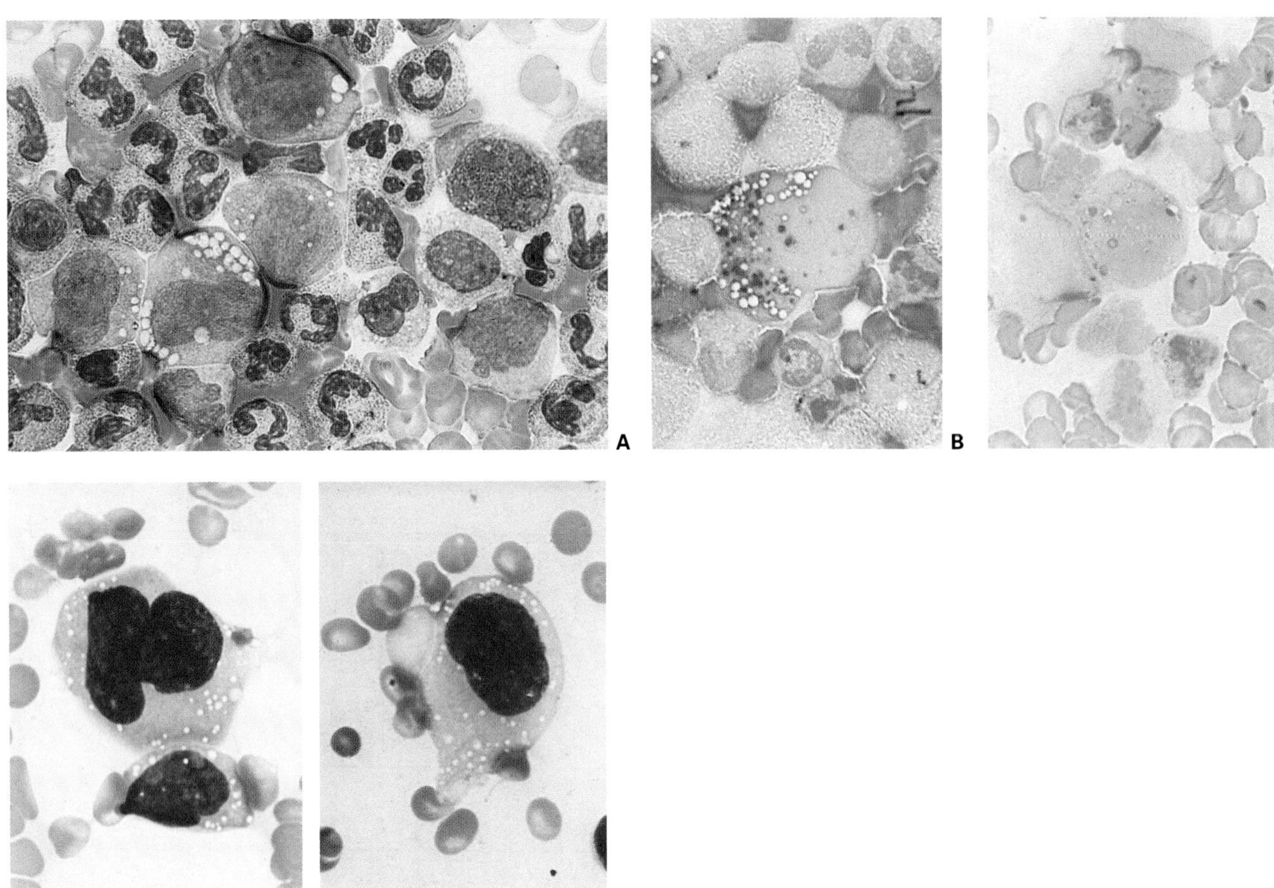

Fig. 5.31 Malignant histiocytosis. **a–c** Blood, 13-year-old boy with multisystem (pulmonary, renal) disorder; malignant cells were ANAE (**b**) and ORO (**c**) positive. Autopsy showed disseminated disease. **d** Marrow, 10-month-old child.

REFERENCES

Ambros I M, Ambros P F, Strehl S et al 1992 MIC2 is a specific marker for Ewing's sarcoma and peripheral primitive neuroectodermal tumors. Cancer 67: 1886–1893

Bain B J 1990 Leukaemia diagnosis. A guide to the FAB classification. Gower Medical Publishing, London

Bain B 1991 Down's syndrome — transient abnormal myelopoiesis and acute leukaemia. Leukaemia and Lymphoma 3: 309–317

Benjamin T, Vogt P K 1991 Cell transformation by viruses. In: Fields B N, Knipe D M (eds) Fundamental virology, 2nd edn. Raven Press, New York, pp 327–330

Bennett J M, Catovsky D, Daniel M-T et al 1991 Proposal for the recognition of minimally differentiated acute myeloid leukaemia (AML-M0). British Journal of Haematology 78: 325–329

Benz-Lemoine E, Brizard A, Huret J-L et al 1988 Malignant histiocytosis: a specific t(2;5)(p23;q35) translocation? Blood 72: 1045–1047

Berndt M C, Kabral A, Grimsley P et al 1988 An acquired Bernard-Soulier-like platelet defect associated with juvenile myelodysplastic syndrome. British Journal of Haematology 68: 97–101

Bloomfield C D, Brunning R D 1985 The revised French-American-British classification of acute myeloid leukemia: is new better? Annals of Internal Medicine 103: 614–616

Brito-Babapulle F, Catovsky D, Galton D A G 1987 Clinical and laboratory features of de novo acute myeloid leukaemia with trilineage myelodysplasia. British Journal of Haematology 66: 445–450

Bunn H F 1986 5q– and disordered haematopoiesis. Clinics in Haematology 15: 1023–1035

Castro-Malaspina H, Schaison G, Passe S et al 1984 Subacute and chronic myelomonocytic leukemia in children (juvenile CML). Cancer 54: 675–686

Cherif D, Der-Sarkissian H, Derré J et al 1992 The 11q23 breakpoint in acute leukaemia with t(11;19)(q23;p13) is distal to those of t(4;11),t(6;11) and t(9;11). Genes, Chromosomes and Cancer 4: 107–112

Chesney P J, Taher A, Gilbert E M F, Shahidi N T 1978 Intranuclear inclusions in megakaryocytes in congenital cytomegalovirus infection. Journal of Pediatrics 92: 957–958

Chessells J M 1991 Myelodysplasia. Baillière's Clinical Haematology 4: 459–482

Cooper P H, Frierson H F, Kayne A L, Sabio H 1984 Association of juvenile xanthogranuloma with juvenile myeloid leukemia. Archives of Dermatology 120: 371–375

Danish E H, Rasch C A, Harris J W 1980 Polycythemia vera in childhood: case report and review of the literature. American Journal of Hematology 9: 421–428

Darbyshire P J, Shortland D, Swansbury G J et al 1987 A myeloproliferative disease in two infants associated with eosinophilia and chromosome t(1;5) translocation. British Journal of Haematology 66: 483–486

Di Sant'Agnese P A, Ettinger L J, Ryan C K et al 1983 Histiomonocytic malignancy. A spectrum of disease in an 11-month-old infant. Cancer 52: 1417–1422

Fitzmaurice R J, Johnson P R E, Liu Yin J A, Freemont A J 1991 Rhabdomyosarcoma presenting as 'acute leukaemia' Histopathology 18: 173–175

Fontana J, Koss W, McDaniel D et al 1987 Histiocytosis X and acute monocytic leukemia. Biologic illustration of the monocyte phagocytic system. American Journal of Medicine 82: 137–141

Foucar E, Rosai J, Dorfman R 1990 Sinus histiocytosis with massive lymphadenopathy (Rosai-Dorfman disease): review of the entity. Seminars in Diagnostic Pathology 7: 19–73

Gay J C, Dessypris E N, Roloff J S, Lukens J N 1984 Juvenile features in adult-type chronic granulocytic leukemia. American Journal of Hematology 16: 99–102

Herrod H G, Dow L W, Sullivan J L 1983 Persistent Epstein-Barr virus infection mimicking juvenile chronic myelogenous leukemia: immunologic and hematologic studies. Blood 61: 1098–1104

Hibi S, Esumi N, Todo S, Imashuku S 1988 Malignant histiocytosis in childhood: clinical, cytochemical and immunohistochemical studies of seven cases. Human Pathology 19: 713–719

Inaba T, Hayashi Y, Hanada R et al 1988 Childhood myelodysplastic syndromes with 11p15 translocation. Cancer Genetics and Cytogenetics 34: 41–46

Innes D J, Hess C E, Bertholf M F, Wade P 1987 Promyelocyte morphology. Differentiation of acute promyelocytic leukemia from benign myeloid proliferations. American Journal of Clinical Pathology 88: 725–729

Kahle L H, Avvisati G, Lamping R J et al 1985 Turnover of alpha-2-antiplasmin in patients with acute promyelocytic leukaemia. Scandinavian Journal of Clinical and Laboratory Investigation 45 (suppl 178): 75–80

Kaneko Y, Frizzera G, Edamura S et al 1989 A novel translocation, t(2;5)(p23;q35), in childhood phagocytic large T-cell lymphoma mimicking malignant histiocytosis. Blood 73: 806–813

Keene P, Mendelow B, Pinto M R et al 1987 Abnormalities of chromosome 12p13 and malignant proliferation of eosinophils: a nonrandom association. British Journal of Haematology 67: 25–31

Look A T, Hayes F A, Shuster J J et al 1991 Clinical relevance of tumor cell ploidy and N-myc gene amplification in childhood neuroblastoma: a pediatric oncology group study. Journal of Clinical Oncology 9: 581–591

McMullin M F, Chisholm M, Hows J M 1991 Congenital myelodysplasia: a newly described disease entity? British Journal of Haematology 79: 340–342

Malone M 1991 The histiocytoses of childhood. Histopathology 19: 105–119

Matutes E, Pombo de Oliveira M, Foroni L et al 1988 The role of ultrastructural cytochemistry and monoclonal antibodies in clarifying the nature of undifferentiated cells in acute leukaemia. British Journal of Haematology 69: 205–211

Mazur E M, Lindquist D L, De Alarcon P A, Cohen J L 1988 Evaluation of bone marrow megakaryocyte ploidy distributions in persons with normal and abnormal platelet counts. Journal of Laboratory and Clinical Medicine 111: 194–202

Mufti G J, Galton D A G 1986 Myelodysplastic syndromes: natural history and features of prognostic importance. Clinics in Haematology 15: 953–971

Nakagawa T, Nishida H, Arai T et al 1988 Hyperviscosity syndrome with transient abnormal myelopoiesis in Down syndrome. Journal of Pediatrics 112: 58–61

Ng C S, Leung W T, Shui W et al 1989 Test and Teach, Number sixty. Pathology 21: 88–89

Niikawa N, Deng H-X, Abe K et al 1991 Possible mapping of the gene for transient myeloproliferative syndrome at 21q11.2. Human Genetics 87: 561–566

Randall D L, Reiquam C W, Githens J H, Robinson A 1965 Familial myeloproliferative disease. American Journal of Diseases of Children 110: 479–500

Reid M M, Saunders P W G, Brown N et al 1992 Alveolar rhabdomyosarcoma infiltrating bone marrow at presentation: the value to diagnosis of bone marrow trephine biopsy specimens. Journal of Clinical Pathology 45: 759–762

Russo P A, Seidman E 1990 An unusual histiocytoid proliferation in infancy. Human Pathology 21: 564–567

Schwartz C L, Cohen H J 1988 Preleukemic syndromes and other syndromes predisposing to leukemia. Pediatric Clinics of North America 35: 853–871

Sheffer R, Cividalli G, Zaharan Y et al 1988 Disturbed patterns of globin chain synthesis in childhood monosomy 7 myeloproliferative syndrome. British Journal of Haematology 68: 357–362

Smith C M, Nesbit M E, McKenna R et al 1979 Transient myeloid metaplasia associated with an unusual hemoglobin in a newborn infant. American Journal of Pediatric Hematology/Oncology 1: 291–299

Stass S A, Lanham G R, Butler D 1984 Auer rods in mature granulocytes: a unique morphologic feature of acute myelogenous leukemia with maturation. American Journal of Clinical Pathology 81: 662–665

Tulliez M, Vernant J P, Breton-Gorius J et al 1979 Pseudo-Chediak-Higashi anomaly in a case of acute myeloid leukemia: electron microscopic studies. Blood 54: 863–871

Van Roy N, Laureys G, Cheng N C et al 1994 1;17 translocations and other chromosome 17 rearrangements in human primary neuroblastoma tumors and cell lines. Genes, Chromosomes and Cancer 10: 103–114

Whang-Peng J, Knutsen T, Theil K et al 1992 Cytogenetic studies in subgroups of rhabdomyosarcoma. Genes, Chromosomes and Cancer 5: 299–310

Zipursky A, Poon A, Doyle J 1992 Leukemia in Down syndrome: a review. Pediatric Hematology and Oncology 9: 139–149

6 Anomalies of leucocyte structure

Abnormalities of leucocyte morphology other than leukaemia and infection, detectable by light microscopy of films of blood and marrow stained by Romanowsky and readily available cytochemical procedures. Most conditions are hereditary. Detection of abnormality in a routine blood film may be the first indication of serious disorder.

Abbreviations and notes

AcPh: acid phosphatase; ANAE: α naphthyl acetate esterase; CAE: chloroacetate esterase; LCAT: lecithin: cholesterol acyltransferase; ML: mucolipidosis; MPO: myeloperoxidase; MPS: mucopolysaccharidosis; NAP: neutrophil alkaline phosphatase; ORO: oil red O; SBB: sudan black B; TC: transcobalamin.

Magnifications: × 750 unless otherwise stated.

Lymphocytes 202
Vacuolation 202
Gasser lymphocytes 208
Giant granules 212
'Black' granules 212
Grey bodies 212
Plasma cells 212
Vacuolation 212
Buhot cells 212
Grey bodies 212
Granulocytes: cytoplasmic anomalies 214
Alder anomaly 214
Sparse, coarse azurophil granules 214
Vacuolation 214
Döhle-like bodies 216
Neutrophil specific granule deficiency 216
Eosinophil specific granule deficiency 218
Peroxidase deficiency in neutrophils and monocytes 218
Giant granulation 220
Grey bodies 220
Other 222
Granulocytes: nuclear anomalies 222
Pelger-Huet 222
Excessive tags 222
Hypersegmentation of neutrophil nuclei 222
Hypersegmentation of eosinophil nuclei 224
Nuclear changes in toxic states 224
Monocytes 224
Marrow 224
Gaucher cells 224
Foamy macrophages 226
Sea-blue histiocytes 232
Striated, sky-blue cells 232
Gasser 'reticulum' cells 234
Hyperphagocytic macrophages 234
Macrophages with blue-staining vacuoles 234
Abnormal osteoblasts 234
Crystals 236

Abnormalities are considered under the following main headings: lymphocytes, plasma cells, granulocytes, monocytes, bone marrow macrophages and macrophage-like cells, bone marrow osteoblasts, crystals in marrow.

Comprehensive coverage of the genetic disorders considered in this chapter is given by Lake (1992) and Scriver et al (1989).

Lymphocytes (Table 6.1)

VACUOLATION OF OTHERWISE NORMAL LYMPHOCYTES (Fig. 6.1)

In blood films, this is most readily recognized in the trails. In genetic syndromes, vacuolation affects only lymphocytes with basophil cytoplasm and spares larger, 'pale' granulated cells (Smith & Collins 1977 and p. 8). The proportion of vacuolated cells is higher in blood than in marrow aspirates.

Unless otherwise stated in descriptions of individual disorders, the vacuoles are negative with standard cytochemical procedures — PAS, SBB, ORO, AcPh, ANAE and β glucuronidase — and do not show metachromasia with toluidine blue. Electron microscopy shows membrane-bound spaces which are usually empty or sometimes contain nondescript membranous fragments.

The proportion of cells vacuolated and the size and number of vacuoles in individual cells vary with the nature of the disorder (Fig. 6.1, Table 6.2). A high proportion is taken as > 20%; absence from a sample of 20 to 30 cells is sufficient to exclude abnormality with reasonable certainty. Vacuolation may be prominent in malignant lymphoblasts (Fig. 4.8).

Table 6.1 Morphologic anomalies of lymphocytes and plasma cells

- Lymphocytes
  - Vacuolation
  - Gasser lymphocytes
  - Giant azurophilic granules
  - 'Black-granuled' lymphocytes
  - 'Grey' bodies
- Plasma cells
  - Abnormal vacuolation
  - Buhot cells

Table 6.2 Vacuolation of otherwise normal lymphocytes

- Affecting a high proportion of cells with vacuoles large and profuse in individual cells
  - Genetic
    - Batten's disease, juvenile (Spielmeyer-Vogt)
    - Mannosidosis I (infantile)
    - Mannosidosis II (juvenile/adult)
    - G_{M1} gangliosidosis I (infantile)
    - Neuraminidase deficiency, dysmorphic*
    - Galactosialidosis
    - Mucolipidosis II (I cell disease)*
    - Aspartylglycosaminuria (some cases)
    - Salla disease
    - Infantile free sialic acid storage
  - Other
    - Coronary vasodilators (not described in children)
- Affecting a high proportion of cells with smaller, fewer vacuoles
  - Wolman's disease
  - Niemann-Pick disease type A*
  - Aspartylglycosaminuria (some cases)
  - Glycogenosis type II, infantile (Pompe)
  - Fucosidosis*
- Affecting only a small proportion of cells
  - Genetic
    - Cholesteryl ester storage disease (adult Wolman's)
    - Neuraminidase deficiency, normosomatic
    - Mucolipidosis III (pseudo-Hurler polydystrophy)*
    - Fucosidosis type II (adult)
    - Glycogenosis type II, juvenile/adult
  - Other
    - Infection
    - Anticoagulant (e.g. EDTA) artefact

*Variable proportion of lymphocytes affected

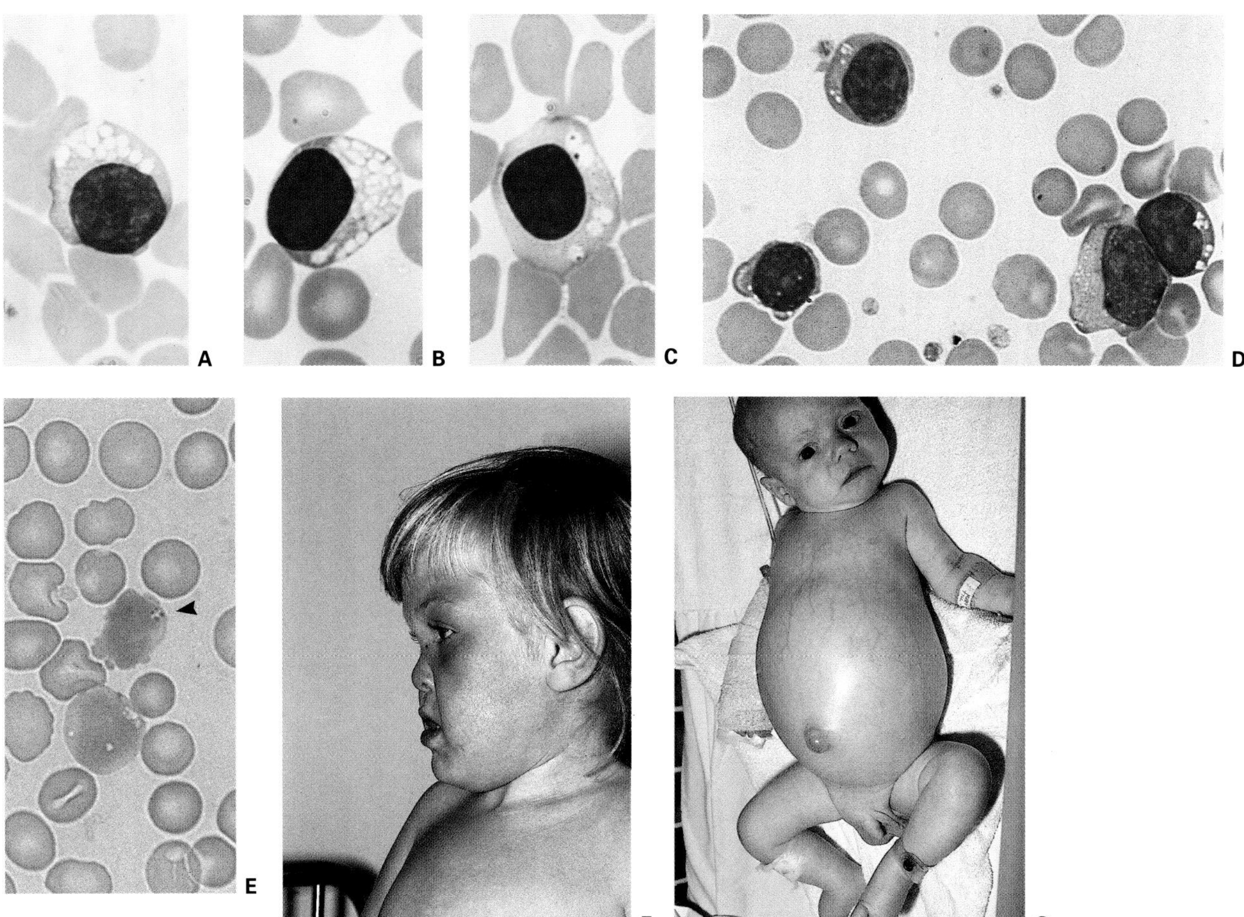

Fig. 6.1 Abnormal lymphocyte vacuolation and some of its causes. **a** Spielmeyer-Vogt lipofuscinosis. **b,c** Mannosidosis juvenile/adult type. **d,e** Wolman's disease; arrow shows ORO positive droplets. **f** 5-year-old girl with mannosidosis. **g** 2-month-old infant with Wolman's disease, abdominal distension from hepatosplenomegaly. **a–c** × 1250; **d,e** × 950

While lymphocyte vacuolation is readily detectable by light microscopy, other lesions can be seen only by electron microscopy, for example granular osmiophilic deposits in infantile (Hagberg-Santavuori) Batten's disease and curvilinear bodies in late infantile (Bielschowsky-Jansky) Batten's disease (Fig. 6.2).

Disorders associated with lymphocyte vacuolation are summarized in Tables 6.2–6.4. Further information is given in the descriptions following. Unless otherwise stated, these disorders have autosomal recessive inheritance. The heterozygous state cannot be identified from lymphocyte morphology.

Batten's disease, juvenile (Spielmeyer-Vogt type neuronal lipofuscinosis)

Onset at 4–5 years of age with increasing blindness (retinitis pigmentosa), disturbed gait and speech, fits, progressive dementia. Survival to 10–25 years. Definitive diagnosis requires rectal biopsy for storage of lipofuscin-like material and 'finger-print' bodies in neurones. Finger-print bodies may also be sought in endothelial and smooth muscle cells and in sweat glands (skin, conjunctiva), where they may be admixed with 'curvilinear' and 'rectilinear' profiles. Enzyme defect not identified.

Mannosidosis

I, infantile

Coarse facies (Fig. 6.1), severe mental retardation. Onset at 3–12 months, survival to 3–10 years. Lymphocyte vacuoles may be PAS positive after celloidin protection, disatase resistant. Foam cells in marrow, vacuolated plasma cells (Fig. 6.7). Definitive diagnosis by acid a mannosidase assay in leucocytes or cultured skin fibroblasts.

II, juvenile/adult

Milder form of I, but deafness more prominent. Onset at 1–4 years, survival to adulthood.

Table 6.3 Blood and marrow changes in storage disorders

	Blood Vacuolated lymphocytes	Foam cells	*Marrow* Sea-blue cells	Vacuolated plasma cells	*Other*
Batten's juvenile	+	–	+	–	
Cholesteryl ester storage	+/–	+	–	–	
Fabry's	–	+/–	+/–	–	
Farber's	–	+/–	–	–	
Fucosidosis I, infantile	+	+	–	–	cell phagocytosis ++, Gasser reticulum cells
Galactosialidosis	+	+	–	+	
Gaucher's	–	+/–	–	–	Gaucher cells
G_{M1} gangliosidosis I	+	+	–	+	abnormal eosinophils
II	–	+	–	–	striated sky-blue cells
Infantile free sialic acid storage	+	+	–	–	abnormal eosinophils, Gasser-like reticulum cells
LCAT deficiency, familial	–	+/–	+	–	
Mannosidosis	+	+	–	+	
Mucolipidosis II (I cell)	+	+	–	+	
Neuraminidase deficiency					
Dysmorphic	+	+	–	–	
Normosomatic	+/–	+/–	–	–	macrophages with blue-staining vacuoles
Niemann-Pick A	+	+	+/–*	–	
B	–	+	++*	+	
C	+/–	+	+/–*	–	
Tangier	–	+	–	–	
Wolman's	+	+	–	–	

+/– = inconstant or only small proportion of cells affected; – = absent or not described;
*Increase with age

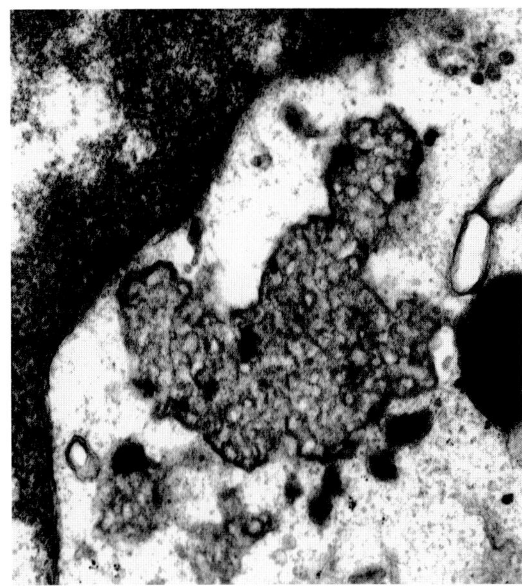

Fig. 6.2 Membrane-enclosed collection of curvilinear bodies in lymphocyte of a 4-year-old boy with late infantile Batten's disease; lymphocytes normal by light microscopy. × 30 000

Table 6.4 Major clinical features of genetic storage disorders

	Psychomotor retardation	Dysostosis	Hepatosplenomegaly	Other
Aspartylglycosaminuria	+/–	+/–	–	lens opacity, acne
Batten's, juvenile	+	–	–	retinitis pigmentosa, late seizures, dementia, tetraplegia
Cholesteryl ester storage	–	–	+	
Fabry's	–	–	–	paraesthesiae, angiectasia, hypohidrosis
Farber's, classic form	+/–	–	+/–	joint deformity, s/c nodules, hoarseness
Fucosidosis I	+	+	+	cardiomegaly
Galactosialidosis				
Infantile	+/–	+	+	oedema
Juvenile	–	+	–	cherry-red spot, corneal opacity, angiokeratomas
Gaucher's	types 2,3	–	+/++	bone pain in types 1 and 3
Glycogenosis II infantile	–	–	liver +	muscle weakness
G_{M1} gangliosidosis I	+	+	+	macular cherry-red spot
II	+	–	–	
Infantile free sialic acid storage	+	+	+	oedema, capillary angiectasia, cardiomyopathy
Mannosidosis, infantile	+	+	+	corneal, lens opacity, deafness
Mucolipidosis II (I cell)	+	+	liver +	corneal opacity, aortic incompetence
III		+/–	+	– corneal clouding
Neuraminidase deficiency				
Normosomatic	–	–	–	macular cherry-red spot, myoclonus
Dysmorphic — congenital	+/–	+	+	oedema (hydrops, ascites, pericardial effusion), corneal opacity
— childhood	+	+	+	macular cherry-red spot; corneal, lens opacity
Niemann-Pick disease A	+	–	++	macular cherry-red spot
B	–	–	+	platelet, lung dysfunction
C	+	–	+/–	neonatal 'hepatitis'; vertical supranuclear ophthalmoplegia
Salla	+	–	–	
Wolman's	+	–	++	adrenal calcification

+/– = mild or inconstant; s/c = subcutaneous

G_{M1} gangliosidosis I (infantile)

Coarse facies, severe psychomotor retardation; macroglossia, hypotonia, macular cherry-red spots in about half of patients; thick, rough, hirsute skin, stiff joints, facial and peripheral oedema; convulsions after about 1 year, later decerebrate rigidity. Onset from birth to infancy, survival to 6 months to 2 years. Definitive diagnosis by assay for acid β galactosidase — histochemical in neutrophils, platelets and lymphocytes, or quantitation in leucocytes or cultured skin fibroblasts; because secondary deficiency occurs in other storage disorders, demonstration of approximately one half normal values in heterozygotes is necessary.

Primary neuraminidase deficiency (sialidosis) (Young et al 1987)

a. With dysmorphism, congenital
Evident at birth. Survival beyond 6 months unusual. Lymphocytes may contain metachromatic granules. Monocyte vacuolation; foam cells in marrow. Urine contains metachromatic sediment (sialoligosaccharides). Definitive diagnosis by assay of acid neuraminidase (sialidase) in cultured skin fibroblasts or (less reliable) leucocytes.

b. With dysmorphism, childhood onset (sialidosis II, ML I)
Onset in early childhood. Coarse Hurler-like facies, mental retardation. Deafness, myoclonus in older children. Survival to < 25 years. Other features, diagnosis as in (a) above.

c. Without dysmorphism (cherry-red spot–myoclonus syndrome, sialidosis type I)
Progressive blindness (macular cherry-red spot, lens opacities), normal appearance and intellect, late dementia. Onset 8–25 years, survival usually to more than 30 years. Diagnosis as for (a) above.

d. Combined deficiency of neuraminidase and *b* galactosidase (galactosialidosis)
Severe form presents at birth with hydrops or ascites, or in infancy with coarse facies, hepatosplenomegaly and dysostosis multiplex.

Milder form presents in early teens with coarse facies, short stature, abnormal gait, myoclonus, failing vision (cherry-red spot, corneal clouding) and angiokeratomas, especially in 'bathing-suit' area; no or mild intellectual impairment, no hepatosplenomegaly. Survival to adulthood. Most patients are Japanese. Vacuolation of plasma cells and nuclei of myeloid cells; foam cells numerous in marrow.

ML II (I cell disease)

Severe Hurler-like dysmorphism and psychomotor retardation. Differences from Hurler MPS include: head not enlarged (may be microcephalic), gingival hyperplasia, no excess mucopolysaccharide in urine. Onset from birth to 1 year. Survival beyond 5–10 years unusual.

Lymphocyte vacuoles may contain purple-staining inclusions. Foam cells in marrow, vacuolated plasma cells and osteoblasts. Coarse refractile inclusions in cultured fibroblasts ('I' for inclusions). Definitive diagnosis:

(i) acid hydrolases (lysosomal enzymes) increased in serum and fibroblast culture fluid but decreased within cells; leakage outside cells due to defect in targeting of lysosomal enzymes to lysosomes
(ii) GlcNAc-phosphotransferase deficiency (leucocytes, cultured fibroblasts).

ML III (pseudo-Hurler polydystrophy)

Milder form of ML II, of later onset (2–4 years) and longer survival (adulthood); some mental retardation in about half. Definitive diagnosis as for ML II.

Fucosidosis

Type I (infantile)
Hurler-like coarse facies. Onset 3–18 months, survival to less than 10 years. Foam cells in marrow and, in some cases, Gasser 'reticulum' cells (Fig. 6.21). Definitive diagnosis by assay of lysosomal α-L-fucosidase in leucocytes or cultured fibroblasts.

Type II (adult)
Milder, with longer survival (adulthood); angiokeratomas, anhidrosis.

Aspartylglycosaminuria

Onset at 1–5 years of coarse facies, sagging coarse skin, mild mental retardation, excitability, clumsiness, hypotonia, microcephaly, acne, sun sensitivity, macroglossia, angiokeratomas. Many patients are Finnish. Survival to adulthood.

Red granules in some lymphocyte vacuoles. Neutropenia in about half. Definitive diagnosis by assay of aspartylglycosaminidase in leucocytes, cultured fibroblasts.

Salla disease

Onset at 3–12 months of moderate to severe psychomotor retardation, mildly coarse facies, hypotonia (later spasticity), ataxia, athetosis, strabismus. Most patients are Finnish. Survival to adulthood. Definitive diagnosis by excess of free sialic acid in urine (5–10 × n) and tissues or tissue cultures. Defect for lysosomal accumulation of sialic acid not identified.

Infantile free sialic acid storage disease

Onset from birth to 3 months of severe psychomotor delay, failure to thrive, cardiomyopathy, ascites (Fig. 6.3), aneurysmal dilatation of capillaries of conjunctiva and elsewhere. Survival beyond 5 years unusual.

Non-metachromatic granules in lymphocytes (Fig. 6.3), granule-poor eosinophils (Fig. 6.11), Alder-like granulation in neutrophils (Fig. 6.8), foam cells and Gasser-like reticulum cells in marrow (Fig. 6.21). Free sialic acid increased in tissues and urine (20–200 × n, cf Salla disease).

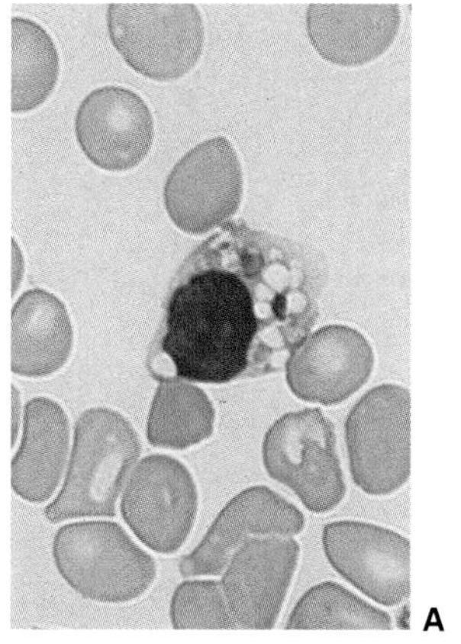

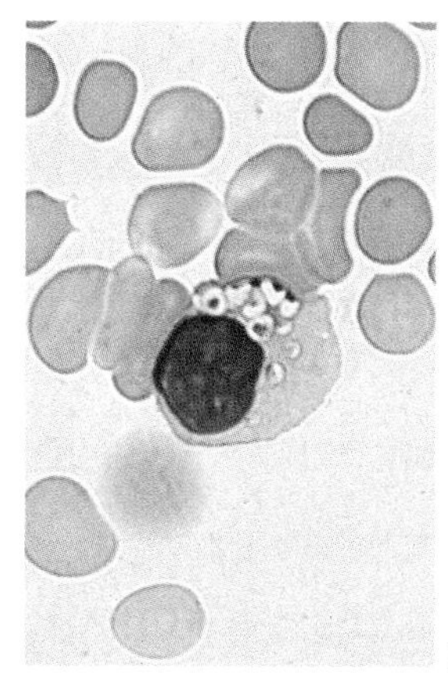

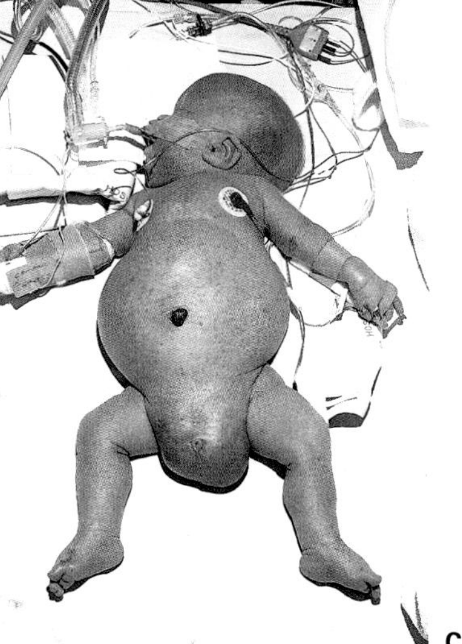

Fig. 6.3 Infantile free sialic acid storage disease. Lymphocytes (blood film) contain coarse azurophilic granules inconstantly related to vacuoles. Hydroceles and abdominal distension from hepatosplenomegaly and ascites.

Wolman's disease

Manifestations are due to accumulation of triglycerides and cholesteryl esters. Onset at less than 1 month of age of diarrhoea, vomiting, inanition, hepatosplenomegaly (Fig. 6.1), calcification and symmetric enlargement of adrenals. Survival to more than 6 months unusual.

Some lymphocyte vacuoles positive with ORO (Fig. 6.1) and SBB. ANAE activity in lymphocytes weak and infrequent (< 10% of cells, normal 70–80%). ANBE activity absent. Foamy ORO positive macrophages in marrow (Fig. 6.18) and occasionally in blood. Acanthocytosis may result from hypo-β lipoproteinaemia (malabsorption). Definitive diagnosis by assay of acid lipase or esterase (histochemical in leucocytes, quantitation in leucocytes, cultured fibroblasts).

Cholesteryl ester storage disease (adult Wolman's)

Milder form of Wolman's, with greater accumulation of cholesteryl esters than of triglycerides. Hepatomegaly; adrenal calcification in occasional cases, premature atherosclerosis. Onset from birth to second decade, most survive to adulthood.

Niemann-Pick disease type A (neurovisceral)

Emaciation, severe psychomotor retardation; spasticity, blindness (cherry-red spot in about 60%), diffuse lung disease. Onset from birth to under 1 year, survival to less than 5 years.

Foam cells numerous in marrow. Definitive diagnosis by sphingomyelinase assay of leucocytes or cultured fibroblasts.

Glycogenosis type II

Infantile (Pompe disease)
Muscle weakness, cardiac failure, macroglossia; muscles firm, enlarged and hypotonic; electromyography usually abnormal even if muscle clinically normal, hepatomegaly but function normal. Onset from birth to 6 months, survival beyond 2 years unusual.

Lymphocyte vacuoles PAS positive after celloidin protection, diastase sensitive (glycogen). Vacuolated plasma cells and osteoblasts in marrow. Definitive diagnosis by acid α-glucosidase assay in muscle, liver, leucocytes.

Juvenile/adult
Milder than infantile, with later onset (some > 15 years) and longer survival. Cardiomegaly, macroglossia infrequent.

GASSER LYMPHOCYTES (Fig. 6.4)

The characteristic granules are densely staining, usually grouped in one part of cell, often coarse, often individually within clear vacuoles, and are metachromatic (some granules in normal, large granular lymphocytes [Fig. 1.2] may be slightly metachromatic). This granulation is more obvious with May-Grünwald-Giemsa than Wright's stains, and (like vacuolation, p. 202) is restricted to lymphocytes with basophil cytoplasm. Unless otherwise stated in summaries below, it affects at least 20% of cells, absence from a sample of 20–30 cells excluding abnormality with reasonable certainty. The cells are most readily detectable by oil-immersion examination of tail-ends of films. The granulation is negative for MPO, SBB, PAS and ORO. In a small proportion of lymphocytes vacuolation is the only abnormality.

Gasser lymphocytes are characteristic of the mucopolysaccharidoses (Fig. 6.5, Table 6.5), excepting Morquio disease.

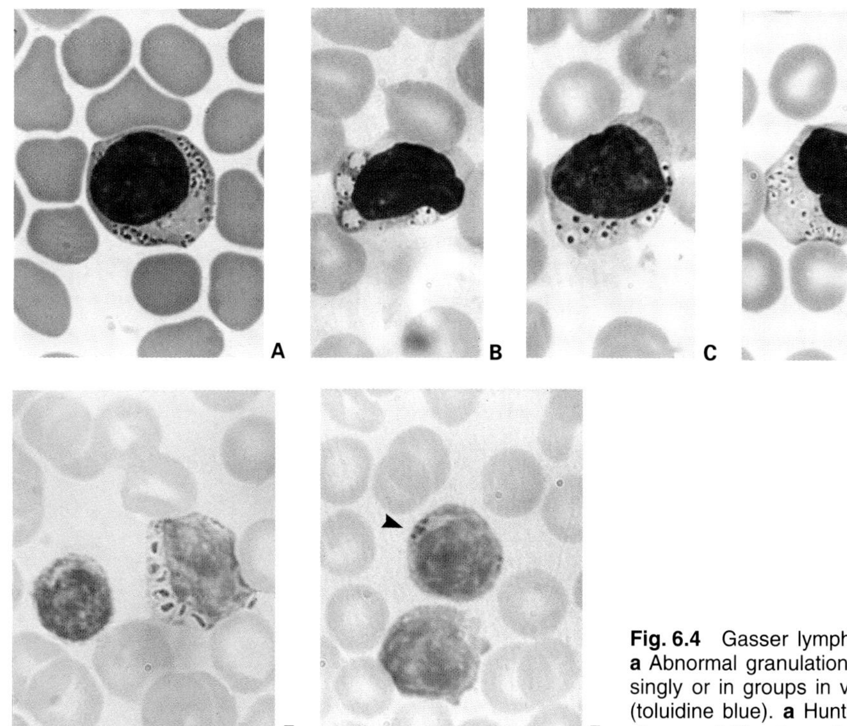

Fig. 6.4 Gasser lymphocytes in blood in mucopolysaccharidoses. **a** Abnormal granulation with minimal vacuolation. **b–d** Granules lying singly or in groups in vacuoles. **e,f** Metachromatic granulation (toluidine blue). **a** Hunter MPS; **b,c,e** Hurler MPS; **d** Sanfilippo disease; **f** Maroteaux-Lamy MPS. All × 1250

Table 6.5 The mucopolysaccharidoses

	Gasser lympho-cytes	Neutro-phils with sparse coarse granules	Gasser reticulum cells	Buhot plasma cells	Psycho-motor retardation	Dysostosis	Hepato-spleno-megaly	Corneal opacity	Other
Hurler, IH	+	–	+	+	+	+	+	+	
Scheie, IS	+	–	+		–	–	–	++	
Hurler-Scheie, IHS	+	–	+		+/–	+		+	receding chin
Hunter, II[1]	+	–	+	+	+	+	–	–	pebblestone skin
Sanfilippo, III	+	–	+	+	+	+/–	+/–	+/–	
Morquio, IV[1]	–	+	+		–	++	liver +	+/–	
Maroteaux-Lamy, VI	+	–	+		–	+	+	+	Alder granulation
Sly, VII[2]	+	–	+	+	+	+	+	+/–	Alder granulation
MSD[3]	+	–	+	+	+	+/–	+	+/–	ichthyosis, optic atrophy, Alder granulation, abnormal eosinophils

[1] Mild forms occur
[2] Milder and more severe forms occur
[3] Multiple sulphatase deficiency
+/– = mild or inconstant; gaps = insufficient information

MPS IH (Hurler) (Fig. 6.5)

Severe dysmorphism and mental retardation; hearing loss, noisy breathing from mural accumulation of mucopolysaccharide, cardiac disease (mucopolysaccharide in muscle, valves and coronary vessels), stiff joints, carpal tunnel syndrome. Onset at 6–24 months, survival beyond 10 years unusual. Autosomal recessive.

Buhot plasma cells (Fig. 6.6), Gasser 'reticulum' cells (Fig. 6.21), and abnormal osteoblasts (Fig. 6.22) in marrow, increased urine mucopolysaccharide. Definitive diagnosis by assay of lysosomal α-L-iduronidase in leucocytes, cultured fibroblasts or serum.

MPS IS (Scheie)

Prominent eye changes (corneal clouding, glaucoma, retinal degeneration), mildly coarse facies, late mucopolysaccharide accumulation in tissues (carpal tunnel, aortic valve). Onset 5–10 years, normal life span. Autosomal recessive.

Gasser lymphocytes usually < 10% of cells; Gasser 'reticulum' cells in marrow, increased urine mucopolysaccharide. Diagnosis as for MPS IH.

MPS IH/S (Hurler-Scheie) (Fig. 6.5)

Intermediate between MPS IH and IS. Receding chin may be characteristic; cervical cord compression from mucopolysaccharide infiltration of dura, but hydrocephalus uncommon. Onset 3–8 years, survival to adulthood unusual. Other features as for MPS IH.

MPS II (Hunter) (Fig. 6.5)

Similar to MPS IH, but slower progression, clear corneas (opacity may be visible on slit-lamp, may have retinal degeneration), 'pebblestone' skin (distinctive for this MPS) and X-linked recessive inheritance. Onset 2–4 years, survival to 10–15 years. Mild forms have normal intelligence, with survival to adulthood.

Definitive diagnosis by iduronate sulphatase assay in leucocytes, cultured fibroblasts or serum.

MPS III (Sanfilippo) (Fig. 6.5)

Severe mental retardation with mild somatic change — hyperactivity, sleep disturbance, athetosis, mild facial coarsening; hirsutism, joint stiffness, stature usually normal. Type A patients (of types A–D) tend to be most severely affected. Onset 2–6 years, survival to adolescence. Autosomal recessive.

Abnormal lymphocytes may be sparse in Romanowsky blood films, but metachromasia usual in high proportion (> 20%) of cells. Buhot plasma cells, Gasser reticulum cells and abnormal osteoblasts in marrow, increased mucopolysaccharide in urine. Definitive diagnosis by assay of 4 enzymes necessary for degradation of heparin sulphate in leucocytes, cultured fibroblasts or (type B only) serum.

MPS VI (Maroteaux-Lamy)

Hurler-like somatic abnormalities but normal intelligence and may survive to adulthood. Cervical cord compression from dural thickening and odontoid dislocation. Autosomal recessive. Definitive diagnosis by assay of N-acetylgalactosamine 4-sulphatase (arylsulphatase B) in leucocytes or cultured fibroblasts.

MPS VII (Sly)

Severe form (rare) presents at birth with hydrops and dysostosis multiplex. Commonest form presents before 4 years with Hurler-like features. Mildest cases present after 4 years with slight skeletal change, normal facies, stature and intelligence, insignificant corneal opacity. Autosomal recessive.

Increased mucopolysaccharide in urine. Definitive diagnosis by β glucuronidase assay (cytochemistry of lymphocytes, granulocytes, monocytes or quantitation in leucocytes, cultured fibroblasts or serum).

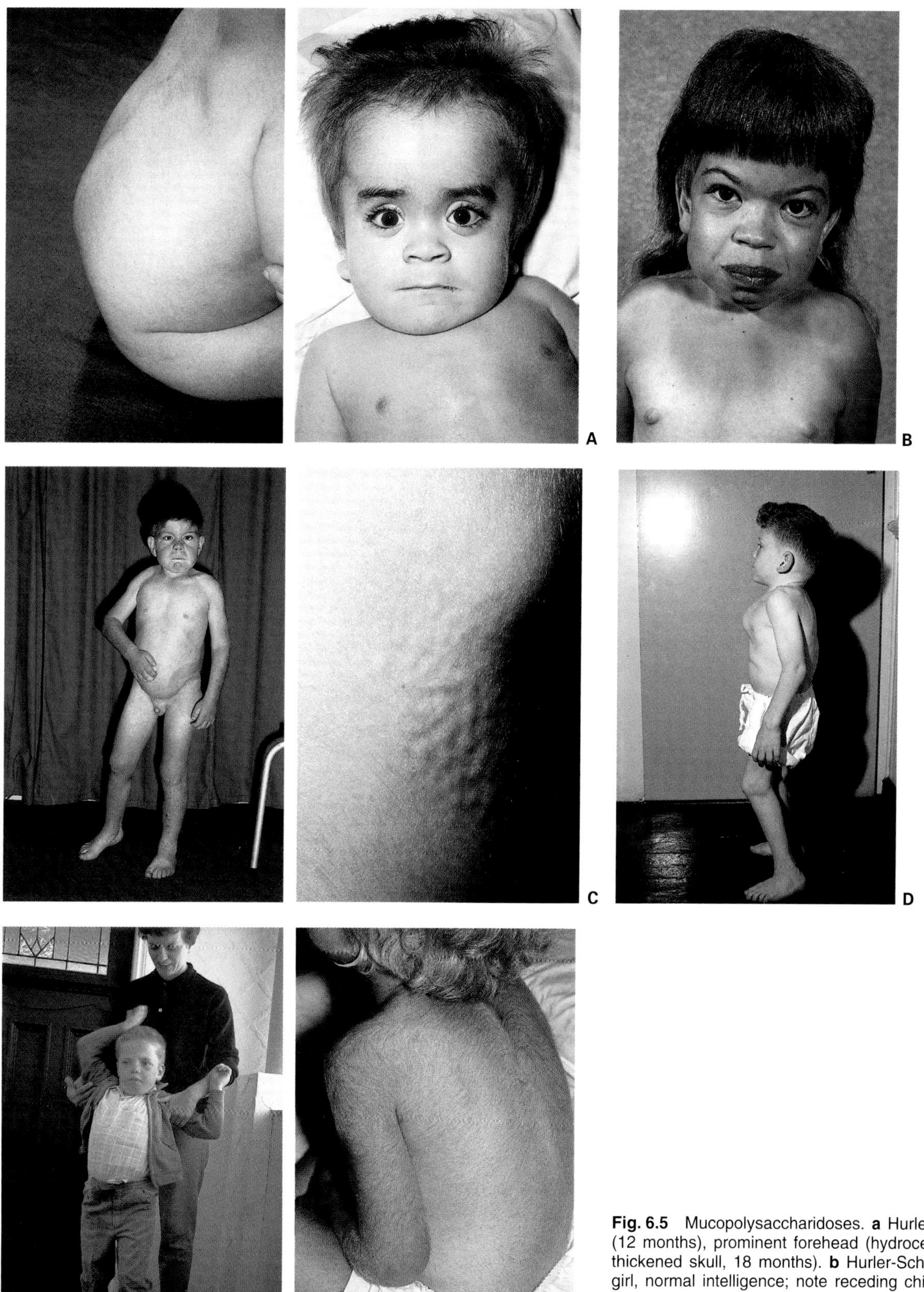

Fig. 6.5 Mucopolysaccharidoses. **a** Hurler, lumbar gibbus (12 months), prominent forehead (hydrocephalus, thickened skull, 18 months). **b** Hurler-Scheie, 11-year-old girl, normal intelligence; note receding chin. **c** Hunter, 6 years, clawed hands, pebblestone skin in scapular region. **d** Morquio, 9-year-old boy, normal intelligence. **e** Sanfilippo, 9-year-old boy with choreoathetosis, large head, coarse facies; hirsutism in 7-year-old girl.

Mucosulphatidosis (multiple sulphatase deficiency, Austin variant of metachromatic leukodystrophy)

Features of both mucopolysaccharidosis and metachromatic leukodystrophy. The common form presents at 6 months–2 years with mild facial coarsening, moderate psychomotor retardation (eventual spasticity), hearing impairment, stiff joints, visual impairment (optic atrophy, retinal degeneration and, in some, cherry-red macula). Rare, severe form manifests at birth with additional features of hydrocephalus and corneal clouding. Autosomal recessive.

Absence of specific granules in eosinophils (Fig. 6.11). Urine mucopolysaccharides increased. Urine shows golden-brown, granular and flocculent metachromatic sediment. A deficiency of 7 sulphatases that degrade mucopolysaccharides and sulphated glycolipids and steroids; most convenient to assay are arylsulphatases A,B,C in leucocytes or cultured fibroblasts.

GIANT GRANULATION (Fig. 6.6)

A characteristic of the Chediak-Higashi syndrome. The enlarged granules are lysosomes formed by granule fusion as a result of membrane abnormality, affecting leucocytes, platelets, Schwann cells and melanocytes (hair, skin, iris, ocular fundus).

Lymphocyte granules are ANAE and AcPh positive and MPO negative. Absence of large granular lymphocytes (Collins et al 1979) may be correlated with deficiency of natural killer cell activity (Abo et al 1982).

Granulocyte abnormality and clinical features are considered on page 220.

'BLACK-GRANULED' LYMPHOCYTES

A possibly genuine anomaly, in which 20–45% of lymphocytes contain black-staining granules, was found in 2 sibs (one with serious anomalies) but not parents. Co-occurrence with normal azurophil granules in the one cell was rare. No abnormality of ultrastructure was found.

GREY-STAINING BODIES

See page 220, and Figure 6.12.

Plasma cells

ABNORMAL VACUOLATION (Fig. 6.7, Table 6.6)

Affected cells may be normal in size or enlarged, resembling foamy macrophages. However, they are not phagocytic, the cytoplasm is more basophilic and nuclear structure more compact.

POLYMORPHOUS INCLUSIONS, OFTEN INDIVIDUALLY WITHIN CLEAR VACUOLES, METACHROMATIC (BUHOT CELLS)

The inclusions are densely staining and appear in the shape of granules, rods, commas, rings, crescents or hollow pears (Fig. 6.7). A small proportion of cells contains vacuoles only. Occur in a variety of mucopolysaccharidoses (Table 6.5). Metachromasia is weak or absent in MPS VII (Sly).

GREY-STAINING BODIES

See page 220.

Table 6.6 Plasma cells: abnormal vacuolation

Mannosidosis
G_{M1} gangliosidosis
Mucolipidosis II (I cell disease)
Galactosialidosis[1]
Glycogen storage disease type II[1]
Niemann-Pick disease type B
Mucolipidosis III (pseudo-Hurler polydystrophy)[2]
Ichthyosis and neutral lipid storage disease[3]

[1] Vacuoles PAS positive, weaker after diastase
[2] Some cells contain coarse inclusions
[3] Vacuoles ORO and sudan III positive

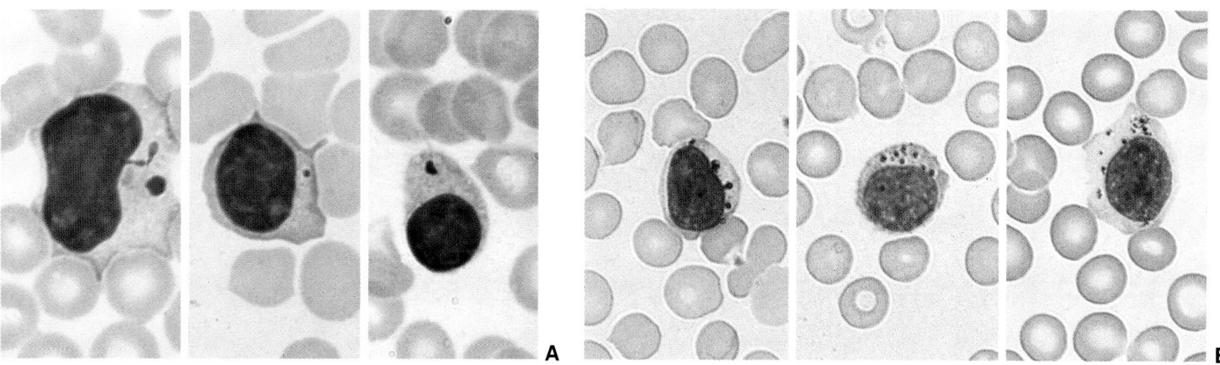

Fig. 6.6 Lymphocytes with abnormal azurophil granulation. **a** Giant granulation, Chediak-Higashi syndrome. **b** 'Black-granuled' lymphocytes; cell at right also contains normal granules. **a** × 1250; **b** × 950

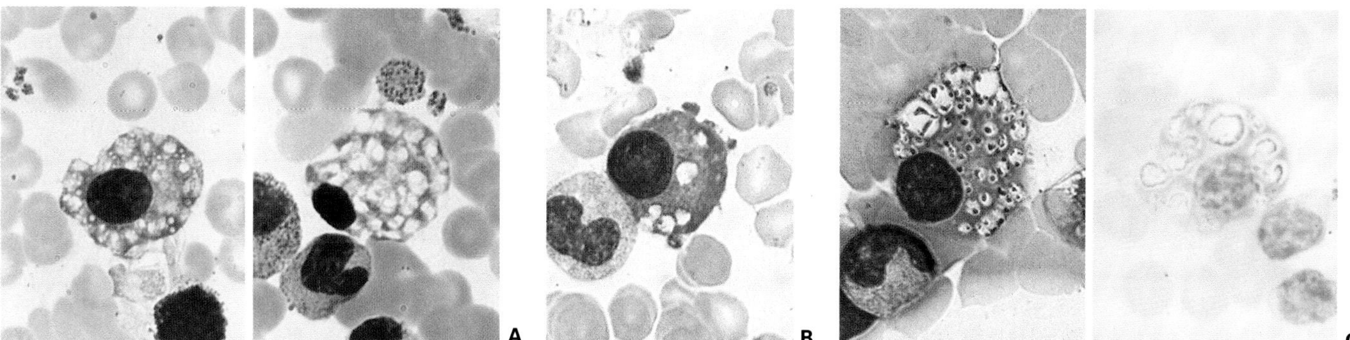

Fig. 6.7 Abnormal plasma cells. **a** Vacuolation, mannosidosis. **b** Vacuolation, Niemann-Pick disease type B. **c** Buhot cells, Sanfilippo MPS (toluidine blue at right). All × 950

Granulocytes: cytoplasmic anomalies (Table 6.7)

ALDER ANOMALY (Fig. 6.8, Table 6.8)

Coarse, densely-staining granulation in neutrophils, anomalous staining of eosinophil granules (violet, green or grey-black, may resemble basophil granules), and unusually coarse or densely staining granules in basophils, monocytes and mast cells. Precursor cells in marrow are also affected. To be distinguished from toxic granulation (finer, often associated with other signs of toxicity, temporary).

SPARSE, COARSE AZUROPHIL GRANULES (Fig. 6.8)

A minority of neutrophils contains a light sprinkling of coarse granules. Rare granules may be metachromatic. Other granulocytes are normal.

Characteristic of MPS IV (Morquio) type A (early onset). Main features (Fig. 6.5): normal intelligence, gross and distinctive skeletal change, mild facial coarsening and corneal clouding, risk of spinal cord compression from odontoid hypoplasia; valvular heart disease. Onset 1–3½ years, survival beyond 30 years unusual. Autosomal recessive. Definitive diagnosis by galactose-6-sulphatase (arylsulphatase A) assay in leucocytes or cultured fibroblasts. Milder forms occur, with no excess of mucopolysaccharide in urine and longer survival.

VACUOLATION

Vacuolation is uncommon as a genetic anomaly. More common causes are toxic states (infection, inflammation, cytotoxics) and artefact of anticoagulation.

Vacuoles of neutral lipid (Jordans anomaly) (Jordans 1953)

Vacuoles are ORO and sudan III positive, stain red with nile blue sulphate and occur in most to all neutrophils, eosinophils, basophils and monocytes and in a proportion of plasma cells, but not in other haemopoietic cells. Absent from myeloblasts and increase with cell maturity from promyelocyte onward.

Ichthyosis and neutral lipid storage disease
(Williams et al 1985)
Triglyceride droplets also in other tissues, e.g. muscle, liver. Main features: ichthyosis, myopathy, ataxia, sensorineural deafness, cataracts, liver dysfunction, variable mental retardation. Evident at birth, autosomal recessive.

Carnitine deficiency
A heterogeneous and incompletely characterized group of disorders in which carnitine deficiency may be genetic or acquired (e.g. renal Fanconi syndrome, haemodialysis, total parenteral nutrition, Roe & Coates 1989). The defect/s in some of the genetic deficiencies is unidentified and the traditional distinction between 'muscle' and 'systemic' deficiency may be artificial. In some there is a defect in carnitine transport across mitochondrial membranes, in others a defect in carnitine synthesis. Jordans anomaly is associated with muscle carnitine deficiency (skeletal and cardiac), less so with systemic deficiency.

Wolman's disease
Lipid vacuoles are inconsistent and infrequent. For other features see page 207.

Neonatal haemochromatosis
Neutrophils with ORO positive vacuoles may occur in neonatal haemochromatosis. In the infant shown in Figure 6.9 vacuolation was associated with nuclear pyknosis/cell death, and vacuolated cells contained (between the vacuoles) fine Perls positive granulation (finer than in adults with haemochromatosis, Yam et al 1968).

Other
ORO positive neutrophils may occur transiently in biliary atresia and following GCSF treatment.

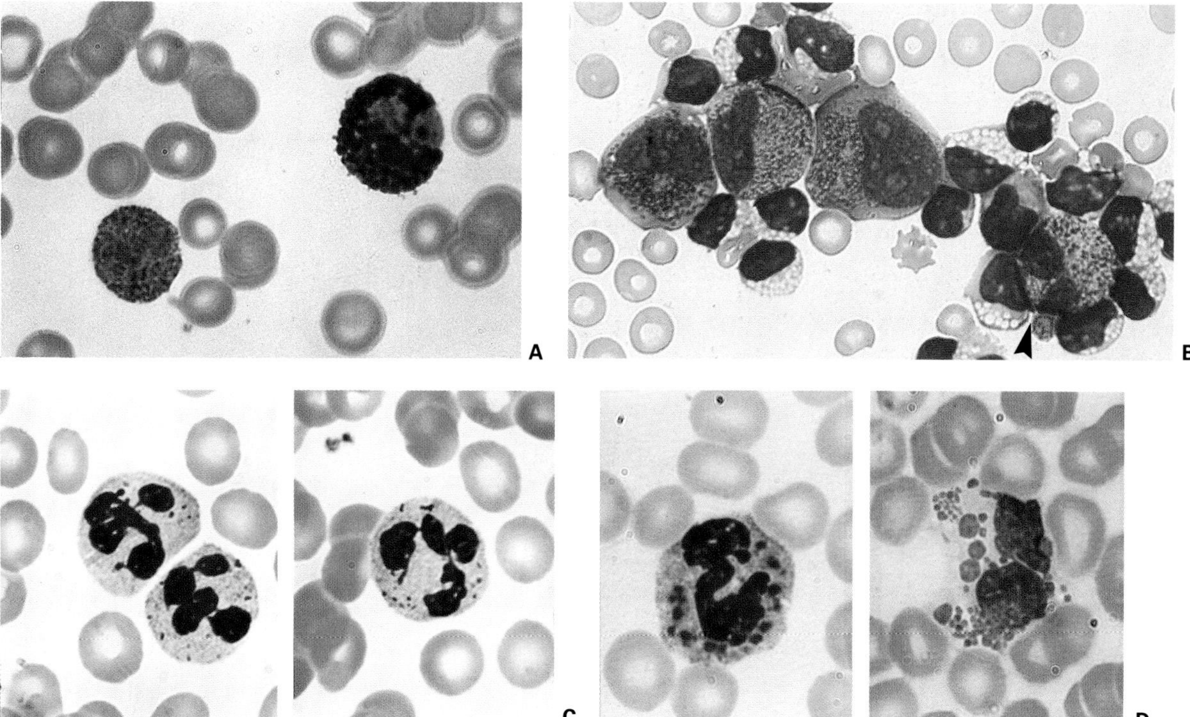

Fig. 6.8 Abnormal granulation in granulocytes. **a** Alder granulation in neutrophil and basophil, Maroteaux-Lamy MPS. **b** Alder-type granulation in neutrophils, most noticeable in stab form (arrow), vacuolated lymphocytes, infantile free sialic acid storage disease, ascitic fluid cytospin. **c** Sprinkling of coarse azurophil granules in neutrophils, Morquio MPS. **d** Giant granulation in neutrophil and eosinophil, Chediak-Higashi syndrome. **a,c,d** × 1250. **d** Courtesy of Dr I Green

Table 6.7 Anomalies of granulocyte cytoplasm

Anomalies of granulocyte cytoplasm
Alder anomaly
Sparse coarse azurophilic granules
Vacuolation
Vacuolation of granulocyte precursors and erythroblasts
Döhle-like bodies
Neutrophil specific granule deficiency
Eosinophil specific granule deficiency
Peroxidase deficiency in neutrophils
Giant granulation in granulocytes and monocytes
Amorphous rounded 'grey' bodies
Haemosiderin
Bilirubin

Table 6.8 Alder granulation

Alder granulation
MPS VI (Maroteaux-Lamy)[1]
MPS VII (Sly)
Multiple sulphatase deficiency
Infantile free sialic acid storage disease[2]
Asymptomatic[3]

[1] Granules metachromatic and birefringent
[2] Partially developed Alder granulation
[3] Existence doubted

Pearson's marrow–pancreas syndrome

(Pearson et al 1979)

Vacuolation of granulocyte and erythroid precursors, ringed sideroblastosis (Fig. 6.9), increased storage haemosiderin, transfusion-dependent macrocytic anaemia, reticulocytopenia; variable neutropenia, thrombocytopenia and splenic atrophy. May evolve to marrow aplasia or leukaemia. A deletion of mitochondrial DNA has been identified (Rotig et al 1989). Possible maternal inheritance.

Presents in infancy with growth failure and refractory steatorrhoea (pancreatic fibrosis). About half die before the age of 3 years, others improve with age.

Differential diagnosis is from other marrow–pancreas syndromes and from hereditary sideroblastic anaemia:

- Shwachman syndrome (p. 50)

No vacuolation or sideroblastosis; marrow hypoplasia earlier and more prominent than in Pearson's.

- Hereditary sideroblastic anaemia (p. 20)

A proportion of erythrocytes is microcytic. No vacuolation or pancreatic insufficiency.

- Atypical cystic fibrosis with marrow hypoplasia (Fig. 2.18)

No vacuolation or sideroblastosis.

DÖHLE-LIKE BODIES

These are usually more sharply defined and larger than Döhle bodies, are not accompanied by toxic changes and are permanent.

May-Hegglin anomaly
Inclusions (Fig. 6.10) usually easily seen, but may be inconspicuous in some cases; occur in granulocytes and monocytes but not lymphocytes; pyroninophilic (reaction abolished by ribonuclease), with distinctive ultrastructure of 7–10 nm filaments oriented in parallel in long axis. Associated with enlarged platelets and, in about one quarter, mild thrombocytopenia (p. 302). Autosomal dominant.

Fechtner's syndrome (Alport's syndrome variant)
(Peterson et al 1985)
Döhle-like inclusions, giant platelets, nephritis (microscopic haematuria to renal failure), sensorineural deafness and congenital blue-spotted ('caerulean') cataracts. The Döhle-like bodies occur in most neutrophils and some eosinophils, are smaller and less intensely staining than in May-Hegglin and consist of segments of rough endoplastic reticulum and ribosome clusters but no filaments (cf May-Hegglin above). Platelets are large; moderate to severe thrombocytopenia common. Autosomal dominant.

Sebastian platelet syndrome
Similar to Fechtner's syndrome but without the clinical abnormalities.

NEUTROPHIL SPECIFIC GRANULE DEFICIENCY (Gallin 1985)

Specific granule deficiency is usually acquired (myeloid leukaemias, burns, infection, normal neonate). The genetic deficiency is more severe and is rare. Main features:

- In stained films cells appear poorly granulated and washed out (MPO-deficient cells appear normal).
- NAP decreased or absent. NAP is not a constituent of specific granules but plasma membrane linked, deficiency being attributed to an anomaly common to both plasma membrane and specific granules.
- Granule ultrastructure consists only of the enveloping vesicle.
- Deficiency of specific granule components, e.g. lactoferrin, TCII, can be shown by biochemical or immunologic methods. Deficiency of TCII in serum may be associated (p. 38).
- Deficiency of defensins (normal component of subpopulation of azurophil granules) accompanies the specific granule defect (Parmley et al 1989).
- Pelgeroid changes — bilobed nuclei of uneven size; micronuclei in some cells.
- Cells are defective in chemotaxis (specific granules produce chemotactic receptors) and in bactericidal capacity (deficiency of lactoferrin, defensins, Ganz et al 1988).
- Neutropenia due to intramedullary destruction may occur.
- Manifests as pyogenic infections, which may be indolent.
- Probably autosomal recessive.

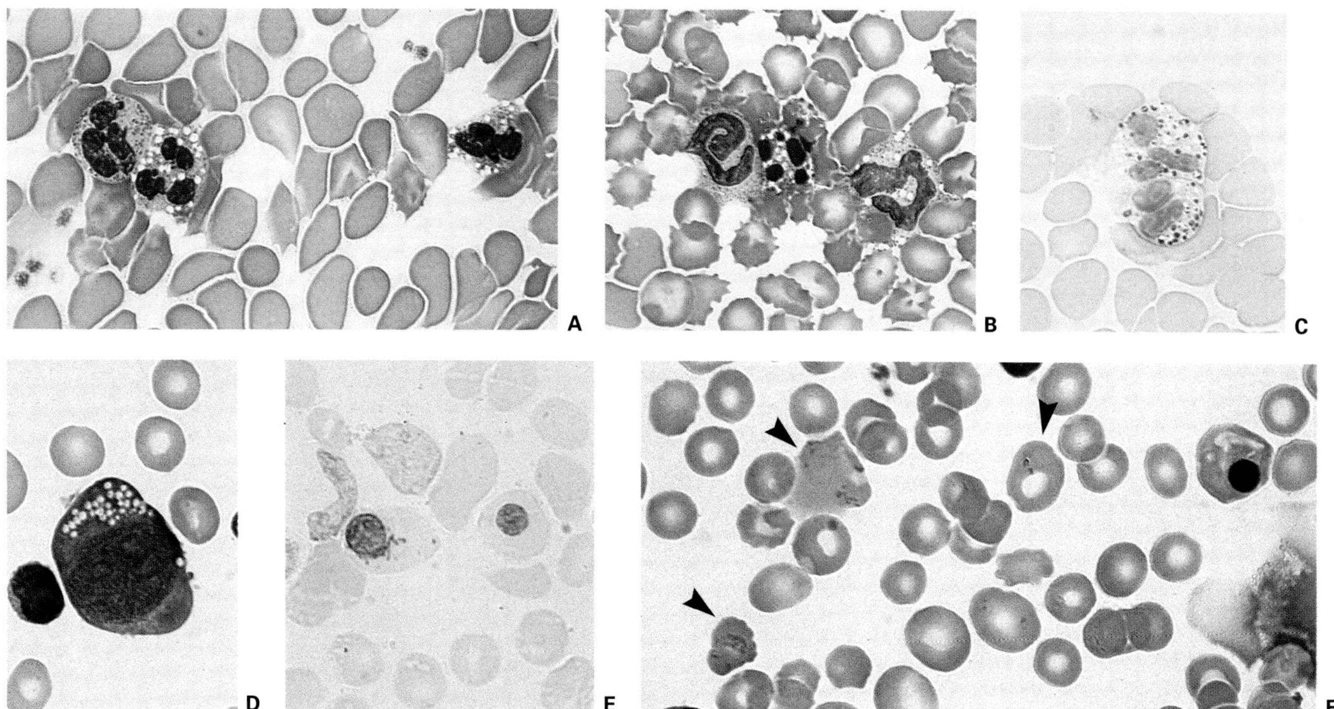

Fig. 6.9 Vacuolated neutrophils. **a–c** Jordans-like abnormality in a 2-day-old infant with haemochromatosis, unanticoagulated blood films. In **a** the 2 vacuolated neutrophils show nuclear pyknosis; in **b** the vacuolated neutrophil in the middle is dead. **c** ORO positive droplets in neutrophils. Fine Perls positive granulation was also noted in vacuolated cells. Vacuolation disappeared by day 10. **d–f** Marrow, Pearson's syndrome, 10-month-old boy. **d** Vacuolated myeloblast. **e** (Perls) 2 erythroblasts, one a ringed sideroblast. **f** Erythroblast with defective haemoglobinization and 3 siderocytes (arrows). Death occurred at 3 years from marrow aplasia. **d–f** $\times$ 950. **d–f** Courtesy of Dr G Tauro

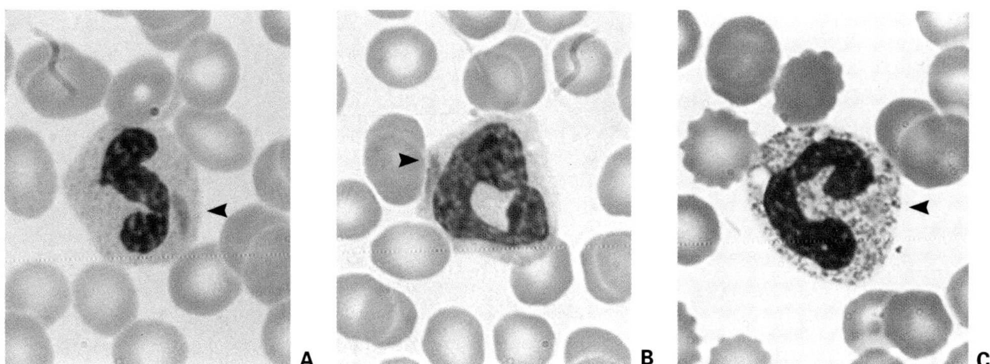

Fig. 6.10 Sabre-shaped Döhle-like bodies in neutrophil (**a**) and monocyte (**b**), May-Hegglin anomaly, vs Döhle body in septicaemia (**c**). All $\times$ 1250

EOSINOPHIL SPECIFIC GRANULE DEFICIENCY (Fig. 6.11)

Occurs in a variety of acquired and inherited disorders (Table 6.9).

In patients receiving colony stimulating factors, clearing of cytoplasm is due more to granule agglutination than to deficiency (Fig. 6.11). Acquired absence of eosinophils (and sometimes basophils) due to Ig-mediated destruction is a rare occurrence in allergic rhinitis/asthma and in thymoma with hypogammaglobulinaemia; the direct antiglobulin test is positive in some cases (Mitchell et al 1983, Nakahata et al 1984).

The inherited disorders in Table 6.9 are rare; the first 3 are considered elsewhere; the last 2 are considered here.

Hereditary deficiency of eosinophil peroxidase (EPO) (Presentey 1968)
EPO normally is localized to the cortex ('matrix') surrounding the crystalloid core of the specific granule. In most cases of EPO deficiency eosinophils appear normal by light microscopy. In some, however, eosinophils or a proportion of them appear deficient in granules and nuclei are hypersegmented — usually 3 lobes, sometimes 4 or 5; precursors in marrow however are normal. Cells do not stain for MPO and SBB, whether they appear granule-deficient or not.

Identification is by conventional cytochemistry or by recognition of anomalous leucocyte peroxidase distribution pattern in automated differential counting systems measuring cell size and peroxidase content. Electron microscopy shows the covering (matrix) of the granule to be thin, and only the periphery instead of all of the crystalloid core to be electron dense. MPO in neutrophils and monocytes is normal. No clinical disease has been linked to EPO deficiency. Inheritance autosomal recessive.

A syndrome of granule-deficient eosinophils, hyperphagocytic macrophages and Michaelis-Gutmann bodies (Fig. 6.11)
The nature of this combination, noted in an infant born with gross splenomegaly, is unknown. The Michaelis-Gutmann bodies (calcospherites, malacoplakia) showed typical ultrastructure and cytochemistry (positive with PAS, sudan black, Perls, von Kossa, pyronin).

The only discernible effect was thrombocytopenia due to hypersplenism. The patient remains well at last follow-up (25 years, splenectomy at 3 weeks). The proportion of granule-poor eosinophils has diminished with age — 90% in infancy, 25% at 25 years. Leucocyte morphology in both parents and 2 sibs is normal.

A profusion of Michaelis-Gutmann bodies has been noted in brain in herpes simplex infection (Ho-Chang et al 1980) and in the retroperitoneum in SLE (Hamdan et al 1982).

PEROXIDASE DEFICIENCY IN NEUTROPHILS AND MONOCYTES (Nauseef 1988)

The peroxidase in neutrophils and monocytes (MPO) differs from that in eosinophils and is under different genetic control. In neutrophils MPO is localized to azurophil (primary) granules (cf EPO, above).

- Acquired deficiency occurs in myeloid leukaemias (M2, M3, M4 especially) and myelodysplasias (Cech et al 1982). Usually a proportion of neutrophils is completely lacking in enzyme (cf genetic partial deficiency below). The gene for MPO lies in 17q in the vicinity of the breakpoint for the t(15;17) of AML M3.
- Activity is diminished by some drugs — sulphonamides, antithyroid drugs, phenothiazines, ascorbic acid.
- MPO deficiency is the commonest inherited disorder of neutrophils (complete deficiency about 1/4000, partial about 1/2000). The partial deficiency affects all or almost all neutrophils, though not necessarily to the same degree. Identification is by standard cytochemical methods (MPO, SBB, Dacie & Lewis 1991) or, for partial deficiency especially, automated flow cytometry using 4-chloro-1-naphthol as substrate (e.g. Hemalog D counter). MPO-deficient bloods will be wrongly identified as neutropenic by automated counters which identify neutrophils cytochemically. EPO is normal.

Morphology of neutrophils and monocytes in stained films is normal (cf specific granule deficiency above).

Surprisingly, bactericidal capacity of MPO-deficient granulocytes is only mildly diminished; killing of fungi (candida, aspergillus) however is severely affected. Patients have little susceptibility to bacterial infection, but there is a risk of disseminated candidiasis if MPO deficiency is associated with diabetes mellitus. Mode of inheritance is uncertain. Simple Mendelian genetics are unlikely and polygenic inheritance has been proposed.

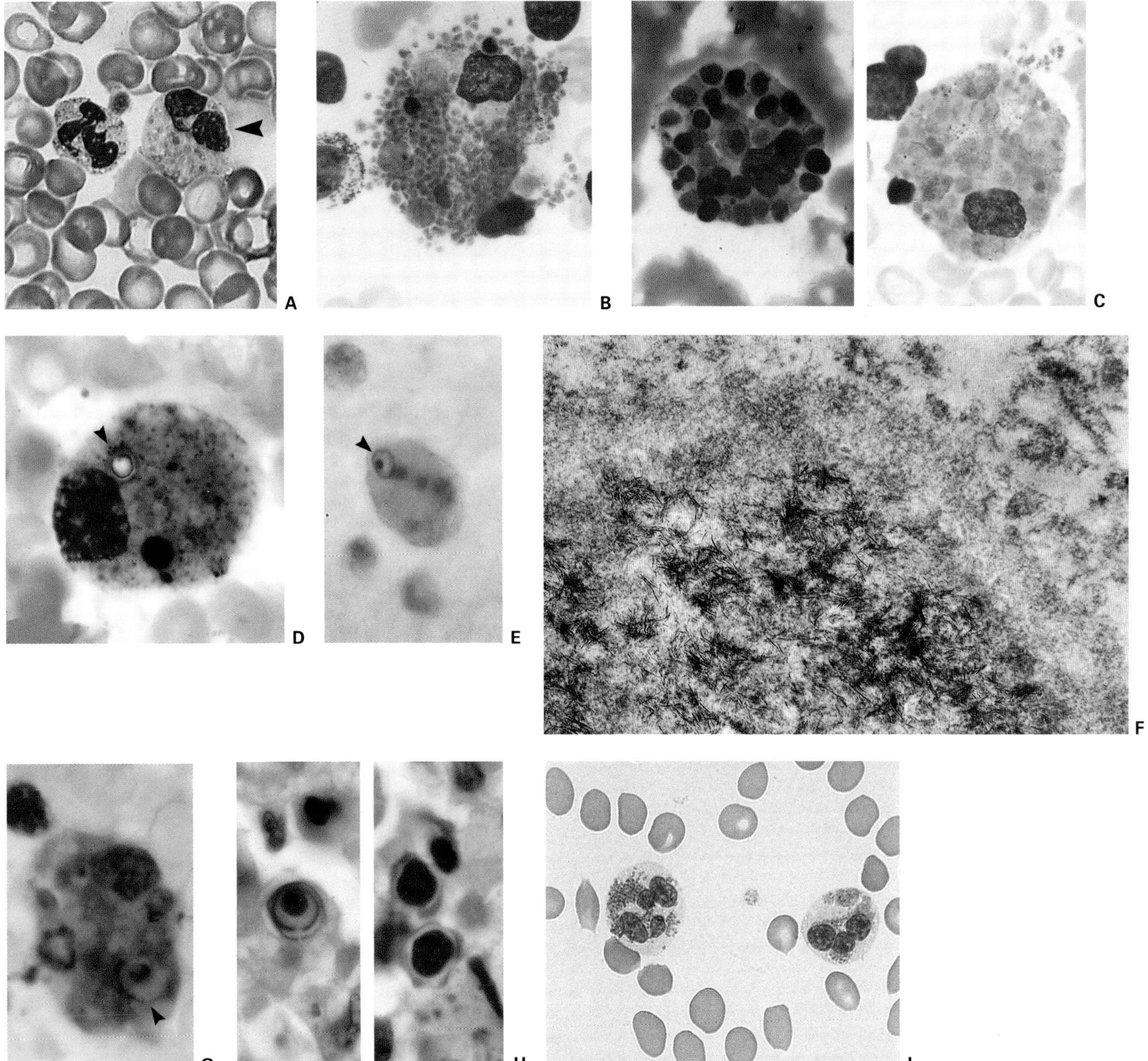

Fig. 6.11 Eosinophil specific granule deficiency. **a** Infantile free sialic acid storage disease, normal neutrophil also in field. **b–g** (Marrow) and **h** (spleen) in a neonate with syndrome of hypogranular eosinophils, 'greedy' macrophages and Michaelis-Gutmann (MG) bodies. **b** Macrophage with profusion of platelets. **c** Macrophages with unidentified nucleated cells, in advanced degeneration in cell at right. **d,e** MG bodies (**e** methyl green-pyronin). **f** MG body, microcrystals of hydroxyapatite. **g,h** Beginning formation of MG bodies around phagocytosed nuclei (**g** PAS, **h** H & E). **i** Granule deficiency and agglutination, GCSF treatment. **b–e**,**g**,**h** × 800; **f** × 36 000

Table 6.9 Eosinophil specific granule deficiency

Acquired
Myeloid leukaemias
Infection
Treatment with colony stimulating factors
Acquired absence of eosinophils
Inherited
Infantile free sialic acid storage disease
G_{M1} gangliosidosis, infantile
Mucosulphatidosis
Hereditary deficiency of eosinophil peroxidase
Syndrome of granule-deficient eosinophils, hyperphagocytic macrophages and Michaelis-Gutmann bodies (?inherited)

• Partial deficiency of MPO has been described in adult onset ceroid lipofuscinosis (Kufs disease). The deficiency was unusual in being detectable by the 4-chloro-1-naphthol substrate method but not by the benzidine-based procedure, and in affecting eosinophils as well as neutrophils (Bozdech et al 1980).

GIANT GRANULATION IN GRANULOCYTES AND MONOCYTES

Chediak-Higashi syndrome (Fig. 6.8)
An unidentified membrane abnormality results in fusion of azurophil and specific granules to form giant granules (Rausch et al 1978). These are positive for MPO, SBB, AcPh and CAE (constituents of azurophil granules) and contain lactoferrin (specific granules). Normal specific granules are sparse and azurophil granules absent. Defects in chemotaxis, mobilization and degranulation are attributed to mechanical impediment imposed by granule size (White & Clawson 1980). These defects, together with neutropenia and deficient natural killer cell activity (p. 212), contribute to susceptibility to infection.

Neutrophil precursors (marrow) contain large, MPO positive, pink to purple staining inclusions, often within vacuoles. Neutropenia and increase in serum muramidase are attributed to intramedullary destruction of precursor cells (Blume et al 1968). Eosinophil precursors may contain giant, densely staining azurophil granules. For the lymphocyte abnormality see page 212 and Figure 6.6.

A minority of platelets may contain large granules. Bleeding is due to deficiency of dense bodies (p. 314) and, in the accelerated phase, thrombocytopenia.

The main clinical features are partial oculocutaneous albinism, cranial and peripheral neuropathy (muscle weakness, ataxia, sensory loss, nystagmus), infection (especially *S. aureus*) and bleeding (see above). In the accelerated phase (usually pre-terminal, first or second decade), organ enlargement and pancytopenia are due to lymphohistiocytic proliferation and haemophagocytosis.

Autosomal recessive. Heterozygotes may show giant granulation in occasional leucocytes, but this is an unreliable test for the carrier state.

Pseudo-Chediak-Higashi granulation
Giant granulation in granulocytes, but not lymphocytes, may occur in myeloid leukaemias (Tulliez et al 1979, Fig. 5.5). Abnormal granules are formed by fusion of azurophil granules and may contain Auer-like microcrystals, which differ from true Auer rods in periodicity of ultrastructure.

GREY-STAINING BODIES

Amorphous, rounded, grey-staining bodies (Fig. 6.12) have been noted in:

• Granulocytes of the 3 types, monocytes and mast cells in an infant with livedo reticularis of the skin and extrahepatic biliary atresia (Smith 1967). Leucocyte morphology in both parents was normal. Inclusions negative by routine cytochemical procedures. The anomaly is not a result of the biliary atresia (absent in 130 control infants).
• Eosinophils and basophils only, as a dominantly inherited, apparently asymptomatic anomaly (Tracey & Smith 1978). Inclusions absent from other haemopoietic cells, including mast cells; mildly positive with some cytochemical procedures (e.g. PAS), distinctive in ultrastructure, and associated with crystals of latticed ultrastructure. (Charcot-Leyden crystals, which may also occur in eosinophils, are not latticed.)
• Granulocytes (all types), monocytes, lymphocytes and plasma cells, from birth in an infant with hepatosplenomegaly, spherocytic haemolysis, thrombocytopenia, neutropenia and infections. These features disappeared and the child is apparently well at the age of 2 years. Inclusions negative with routine cytochemistries. Electron microscopy showed a ribosomal type composition without identifiable organelles (Willoughby M L 1975, personal communication).

In a (possibly) similar case, inclusions identified as collections of actin microfilaments occurred in all haemopoietic cells, but mainly granulocytes in a 13-month-old boy with transfusion-dependent anaemia, splenomegaly, grey skin discoloration and intermittent neutropenia and thrombocytopenia. Clinical abnormalities resolved spontaneously at about 18 months but inclusions have persisted (Ribeiro et al 1994).

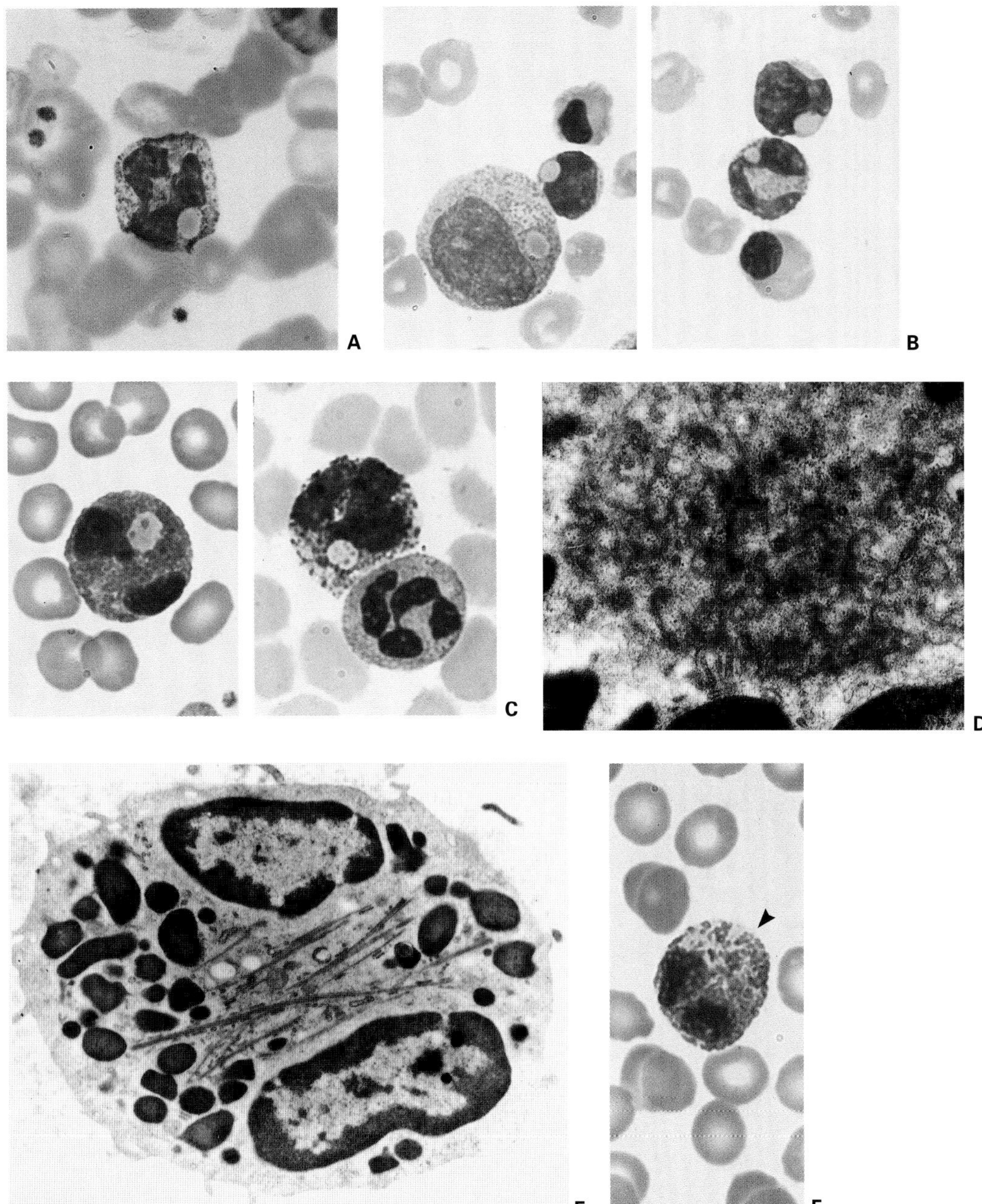

Fig. 6.12 'Grey' body inclusion anomalies. **a** Neutrophil in an infant with livedo reticularis of skin and intrahepatic biliary atresia; no other family members affected. **b** (Buffy coat): inclusions in lymphocytes and granulocytes but not erythroblasts, a temporary phenomenon in an infant with spherocytic haemolysis, thrombocytopenia, neutropenia and infections. **c-f** Dominantly-inherited, apparently asymptomatic anomaly. **c** Eosinophil and basophil, each with a single inclusion, normal neutrophil. **d** Part of inclusion, showing bilaminar membrane arcs, absence of enclosing membrane. **e** Eosinophil containing crystals. **f** Eosinophil containing unstained splinters, possibly crystals. **a,c,f** × 1200; **b** × 1000; **d** × 20 000; **e** × 6500. **b** Courtesy of Dr M Willoughby. **d** Reproduced with permission from Tracey R, Smith H 1978 An inherited anomaly of human eosinophils and basophils. Blood Cells 4: 293 (Fig. 3b). Copyright Springer-Verlag

OTHER INCLUSIONS

Neutrophils and/or monocytes may contain haemosiderin (brown-yellow staining, often refractile, Fig. 6.13) and bilirubin (yellow-green to green-black, Fig. 6.15).

Granulocytes: nuclear anomalies
(Table 6.10)

PELGER-HUET ANOMALY

● Pelgerization is most commonly acquired, occurring especially in myeloid leukaemias, myelodysplasias, bilineage ALL (Fig. 4.4), toxic states (Fig. 7.6) and colchicine poisoning (Fig. 6.14).

● The inherited anomaly may be heterozygous or homozygous and affect all or only some (5–20%) cells. In the common, heterozygous state, neutrophil nuclei have rod, dumb-bell, peanut or pince-nez shapes (Fig. 6.14), and eosinophil nuclei ≯ 2 lobes; abnormality is not readily recognizable in basophils. In the rare homozygote, most cells have rounded nuclei (Stodtmeister forms).

Inheritance is autosomal dominant, with some rare exceptions (following). The common, heterozygous state is not convincingly linked to any clinical illness. Associations have however been suggested with: (i) muscular dystrophy; (ii) a syndrome of episodic fever and abdominal pain (thought to be autosomal recessive because of an intermediate degree of Pelgerization in one parent available for study, Murros & Konttinen 1974); (iii) a syndrome of leucopenia and infections, probably X-linked (Heyne 1976).

The homozygous state appears to be usually lethal in utero.

● Pelgerization is conspicuous in inherited neutrophil specific granule deficiency (p. 216).

Table 6.10 Abnormalities of granulocyte nuclei

Pelger-Huet and like anomalies
Excessive tags
Hypersegmentation of neutrophil nuclei
Hypersegmentation of eosinophil nuclei
Chromomeres
Toxic states

EXCESSIVE TAGS (Fig. 6.14)

Short projections, with head as wide as or slightly wider than the attachment stalk, to be distinguished from drumsticks (larger mass of dense chromatin, attached by short filament) and clubs (larger than drumstick, longer filament). The chromatin may be coarse and lumpy and separation of lobes indistinct.

Occurrence of 2 or more tags in > 15% of neutrophils is characteristic of trisomy 13, whether isolated or as part of triploidy. Hereditary persistence of nuclear appendages is described as an autosomal dominant, asymptomatic defect, but its status as a genuine, independent anomaly is uncertain.

HYPERSEGMENTATION OF NEUTROPHIL NUCLEI (Table 6.11)

The normal mean lobe count, after the neonatal period, is 2.8 (2.5–3.1). Only the last 2 in Table 6.11 are considered here. Others are discussed elsewhere.

● Hereditary constitutional hypersegmentation — mean lobe count approximately 4, but cells normal in size. Asymptomatic, autosomal dominant.

● Hereditary giant neutrophils (macropolycytes) — 5–15% of neutrophils abnormally large, with 6–10 lobes (probably tetraploid, Fig. 6.14). Normally up to 2 cells per 1000, slightly more in a variety of illnesses, including cytotoxic exposure. Asymptomatic, autosomal dominant, but only the heterozygous state is known.

Table 6.11 Hypersegmentation of neutrophil nuclei

Toxic states
Megaloblastosis[1]
Triploidy[2]
Myelokathexis
Neutropenia and hypogammaglobulinaemia with abundant, abnormal neutrophils in marrow
Lightsey anomaly[3]
Iron deficiency (uncommon)
Hereditary constitutional hypersegmentation
Hereditary giant neutrophils (macropolycytes)

[1] Benign or as a part of myeloid leukaemia/myelodysplasia
[2] Sadowitz et al 1984
[3] Neutropenia with gigantism and multinuclearity of marrow neutrophils

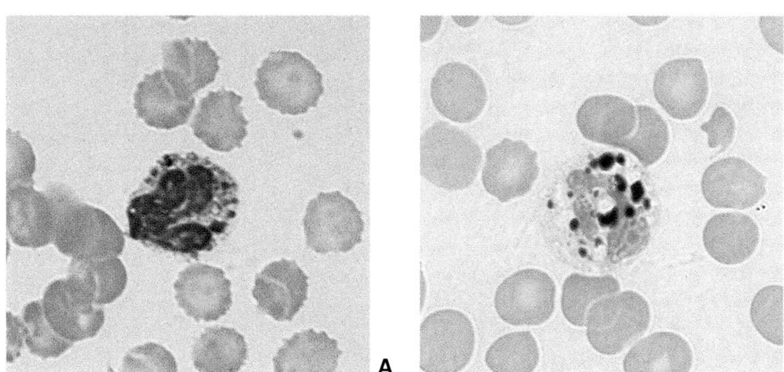

Fig. 6.13 Haemosiderin in neutrophils (Perls, right), infant with histiocytosis receiving frequent blood transfusions. × 950

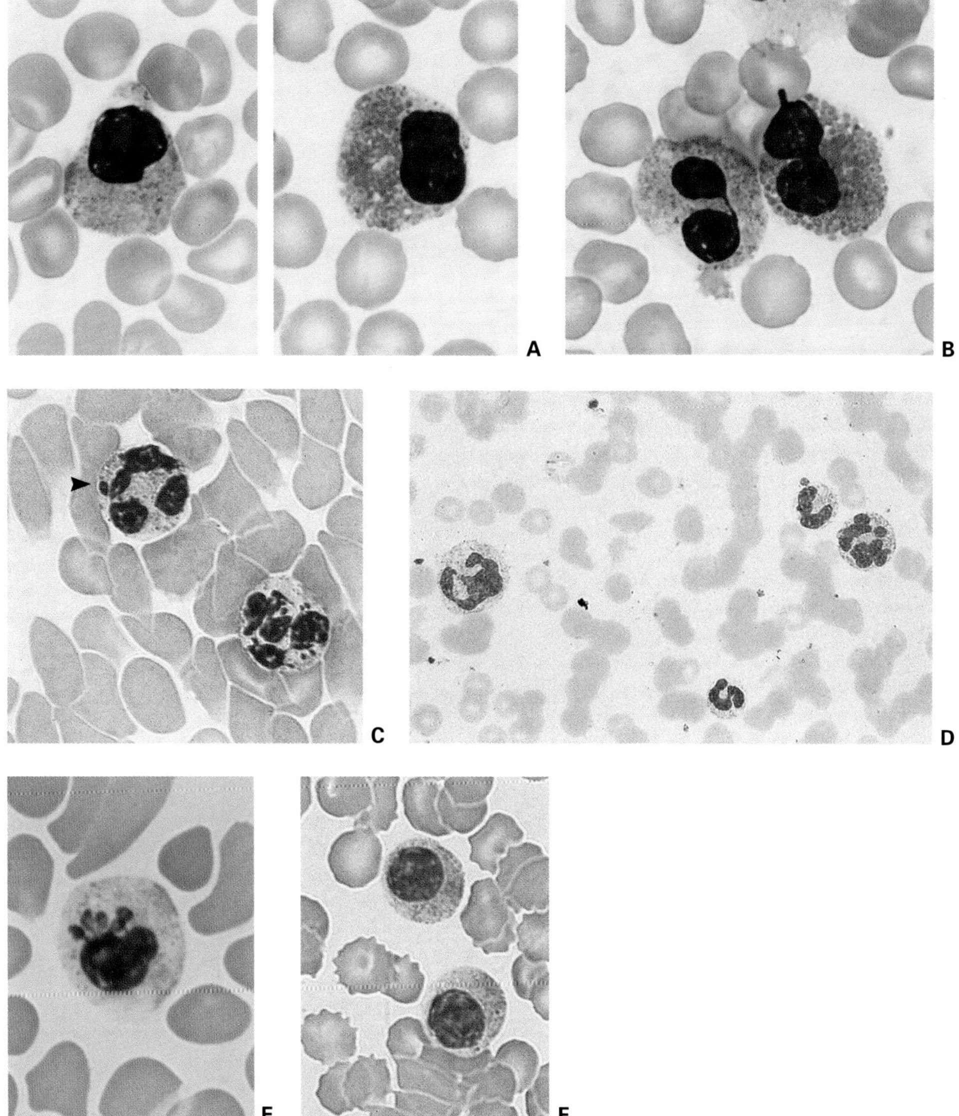

Fig. 6.14 Nuclear abnormalities in granulocytes. **a,b** Pelger-Huet anomaly, heterozygote, fields from same blood film. Peanut-shaped nuclei in neutrophils (**a**); stab eosinophil, neutrophil with pince-nez nucleus (**b**). **c** Nuclear tags (drumstick arrowed) in 1-day-old female infant with trisomy 13. **d** Hereditary giant neutrophils, 2 macropolycytes and 2 normal neutrophils. **f,g** Colchicine poisoning, nuclear extrusions (**f**) and Pelgerization (Stodtmeister forms, **g**). **a,b** × 1300; **c** × 950; **d** × 500; **e** × 1100; **f** × 950

HYPERSEGMENTATION OF EOSINOPHIL NUCLEI

Normal mean lobe count is approx 2.5 — about two thirds of cells have 2 lobes, one third 3, with rare cells containing 4 lobes or an unsegmented nucleus. Hypersegmentation occurs in: megaloblastosis, hereditary deficiency of eosinophil peroxidase (Presentey anomaly, p. 218) and hereditary hypersegmentation (asymptomatic, probably autosomal dominant).

NUCLEAR CHANGES IN TOXIC STATES

- Infection, treatment with cytotoxics

See page 257.

- Heat stroke, hyperpyrexia

'Botryoid' nuclei (shrinkage, pyknosis, clustering of lobes), often with fragmentation and chromomere formation, may occur in heat stroke and hyperpyrexia (Hernandez et al 1980). Changes disappear within 24 hours after removal from injury.

- Colchicine poisoning

Extrusions, chromatin damage and Pelgerization may be noted (Fig. 6.14).

Table 6.12 Abnormal macrophages and macrophage-like cells in bone marrow

Gaucher cells
Foamy macrophages
Sea-blue cells
Striated sky-blue cells
Gasser 'reticulum' cells
Hyperphagocytic macrophages
Macrophages with blue-staining vacuoles

Monocytes

Monocytes are rarely affected in isolation from other blood leucocytes:

- Polymorphous, metachromatic inclusions in mucopolysaccharidoses (Fig. 6.15).
- Alder granulation in MPS VI and VII.
- Giant granulation in Chediak-Higashi syndrome. Yellow or orange-yellow coloration may cause confusion with erythrocyte fragments; like giant granules in neutrophils, are formed by fusion and contain components (MPO, AcPh, muramidase) which normally are distributed in separate types of granule.
- Döhle-like bodies in May-Hegglin anomaly (Fig. 6.10).
- Vacuolation. Usually a toxic or reactive change (Fig. 7.13), but may be noted in inherited disorders with foamy macrophages in marrow (e.g. Wolman's disease) and in association with granulocyte vacuolation in Jordans anomaly (p. 214).
- Bilirubin (Fig. 6.15).
- Grey-staining inclusions (p. 220).
- Toxic changes, e.g. vacuolation, Döhle bodies.
- Crystals in histiocytoses (Fig. 5.30).
- Hyperphagocytic macrophages (Fig. 6.11).

Bone marrow macrophages and macrophage-like cells

These are considered in the order of listing in Table 6.12.

GAUCHER CELLS

'Typical' Gaucher cells (often in the minority in marrow), have one or more nuclei, often eccentric, and cytoplasm of striped, 'crumpled tissue paper' or 'jumbled tooth-picks' texture (Fig. 6.16). Parts of cells may be foamy rather than striated. Inclusions of leucocytes and erythrocytes occur in occasional cells. Cells are positive for AcPh (diminished by tartrate), ANAE (fluoride resistant), β glucuronidase, PAS (mild to moderate only), and (rare cells) Perls, interpreted as indicating an origin of storage cerebroside from phagocytosed erythroid cells; negative for fat stains. Electron microscopy shows cerebroside in the form of spiralled tubules 30–75 nm wide.

Gaucher's disease

Three clinical types are recognized:

- Type I (adult, non-neuronopathic chronic): bone lesions, splenomegaly, lesser hepatomegaly, bleeding from thrombocytopenia, platelet dysfunction and (unexplained) Factor IX deficiency. No neurologic disease.
- Type II (infantile, acute neuronopathic): failure to thrive, marked hepatosplenomegaly and psychomotor retardation, brain stem dysfunction (retroflexion of head, trismus, strabismus). Cerebroside accumulates in neurones, which are phagocytosed. Survival beyond 2 years unusual.
- Type III (juvenile, subacute neuronopathic): psychomotor retardation dominant; ataxia, myoclonus, spasticity, supranuclear palsy of horizontal gaze, seizures; bone changes, splenomegaly. High proportion Swedes (Norrbottnian Gaucher disease). Gaucher cells accumulate in Virchow-Robin space but neurones normal.

Features common to all types are:

- Gaucher cells usually in profusion in marrow but most profuse in infantile type. Cells may be more profuse in crush than smear of aspirate.
- Increase in serum acid phosphatase, tartrate stable.
- Hypersplenism, causing thrombocytopenia or pancytopenia, but Hb rarely < 8 g/dl.
- Autosomal recessive.
- Definitive diagnosis by glucocerebrosidase assay in leucocytes or cultured skin fibroblasts.

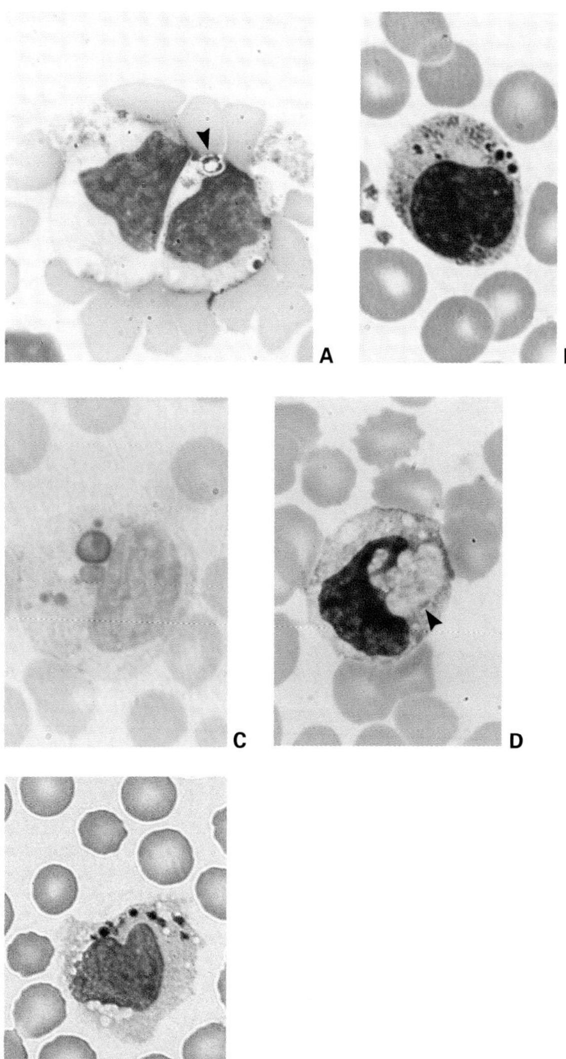

Fig. 6.15 Monocytes with inclusions. **a** (Hurler MPS), **b,c** (Maroteaux-Lamy MPS): densely staining circle (arrow) and granules, some individually within vacuoles; inclusions are metachromatic (**c**, toluidine blue). **d,e** Bilirubin in monocytes, severe jaundice from biliary obstruction. **a–d** × 1200; **e** × 950

Other disorders

Gaucher and Gaucher-like cells (Figs 6.16, 4.16) are usually sparse in conditions other than Gaucher's disease — thalassaemia major, HIV infection, congenital dyserythropoietic anaemias (especially type II), Shwachman's syndrome, cytotoxic treatment and malignancy (ALL, Hodgkin's disease, chronic myeloid leukaemia). Occurrence in these disorders is attributed to overloading of normal enzymic mechanisms for handling products of cell breakdown. In some instances structure is indistinguishable by both light and electron microscopy from true Gaucher cells (Zaino et al 1971); in others ultrastructure is one of fibrils rather than tubules (Lee & Ellis 1971), or other differences are noted (Fig. 6.16). In HIV infection and immunodeficient states, a pseudo-Gaucher appearance may result from phagocytosis of Ziehl-Neelsen-positive mycobacteria (Solis et al 1986).

FOAMY MACROPHAGES

To be distinguished from normal fat cells (Fig. 6.18, nucleus more eccentric, a proportion of vacuoles large; ORO positive, no cell inclusions), Gaucher and Gaucher-like cells (Fig. 6.16) and vacuolated plasma cells (Fig. 6.7). Foamy macrophages are a common abnormality in marrow but diagnostic significance is limited unless they are present in profusion and possessed of distinctive cytochemistry.

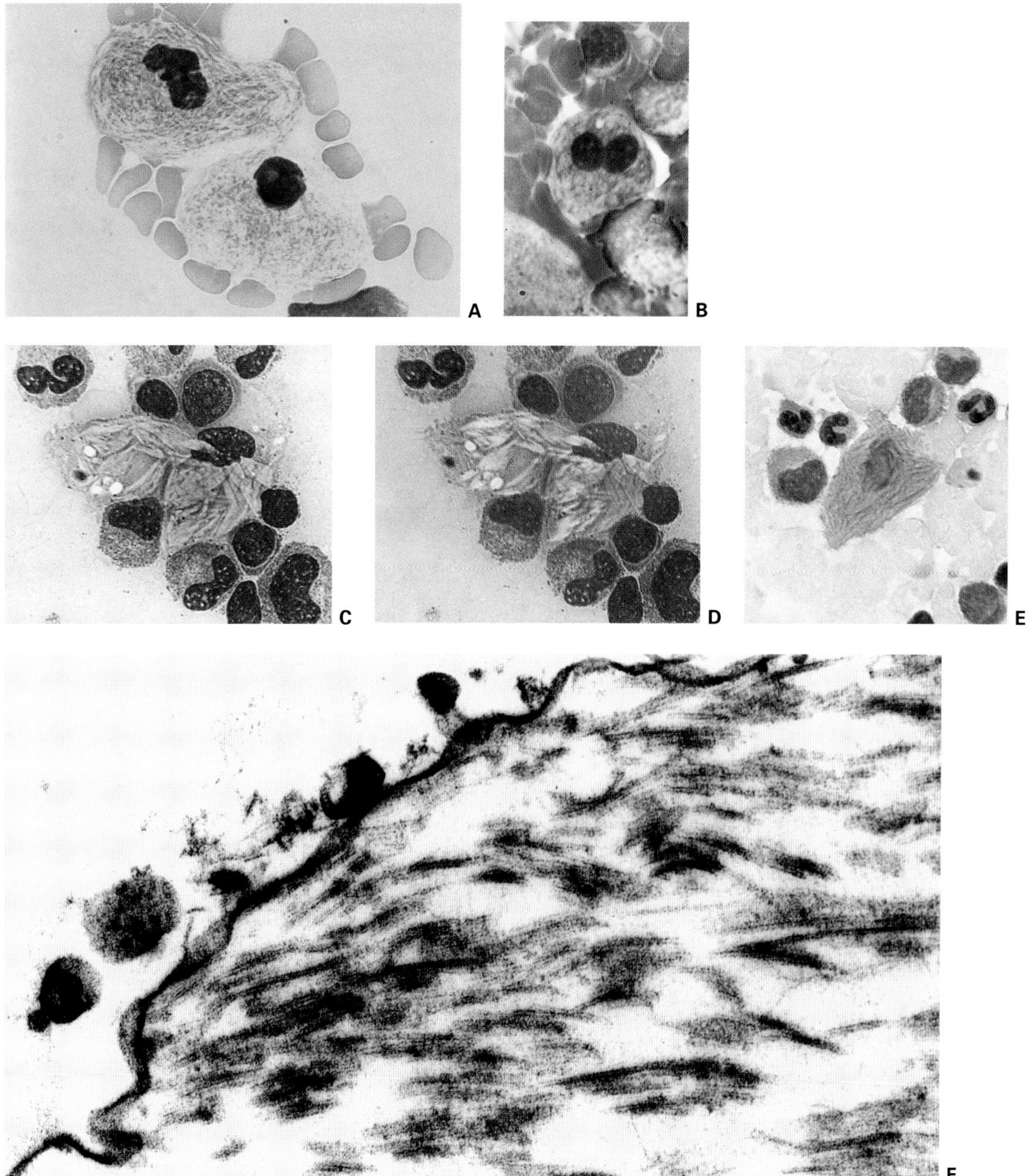

Fig. 6.16 Gaucher (**a**) and Gaucher-like (**b–f**) cells in marrow aspirates. **a** Gaucher disease type I, 5-year-old girl presenting with bruising from thrombocytopenia. **b** 18-month-old child with Shwachman's syndrome. **c–f** ALL t(4;11) in remission 2 months after diagnosis. **c** Romanowsky. **d** Same cell in polarized light. **e** PAS, reaction stronger than in true Gaucher cells. **f** Straight tubules approx 16 nm wide (true Gaucher tubules are spiralled and wider); × 60 000.

Disorders with foamy macrophages in profusion in marrow

These are listed, with cell characteristics, in Table 6.13 and illustrated in Figures 6.17 and 6.18. Other features of inherited disorders are summarized in Tables 6.3 and 6.4. Descriptions below are of disorders not considered elsewhere in this chapter.

Niemann-Pick disease type B ('adult')
Main clinical features: splenomegaly, later hepatomegaly; lung dysfunction (diffuse infiltration), thrombocytopenia or pancytopenia (hypersplenism), bleeding (liver cirrhosis, decreased liver coagulation factors, thrombocytopenia, platelet dysfunction), pingueculae. Psychomotor dysfunction absent or mild, retinal cherry-red spot in rare cases. Onset from 6 months to more than 20 years. Autosomal recessive. Definitive diagnosis by sphingomyelinase assay (leucocytes, cultured fibroblasts).

Niemann-Pick disease type C (Pentchev et al 1995)
A heterogeneous disorder. Main features: history of neonatal hepatitis and splenomegaly of unknown nature lasting up to 6 months (may be fatal), progressive mental retardation, vertical supranuclear ophthalmoplegia (impairment of downward gaze), splenomegaly, lesser hepatomegaly, seizures, myoclonus. Autosomal recessive. Definitive diagnosis by impaired cholesterol esterification in cultured fibroblasts, characteristic intense perinuclear fluorescence after staining with filipin (intralysosomal cholesterol).

Table 6.13 Disorders with foam cells profuse in marrow[1]

	Foam cells[2]
Inherited	
Niemann-Pick A	sphingomyelin + variable amount ceroid fairly uniform in size, occasional giant vacuoles; no cell inclusions; SBB mild pos, stained cells red birefringent (may be specific); acid haematein and ferric-haematoxylin pos; green-yellow fluorescence in UV
B	vacuolation as in type A, no cell inclusions
C	may contain cell inclusions, vacuoles variable in size and number; not birefringent
Wolman's	pos for ORO, SBB (neutral fat), Nile blue (free fatty acids); birefringent (acicular crystals, Maltese cross, cholesteryl esters)
Cholesteryl ester storage (adult Wolman's)[3]	ORO, SBB pos, cells less profuse than in Wolman's
G_{M1} gangliosidosis I (infantile)	ORO, SBB neg
Chylomicronaemia	fine foam, ORO, SBB pos
Tangier[3]	cholesteryl esters; ORO, SBB pos, birefringent (Maltese cross)
Mannosidosis[3]	PAS pos if celloidin protected
Fucosidosis, infantile[3]	prominent cell phagocytosis
Neuraminidase deficiency, dysmorphic	PAS pos
Galactosialidosis	PAS pos
Infantile free sialic acid storage	rbc phagocytosis may be prominent
Mucolipidosis II (I cell disease)	
Other	
Chylomicronaemia	fine vacuoles, ORO, SBB pos
Fat necrosis	ORO pos

[1] Other characteristics of inherited disorders summarized in Tables 6.3, 6.4
[2] Foam cells usually AcPh positive (around vacuoles)
[3] Foam cells sparse in some cases
pos = positive; neg = negative

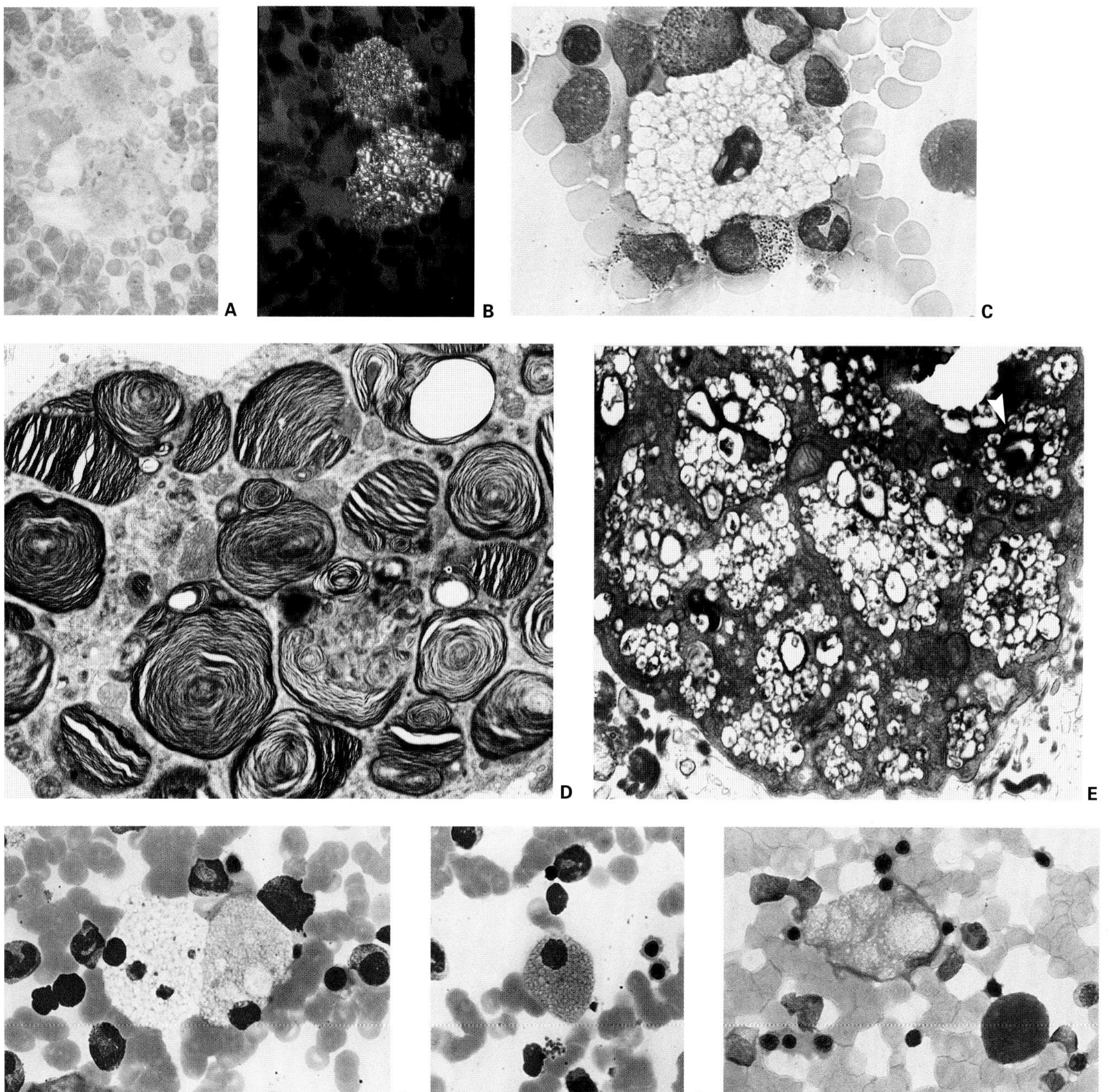

Fig. 6.17 Foam cells in marrow, Niemann-Pick disease. **a,b** Type A. **a** SBB. **b** Same cell, red fluorescence in polarized light. **c,d** Type B, absence of cell inclusions, lamellar ultrastructure. **e–h** Type C. **e** Groups of membranous bodies, some with more than one layer. **f** One of the macrophages contains cell inclusions. **g** Blue foam cell. **h** (PAS): larger cell has weak reaction typical of foam cells in this disorder; smaller, intensely stained cell is a blue foam cell; these were also SBB and ORO positive and autofluorescent in UV; there were no classic (granular) sea-blue cells. **a,b** × 300; **d** ×10 000; **e** × 12 000; **f–h** × 500. **a,b** Reproduced with permission from Hann I M et al 1990 Colour atlas of paediatric haematology, Oxford University Press

Chylomicronaemia (Figs 6.18, 6.19, 4.14, 3.23)
Chylomicronaemia may be visible as a 'tomato-sauce' appearance of whole blood or as a milky appearance of plasma (may separate to surface after refrigeration overnight), and may be evident in blood films. Spurious increase in Hb readings is common, and smudge cells may result in spurious leucopenia. Inherited causes include lipoprotein lipase deficiency and type I glycogenosis (von Gierke's disease). Chylomicronaemia is, however, more commonly acquired (intravenous lipid alimentation, nephrosis, diabetes mellitus, haemolytic-uraemic syndrome, pancreatitis, steroid treatment, malignancy, SLE).

Tangier disease
Tissue discoloration and enlargement due to accumulation of cholesteryl esters — hyperplastic, orange tonsils and adenoids, mild splenomegaly and lymph node enlargement, recurring neuropathy, corneal infiltration (slit-lamp). Little, if any, shortening of life span. Autosomal recessive. Definitive diagnosis by gross decrease or absence of serum apolipoprotein A-I and high-density lipoproteins.

Marrow fat necrosis
Finely foamed cells may be noted at a site from which marrow has already been aspirated within the preceding week; attributed to trauma-induced necrosis of marrow fat cells (Wong & Chan 1989).

Disorders with foamy macrophages sparse in marrow

These are listed, with cell characteristics, in Table 6.14. Other features of inherited disorders are summarized in Tables 6.3 and 6.4. Descriptions below are of disorders not considered elsewhere in this chapter.

Fabry's disease
Manifestations are due to accumulation of glycosphingolipid, especially in vascular endothelium: painful burning paraesthesiae, especially hands and feet, often with fever and increased ESR (may mimic rheumatic fever), angiectasia of skin (especially between umbilicus and knees) and mucosae, corneal and lens opacities, hypohidrosis (sweat, tears, saliva); in older patients, proteinuria, renal failure, vascular disease, especially coronary, cerebral. No splenomegaly. In heterozygous females commonest abnormality is corneal dystrophy. X-linked recessive. Diagnosis by α galactosidase assay (plasma, leucocytes).

Table 6.14 Disorders with foamy macrophages sparse in marrow

	Foam cells
Inherited	
Fabry's	glycosphingolipid; PAS pos, birefringent (Maltese cross)
Familial hypercholesterolaemia	ORO pos, birefringent
Farber's lipogranulomatosis	pos PAS, weak SBB, birefringent
Familial LCAT deficiency	
Neuraminidase deficiency, normosomatic[1]	blue-staining vacuoles, PAS pos
Other	
Infection, toxic states	foam cells profuse in some cases
Thrombocytopenias due to platelet destruction	
Drugs	
Cytotoxics	
Steroid	ORO pos (hypertriglyceridaemia)
Malignancy (involving marrow or not)	foam cells may be prominent in T lymphoma

[1] Cherry-red spot–myoclonus syndrome, sialidosis I
pos = positive

Familial hypercholesterolaemia
Main features: cholesterol xanthomas of skin and tendons, especially Achilles and dorsal hand, premature atherosclerosis of coronary, cerebral and peripheral vessels, aortic valve stenosis, premature arcus corneae. Autosomal dominant with gene dosage effect.

Farber's lipogranulomatosis
Manifestations are due to accumulation of ceramide and glycolipid, with granuloma formation and, later, fibrosis.

Most common type manifests at under 4 months with painful joint deformity and swelling, subcutaneous nodules around joints and over pressure areas, hoarseness (laryngeal granulomas), lung dysfunction and variable hepatomegaly, psychomotor retardation, cardiac dysfunction and pale cherry-red spot in retina.

Fulminant 'neonatal visceral' form has dominant hepatosplenomegaly, corneal opacities; it may mimic malignant histiocytosis.

Neurologic progressive form has dominant psychomotor retardation after the first year and, often, macular cherry-red spot. Autosomal recessive. Diagnosis by acid ceramidase assay (leucocytes, cultured fibroblasts).

Infection, toxic states
Foam cells are rarely profuse (Fig. 6.18). When phagocytosis of erythrocytes and nucleated elements is prominent, a designation of infection-associated haemophagocytosis (p. 267) may be appropriate.

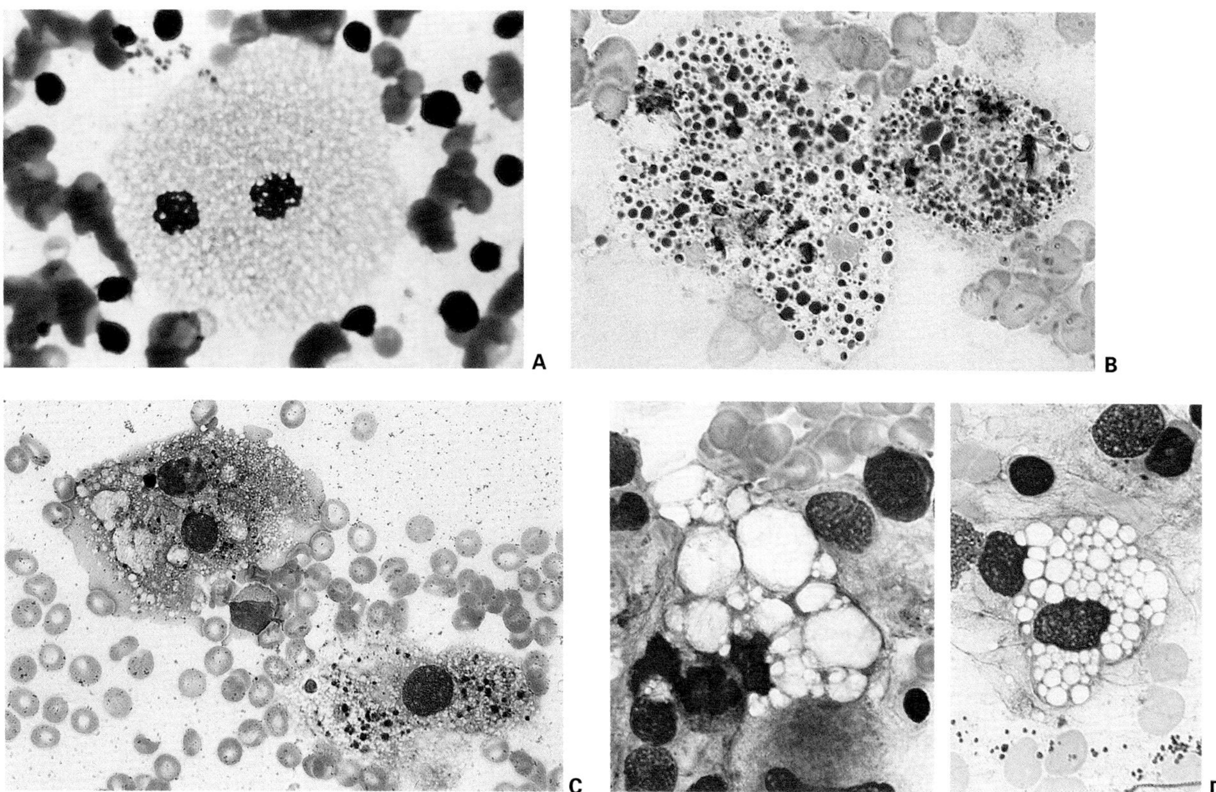

Fig. 6.18 Foam cells vs normal fat cells in marrow. **a** Finely foamed macrophage, hyperchylomicronaemia, lipoprotein lipase deficiency. **b** 2 macrophages, ORO, Wolman's disease. **c** Candidiasis during remission induction for ALL. **d** Normal fat cells. **a,c** × 500; **b** × 630; **d** × 750

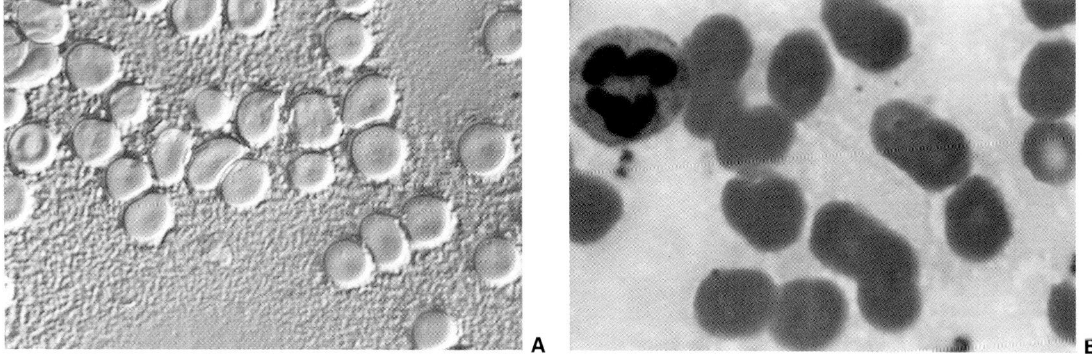

Fig. 6.19 Hyperchylomicronaemia. **a** Nephrosis, untreated blood film, Normanski optics. **b** Haemolytic-uraemic syndrome, routinely stained blood film, showing 'moth-eaten' background. **a** × 800; **b** × 1300

SEA-BLUE CELLS (SEA-BLUE HISTIOCYTES)

The sea-blue material stains blue or blue-green with Romanowsky, and is usually in the form of coarse granules, less often as diffuse blue coloration of foam cells (Fig. 6.20). Granulation tends to be coarser and more profuse in inherited than in non-inherited disorders. Sea-blue material is not a homogeneous species (Fig. 6.20). In inherited disorders it usually has the characteristics of ceroid (lipofuscin) — yellow unstained, bright yellow autofluorescence in UV, strongly positive with PAS (before and after diastase), SBB (grey-black rather than the brown of myeloid cells) and AcPh (in some granules tartrate resistant); positive with ORO, acid-fast with Ziehl-Neelsen, not birefringent. Negative with Feulgen, MPO, Perls, not metachromatic with toluidine blue.

Sea-blue cells may be associated with foam cells, and blue foam cells may be regarded as intermediate between the two (Fig. 6.20). In inherited disorders sea-blue cells tend to increase with age and may be absent from marrow when present in other body sites such as spleen.

Sea-blue material is regarded as an end product of leucocyte breakdown, accumulation being due to either a defect in handling mechanism (e.g. Niemann-Pick disease) or overloading of normal handling mechanisms (e.g. leukaemia).

Causes are listed in Table 6.15. Other characteristics of inherited disorders are summarized in Tables 6.3 and 6.4. Descriptions following are of disorders not considered elsewhere in this chapter.

Table 6.15 Sea-blue histiocytes in marrow

Profuse
Niemann-Pick type B[1]
Hermansky-Pudlak
Sparse
Inherited
Batten's disease, juvenile (Spielmeyer-Vogt)
Niemann-Pick type A[1]
type C[1,2]
Hallervorden-Spatz disease
Familial LCAT deficiency
Fabry's disease
Thalassaemia major
Congenital dyserythropoietic anaemias (II especially)
Other
Thrombocytopenias due to platelet destruction
Leukaemias, non-haemopoietic malignancy (involving marrow or not)

[1] Sea-blue cells more numerous in older patients; foam cells dominate in younger patients
[2] Granules may stain pale blue

Hermansky-Pudlak syndrome (albinism with haemorrhagic diathesis)
Main features: oculocutaneous albinism (photophobia, nystagmus, decreased visual acuity), bleeding tendency, usually mild (platelet storage pool deficiency), other manifestations due to fibrosis and granuloma formation provoked by ceroid in tissues (fibrotic restrictive lung disease, granulomatous colitis and gingivitis, renal failure, cardiomyopathy). Autosomal recessive. Specific defect not identified. Ceroid in urine sediment (fluorescent in UV) and deficiency of platelet dense bodies (electron microscopy) may help in diagnosis.

Familial LCAT deficiency
Sea-blue cells more profuse in spleen than marrow. Main manifestations (due to accumulation of unesterified cholesterol and phosphatidyl choline): corneal opacities, mild normocytic anaemia with target cells (decreased erythrocyte survival), proteinuria (renal failure in some patients, foam cells in glomeruli), premature atherosclerosis, xanthomas occasionally, usually no hepatosplenomegaly. Autosomal recessive. Diagnosis by assay of LCAT in plasma.

STRIATED SKY-BLUE CELLS

Blue-staining cells with finely-striated cytoplasm reminiscent to a degree of Gaucher cells occur in small numbers in marrow in G_{M1} gangliosidosis II (late infantile). Moderately positive with PAS, not autofluorescent (see Hann et al 1990).

G_{M1} gangliosidosis II is later in onset, milder and slower in course than type I (p. 206); ataxia and clumsiness, beginning at about 1 year, are usually the first symptoms. Psychomotor retardation progresses to seizures, spasticity and decerebrate rigidity. Facies usually normal, cornea and retina normal, though late blindness common, usually no hepatosplenomegaly or bone changes. Survival beyond 10 years unusual.

Diagnosis as for type I.

Fig. 6.20 (facing page) Sea-blue cells. **a–d** Niemann-Pick disease type B. **b** Ultrastructure of granulated sea-blue cells; granules contain lipid droplets, and in some, myelin figures. **c** Blue foam cell and typical foam cell. **d** (Blue foam cell): lipid droplets scattered diffusely among myelin figures. **e,f** ALL, pre-treatment; ultrastructure shows elongated granules containing lipid droplets and fine (5–8 nm) fibrils (arrow). **a,e** × 750; **c** × 500; **b,f** × 10 000; **d** ×15 000

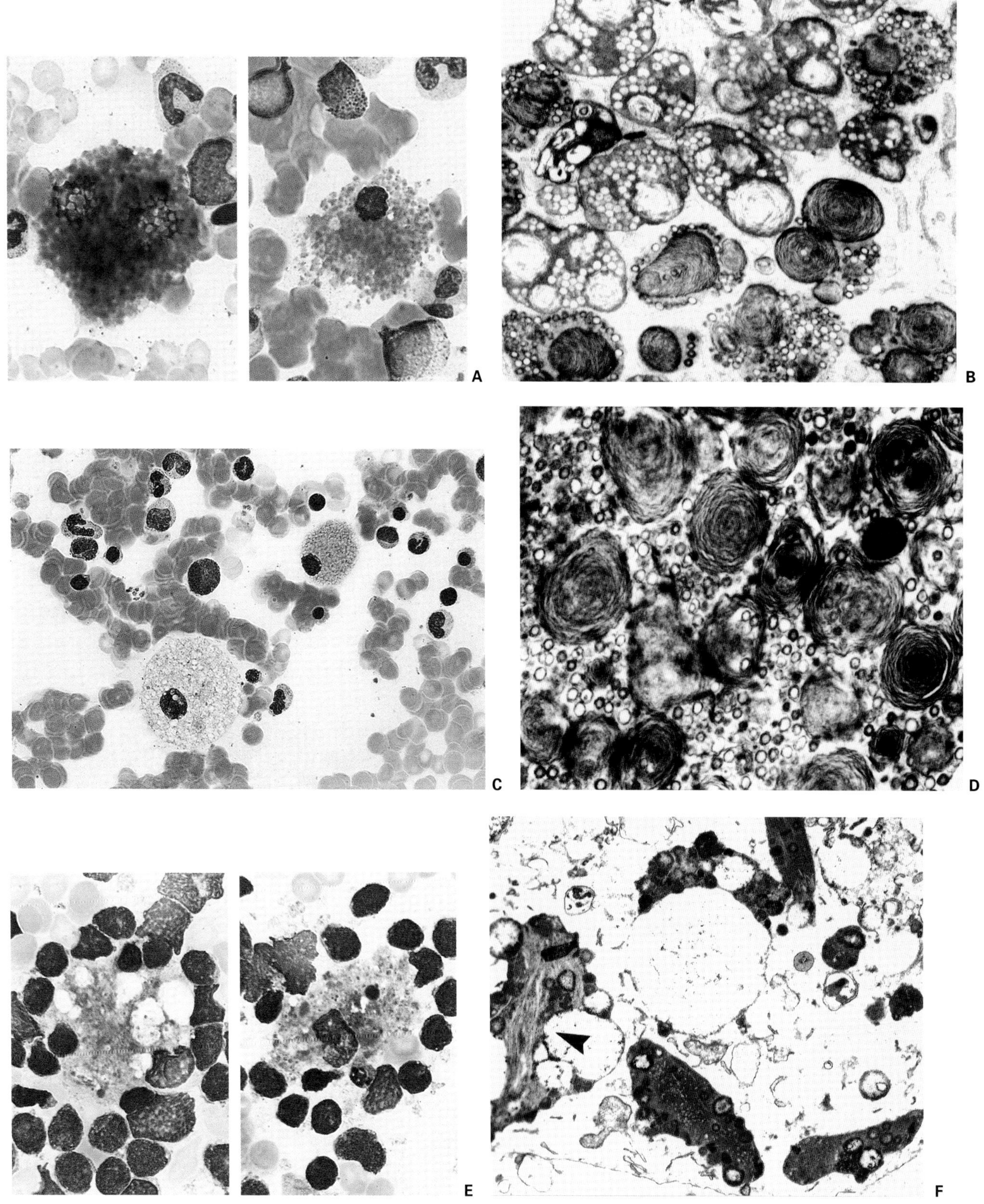
A
B
C
D
E
F

GASSER TYPE 'RETICULUM' CELLS
(Fig. 6.21)

Characterized by a profusion of intensely basophilic granules or coarser bodies, lying individually in clear vacuoles, which may cover or obscure the nucleus, purple-red metachromasia with toluidine blue, negative with PAS and SBB. The cells do not contain corpuscular inclusions and do not appear to be macrophages, though metachromatic inclusions may occur within macrophages in marrows which contain Gasser cells. Most profuse in and around bone fragments, may increase with age.

To be distinguished from mast cells — mast cell granules finer, more closely packed, do not lie individually in clear vacuoles, tend not to overlie or obscure nucleus and metachromasia more reddish with toluidine blue.

Occurrence:

- Mucopolysaccharidoses, but may be sparse in IS (Scheie); metachromasia is weak or absent in VII (Sly). May occur in marrow when Gasser lymphocytes (p. 208) are sparse or absent in blood. Also occur in tissues other than marrow, e.g. subcutaneous.
- Fucosidosis.
- Mucosulphatidosis.
- Infantile free sialic acid storage disease. Cells contain metachromatic inclusions, but unlike Gasser cells show some foaming.

SYNDROME OF HYPERPHAGOCYTIC MACROPHAGES, MICHAELIS-GUTMANN BODIES AND GRANULE-POOR EOSINOPHILS

See page 218.

MACROPHAGES WITH BLUE-STAINING VACUOLES

These macrophages have some resemblance to vacuolated plasma cells, but PAS is strongly positive, and AcPh strongly positive at periphery of vacuoles (see Hann et al 1990). They occur in small numbers in marrow in primary neuraminidase deficiency without dysmorphism (sialidosis type I, p. 206).

Bone marrow osteoblasts (Fig. 6.22)

Abnormality is often associated with abnormal bone structure in genetic disorders:

- densely staining metachromatic granules in mucopolysaccharidoses
- abnormal granulation in infantile free sialic acid storage disease and ML II (I cell disease)
- vacuolation in glycogen storage disease II infantile (Pompe, vacuoles strongly positive with PAS, diastase sensitive), and in ML II.

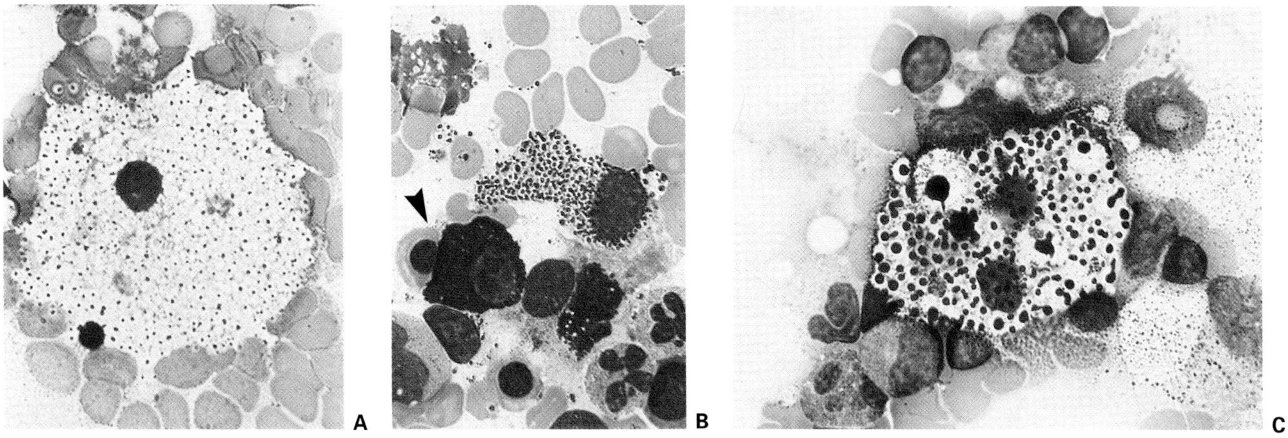

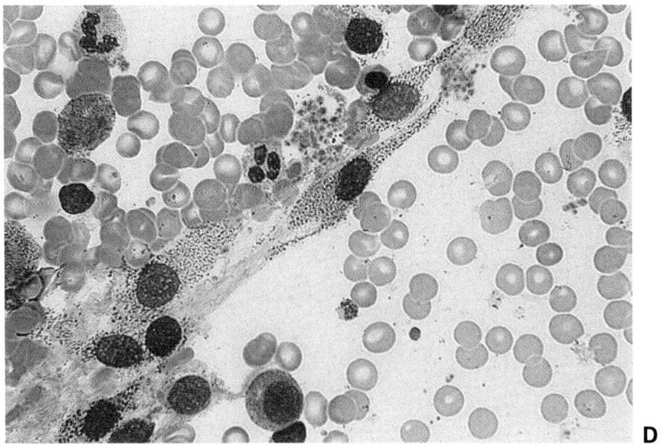

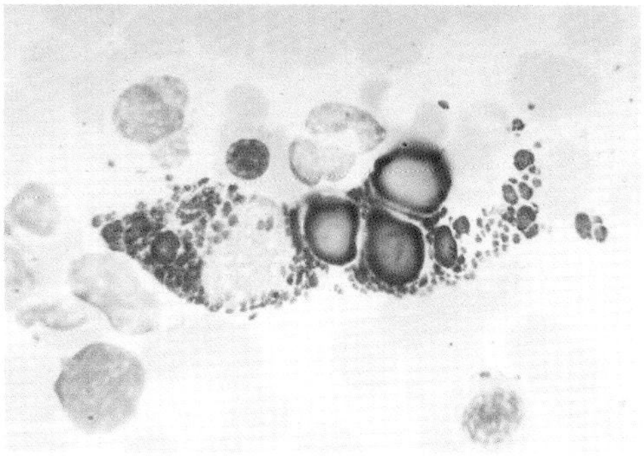

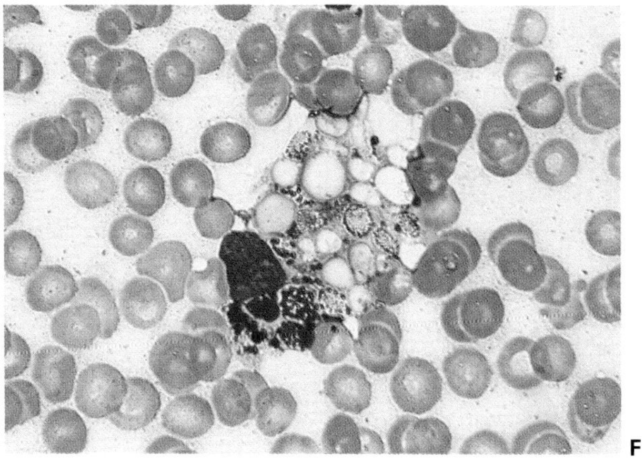

Fig. 6.21 Gasser and Gasser-like 'reticulum' cells in marrow. **a** Finely granuled cell. **b** Gasser cell with medium-sized granules vs mast cell (arrow). **c** Coarse granulation. **d** Syncytium of Gasser cells. **e** Metachromasia of inclusions, toluidine blue. **f** Gasser-like cell containing clear vacuoles and 'necklace' inclusions; solid inclusions were metachromatic with toluidine blue. **a,e** Hurler MPS; **b–d** Sanfilippo MPS; **f** infantile free sialic acid storage disease. All × 750 except **d** × 480, e × 1000

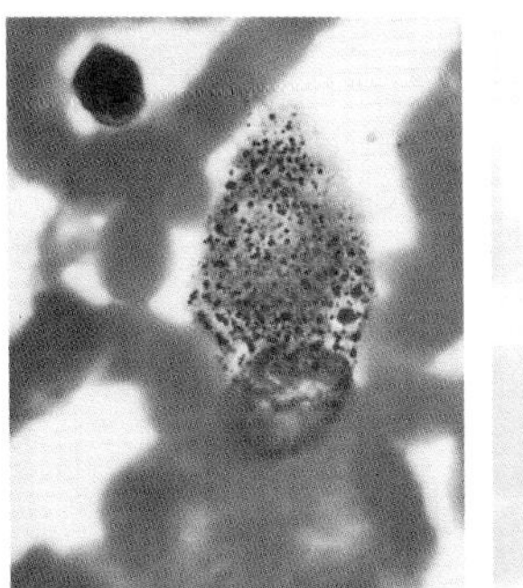

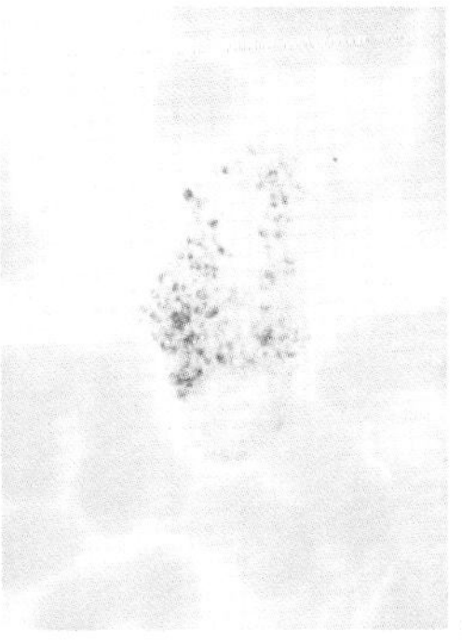

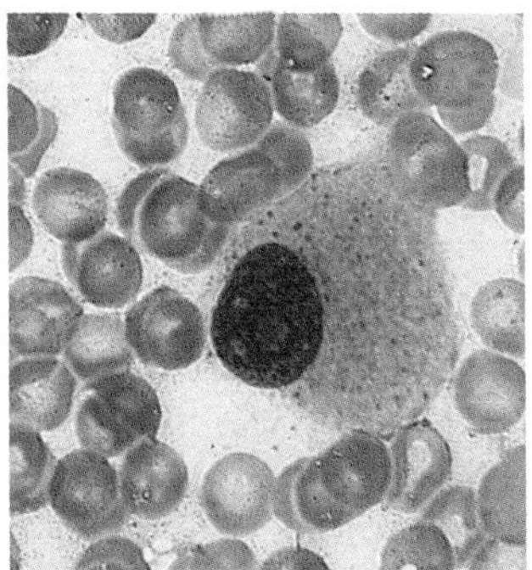

Fig. 6.22 Abnormal osteoblasts in marrow. **a** Abnormal granulation, metachromatic with toluidine blue (right), Hurler MPS. **b** Abnormal, fine granulation, infantile free sialic acid storage disease.

Crystals in marrow (Table 6.16, Fig. 6.23)

Some types of crystal are normal, some are contaminants and others pathologic. Some crystals (e.g. oxalate) occur in bone but not in marrow. Crystals may on occasion be noted in blood monocytes (Fig. 5.30).

- Neutral fat

Crystallization is an artefact of cooling.

- Starch

A common contaminant (surgical glove powder). Refractile pale-blue coloration in Romanowsky films, 'hot-cross bun' in polarized light.

- Cystine

Crystals are most readily detected in fluid preparations of anticoagulated (e.g. EDTA) marrow viewed in polarized light, occurring within macrophages as rectangles ('bricks'), squares, hexagons and needles. Rectangular shapes are more consistently birefringent than other shapes; soluble in 10% ammonia and dilute mineral acid pH 5.5 (and water), not autofluorescent. Soluble to some extent in routine haematologic stains but not difficult to detect in stained marrow films (Fig. 6.23). Crystal-containing macrophages are most profuse in and around fragments.

Diagnostic of cystinosis. Main features: onset at 6–12 months of renal tubular Fanconi syndrome (failure to thrive, polyuria, acidosis, vomiting, rickets, retarded growth, progressive renal failure), corneal crystals (slit-lamp), poor muscle function (carnitine loss in urine contributes), hypohidrosis, light skin and hair, normal intelligence. Benign form manifests in adulthood with corneal crystals but no renal involvement. Autosomal recessive. Definitive diagnosis by increased cystine content in leucocytes, cultured fibroblasts.

- Charcot-Leyden crystals (Smith & Forbes 1972)

Compass-needle (view in elevation of hexagonal dipyramid), needle, boat and rhombohedral shapes, 4–20 μm long, staining grey or orange-grey, not birefringent or autofluorescent, negative with standard cytochemical procedures. Ultrastructure not latticed (crystalloid within specific granules of eosinophils often is). May be accompanied by orange-staining masses derived from phagocytosed eosinophils. Occur in macrophages, eosinophils of normal or abnormal structure, and other granulocytes (Fig. 5.6). Crystals may be noted in:

(i) gross benign eosinophilias (Fig. 6.23)
(ii) AML and myelodysplasias with dysplasia of granulocytes (Figs 5.4, 5.6)
(iii) marrow necrosis (Fig. 4.13).

- Auer rods

Derived by phagocytosis of leukaemic cells (Fig. 5.7).

- Tyrosine

Broom-shaped birefringent crystals may be noted in tyrosinaemia type I in marrow taken into anticoagulant and let stand 24–48 h (Jaiswal et al 1968). Main features are renal tubular dysfunction and vitamin D-resistant rickets.

Table 6.16 Crystals which may be seen in films of bone marrow aspirate

Neutral fat
Starch
Cystine
Charcot-Leyden
Auer rods
Tyrosine
Other

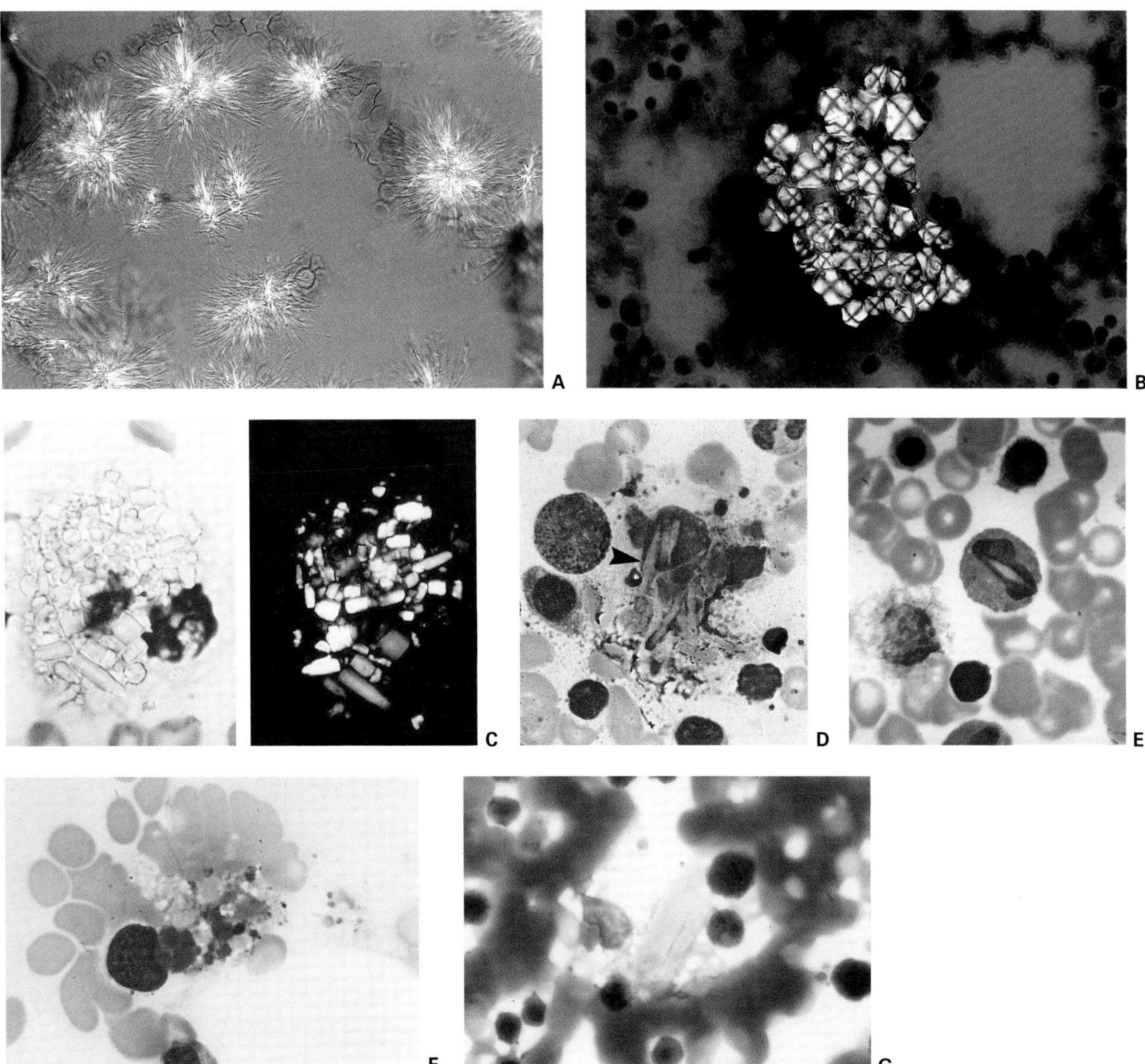

Fig. 6.23 Crystals in marrow aspirates. **a** Neutral fat, crystals in adipocytes (polarized light). **b** Starch (polarized light). **c** Cystine, same cell, Romanowsky and polarized light; most of the crystals are birefringent. **d–f** Benign gross eosinophilia, Charcot-Leyden crystals in macrophage and eosinophil; orange masses derived from phagocytosed eosinophils in macrophage (**f**). **g** Unidentified crystal in macrophage, mannosidosis juvenile/adult type. **a,b** × 310; **c** × 1000; **d–g** × 750

REFERENCES

Abo T, Roder J C, Abo W, Cooper M D 1982 Natural killer (HNK-1+) cells in Chediak-Higashi patients are present in normal numbers but are abnormal in function and morphology. Journal of Clinical Investigation 70: 193–197

Blume R S, Bennett J M, Yankee R A, Wolff S M 1968 Defective granulocyte regulation in the Chediak-Higashi syndrome. New England Journal of Medicine 279: 1009–1015

Bozdech M J, Bainton D F, Mustacchi P 1980 Partial peroxidase deficiency in neutrophils and eosinophils associated with neurologic disease. Histochemical, cytochemical and biochemical studies. American Journal of Clinical Pathology 73: 409–416

Cech P, Schneider P, Bachmann F 1982 Partial myeloperoxidase deficiency. Acta Haematologica 67: 180–184

Collins R, Wilson R, Bates J, Smith H 1979 A distinctive population of lymphocytes in human blood (abstract). Australian Paediatric Journal 15: 290

Dacie J W, Lewis S M 1991 Practical haematology, 7th edn. Churchill Livingstone, Edinburgh

Gallin J I 1985 Neutrophil specific granule deficiency. Annual Review of Medicine 36: 263–274

Ganz T, Metcalf J A, Gallin J I et al 1988 Microbicidal/cytotoxic proteins of neutrophils are deficient in two disorders: Chediak-Higashi syndrome and 'specific' granule deficiency. Journal of Clinical Investigation 82: 552–556

Hamdan J A, Ahmad M S, Sa'adi A R 1982 Malacoplakia of the retroperitoneum in a girl with systemic lupus erythematosus. Pediatrics 70: 296–299

Hann I M, Lake B D, Pritchard J, Lilleyman J 1990 Colour atlas of paediatric haematology, 2nd edn. Oxford University Press, Oxford, Figs 16.21, 16.31–33

Hernandez J A, Aldred S W, Bruce J R et al 1980 "Botryoid" nuclei in neutrophils of patients with heatstroke. Lancet 2: 642–643

Heyne K 1976 Konstitutionelle familiäre Leukocytopenie mit partieller Pelger-anomalie und ossärer Entwicklungsverzögerung. European Journal of Pediatrics 121: 191–201

Ho-Chang C, Nigro M A, Perrin E V 1980 Cerebral malakoplakia and neonatal herpes simplex infection. Archives of Pathology and Laboratory Medicine 104: 494–495

Jaiswal R B, Bhai I, Nath N 1968 Tyrosine crystals in bone marrow. Lancet 1: 1254–1255

Jordans G H W 1953 The familial occurrence of fat containing vacuoles in the leukocytes diagnosed in two brothers suffering from dystrophia musculorum progressiva (ERB). Acta Medica Scandinavica CXLV (fasc VI): 419–423

Lake B D 1992 Lysosomal and peroxisomal disorders. In: Adams J H, Duchen L W (eds) Greenfield's neuropathology, 5th edn. Edward Arnold, London, ch 12

Lee R E, Ellis L D 1971 The storage cells of chronic myelogenous leukemia. Laboratory Investigation 24: 261–264

Mitchell E B, Platts-Mills T A E, Malkovska V, Webster A D 1983 Acquired basophil and eosinophil deficiency in a patient with hypogammaglobulinaemia associated with thymoma. Clinical and Laboratory Hematology 5: 253–257

Murros J, Konttinen A 1974 Recurrent attacks of abdominal pain and fever with familial segmentation arrest of granulocytes. Blood 43: 871–874

Nakahata T, Spicer S S, Leary A G et al 1984 Circulating eosinophil colony-forming cells in pure eosinophil aplasia. Annals of Internal Medicine 101: 321–324

Nauseef W M 1988 Myeloperoxidase deficiency. Hematology/Oncology Clinics of North America 2: 135–151

Parmley R T, Gilbert C S, Boxer L A 1989 Abnormal peroxidase-positive granules in 'specific granule' deficiency. Blood 73: 838–844

Pearson H A, Lobel J S, Kocoshis S A et al 1979 A new syndrome of refractory sideroblastic anaemia with vacuolization of marrow precursors and exocrine pancreatic dysfunction. Journal of Pediatrics 95: 976–984

Pentchev P G, Vanier M T, Suzuki K, Patterson M C 1995 Niemann-Pick disease type C: a cellular cholesterol lipidosis. In: Scriver C R, Beaudet A L, Sly W S, Valle D (eds) The metabolic and molecular bases of inherited disease, 7th edn. McGraw-Hill, New York, ch 85

Peterson L C, Rao K V, Crosson J T, White J G 1985 Fechtner syndrome — a variant of Alport's syndrome with leucocyte inclusions and macrothrombocytopenia. Blood 65: 397–406

Presentey B-Z 1968 A new anomaly of eosinophil granulocytes. American Journal of Clinical Pathology 49: 887–890

Rausch P G, Pryzwansky K B, Spitznagel J K 1978 Immunochemical identification of azurophilic and specific granule markers in the giant granules of Chediak-Higashi neutrophils. New England Journal of Medicine 298: 693–698

Ribeiro R C, Howard T H, Brandalise S et al 1994 Giant actin inclusions in hematopoietic cells associated with transfusion-dependent anemia and grey skin discoloration. Blood 83: 3717–3726

Roe C R, Coates P M 1989 Acyl-CoA dehydrogenase deficiencies. In: Scriver C R, Beaudet A L, Sly W S, Valle D (eds) The metabolic basis of inherited disease, 6th edn. McGraw-Hill, New York, ch 33

Rotig A, Colonna M, Bonnefont J P et al 1989 Mitochondrial DNA deletion in Pearson's marrow/pancreas syndrome. Lancet 1: 902–903

Sadowitz P D, Balcolm R, Gordon L 1984 Abnormal hematologic findings in triploidy. Clinical Pediatrics 23: 641–643

Scriver C R, Beaudet A L, Sly W S, Valle D (eds) 1989 The metabolic basis of inherited disease, 6th edn. McGraw-Hill, New York

Smith H 1967 Unidentified inclusions in haemopoietic cells, congenital atresia of the bile ducts and livedo reticularis in an infant: a new syndrome? British Journal of Haematology 13: 695–705

Smith H, Collins R J 1977 A population of lymphocytes in human blood distinctive in morphology and other characteristics. Journal of Clinical Pathology 30: 243–249

Smith H, Forbes I M 1972 Charcot-Leyden crystals in human bone marrow. Pathology 4: 279–294

Solis O G, Belmonte A H, Ramaswamy G, Tchertkoff V 1986 Pseudogaucher cells in mycobacterium avium intracellulare infections in acquired immune deficiency syndrome (AIDS). American Journal of Clinical Pathology 85: 233–235

Tracey R, Smith H 1978 An inherited anomaly of human eosinophils and basophils. Blood Cells 4: 291–298

Tulliez M, Verrant J P, Breton-Gorius J et al 1979 Pseudo-Chediak-Higashi anomaly in a case of acute myeloid leukemia: electron microscopic studies. Blood 54: 863–871

White J G, Clawson C C 1980 The Chédiak-Higashi syndrome: the nature of the giant neutrophil granules and their interactions with cytoplasm and foreign particulates. American Journal of Pathology 98: 151–196

Williams M L, Koch T K, O'Donnell J J et al 1985 Ichthyosis and neutral lipid storage disease. American Journal of Medical Genetics 20: 711–726

Wong K F, Chan J K G 1989 Foamy histiocytes in repeat marrow aspirates. Pathology 21: 153–154

Yam L T, Finkel H E, Weintraub L R, Crosby W H 1968 Circulating iron-containing macrophages in hemochromatosis. New England Journal of Medicine 279: 512–514

Young I D, Young E P, Mossman J et al 1987 Neuraminidase deficiency: case report and review of the phenotype. Journal of Medical Genetics 24: 283–290

Zaino E C, Rossi M B, Pham T D, Azar H A 1971 Gaucher's cells in thalassemia. Blood 38: 457–462

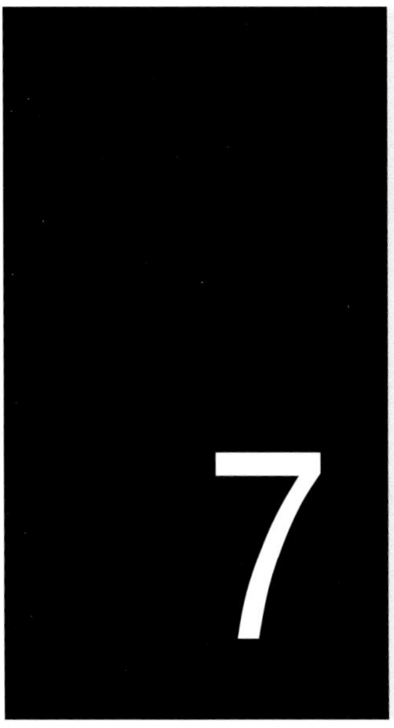

7 Benign change in leucocytes: leucocytosis, leucopenia, infection

Benign changes in leucocyte numbers and leucocyte changes in infection (malignancies considered in Chs 4 and 5 and genetic anomalies in Ch. 6).

Abbreviations

AcPh: acid phosphatase; ALL: acute lymphoblastic leukaemia; ANAE: α naphthyl acetate esterase; C: complement; EBNA: Epstein-Barr virus nuclear antigen; H & E: haematoxylin and eosin; MPD: myeloproliferative disease; MPO: myeloperoxidase; NAP: neutrophil alkaline phosphatase; SCID: severe combined immunodeficiency; TAR: thrombocytopenia absent radius; VCA: viral capsid antigen.

Neutropenia, transient 240

Neutropenia, chronic 240
Cyclic 240
Kostmann 242
Lazy leucocyte syndrome 244
With abnormal marrow neutrophils 244
As part of genetic syndrome 244
Antibody-induced 244
  Alloimmune 244
  Autoimmune 245
Marrow infiltration/replacement 247
Deficiency of haematinics 247
Drugs 248
Sequestration 248

Neutrophilia 248

Lymphocytosis 250

Atypical lymphocytosis 252
  Infectious mononucleosis 252

Lymphopenia 254

Eosinophilia 255

Eosinopenia 257

Qualitative changes in infection 257
Toxic neutrophils 258
Phagocytic neutrophils 260
  Intracellular organisms 260
Cell death 264
Monocytes/macrophages 265
  Blood 265
  Marrow 266
  Infection-associated haemophagocytosis 267

Multinucleate cells 268

Neutropenia, transient

Neutropenia is occasionally spurious:

- clotting in sample (likely to depress counts of all cell types rather than neutrophils only)
- MPO deficiency (neutropenia wrongly identified by counters, e.g. Hemalog D, which recognize neutrophils cytochemically)
- aggregation, in some cases EDTA-induced (Epstein & Kruskall 1988)
- cell fragility (smudging) in chylomicronaemia (p. 230).

Neutropenia in childhood (Table 7.1) is most commonly due to infection, especially viral. Neutropenia is usually not severe ($> 0.2 \times 10^9/l$) and usually begins to recover within 5 days, rarely not for 2–3 weeks. Destruction may be due to direct effect or immune mechanism (p. 246). Morphologic evidence in blood films of antibody/opsonic effect includes agglutination (Fig. 3.5, Guibaud et al 1983) and phagocytosis of neutrophils by monocytes (Fig. 7.13) or rarely neutrophils. The marrow appears normal or shows 'maturation arrest' at the myelocyte/stab stage or, rarely, destruction (Fig. 2.17). In a high proportion the organism is not identified (or sought). Recovery of count after treatment with antiviral agents, e.g. ganciclovir, suggests a viral cause.

Mechanisms for neutropenia in sepsis include destruction by endotoxin or phagocytosed organisms and agglutination by activated complement components, e.g. 5a (Nathan 1987). The marrow may be depleted of granulocytes, especially in the neonate (Christensen & Rothstein 1980). Transient neutropenia associated with burns and haemodialysis is attributed to agglutination by activated C5.

Neutropenia, chronic (more than 3 months)

Less frequent than transient neutropenia. An empiric classification has been given (Tables 7.3–7.6), as in many cases the mechanism is unknown. A suggested schema for initial investigation is given in Table 7.2.

CYCLIC NEUTROPENIA (Dale & Hammond 1988)

Periodicity of infections, especially upper respiratory and oral, should suggest the diagnosis. The cycling period is usually 19–21 days; neutropenia lasts for 3–6 days, with complete absence for 1–3 of these. In neutropenic phases, patients feel unwell from fever and infection, especially staphylococcal and streptococcal. Oral infection may be associated with cervical lymphadenopathy. Monocytes are usually increased in neutropenic phases, but infection is nevertheless a problem, as monocytes are less efficient than neutrophils in tracking and destroying bacteria. Monocytes, lymphocytes, eosinophils and platelets also show some cycling (usually from normal to above normal), while reticulocytes cycle from above to below normal. An increase in large granular lymphocytes is often noted in cases of adult onset.

In neutropenic phases the marrow shows 'maturation arrest' at the myelocyte stage. Increase in mature forms and paucity of precursors precede by some days increase in neutrophils in blood.

In some cases oscillations tend to dampen over the years and evolve to chronic neutropenia. The condition does not appear to predispose to leukaemia, though cyclic neutropenia may rarely be a harbinger of ALL (Lensink et al 1986) or myelodysplasia (p. 176).

In most cases, especially those of adult onset, inheritance cannot be discerned. In familial cases (about one third), transmission is autosomal dominant with variable penetrance.

The defect appears to reside in the stem cell/committed progenitor cell, as it is transmissible by transplantation in humans and can be cured in affected animals (collie dogs) by transplantation of normal marrow.

Differential diagnosis

A degree of cycling may be noted in neutropenias such as Shwachman's syndrome and monosomy 7 MPD. Cycling, however, usually does not have the predictability of true cyclic neutropenia.

Table 7.1 Neutropenia: transient

Infection
- Viral (including HIV)
- Bacterial
  - Pyogenic infection (staphylococcus, streptococcus, coliforms, meningococcus, haemophilus), if severe
  - Brucella, typhoid, paratyphoid[1]
- Tularaemia[1]
- Malaria, occasional cases[1]

Burns
Haemodialysis
Drugs (Table 7.9)

[1] Neutropenia may be chronic

Table 7.2 Chronic neutropenia: initial assessment

Clinical history, age at onset, physical examination
Blood values
Blood film
Neutrophil count, once or twice weekly for 6 weeks
Bone marrow
- Aspirate
  - Morphology
  - Karyotype
- Trephine biopsy
- Electron microscopy

Serum
- Immunoglobulins
- Complement components
- Autoimmune screen
- B_{12}, folate
- Viral serology
- Antigranulocyte antibodies

Lymphocyte subsets
As appropriate: tests for disorders in Tables 7.3–7.6

Table 7.3 Chronic isolated neutropenia in childhood — inherited[1]

No other anomalies
- Cyclic
- Kostmann
- Lazy leucocyte syndrome
- With abnormal marrow neutrophils: myelokathexis and others

As part of genetic syndrome
- With visible somatic anomalies (Table 7.4)
- Without visible somatic anomalies (Table 7.5)

[1] Neutropenia usually congenital

Table 7.4 Genetic syndromes with visible somatic anomalies which may be associated with neutropenia

	Main clinical features	References
Shwachman	exocrine pancreatic insufficiency, metaphyseal dyschondroplasia, growth retardation. See also p. 50	Aggett et al 1980
Fanconi	abnormal pigmentation, short stature, thumb and radius anomalies, abnormal head/face, hypogonadism. See also p. 48 and Fig. 2.18	Alter 1993
Dyskeratosis congenita	skin: reticular hyperpigmentation, depigmentation, atrophy; hair loss, nail dystrophy, leukoplakia, dental dystrophy. See also p. 48 and Fig. 2.18	Jacobs et al 1984
Chediak-Higashi	partial oculocutaneous albinism, bacterial infections, esp *S. aureus*, gingivitis and periodontitis, cranial and peripheral neuropathies, hepatosplenomegaly. See also p. 220 and Fig. 6.8	Blume & Woff 1972
Cartilage-hair hypoplasia	short-limbed dwarfism, fine hair, infections, esp varicella	Wilson et al 1978
Cohen	non-progressive psychomotor retardation, microcephaly, short stature, delayed puberty, hypotonia, joint hypermobility, peculiar facies and teeth, myopia, narrow hands and feet, not infection-prone	Norio et al 1984
Hernández	dystrophy of nails and hair, mild mental retardation,	Hernández et al 1979
—	microcephaly, psychomotor retardation, retinitis pigmentosa, marrow normal by light microscopy	Fanning al 1994

Table 7.5 Genetic syndromes without visible somatic anomalies which may be associated with neutropenia

	Main features	References
Neutropenia with immunodeficiency[1]		
X-linked agammaglobulinaemia		Kozlowski & Evans 1991
dysgammaglobulinaemia type 2	0 IgG, IgA, n to ↑ IgM	Ackerman 1964 Lonsdale et al 1967
—	hyper-IgA, eosinophilia, defective neutrophil chemotaxis, T, B cell function	Björkstén & Lundmark 1976
Reticular dysgenesis	hypogammaglobulinaemia, lymphopenia (imperceptible tonsils, impalpable lymph nodes, no thymus on X-ray). Marrow depleted of granulocytes, lymphocytes. AR	Roper et al 1985
	mild variant described	Gasparetto et al 1994
—	lymphopenia, T cell deficit, partial Pelgerization, benign course, X-linked recessive	Heyne 1976
Organic acidaemias: isovaleric, propionic, methylmalonic	recurrent metabolic acidosis, often with vomiting; variable mental retardation; odour of 'sweaty feet' in isovaleric acidaemia; thrombocytopenia/pancytopenia in acidotic episodes of isovaleric acidaemia	Hutchinson et al 1985 Sweetman 1989 Rosenberg & Fenton 1989
Glycogen storage 1b	hypoglycaemia, convulsions, failure to thrive, infections, bleeding, hepatomegaly	Ambruso et al 1985

AR = autosomal recessive; n = normal
[1] Neutropenia may be a result rather than a cause of infection, as neutropenia appears to be infrequent in those treated with immunoglobulin

Table 7.6 Chronic isolated neutropenia in childhood — acquired

- Alloimmune
- Autoimmune[1]
- Infection
  - Virus
  - Other[2]
    - Brucellosis
    - Typhoid, paratyphoid
    - Malaria
    - Leishmaniasis
- Marrow pathology[2]
  - Leukaemia
    - Monosomy 7 MPD
    - Pre-ALL
  - Neuroblastoma
  - Hypoplasia
  - Myelosclerosis
  - Osteopetrosis
- Deficiency of haematinics[2]
  - Folate, B_{12}
  - Copper
- Drugs
  - Immune
  - Non-immune
- Sequestration
  - Spleen[2]
  - Marrow macrophages

[1] In neonates passive transfer may occur from a mother with autoimmune disease
[2] Usually with other cytopenias

KOSTMANN'S SYNDROME (INFANTILE GENETIC AGRANULOCYTOSIS)

(Kostmann 1975)

Neutrophils are persistently lower than $0.3 \times 10^9/l$; bacterial infections are frequent and severe (Fig. 7.1) and are the usual cause of death. There is often a 'compensatory' monocytosis which, even if striking (in a personal case to $14.6 \times 10^9/l$), assists little in ameliorating infection because of the inefficiency of monocytes in handling infection. The marrow is cellular, usually with maturation arrest at the promyelocyte/myelocyte stage, or in some cases normal maturation. Electron microscopy shows dysgranulopoiesis in some cases (?subclass of disease, Parmley et al 1980).

A deficiency in responsiveness to granulocyte colony stimulating factor (GCSF) is likely (Moore 1991), which can however be overridden in vivo by administration of GCSF. Evolution to (myeloid) leukaemia may occur (Rosen & Kang 1979). Inheritance is autosomal recessive.

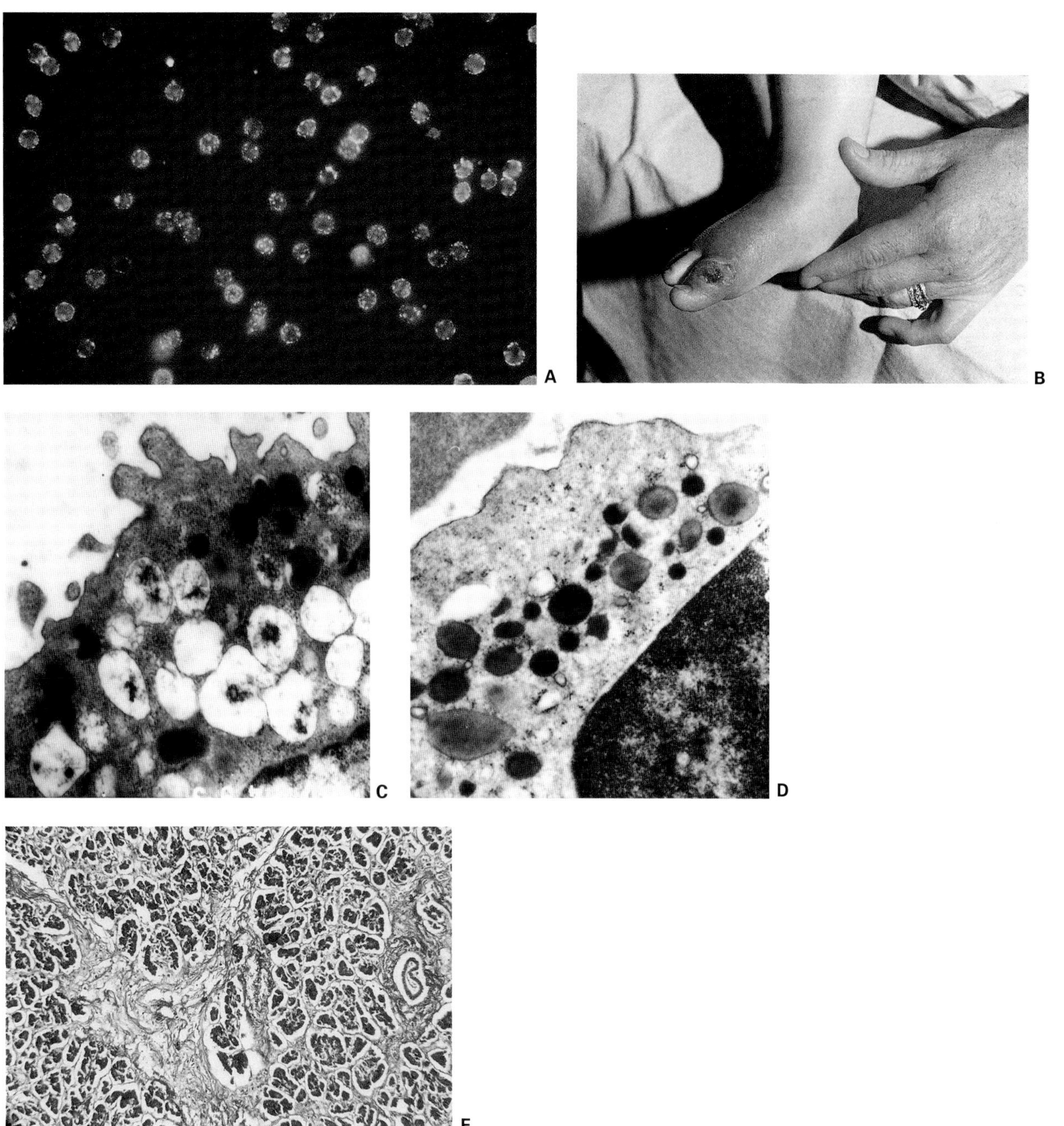

Fig. 7.1 Neutropenias. **a** Neonatal alloimmune, maternal serum reacted with paternal neutrophils (specificity anti-NA2). **b** Kostmann's, 2-year-old boy, infection with inflammation but little pus formation. **c–e** With abnormal granule structure and pancreatic fibrosis, presenting at 2 months. **c** Degenerate granules in neutrophil myelocyte, compared with normal (**d**). **e** Pancreas, haematoxylin-van Gieson (collagen red). **a** × 300; **c,d** × 20 000; **e** ×60. **a** Courtesy of Dr R Minchinton

LAZY LEUCOCYTE SYNDROME

A rare, chronic neutropenia (< $0.2 \times 10^9/l$) with morphologically normal marrow and severe curtailment of chemotaxis and random mobility of neutrophils (Miller et al 1971). Neutropenia shows no response to intravenous adrenalin and subnormal response to Pneumococcus polysaccharide. An abnormality of surface configuration may make the cell rigid (Pinkerton et al 1978). A similar disorder may occur as a temporary (< 12 months) phenomenon (Yoda et al 1980).

NEUTROPENIAS WITH ABNORMAL MARROW NEUTROPHILS

Myelokathexis (Zuelzer 1964; kathexis = retention)
A rare neutropenia (chronic, non-cycling) associated with, and attributed to, abnormality of segmented neutrophils in marrow which are abundant but show signs of degeneracy (nuclear pyknosis, hypersegmentation with slender connecting filaments, cytoplasmic vacuolation). Neutrophils show variable impairment of function (decreased NAP, impaired dye exclusion, mobility and phagocytosis). MPO is normal. Count increases in infection and after injection of GCSF (Weston et al 1991). Possible variants include familial occurrence (father, daughter) with hypogammaglobulinaemia (Mentzer et al 1977), and association with growth retardation and dysmorphism (Plebani et al 1988).

Neutropenia with gigantism and multinuclearity of marrow neutrophils (Lightsey et al 1985)
Marrow promyelocytes contain up to 4 nuclei, and segmented neutrophils up to 16. Some cells are hypogranular and others hypergranular. Cells are severely deficient in lactoferrin (specific granules). The abnormalities impair survival in marrow and are attributed to aberration of centrioles. Karyotype is normal.

Blood neutrophils by contrast are normal. Increase is inconstant in infection and minimal after adrenalin and dexamethasone.

Neutropenia with large, binucleate, tetraploid neutrophils and monocytes in marrow (Mamlok et al 1987)
The proportion of binucleate cells increases with maturity (metamyelocytes 42%, segmented 100%). Other leucocytes are normal. Neutropenia is attributed to impaired egress of abnormal cells from marrow. Binucleate cells are rare (< 1%) in blood.

- In a personally observed case, neutropenia was associated with abnormal granule structure and pancreatic fibrosis (Fig. 7.1).

NEUTROPENIA AS PART OF A GENETIC SYNDROME (Tables 7.4, 7.5)

Neutropenia in these disorders is due to a variety of mechanisms:

- precursor cell deficiency, e.g. Fanconi, Shwachman, cartilage-hair hypoplasia
- intramedullary destruction, e.g. Chediak-Higashi (abnormal myeloid precursors in marrow, increased serum muramidase in absence of monocytosis or decreased survival of blood neutrophils)
- suppression of myeloid maturation, e.g. by organic acids and glycine in organic acidaemias.

ANTIBODY-INDUCED NEUTROPENIAS

Antibodies to neutrophil-specific antigens are an important cause of neutropenia (Minchinton & Waters 1984). Antigens shared with other cell types (e.g. HLA) do not appear to be significant in neutropenia. Serum may be tested against a panel of neutrophils of known phenotype or against films of marrow aspirate. Serum should be tested fresh, but if delay in transport to a reference lab is likely, blood should be taken into citrate-phosphate-dextrose-EDTA solution. Serum or plasma should be heated before application, to remove complement which interferes with antibody binding. Marrow films should be fresh, or stored at –30°C till use and fixed with paraformaldehyde at time of testing (McCullough et al 1988, Minchinton R M 1994, personal communication). Antibody is demonstrable on more mature stages (metamyelocyte onward) in mild to moderate neutropenias, and on myelocytes and promyelocytes as well, in severe neutropenias (Harmon et al 1984).

Alloimmune neutropenias

Two important types in childhood:

Alloimmune neutropenia of infancy (Minchinton & McGrath 1987)
Estimates of incidence vary from 1/200 to 3% of neonates. Neutropenia is severe ($0–0.5 \times 10^9/l$), often with a 'compensatory' monocytosis. In infected infants antibody should be sought if neutropenia is excessive for the infection (neutropenia is unlikely unless bacterial infection is severe).

Antibodies (IgG) are directed against one of the normal cell-specific antigens (well represented on cord neutrophils), most commonly NA1, NA2, NB1, NC1 and 9a. Rarely, the mother has no NA specific neutrophil antigens (NA null, CD16 negative) and as a consequence reacts to any NA (NA1, NA2) antigens on fetal neutrophils. Immunization is usual with the first child.

Because of paucity of cells, realistic testing can be done only for antibody in the mother's serum which reacts with the father's but not with her own neutrophils (Table 7.7, Fig. 7.1).

Marrow examination excludes the unlikely occurrence of leukaemia as the cause of isolated neutropenia. Cellularity is variable. Stages from metamyelocyte onward may be normally represented, deficient or absent. 'Maturation arrest' is due to destruction of mature forms and not to suppression of maturation.

Neutropenia persists for 3 weeks to 3 months depending on rate of catabolism of antibody. Mortality (bacterial septicaemia) is about 5%.

Febrile, non-haemolytic transfusion reactions
Common but rarely investigated. Most are due to reaction of recipient antibodies with transfused incompatible leucocytes.

Autoimmune neutropenias (Table 7.8)

The commonest in childhood is autoimmune neutropenia of infancy.

Autoimmune neutropenia of infancy ('chronic benign') (Lyall et al 1992)
Neutropenia is severe ($0–0.5 \times 10^9/l$); however there is no excess of infections compared with normal children of the same age. The count increases with infection and urticaria, especially in the recovery period; there is little or no response to adrenalin (draws cells from marginating pool), variable response to steroid (enhances release from marrow), and good response to intravenous immunoglobulin (usually temporary, occasionally permanent, effect attributed to Fc receptor blockade and decreased synthesis of antibody). 'Compensatory' monocytosis is common, so that usually total leucocyte count is within normal limits.

Marrow examination is recommended to exclude the rare possibility of leukaemia as a cause of isolated neutropenia. Myeloid hyperplasia is usual; mature forms (bands and segmented) are normally represented or deficient ('maturation arrest').

Table 7.7 Alloimmune neonatal neutropenia: diagnosis[1]

Combination	Result
Maternal serum + paternal granulocytes	pos
Maternal serum + maternal granulocytes	neg[2]
Baby serum[3] + paternal granulocytes	pos
Baby serum[3] + baby neutrophils[4]	pos
Maternal serum + baby neutrophils[4]	pos

[1] After Minchinton & McGrath 1987
[2] To exclude maternal autoimmune neutropenia, e.g. SLE
[3] Collected while neutropenic
[4] Collected when numbers become normal

Table 7.8 Autoimmune neutropenias of childhood

Autoimmune neutropenia of infancy ('chronic benign')
Viral infection
Autoimmune disease
SLE
Felty
Passive transfer from mother with autoimmune disease, e.g. SLE
With autoimmune haemolysis and thrombocytopenia (Evans syndrome)
Bone marrow transplantation
Drugs (some)
T lymphocytosis with neutropenia

Median age at detection is approximately 8 months (range 3–30). Blood counts shortly after birth have been normal. Girls are more often affected than boys (1.5/1).

The antibody is IgG, with some IgM in occasional cases. Specificity is usually for NA1 or NA2; in some cases the target antigen cannot be identified. Evidence of parvovirus infection (PCR on marrow cells, serology) was obtained in a majority of cases by McClain et al (1993); the occurrence of neutropenia rather than the usual erythroblastopenia may be due to altered immune response, the antibody recognizing myeloid cells as well as virus.

Neutropenia is self-limiting with a median duration of 30 months (range 6–60), 95% recovering by 4 years. There are no known long-term immune or other effects.

Viral infection
Antineutrophil antibodies have been detected in some viral infections, e.g. infectious mononucleosis (Schooley et al 1984), HIV (Klaassen et al 1991) and parvovirus infection (McClain et al 1993). Neutropenia, however, occurs in only a minority of those with antibody (Schooley et al 1984). The target antigen is not clear — it does not appear to be one of the known polymorphous, neutrophil-specific antigens, NA1, NA2, etc. Neutropenia is only occasionally (< 1%) severe and prolonged enough in itself to predispose to bacterial infection (Stevens et al 1979).

Autoimmune disease
- SLE

Antineutrophil antibodies are detectable in about 50% of patients. The antibody does not have specificity for known polymorphous neutrophil-specific antigens and is distinct from the anti-DNA present in most cases (Fig. 7.12, Shastri & Logue 1993).

Neonatal lupus syndrome (Lancet Leader 1987, McCune et al 1987) is a risk if the mother has SLE (not necessarily symptomatic in the pregnancy). Major manifestations are cutaneous lupus (not manifest at birth but becoming so within 2 months) and complete heart block (at birth), usually one or the other, occasionally (< 10%) both. Skin lesions resolve usually within 6 months, but the heart block almost always is permanent. Some infants have, singly or in combination, neutropenia, thrombocytopenia or autoimmune haemolysis.

- Felty's syndrome (rheumatoid arthritis, splenomegaly and neutropenia)

Rare in childhood. The neutropenia is of complex causation (Joyce et al 1980): (i) neutrophil antibodies demonstrable in most cases, (ii) hypersplenism, most patients showing sustained improvement in count after splenectomy, (iii) inadequate compensatory marrow production.

Evans syndrome
Autoimmune thrombocytopenia and haemolysis without detectable underlying cause such as viral infection or SLE (Pui et al 1980). Autoimmune neutropenia also occurs in some cases. Antibodies to the various cell lines are different (Pegels et al 1982).

Marrow transplantation (Minchinton & Waters 1985)
Antibodies to neutrophils (and platelets) occur frequently after marrow transplant (allogeneic or autologous). Antibodies post-allogeneic transplant can be shown by immunoglobulin allotyping to be of donor origin, i.e. antibody against engrafted cells is autoimmune, whether allogeneic or autologous.

Drug-immune neutropenia (Stroncek 1993, Table 7.9)
Rare in childhood.

- In most cases the condition is drug-specific; in contrast to drug-specific haemolysis (p. 76), antibody will not simply react with pre-treated granulocytes, but only when serum, drug and neutrophils are incubated together.
- True autoantibody, comparable to methyl dopa immune haemolysis (p. 76); though autoimmune, antibody cannot be detected in serum after withdrawal of the drug.

Usually antibody is active against both mature and immature cells, in a minority against only precursor or only mature cells. The nature of the target antigen/s is for the most part unknown; the specific neutrophil series (NA1, NA2, etc) is not involved. For quinine, at least, it is a membrane glycoprotein. Antibodies from different drugs occasionally cross-react (e.g. quinine, quinidine).

Neutropenia affects only a minuscule proportion of those exposed, and is unpredictable in occurrence and course. Usually onset is abrupt, 1–5 weeks after start of treatment, sooner (or immediately) after re-exposure. Neutropenia lasts usually for 1–4 weeks after withdrawal of the drug, occasionally as briefly as 1 day. It may be severe enough to cause serious infection.

Marrow may be grossly depleted of neutrophils in general or show 'maturation arrest' at the myelocyte/metamyelocyte stage, with or without hyperplasia of precursor cells.

In some cases antibody is generated against platelets as well as neutrophils (different antibodies), and rarely against other cells, e.g. erythrocytes and T lymphocytes in a haemolytic-uraemic-like syndrome attributed to complement-mediated activation and adhesion of neutrophils to endothelium (quinine, Stroncek et al 1992).

T lymphocytosis with neutropenia (Murray & Lilleyman 1983, Herrod et al 1985)
Rare in childhood. Neutropenia (antibody demonstrable in some cases) with substantial increase in normal mature lymphocytes (CD8 suppressor/cytotoxic; large granular lymphocytes in some cases). Lymphocytosis may first manifest or become more obvious after splenectomy (for other reasons) and may affect marrow. Karyotype normal. May be associated with polyclonal hyperimmunoglobulinaemia. Blood otherwise normal, no anaemia or thrombocytopenia. Chronic (years) with little effect on health. Spleen may be moderately enlarged. Evidence of EBV infection is found in some cases.

MARROW INFILTRATION/REPLACEMENT

(Table 7.6)

Neutropenia is rarely the only finding. In monosomy 7 MPD, however, neutropenia, with or without macrocytosis, may be a prodrome over many years to overt disease. Rarely, neutropenia is a prodrome to ALL (Shepherd et al 1988).

DEFICIENCY OF HAEMATINICS

- Folate, B_{12} deficiency

- Copper deficiency (Zidar et al 1977, Tanaka et al 1980)

A rare cause. Neutropenia is an important and early characteristic, usually severe ($< 0.5 \times 10^9/l$); marrow usually shows vacuolation of precursor cells and 'maturation arrest' at myelocyte/metamyelocyte stage. Anaemia is usually severe (to about 4.5 g/dl) and macrocytic, with megaloblastosis, vacuolated erythroblasts and ringed sideroblasts (10–15% of cells) in marrow. The genesis of these changes is obscure; they do not occur in the best-known copper deficiency in man (Menkes kinky hair syndrome). Possible mechanisms include defective synthesis of cytochrome oxidase and ascorbic acid oxidase, which keep copper in the reduced state. Treatment with copper produces rapid and striking response.

Deficiency is most likely to occur in infants with prolonged diarrhoea and malnutrition, and in those on prolonged total parenteral nutrition without copper supplementation. Deficiency may, however, occur without obvious cause in infants who are thriving.

Table 7.9 Paediatric drugs which may be associated with immune neutropenia[1]

Anti-arrhythmic
Aprinidine HCl
Flecanide acetate[2]
Procainamide
Quinidine
Antibiotics
Penicillin and derivatives
Ampicillin
Amoxycillin
Dicloxacillin
Nafcillin
Oxacillin
Cephalosporins
Cephradine
Cefotaxime
Ceftazidime
Cefuroxime
Sulphonamides
Sulphamethoxazole
Sulphathiazole
Sulphafurazole
Sulphapyridine
Antimalarial
Amodiaquine
Chloroquine
Quinine
Analgesic/anti-inflammatory
Amidopyrine
Aminosalicylic acid
Diclofenac
Ibuprofen
Propyphenazone
Antithyroid
Propylthiouracil[2,3]
Carbimazole
Methimazole
Other
Phenytoin
Chloral hydrate
Gold thiomalate
Levamisole[3]

[1] Adapted from Stroncek 1993
[2] Neutropenia may not occur till months or years after exposure
[3] True autoimmune in some cases

DRUGS AND NEUTROPENIA

Selective granulocytopenia as an idiosyncratic, unpredictable effect of drugs is rare in childhood, though it is possible with a large variety of drugs (Young & Vincent 1980). Mechanisms include personal idiosyncrasies in pharmacokinetics, sensitivity of myeloid precursors and immune response. Drugs with potential for immune destruction are listed in Table 7.9. The same drug may produce granulocytopenia by different mechanisms in different patients and possibly even at different times in one patient.

NEUTROPENIA DUE TO SEQUESTRATION

- Hypersplenism (e.g. biliary atresia, liver cirrhosis, cavernous transformation of portal vein).
- Hyperphagocytosis of band and segmented forms by marrow macrophages is a rare cause of isolated neutropenia (Parmley et al 1981; cf haemophagocytosis, in which macrophages contain a variety of inclusions). There is no evidence of neutrophil antibody, no or slight increase in serum muramidase, no response to adrenalin (marginating pool) but good response to hydrocortisone (marrow reserve).

Neutrophilia

Except for the first weeks of life (Table 1.13) the upper limit of normal is approximately 7.5 × 10^9/l. Rarely, artefactually high counts may be obtained by automated particle counters:

(i) Precipitation of cryoprotein on cooling. Error revealed by examination of stained film. Examine fluid prep by subdued light or phase contrast for crystals.
(ii) Incomplete lysis of erythrocytes. Examination of stained film will reveal error.

Neutrophilia (Table 7.10) has little value in specific diagnosis, with some exceptions considered below.

Infection
As a general rule, neutrophilia is more likely in bacterial than in viral infection. However, neutrophilia is not infrequent in the early stages of viral infection and neutropenia may occur in severe bacterial infection. The neutrophil count (and other 'routine' characteristics) is of value in assessing the likelihood of appendicitis in children admitted to surgical wards with abdominal pain (Table 7.11). All characteristics examined in this study were useful in discrimination, i.e. they were reasonably common in, and reasonably specific for, appendicitis. The most useful and easily obtained is the neutrophil count — a value of 15 × 10^9/l is a useful cut-off. The difference in frequency of atypical ('viral') lymphocytes is an indication of the high frequency of viral infection in non-surgical abdominal pain.

Substantial neutrophilia (> 50 × 10^9/l) is not infrequent in bacterial infection, especially bacterial pneumonia, empyema, bacterial meningitis, septicaemia, urinary tract infection and bacterial endocarditis, and is characteristic of the rare genetic deficiency of integrin adhesion molecules on neutrophils and lymphocytes (delayed separation of umbilical cord, severe bacterial infections, periodontitis, gingivitis, poor pus formation).

Leukaemoid reactions
For those which mimic AML M2 see page 150, M3 page 156, M4 page 158. For TAR syndrome see page 300, and Randall's syndrome, page 172.

Sweet's syndrome (acute febrile neutrophilic dermatosis) (Krilov et al 1987)
A rare syndrome of unknown cause, characterized by high neutrophilia, raised, tender, erythematous plaques and bullae in the skin, spiking fevers and often arthralgia, myalgia and headache. May occur without underlying disease or in association with leukaemia, usually myeloid (in remission and not in a neutropenic phase). Diagnosis requires skin biopsy (dermal infiltration with mature neutrophils, oedema, vesiculation). Without treatment, resolves spontaneously in weeks; no response to antibiotics, but prompt relief from steroids.

Familial neutrophilia (Herring et al 1974)
A familial, lifelong, substantial (to 62 × 10^9/l) neutrophilia of segmented and, to a lesser degree, stab forms. Neutrophils are normal in morphology and function. NAP may be increased. Associated features include increased incidence of chromatid breaks in blood chromosomes, Gaucher-like cells in marrow and spleen, thickening of skull bones (widening of diploë) and hepatosplenomegaly. Regarded as inherited, autosomal dominant.

Table 7.10 Benign neutrophilia: a selection

Artefact
Infection[1]
Inflammation
  Kawasaki
  Inflammatory bowel disease
    Crohn's
    Ulcerative colitis
  Rheumatoid arthritis
  SLE
  Histiocytosis
Tissue necrosis (e.g. hepatic)[1]
Leukaemoid reactions[1,2]
  Viral infection (may mimic e.g. AML M2, M3, M4)
  TAR syndrome
  Randall's syndrome
  Disseminated tuberculosis
Non-haemopoietic malignancy
Post-splenectomy
Drugs
  Steroid
  Ranitidine
  Leucocyte stimulating factors[1]
    Colony stimulating factors
    Interleukins
  Lithium
Stress
  Vomiting
  Convulsions
  Hypoxia, near-drowning
  Acidosis — diabetic, other
  Post-operative
Sweet's syndrome
Familial[1]

[1] Count often exceeds 50 × 10^9/l
[2] Non-leukaemic shift to left, including myeloblasts
Note: Placement of some disorders, e.g. Kawasaki, histiocytosis, is tentative

Table 7.11 Haematology of appendicitis (n = 50)[1] vs non-surgical abdominal pain (n = 50)[2]

		Sensitivity[3]	Specificity[4]
Total leucocytes, × 10^9/l	≥ 15.0	29/50	43/50
	≥ 20.0	15/50	48/50
	≥ 25.0	7/50	50/50
	≥ 30.0	1/50	50/50
Neutrophils, × 10^9/l	≥ 15.0	25/50	48/50
	≥ 20.0	7/50	49/50
	≥ 25.0	3/50	50/50
	≥ 30.0	1/50	50/50
Neutrophils, shift to left, %	≥ 10.0	17/49	37/50
	≥ 20.0	11/49	50/50
	≥ 30.0	4/49	50/50
Atypical lymphocytes: 0 in 200 leucocytes		13/50	48/50
ESR, mm in 1 h	> 30	5/31	38/38

[1] Histologically proven
[2] Admitted to surgical wards with abdominal pain — 46 with various diagnoses discharged without laparotomy, 4 with histologically normal appendix removed
[3] Sensitivity = proportion of patients with positive test
[4] Specificity = proportion of controls with negative test

Lymphocytosis (Table 7.12)

Lymphocytosis is used here to denote an increase in normal lymphocytes, in contrast to atypical lymphocytes of viral infection and blastic lymphocytes of ALL. For normal values see Table 1.14.

Pertussis
Lymphocytosis may be extreme (to about $200 \times 10^9/l$) and affects small, 'dark' lymphocytes and not large granular forms. Rieder forms (cleft nuclei) are not of value in diagnosis. A presence of atypical lymphocytes may be an indication of associated viral infection such as CMV. Neutrophilia suggests secondary bacterial infection and may be a sign of poor prognosis (Fig. 7.2).

Lymphocytosis is due to a factor binding to cells to inhibit their traffic from blood to lymph nodes (Morse & Barron 1970). Marrow lymphocytes are not increased (Landolt 1945).

In children with cough, lymphocytosis is more common in those with than those without pertussis, especially if the count exceeds $15 \times 10^9/l$ (Table 7.13). However, the diagnostic utility of lymphocytosis is limited by insensitivity, especially at that age (first year) when pertussis may be severe or fatal and a rapid aid to diagnosis would as a consequence be welcome.

Viral infection
A mild increase in normal lymphocytes occurs in a minority of children with viral infections. Increase in atypical lymphocytes (p. 252) is more common and more characteristic.

Infectious lymphocytosis (Smith 1941)
The increase in lymphocytes is of mature cells, as in pertussis, and may be substantial (in one of our cases to $160 \times 10^9/l$). The lymphocytes mark as T cells, mainly CD4 (helper/inducer), though T cell function overall may be deficient (Bertotto et al 1985). There is no anaemia or thrombocytopenia; eosinophils may be increased. The marrow may be normal, or show lymphocytosis. Karyotype is normal. Distinction from other causes of lymphocytosis requires clinical information and exclusion of pertussis. Lymphocyte count returns to normal usually within 2 weeks (up to 7).

The condition is sporadic or epidemic, affects infants predominantly, and may be asymptomatic or produce a mild febrile illness, with pharyngeal or upper respiratory infection, rash, and infrequently meningeal irritation or abdominal symptoms. There is no pertussis-like cough. A viral aetiology is suspected, with an incubation period of 12–21 days.

Omenn's syndrome (Omenn 1965, Fig. 7.2)
A rare, often familial immunodeficiency with onset in infancy (2 days–3 months) of extensive skin disease (erythroderma, eczema, thickening), diarrhoea, bacterial and fungal infections, hepatosplenomegaly, failure to thrive and death in 2–6 months. Eosinophilia (to about $30 \times 10^9/l$) is consistent and lymphocytosis frequent. Severe lymphocyte depletion however occurs in lymph nodes and thymus; Langerhans-like cells (S100 protein positive, no Birbeck bodies) may be increased in lymph nodes (Ruco et al 1985). Serum IgE may be increased.

The syndrome may be a graft vs host reaction in a primary cellular immunodeficiency, with persistence and proliferation of maternal cells in lymphoid organs, but this has not been confirmed (Heyderman et al 1991).

Leukaemias
An increase in cells morphologically indistinguishable from lymphocytes (?stem cells) may occur in chronic myeloid leukaemias (Fig. 5.17). For chronic lymphocytic leukaemia see page 140.

Unexplained lymphocytosis
Transient (days to 4 weeks) unexplained lymphocytosis is not uncommon in childhood. Lymphocytosis is usually only modest ($< 20 \times 10^9/l$). Some cases are associated with physical stress such as airway obstruction.

Occasionally more persistent lymphocytosis (months) is unexplained. Viruses such as HTLV 1 (Ehrlich et al 1988) may account for some of these cases.

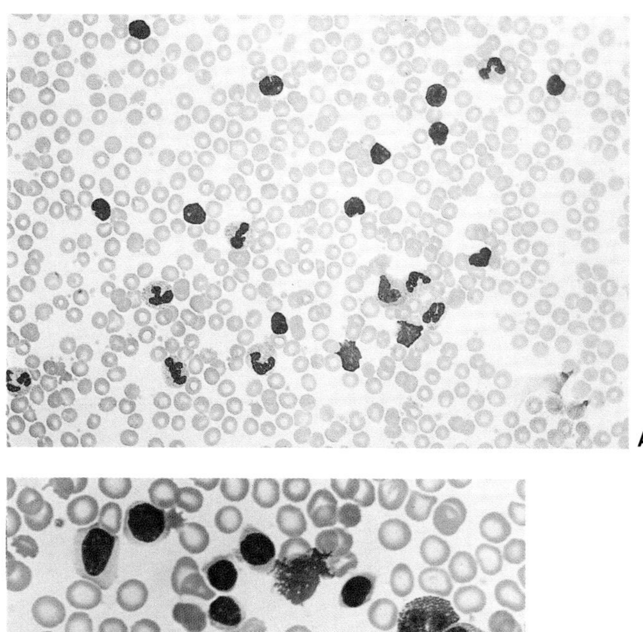

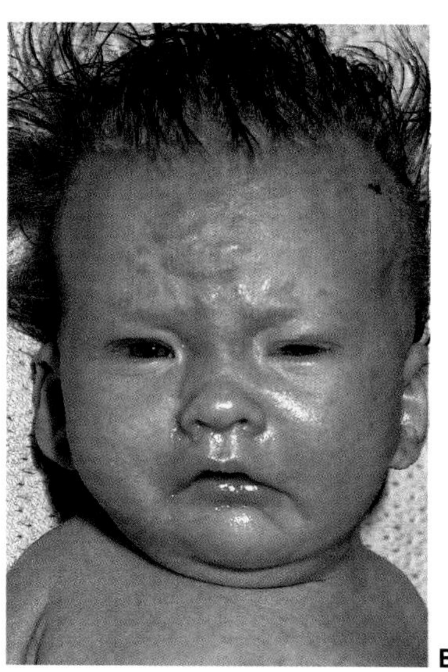

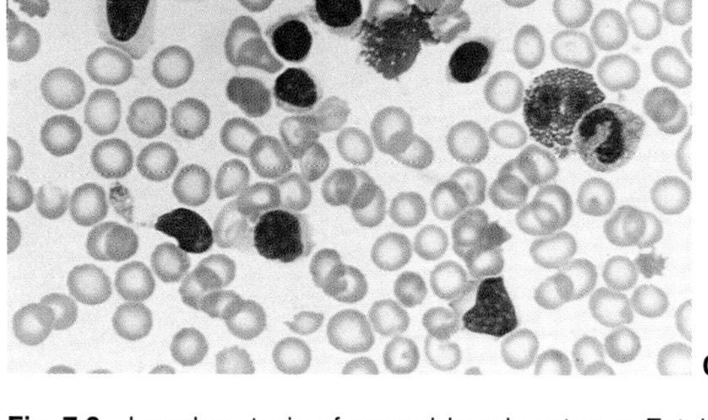

Fig. 7.2 Lymphocytosis of normal lymphocytes. **a** Fatal pertussis in 3-month-old infant, lymphocytosis (42 × 10^9/l); neutrophilia (66 × 10^9/l) due to secondary infection. **b**,**c** Omenn's syndrome, erythroderma and skin thickening (which were generalized), blood film showing lymphocytosis (34 × 10^9/l) and eosinophilia (6.7 × 10^9/l). **a** × 200; **c** × 500. **a** Courtesy of Dr J O'Duffy

Table 7.12 Lymphocytosis (of normal lymphocytes) in childhood

Pertussis
Viral infection
Infectious lymphocytosis
Omenn's syndrome
Leukaemias
Chronic myeloid[1]
Chronic lymphocytic
Acute graft vs host disease
T lymphocytosis with neutropenia
Unexplained

[1] Increase in normal-appearing lymphoid cells (presumably stem cells) as part of the leukaemia

Table 7.13 Lymphocytosis (of normal lymphocytes) in children with troublesome cough

Lymphocytes × 10^9/l ≥	**< 1 yr 15.0 No**	**%**	**1–4 yr 9.0 No**	**%**	**4–8 yr 7.0 No**	**%**	**8–14 yr 6.0 No**	**%**	**> 14 yr 4.5 No**	**%**	**Total No**	**%**
Pertussis												
positive[1]	8/31	27	9/15	60	10/19	53	2/8	25	0 cases		29/73	40
negative[2]	1/23	5	2/14	14	0/8	0	0/2	0	0/3	0	3/50	6
											P < 0.001	

Counts ≥ 15.0 × 10^9/l: pertussis pos 19/73
neg 1/50
P < 0.001

12 with pertussis followed (for 2–13 days):
in 8, both counts high
in 2, both counts normal
in 2, count high at first, then normal

[1] Nasopharyngeal aspirate within 5 days of blood examination positive by culture or direct immunofluorescence
[2] Nasopharyngeal aspirate negative by both culture and immunofluorescence, and serum negative for Bordetella antibody IgG, A, M

Atypical lymphocytosis (atypical, reactive or viral lymphocytes) (Figs 7.3, 4.2, 4.18)

Although a proportion of cells in any individual is likely to be immature or blastic, atypical lymphocytes should not be confused with leukaemic lymphoblasts. Typical morphology and a spectrum of maturity are in contrast to the more uniform, monoclonal appearance of leukaemic lymphoblasts (Fig. 4.5). However, in occasional cases of viral infection, the degree of cell immaturity may raise a suspicion of leukaemia (Fig. 4.18). Degenerate or dead forms may be noted (see leucocyte death, p. 264). Atypical lymphocytes are for the most part activated T cells (Pattengale et al 1974) with a minority, transformed B cells.

Other changes which may be noted in these films (discussed elsewhere) include: neutropenia, neutrophilia, immune spherocytosis, thrombocytopenia (isolated or part of pancytopenia or intravascular coagulation such as purpura fulminans) and phagocytic monocytes.

The morphology of atypical lymphocytes has little value for specific diagnosis. In measles and rubella, the cells tend to be larger and more basophilic ('plasmacytoid') than in the generality of viral infections (Fig. 7.3). Among specific (or apparently specific) changes in haemopoietic cells in viral infection are inclusion-containing multinucleate cells in marrow in CMV infection (Fig. 5.9) and intranuclear inclusions in histologic sections of erythroblasts in parvovirus infection (Anand et al 1987).

The number of atypical lymphocytes in a film has some value for diagnosis (Tables 7.14, 7.15).

Infectious mononucleosis

Atypical lymphocytes are usually profuse (> 10% of leucocytes); counts occasionally are extreme (to 50 × 10^9/l).

Destructive/proliferative effects of the virus are more severe and often fatal in conditions of genetic susceptibility to the virus, such as X-linked lymphoproliferative syndrome (Duncan's syndrome after the first kindred, Purtilo et al 1977, Table 7.16, Fig. 7.4).

Table 7.14 Atypical (reactive) lymphocytes: slight to moderate increase[1]

Most types of viral infection
Conditions which in most cases are probably viral
'Irritable' hip
Intussusception[2]
Mesenteric adenitis
Non-viral
Mycoplasma
Malaria
Toxoplasmosis
Typhoid
Brucellosis
Scarlatina
Kawasaki[3]
Non-infective
Serum sickness
Dilantin sensitivity

[1] Small numbers are a normal finding, especially in the first years of life, though presumably an indication of subclinical viral infection
[2] Yunis et al 1975
[3] Precise nature unknown

Table 7.15 Atypical (reactive) lymphocytes in profusion

Infectious mononucleosis
Cytomegalovirus
Viral hepatitis, pre-icteric phase
Measles[1]
Adenovirus[1]
Echovirus[1]
Unidentified infection[2]

[1] Profuse in minority only
[2] Fall in numbers may be obtained with IV immunoglobulin or ganciclovir

Table 7.16 Haematologic effects of Epstein-Barr virus[1]

Infectious mononucleosis
Atypical lymphocytosis
Immune: neutropenia, agranulocytosis
neutrophil agglutination
Leucocyte death
Immune haemolysis (anti-i, rarely N)
Immune thrombocytopenia
Haemophagocytosis — blood, marrow
Erythroblastopenia
Global marrow destruction
Benign lymphoblastosis
Chronic myelomonocytosis
B lymphocytes
Destruction: acquired hypogammaglobulinaemia
Proliferation
Lymphoma

[1] Effects more severe or fatal in X-linked lymphoproliferative syndrome

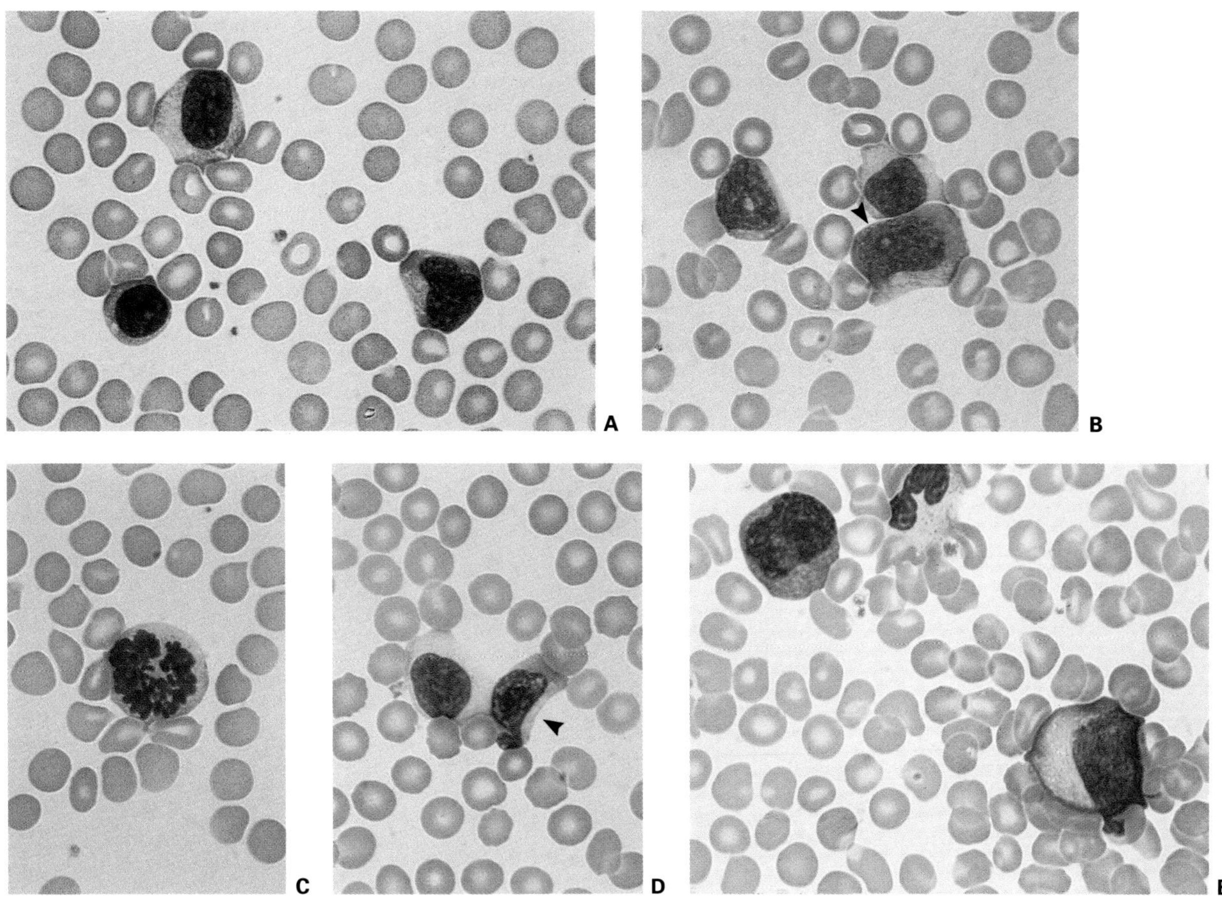

Fig. 7.3 Atypical lymphocytes in infectious mononucleosis (**a–d**) and measles (**e**). **a** 2 atypical lymphocytes and a normal lymphocyte. **b** Blastic cell with nucleolus. **c** Atypical lymphocyte in mitosis. **d** 2 atypical lymphocytes, one dead (arrow). **e** Larger, 'plasmacytoid' cells in measles. All × 750

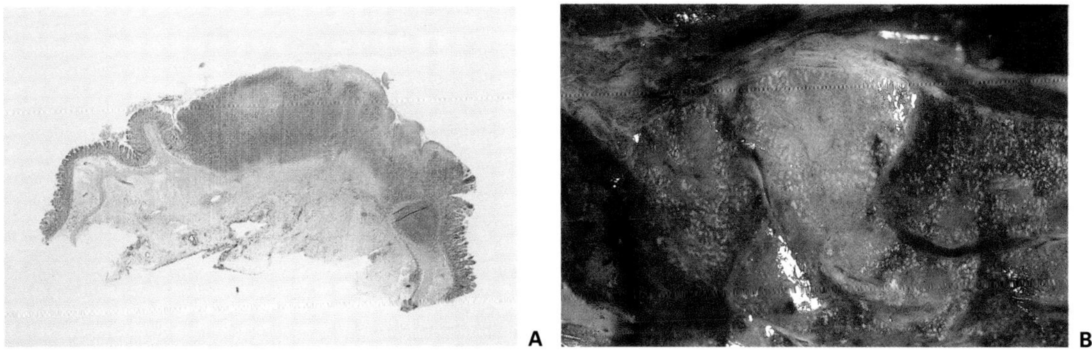

Fig. 7.4 X-linked lymphoproliferative (Duncan's) syndrome, 2 manifestations in the same boy. **a** Age 4 years, lymphoma of ileum, H & E × 2. **b** Age 6 years, death from fulminant infectious mononucleosis; lung contains a mass (centre), composed of atypical lymphocytes; similar masses in liver.

The traditional Paul-Bunnell test is fairly sensitive and specific for diagnosis (Table 7.17, Fleisher et al 1983, Dacie & Lewis 1991). A positive reaction is occasionally obtained in other infections such as CMV, rubella and malaria; a false negative is occasionally obtained if plasma is used instead of serum. The 'IM' antigen on sheep erythrocytes is inactivated by papain and other proteolytic enzymes; antibody remaining after absorption of serum with papain-treated sheep erythrocytes appears to be specific for infectious mononucleosis (Robinson & Smith 1966).

Heterophile titres rise at about 4–6 days, peak at 2–3 weeks and remain positive for 4–5 months. Occasionally a positive result is not obtained for weeks to months or the test is positive only transiently. For unknown reasons, a positive result is rarely obtained in children under 5 years known to be infected with EBV.

Definitive diagnosis may be made by viral serology. VCA-IgM lasts 4–8 weeks, VCA-IgG rises at about the same time but is lifelong. EBNA-IgG rises after 3–4 weeks and is lifelong. Raised VCA-IgM is therefore an indication of recent infection, raised VCA-IgG or EBNA-IgG with normal IgM indicates past infection (Schooley & Dolin 1990).

Lymphopenia (Table 7.18)

Except for immunodeficiency states, lymphopenia is of little clinical significance. Those conditions not described elsewhere are summarized here.

Severe combined immunodeficiency

In addition to classic types, lymphopenia may occur in deficiencies of adenosine deaminase and purine nucleoside phosphorylase. Main clinical features are: failure to thrive, severe infection (viral, bacterial, fungal, Pneumocystis), dermatitis, encephalopathy and other neurologic disturbances; IgG, A and M are grossly diminished in most types of SCID. Erythrocytes, leucocytes and platelets may be damaged by immune effect. Most types autosomal recessive, some X-linked recessive.

Di George syndrome

Main features (result of maldevelopment of 3rd and 4th pharyngeal pouches) are abnormalities of: facies, heart (right sided aortic arch, tetralogy of Fallot, other anomalies), thymus (absent or small on X-ray, T cell deficiency, infections, lymphocyte count variable, often lymphopenia) and parathyroid (hypoparathyroidism, hypocalcaemia, convulsions in first days of life). Genetics uncertain, may be an embryopathy.

Ataxia telangiectasia

Defect in DNA repair of unknown nature. Main features: unsteady gait (cerebellar, onset in first years), bacterial and viral sinopulmonary infections, telangiectasia (onset in late childhood, conjunctiva, skin), hypersensitivity to UV and other radiation, drooling, growth failure, delayed puberty, often late mental retardation.

Table 7.17 Heterophile antibodies: reaction with sheep (or horse[1]) red cells

	Untreated serum	After absorption of serum with: guinea pig kidney	ox red cells
Infectious mononucleosis	+++	+++	0
Normal serum (Forssman)	+	0	+

[1] May be more sensitive

Table 7.18 Lymphopenia in childhood

- Infection
  - Any kind; viral rather than bacterial
- Stress
  - Burns
  - Vomiting
  - Convulsions
- Drugs
  - Steroid
  - Adrenalin
  - Antilymphocyte antibodies
  - Immunosuppressants
  - Cytotoxics[1]
- Irradiation[1]
- Immune disease or immune component of disease
  - SLE
  - Crohn's disease
  - Hodgkin's disease
- Marrow failure[1]
  - Aplasia
  - Leukaemia
- Immunodeficiency[1]
  - Genetic
    - Severe combined
    - Di George
    - Ataxia telangiectasia
    - Wiskott-Aldrich
    - Intestinal lymphangiectasia
    - Transcobalamin II deficiency
    - Nezelof
    - Reticular dysgenesis
  - Acquired
    - Chronic graft vs host disease
    - HIV infection

[1] Usually with other cytopenias

Serum IgA and IgE decreased, α fetoprotein increased, lymphocyte function deficient, translocations involving 7 and 14 common. Risk of malignancy (lymphoproliferative, epithelial). Autosomal recessive.

Intestinal lymphangiectasia
Protein-losing enteropathy results in loss of both cells (lymphopenia of T cells) and protein (variable, occasionally severe reduction in serum IgG and IgA; IgM tends to remain normal). Infection is not a major problem however (Gurbindo & Seidman 1991).

Nezelof's syndrome
Cellular immunodeficiency with abnormal immunoglobulin synthesis. Main features: susceptibility to infection (viral, bacterial, fungal), deficient T cell function; serum IgA, G and M normal but production of some specific antibodies (e.g. tetanus toxoid) deficient; IgE may be increased. X-linked and autosomal recessive patterns of inheritance.

Eosinophilia

The diagnostic significance of eosinophilia is related to some extent to its degree (Table 7.19). The division in the table is not absolute, however: eosinophilia may for example be gross in some disorders (e.g. Hodgkin's disease) in which it is usually mild. Charcot-Leyden crystals may occur in gross eosinophilias (p. 236).

Table 7.19 Eosinophilia in childhood

	Usually < 3.0 × 10⁹/l	Usually > 3.0 × 10⁹/l
Allergic	asthma[1] eczema allergy to plastic tubing[2] toxic epidermal necrolysis pemphigus	acute allergies (milk-protein colitis, Stevens-Johnson, angioneurotic oedema, serum sickness) eosinophilic gastroenteropathy
Parasitic	most gastrointestinal parasites hydatid *Schistosoma*	Löffler syndrome Angiostrongylus[3] *Toxocara* *Trichuris* *Ascaris* *Strongyloides* *Ancylostoma* filariasis
Fungal	pulmonary aspergillosis, candidiasis	coccidioidomycosis
Drugs		
Immune	SLE rheumatoid inflammatory bowel disease some immunodeficiencies e.g. Wiskott-Aldrich	polyarteritis Omenn's syndrome syndrome of recurrent pruritis, oedema, ↓C 1,3,4[4]
Other	Job's (Buckley's) syndrome acute graft vs host disease ALL, pre-ALL AML M2Eo, M4Eo Hodgkin's disease radiation therapy histiocytosis[5] familial	CML adult type eosinophilic leukaemia Idiopathic

[1] Eosinophils (and lymphocytes) are decreased by IV steroid treatment of an attack
[2] Nasogastric, cerebral ventricle, peritoneal dialysis
[3] Helminths which invade the central nervous system produce eosinophilia in cerebrospinal fluid as well as blood (Kuberski 1979)
[4] Geha & Akl 1976
[5] Eosinophilia unusual (Fig. 5.30)

Gross, chronic (> 6 months) eosinophilia of any causation is likely to result in the hypereosinophilic syndrome, in which organ dysfunction is caused by physical effects of tumorous collections of eosinophils and release from eosinophils of substances damaging to endothelium (Alfaham et al 1987, Weller & Bubley 1994). Inhibition of endothelial thrombomodulin by eosinophil major basic protein is a mechanism for damage (Slungaard et al 1993). The most prominent effects are cardiopulmonary (eosinophilic pneumonia, cardiac mural thrombosis, endocardial fibrosis, mitral and tricuspid valve dysfunction, heart failure, Fig. 7.5).

Some of the conditions listed in Table 7.19 are described further below. Eosinophilia in leukaemias and eosinophilic leukaemia are considered in Chapters 4 and 5.

- Allergic states

Milk-protein colitis is an allergic reaction to human or cow's milk (in formula or, if breast-fed, in mother's diet) which results in loss of eosinophils and blood from the bowel. Prompt resolution follows change in diet, though it tends to subside spontaneously over some months, due to acquisition of tolerance, even if the diet is not changed (Cleghorn G J 1994, personal communication).

In eosinophilic gastroenteropathy, infiltration of stomach and intestine causes vomiting, abdominal pain and occasionally obstruction of bowel or appendix; protein-losing enteropathy results in loss of albumin (ascites, oedema) and blood (iron deficiency anaemia). It affects young adults rather than children and is thought to be a sensitivity to agents known (e.g. foods) or unknown (Kirschner 1991).

The eosinophilia often seen in premature neonates may in part be due to intubation (Bhat & Scanlon 1981). The eosinophilia in cerebrospinal fluid of children with shunts for hydrocephalus (Fig. 7.5) is usually not associated with blood eosinophilia (Kennedy & Singer 1988).

- Parasitic infestation

In Löffler syndrome (pulmonary infiltrates with eosinophilia, PIE syndrome, Howard 1990), lung infiltration is due to the pulmonary sojourn in the migratory life cycle of nematodes (e.g. *Ascaris, Trichuris, Toxocara,* filaria), or is an allergic reaction to aspergillosis. Asthma is likely to be prominent in cases due to aspergillus. The disorder typically is self-healing (usually < 1 month).

- Drugs

Drugs which cause eosinophilia (in only few persons exposed and rarely severe) include aspirin, cyclophosphamide, penicillin, sulphonamides, cephalosporins, nitrofurantoin, phenytoin and antihypertensives. Eosinophilia is not uncommon in marrow (rather than blood) of children receiving cytotoxics for leukaemia.

- Other causes

Job's syndrome (Buckley's syndrome, hyper-IgE syndrome with recurrent infections, Geha & Leung 1989) is a rare immunodeficiency characterized by infections of respiratory tract and skin, eczematoid dermatitis, coarse facies, eosinophilia and extreme increase in serum IgE. 'Cold' abscesses containing eosinophils and necrotic material, but few neutrophils, are characteristic. T cell function is deficient and neutrophil chemotaxis impaired (explaining the neutrophil lack in abscesses), but the basic defect is unknown.

It is not clear if the rare familial eosinophilia is inherited or is a familial reaction to a shared pathogen (Naiman et al 1964, Fig. 7.5c). Splenectomy in one patient was followed by return of count to normal.

In a significant proportion of cases, a cause for eosinophilia is not found. A personal case, who was clinically well, had splenomegaly, polyclonal increase in serum IgG, monoclonal IgM paraprotein, marrow eosinophilia with normal karyotype, and serologic evidence of past infection with EBV. Abnormalities resolved slowly over 2 years. The highest eosinophil count was $5.5 \times 10^9/l$.

Eosinopenia, apparent absence of eosinophils

Eosinopenia, usually with lymphopenia, is a temporary (days) effect of high dosage steroid, especially intravenous. For acquired absence of eosinophils see page 218.

Qualitative changes in leucocytes in infection

Appraisal of leucocyte numbers and morphology usually gives some indication of the likelihood of infection, its broad nature (bacterial vs viral) and occasionally the precise cause. Quantitative changes are considered elsewhere. Changes in morphology (Table 7.20) are considered here.

Table 7.20 Qualitative changes in leucocytes in infection

- Neutrophils
  - Shift to left
  - Toxic granulation
  - Degranulation
  - Döhle bodies
  - Vacuolation
  - Pelgeroid change
  - Chromomeres
  - Gigantism
  - Phagocytosis of:
    - leucocytes
    - erythroblasts/cytes
    - organisms
  - Cell death, fragmentation
  - Agglutination
  - NAP usually ↑ in bacterial infection, ↓ in viral
- Lymphocytes
  - Cell death, fragmentation
- Monocytes/macrophages
  - Vacuolation, enlargement, activation, Döhle-like bodies
  - Phagocytosis of:
    - leucocytes
    - erythroblasts/cytes
    - organisms
  - Chromomeres
  - Cell death, fragmentation
  - Transformation to 'histiocytes'
  - Infection-associated haemophagocytosis (marrow, blood)
- Giant cells with intranuclear inclusions (marrow, CMV infection)

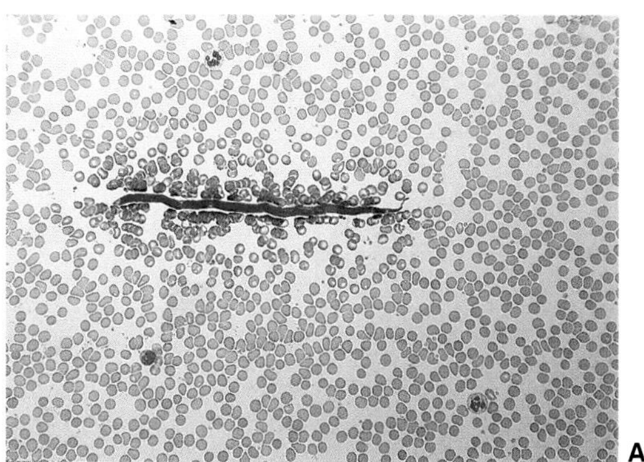
A

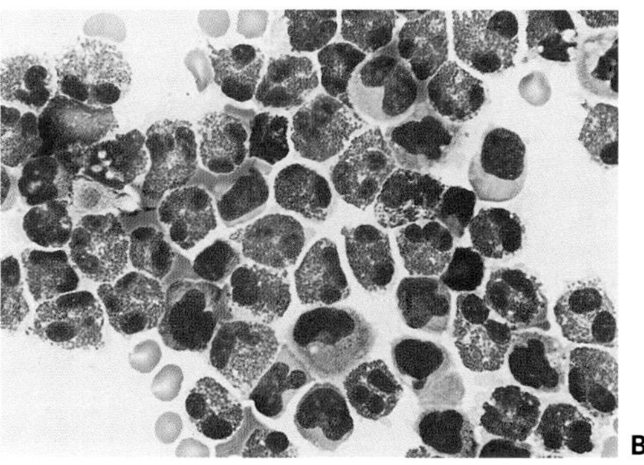
B

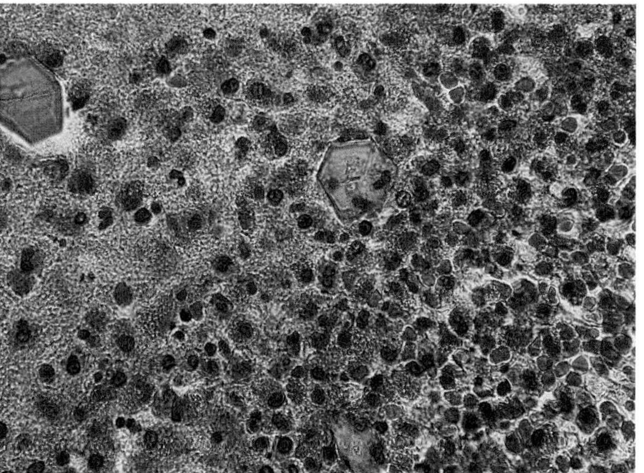
C

Fig. 7.5 Eosinophilia. **a** Microfilaria (*Loa loa*) in blood, eosinophils 1.4×10^9/l. **b** Eosinophilia in cerebrospinal fluid (leucocyte count 4500/cm^3) due to plastic tubing inserted for drainage of subdural haematoma. **c** Thrombus with eosinophils and Charcot-Leyden crystals on porcine replacement of mitral valve in a 14-year-old boy with idiopathic eosinophilia (8–22 $\times 10^9$/l) from birth. A younger brother also has chronic eosinophilia, but of lesser degree. **a** × 160; **b** × 500; **c** H & E × 480. **c** Courtesy of Dr N Johnson

TOXIC CHANGE IN NEUTROPHILS (Fig. 7.6)

Toxic change is characterized by various combinations of the abnormalities listed in Table 7.20. When an apparently toxic change occurs in isolation, e.g. shift to left or heavy granulation, suspicion should be raised of mimicry (Table 7.21).

Toxic change in neutrophils, in combination with other abnormalities in the film, is a useful guide in distinction of bacterial from viral infection (Table 7.22). However, toxic change per se is not specific for infection (Table 7.25). A quantification of toxic change has been devised (Zipursky et al 1976, Table 7.23); this may be combined with other leucocyte changes and the platelet count to produce a score for risk of sepsis in the neonate, in whom (more so than in older children) infection is likely to produce rapid deterioration (Rodwell et al 1988, Table 7.24). However, C reactive protein levels on 2 successive days appear to be more useful than morphologic assessment (if readings can be obtained rapidly); sepsis is likely if values are raised on day 1 and/or day 2, and can be confidently excluded if values are normal on both days (Wagle et al 1994).

Table 7.21 Differential diagnosis of toxic changes in neutrophils

Change	Differential diagnosis
Toxic granulation	Alder granulation (p. 214)
Degranulation	genetic disorder (p. 216) myeloid leukaemias
Döhle bodies	Döhle-like bodies in May-Hegglin, Fechtner and Sebastian syndromes (p. 216)
Vacuolation	anticoagulant/storage artefact Jordans anomaly (p. 214)
Giant neutrophils	hereditary giant neutrophils (p. 222)
Pseudo-Pelgerization	true Pelger anomaly (p. 222)
Cell death	anticoagulant/storage artefact

Table 7.22 Common changes in leucocytes in bacterial and viral infection

	Bacterial infection	Viral infection
Neutrophilia	common	uncommon
Neutropenia	in severe infection	common
Toxic change in neutrophils	common, often severe	slight; marked in some infections, e.g. measles
Atypical lymphocytes	small numbers or absent	increased
Organisms in leucocytes	sometimes	0

Table 7.23 Quantitation of toxic change in neutrophils[1,2]

	% cells affected	Score
Vacuolation, Döhle bodies	0	0
	< 25	+
	25–50	2+
	51–75	3+
	> 75	4+
Toxic granulation	normal granulation	0
	slight toxic granulation	+
	approx 50% cells affected	2+
	toxic granules most cells	3+
	gross; nucleus obscured by toxic granules	4+

[1] After Zipursky et al 1976
[2] For use with Table 7.24

Table 7.24 Haematologic scoring system for sepsis in the neonate[1]

	Abnormality
Total neutrophil count[2,3]	↑ or ↓
Immature/total neutrophil ratio[2]	↑
Immature/mature neutrophil ratio	≥ 0.3
Immature neutrophil count[2]	↑
Total leucocyte count	↓ or ↑ ($\leq 5.0 \times 10^9$/l or ≥ 25.0, 30.0 or 21.0 at birth, 12–24 h and day 2 onward respectively)
Toxic change in neutrophils[4]	≥ 3+ for vacuolation, toxic granulation or Döhle bodies
Platelets	$\leq 150 \times 10^9$/l

Each feature has a score of 1. A total score of ≥ 3 is strong evidence for, and ≤ 2 is strong evidence against sepsis
[1] Rodwell et al 1988
[2] From reference ranges of Manroe et al 1979
[3] If no mature neutrophils in film, score 2 rather than 1 for abnormal total count
[4] Quantitation by criteria of Zipursky et al 1976 (Table 7.23)

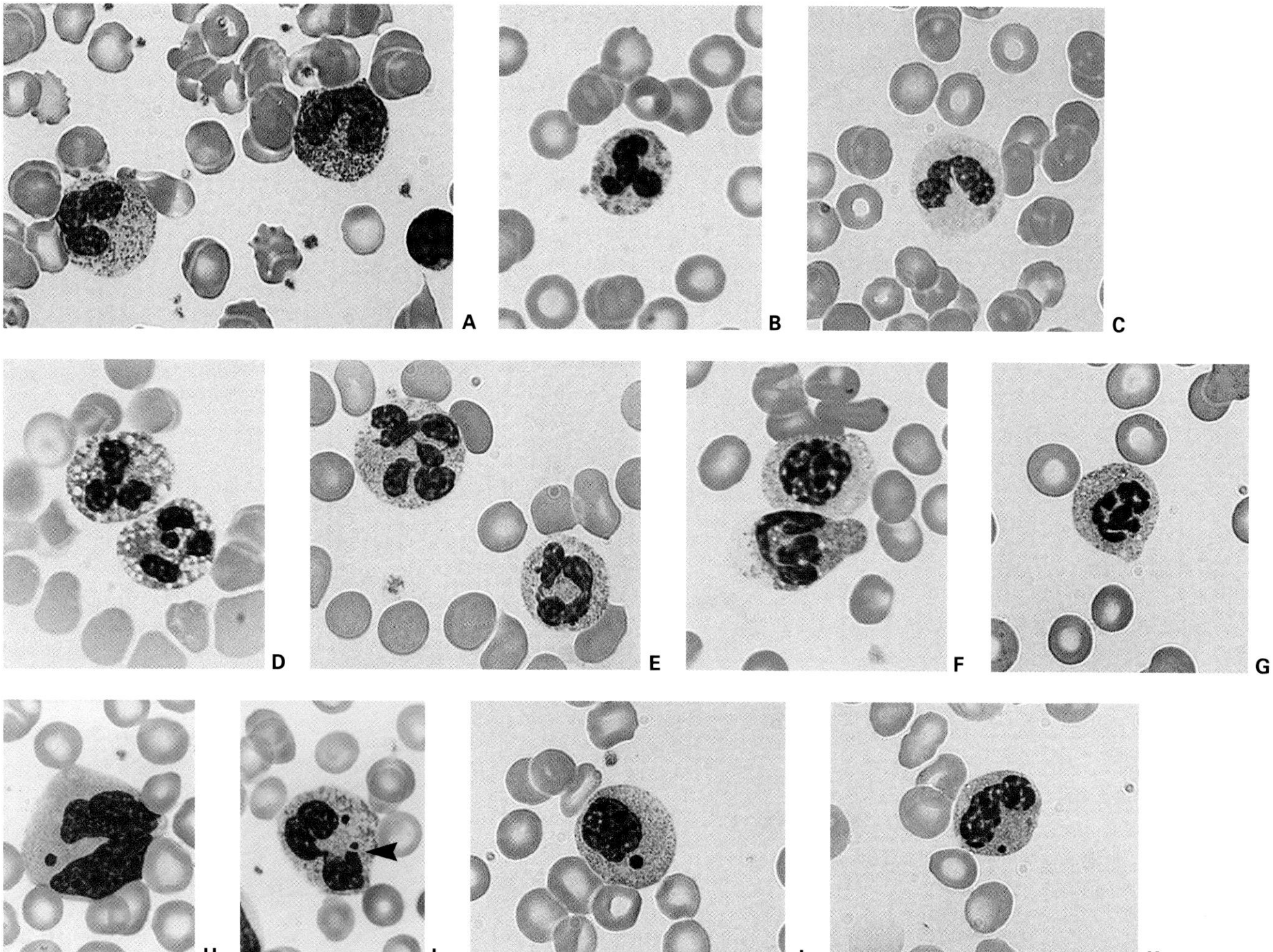

Fig. 7.6 Toxic changes in neutrophils and monocyte. **a** Toxic granulation. **b** Döhle bodies. **c** Döhle bodies + degranulation. **d** Vacuolation. **e** Hypersegmentation, enlargement. **f,g** Pelgeroid change. **h–k** Stages in chromomere formation (monocyte, neutrophils) from degeneration of part of nucleus (arrow) to free-lying nuclear fragment. All × 950

Table 7.25 Toxic change in neutrophils. Some causes other than infection

Collagen disease
Rheumatoid arthritis
SLE
Other vasculitides
Kawasaki
Stevens-Johnson
Inflammatory bowel disease
Crohn's
Ulcerative colitis
Near-drowning[1]
Heat stroke
Tissue necrosis
Hepatic
Necrotizing enterocolitis[2]
Burns[1]
Drugs
Colony-stimulating factors
Cytotoxics

[1] Added infection common
[2] Septicaemia from normal gut flora a significant component

PHAGOCYTOSIS BY NEUTROPHILS

• Of cells (leucocytes, erythroblasts, erythrocytes)
Phagocytic neutrophils are less conspicuous than phagocytic monocytes, which accompany them (see below).

• Of organisms
Careful and systematic examination of the film with a low to medium power objective (×10–×25) for 5–10 minutes will detect organisms in a significant proportion of cases of septicaemia, especially those with severe effects such as circulatory shut-down. On the other hand, blood from an indwelling venous line may contain a profusion of organisms (from colonization) with surprisingly mild accompanying symptoms.

Optimal parts of the film for search are edges and tails (Fig. 7.7). Infected leucocytes are more numerous in films of the first drop of blood from the previously unmanipulated ear-lobe (because of trapping in capillary bed, Smith 1966), and in films of buffy coat (Rodwell et al 1989). Densely-staining organisms (e.g. cocci) are more readily visible than the pale-staining organisms (Gram-negative rods).

Criteria for acceptability of organisms in films as genuine evidence of septicaemia are summarized in Table 7.26; descriptions and illustrations are given in Table 7.27 and Figures 7.8–7.11.

Table 7.26 Organisms in blood films: acceptability as genuine evidence of septicaemia

At least a proportion intracellular; appearances must be typical. Intracellular organisms are unequivocal evidence of septicaemia only in films of capillary blood or films of venous blood made directly from needle (skin organisms may rarely be phagocytosed by leucocytes in venous samples in the interval before films are made)
Disregard: inclusions in lymphocytes infected skin squames, epidermal cells
Differential diagnosis Granules in basophils: more variable in size and shape than cocci, often hollow, no characteristic grouping, no capsule, paler than most cocci, no or minimal staining with Gram Toxic granules Coarse azurophil granules Nuclear appendages Chromomeres (detached, pyknotic nuclear fragments) Phagocytosed nuclear fragments

Table 7.27 Characteristics of bacteria in Romanowsky-stained blood films[1]

N. meningitidis	plump cocci, a proportion in pairs, with some flattening of opposed faces, intense blue-black. *N. gonorrhoeae* indistinguishable in morphology — rare in childhood and clinical features different. Gram negative
S. pneumoniae	fine cocci, some slightly elongated, most in pairs, with clear space (capsule) around; intense, almost black staining. Infection may be heavy post-splenectomy
S. aureus	coarse cocci, usually in small groups, but may be single, in pairs or short chains (to about 4), red-brown to violet or almost black, no capsule
β haemolytic streptococci	fine cocci in groups or chains, intense violet to almost black
Coliforms	small to large rods, grey to grey-pink, Klebsiella often encapsulated. Organisms usually not profuse in individual cells and infected cells usually sparse
H. influenzae	small rods or coccobacilli, often encapsulated, usually not profuse
Clostridia	large rods, often square ended; grey to grey-pink, no capsule

[1] Gram and PAS stains may be useful on spare films if infected cells plentiful

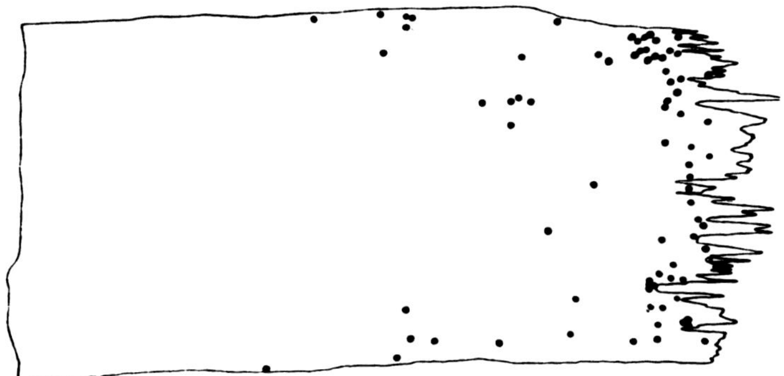

Fig. 7.7 Distribution of infected leucocytes in ear-lobe blood film, meningococcal septicaemia. Reproduced with permission, from Australasian Annals of Medicine, 1966, 15: 218, copyright.

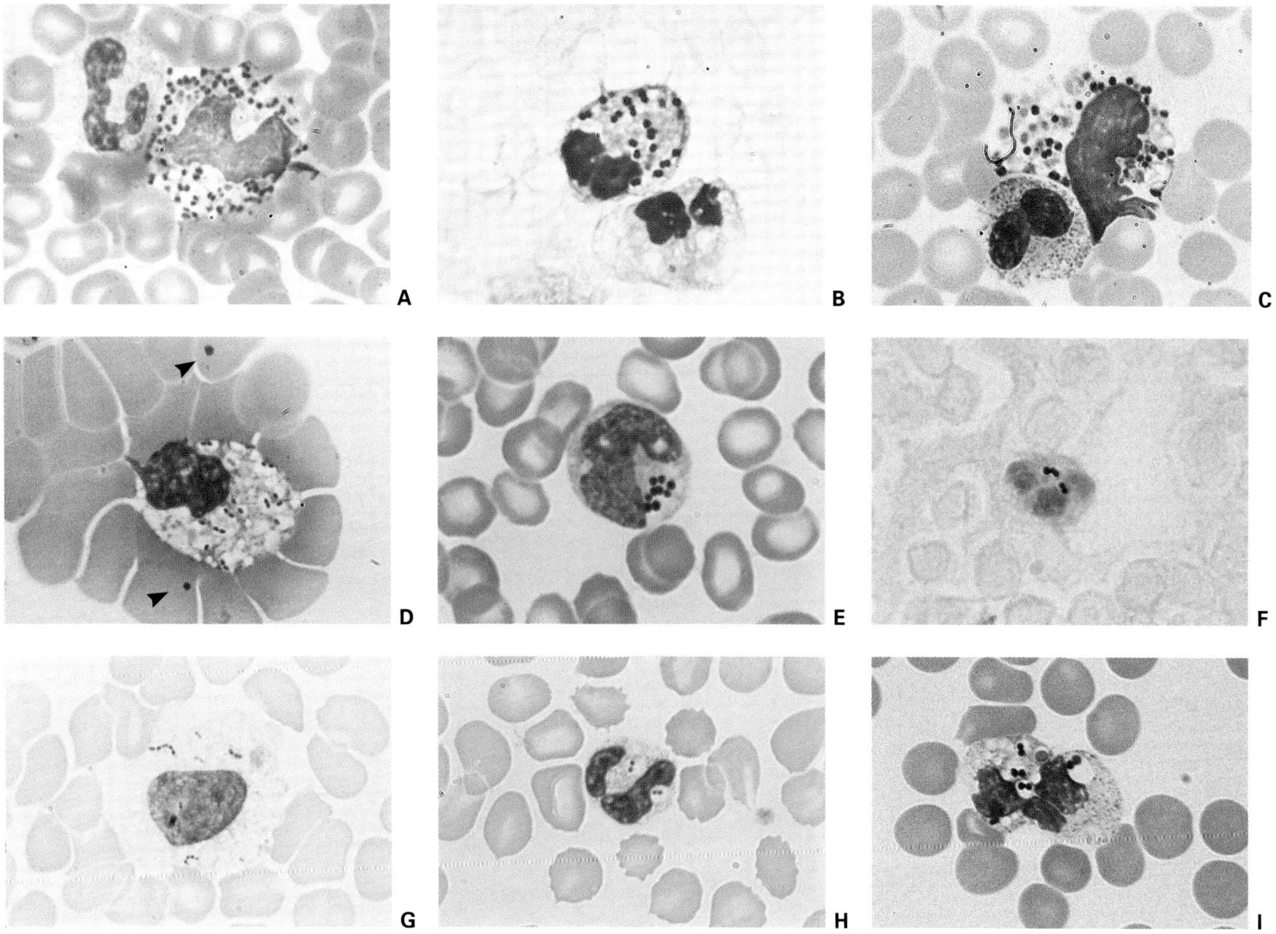

Fig. 7.8 Organisms in plain blood films — cocci. **a–c** *N. meningitidis* (**b**, Gram stain); note degenerate forms in **c**. **d** *Strep. pneumoniae*; note Howell-Jolly bodies (post-splenectomy). **e,f** *S. aureus* (**f**, Gram stain). **g,h** Streptococci. **i** *Aerococcus viridans*. All × 950

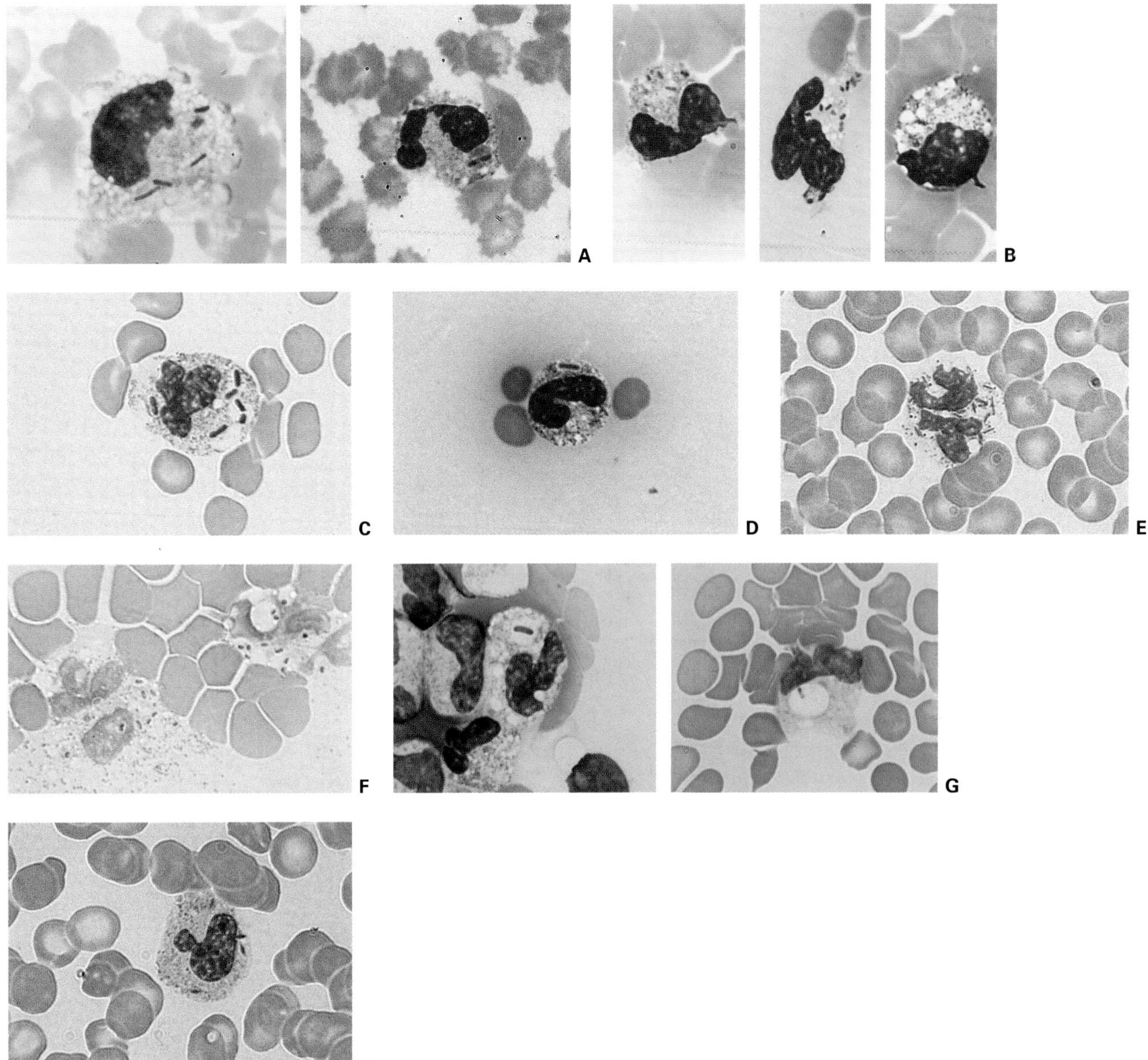

Fig. 7.9 Organisms in plain blood films — bacilli or coccobacilli. **a** *E. coli.* **b** *H. influenzae.* **c** *Lactobacillus sp.* **d** *Cl. perfringens* (note haemoglobin leakage around erythrocytes). **e** *Capnocytophaga canimorsus* (dog-bite). **f** *Acinetobacter sp.* **g** *Klebsiella pneumoniae* (capsule around organism in left frame). **h** Atypical *mycobacterium sp.* (HIV infection). All × 950

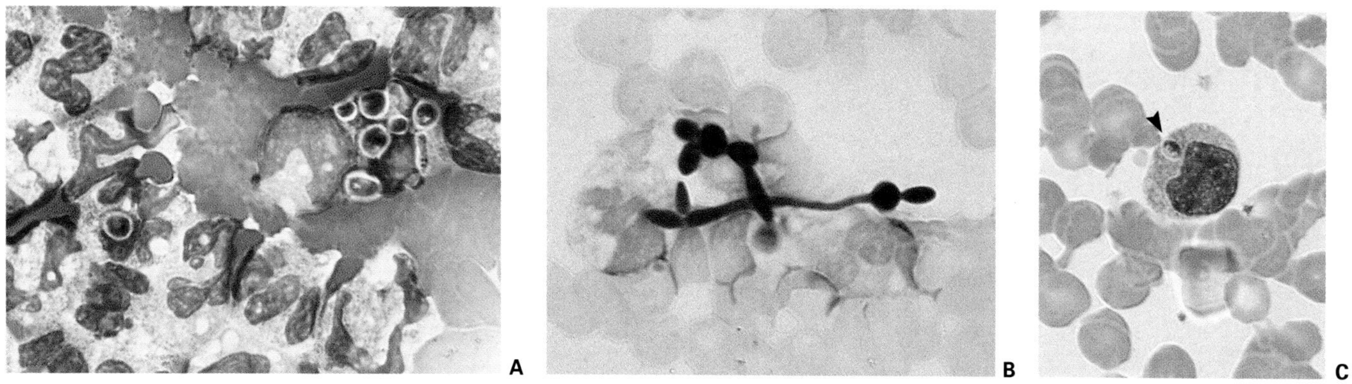

Fig. 7.10 Organisms in plain blood films. **a,b** Candida sp. (**b**, PAS). **c** *Histoplasma capsulatum* (HIV infection). All × 950

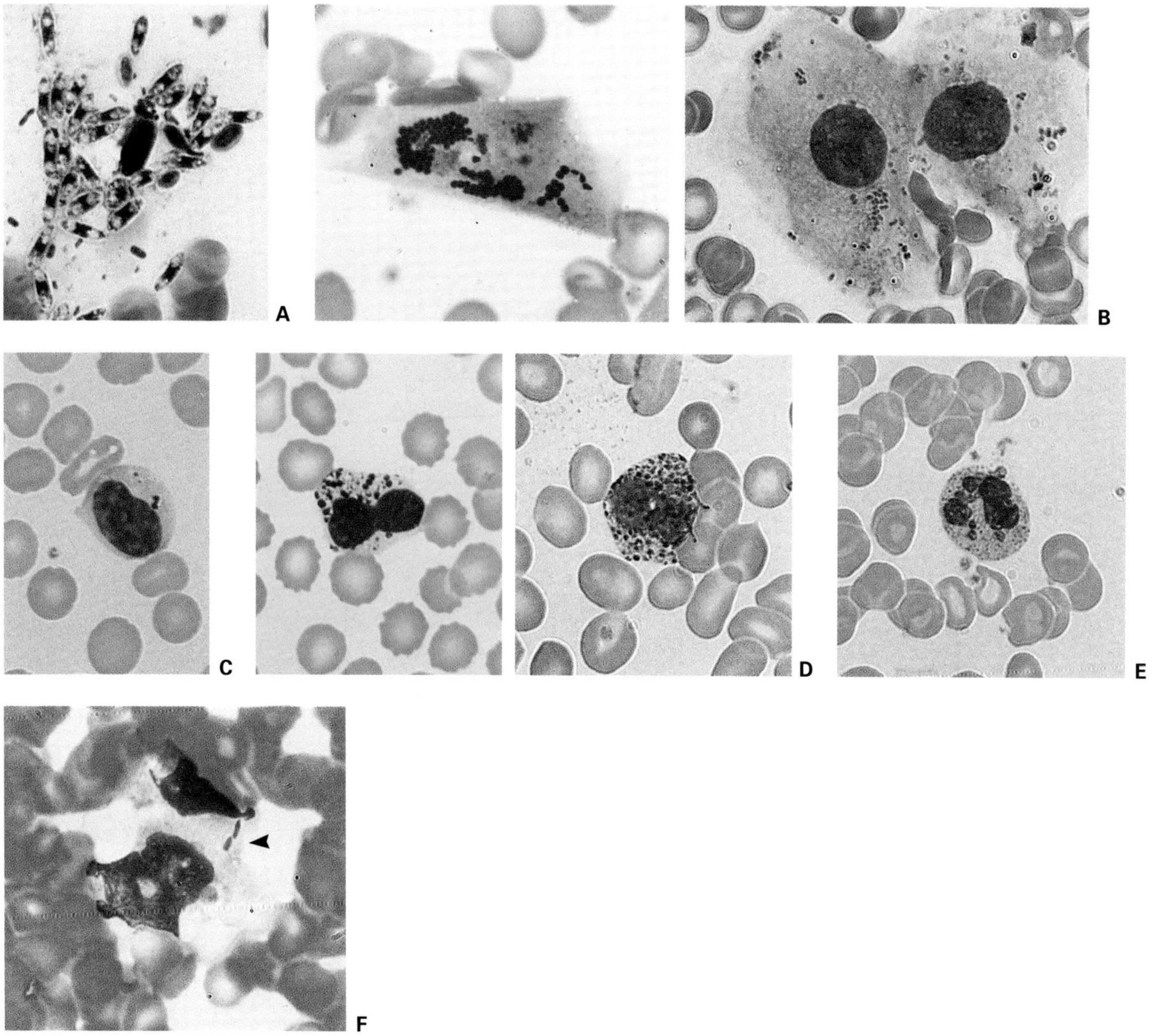

A B C D E F

Fig. 7.11 Structures in plain blood films which may be misinterpreted as evidence of septicaemia. **a** Organisms in staining fluid. **b** Infected skin squame and squamous cells. **c** Azurophil granules in lymphocyte. **d** Granules in basophils. **e** Nuclear appendages in neutrophil. **f** Unidentified rods in monocyte, negative blood cultures. All × 950

CELL DEATH (Fig. 7.12)

Death (apoptosis) of leucocytes is common in infection. Because anticoagulation and storage also cause damage, cell death is most reliably assessed in films made directly from vein, finger or ear.

The process affects leucocytes in general. Whole cells as well as fragments may be observed. Though the phenomenon may be noted in non-infective conditions such as malignancy and SLE, in childhood it almost always is a result of infection and may be striking in viral infections such as infectious mononucleosis, measles and neonatal herpes (Smith 1965, 1969); in viral infection death may affect atypical lymphocytes as well as normal leucocytes (Fig. 7.3).

Possible mechanisms include immune effect, interleukin-2 starvation as a result of cell hyperactivity (Bishop et al 1985) and invasion by virus (Smith 1969). Dead cells are a stimulus to phagocytosis by monocytes/macrophages and neutrophils (see below).

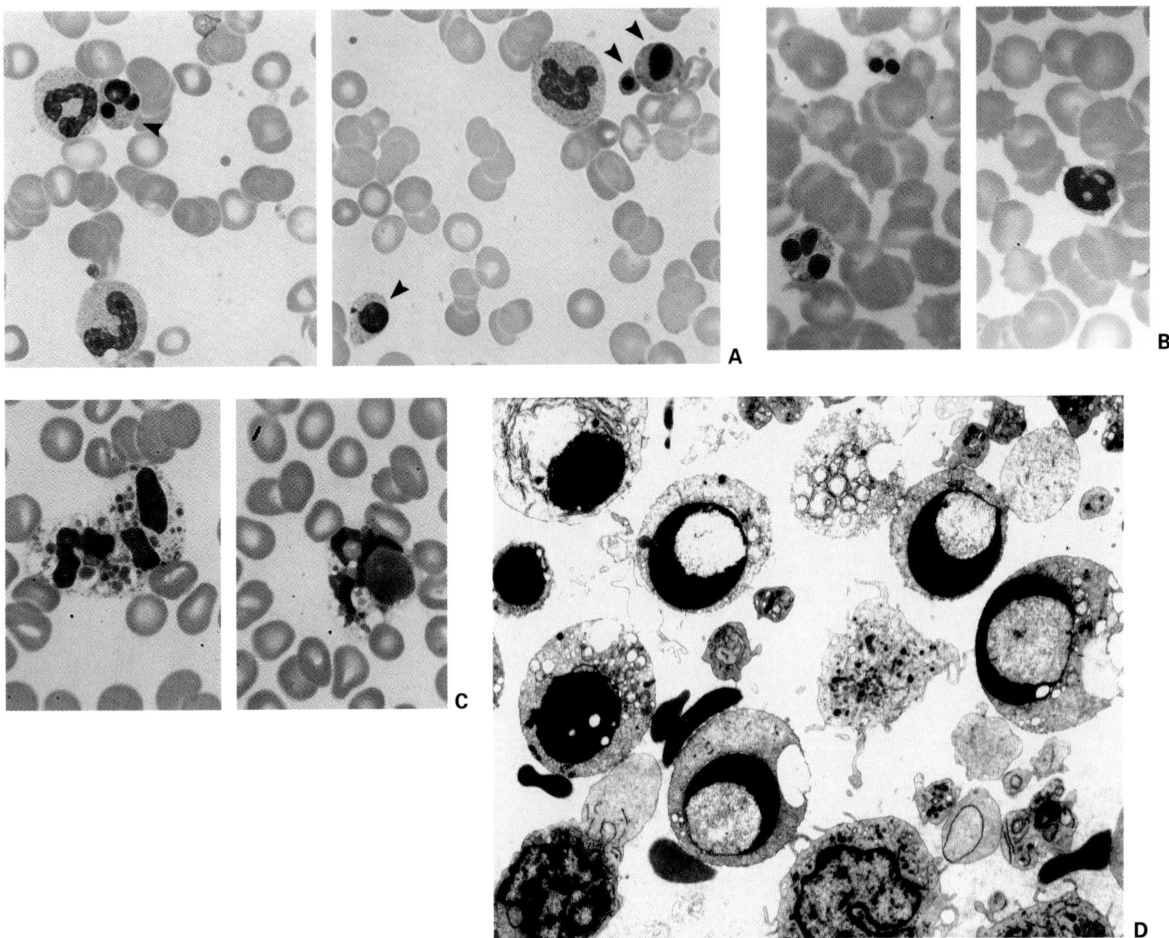

Fig. 7.12 Leucocyte death. **a** *Strep. sanguis* endocarditis; arrows show degenerate neutrophil and neutrophil fragments. **b** Neonatal herpes simplex infection, dead neutrophils in left frame, dead lymphocyte in right. **c** Degenerate neutrophils containing LE material, SLE. **d** Buffy coat, measles, field of lymphocytes, most of which are apoptotic. **a–c** Plain blood films, unanticoagulated × 750; **d** × 3500

MONOCYTES/MACROPHAGES IN INFECTION

Substantial changes may be noted in blood and marrow.

Blood

- Monocytosis is common in infection, especially chronic bacterial infection. Activation, with vacuolation, enlargement and pseudopodial formation is frequent (Fig. 7.13g).
- Phagocytosis of leucocytes or leucocyte fragments and (infrequently) erythroblasts may be noted in bacterial and viral infections (Fig. 7.13). Phagocytic cells are more frequent in films of first-drop ear-lobe blood, because of trapping of larger cells in the capillary bed. An increase in dead leucocytes (above) is a stimulus to phagocytosis (Smith 1965). Occasional erythrocytes may be phagocytosed, but they are not the dominant inclusion, as in immune haemolysis (Fig. 3.5).

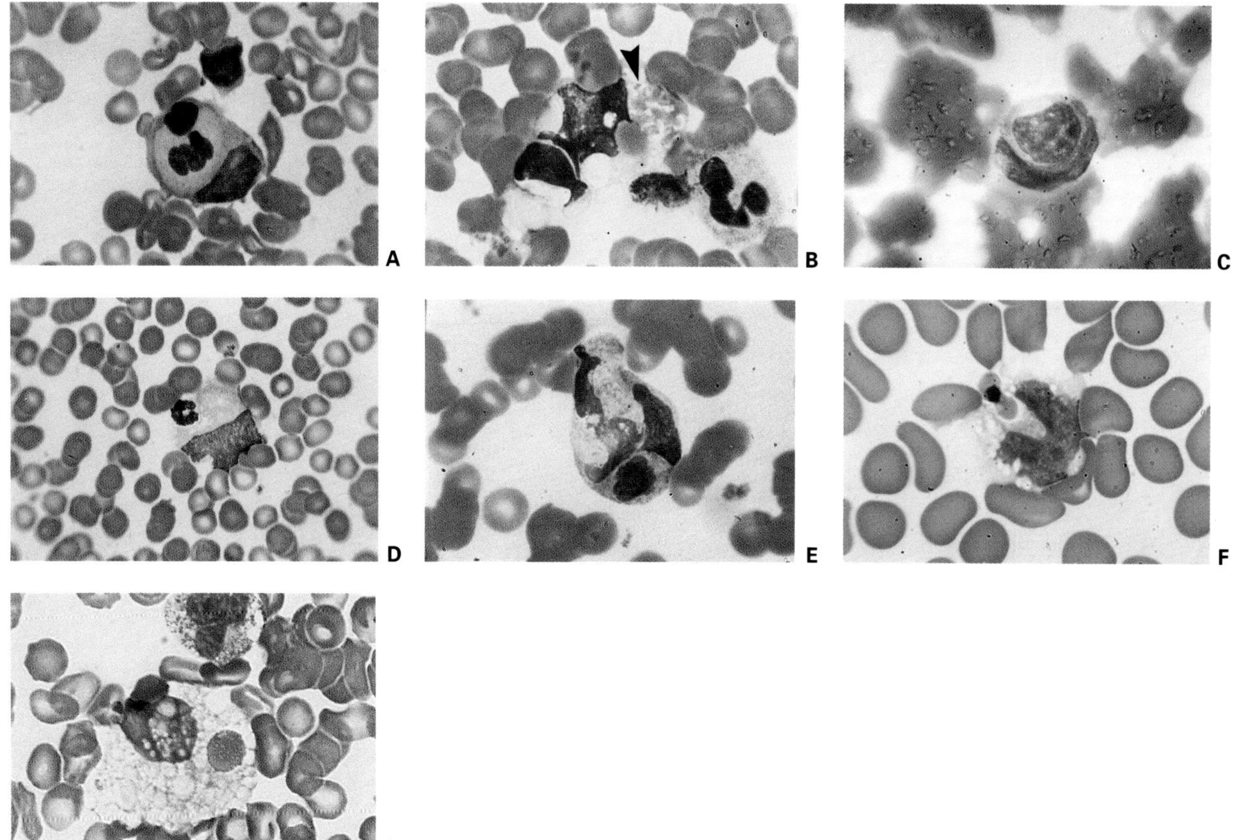

Fig. 7.13 Phagocytic monocytes in plain blood films. **a–d** Infectious mononucleosis. **a** Neutrophil inclusion. **b** Inclusions of lymphocyte, erythrocyte and (arrow) neutrophil in advanced degeneration. **c** Inclusion of atypical lymphocyte. **d** Degenerate neutrophil adherent to monocyte. **e** Neutrophil in process of phagocytosis by a monocyte which already contains a neutrophil, subacute bacterial endocarditis, numerous blood cultures sterile. **f** Erythroblast in process of phagocytosis by monocyte, streptococcal septicaemia. **g** Active, vacuolated monocyte containing an erythrocyte, *Klebsiella pneumoniae* septicaemia. **a–f** ear-lobe films; **g** heel-prick (neonate). All $\times$ 750

- In chronic infection, especially subacute bacterial endocarditis, hypertrophied macrophages ('histiocytes') may be noted, sometimes in spectacular numbers, in ear-lobe but not venous blood (van Nuys 1907, Smith 1964, Fig. 7.14); the cytoplasm is basophilic, there is often evidence of motility and nuclei are large, with open, ropey texture. Distinction is to be made from endothelial cells. Histiocytes may occur in chronic bacteraemia when repeated blood cultures are sterile.
- Organisms may be noted in blood monocytes as well as in neutrophils in septicaemia (Figs 7.8–7.10).

Marrow

Organisms

Marrow examination is useful for diagnosis of histoplasmosis, leishmaniasis, tuberculosis and toxoplasmosis (Fig. 7.15). Fungi and malarial parasites may also occur in marrow macrophages. Symptoms which justify marrow examination include chronic anaemia, thrombocytopenia or pancytopenia, unexplained fever or unexplained splenomegaly or hepatosplenomegaly.

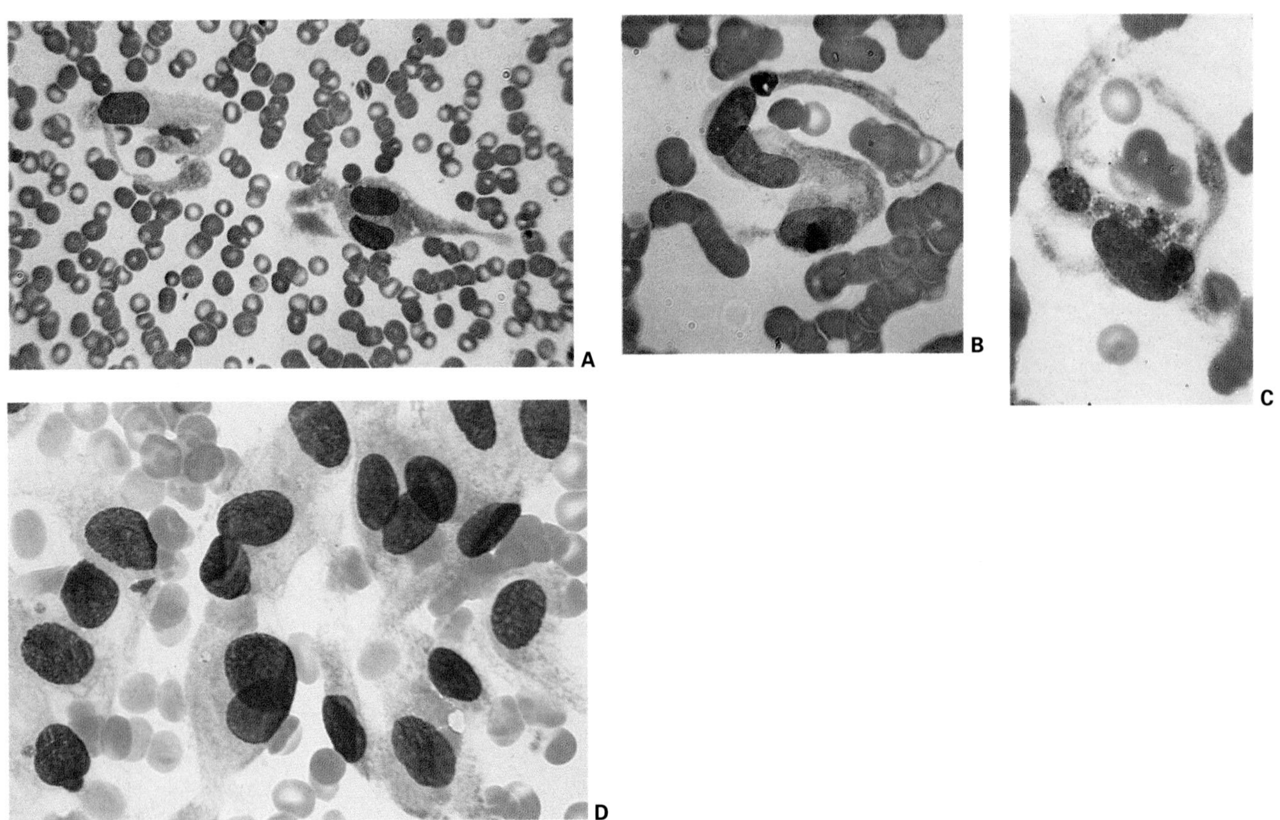

Fig. 7.14 'Histiocytes' in ear-lobe blood films (**a–c**) compared with normal endothelial cells (**d**). Subacute bacterial endocarditis, numerous blood cultures sterile (same patient as 7.13e). **a** × 380; others × 750

Infection-associated haemophagocytosis (Suster et al 1988)

The marrow counterpart of the macrophage/ phagocytic monocyte phenomenon in blood (above). It is customary to separate this from haemophagocytic lymphohistiocytosis (familial and sporadic). However, they are indistinguishable in clinical features and pathology (Janka 1989, Malone 1991), and both may be regarded as a non-specific reaction to a variety of causes, via a common mechanism of corpuscular cell death as a stimulus to phagocytosis. Recognized causes include infection (bacterial, viral), recent blood transfusion, autoimmune disease (e.g. SLE), and some malignancies (e.g. T lymphoma). In a significant proportion of cases however, including the familial, a cause is not identified.

A combination of clinical and cellular abnormalities is required for diagnosis:

(i) Clinical features

Fever, rash, jaundice, hepatosplenomegaly, lymphadenopathy, meningeal irritation, pancytopenia, abnormal liver function, hypofibrinogenaemia (liver dysfunction, intravascular coagulation) and hypertriglyceridaemia occur in various combinations. The sporadic disorder tends to affect older children and recover in 1–8 weeks. Familial cases present in the first 5 years, usually in the first 6 months, are thought to have autosomal recessive inheritance and are likely to be fulminant and fatal. The syndrome is more severe in immunodeficiency states.

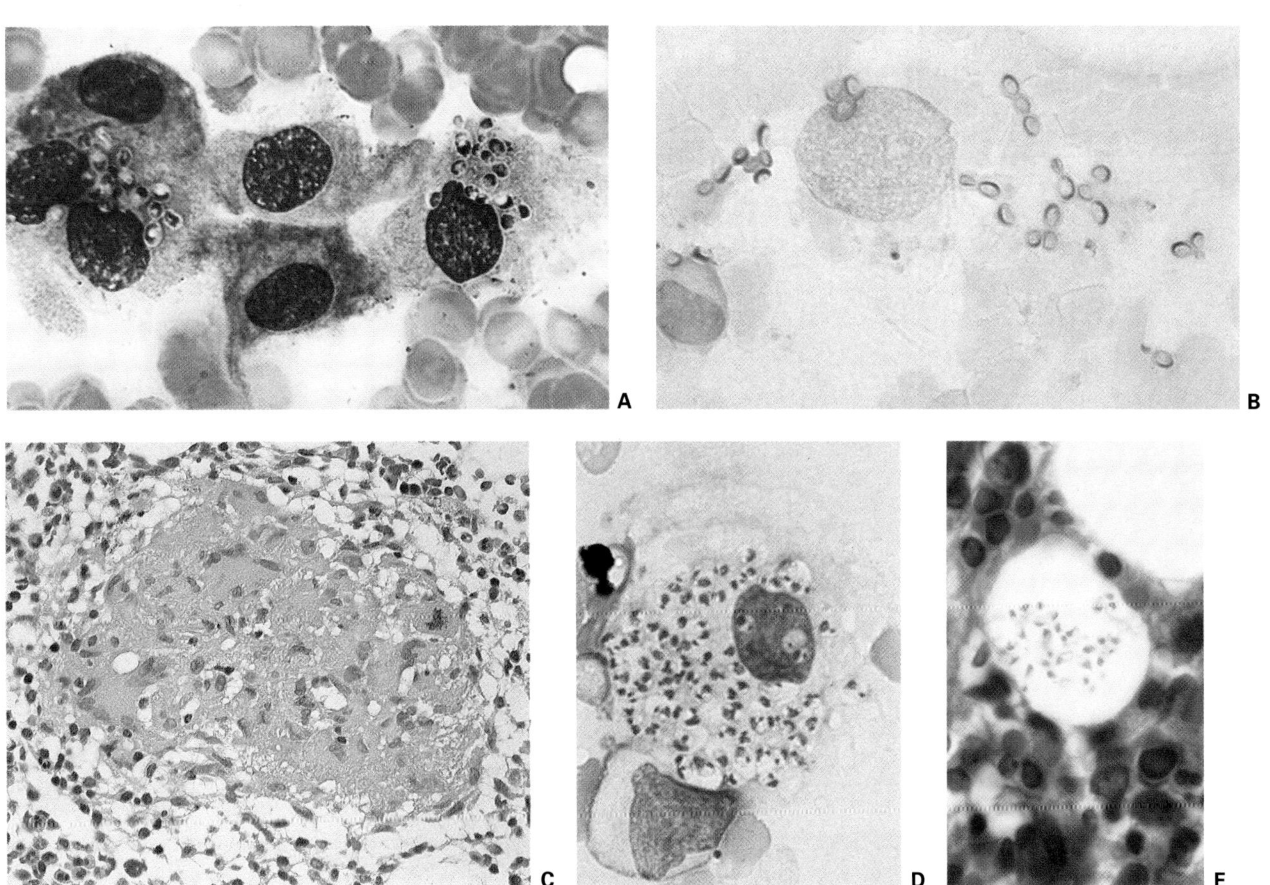

Fig. 7.15 Infections which may be detectable in marrow. **a,b** *H. capsulatum*, Romanowsky and PAS. **c** Tuberculosis, trephine biopsy, H & E; acid-fast bacilli demonstrated in tubercle. **d** Kala-azar (*Leishmania donovani*). **e** Toxoplasmosis, trephine biopsy, H & E. All × 950, except **c** × 330. **d** Courtesy of L Bramich. **e** Courtesy of Dr I D Perel

(ii) Macrophage hypertrophy and excess (Fig. 7.16)
In marrow a profusion of macrophages with variable depletion of other elements is characteristic. Phagocytosis (of nucleated cells and some erythrocytes) is usually but not always conspicuous, foaming being more prominent than phagocytosis in some cases. The cells are positive for ANAE and AcPh.

Differential diagnosis:

- Langerhans cell histiocytosis

In most cases of Langerhans cell histiocytosis the marrow shows, as the only abnormality, basophilic, hypertrophied macrophages in small numbers, with unobtrusive phagocytosis (Fig. 5.29). Langerhans cells (Fig. 5.29) are usually smaller than macrophages, non-phagocytic, and negative for ANAE and AcPh. If tissue is available for histologic section, distinction can also be made on other characteristics (Table 5.14).

- Genetic storage disorders

A profusion of foamy macrophages (Fig. 7.16) may raise a suspicion of storage disorder such as Niemann-Pick disease. The chronicity, other clinical features and appropriate enzyme analysis of blood leucocytes and cultured skin fibroblasts should prevent misidentification.

MULTINUCLEATE CELLS WITH INTRANUCLEAR INCLUSIONS

These occur in occasional cases of CMV infection (Fig. 5.9).

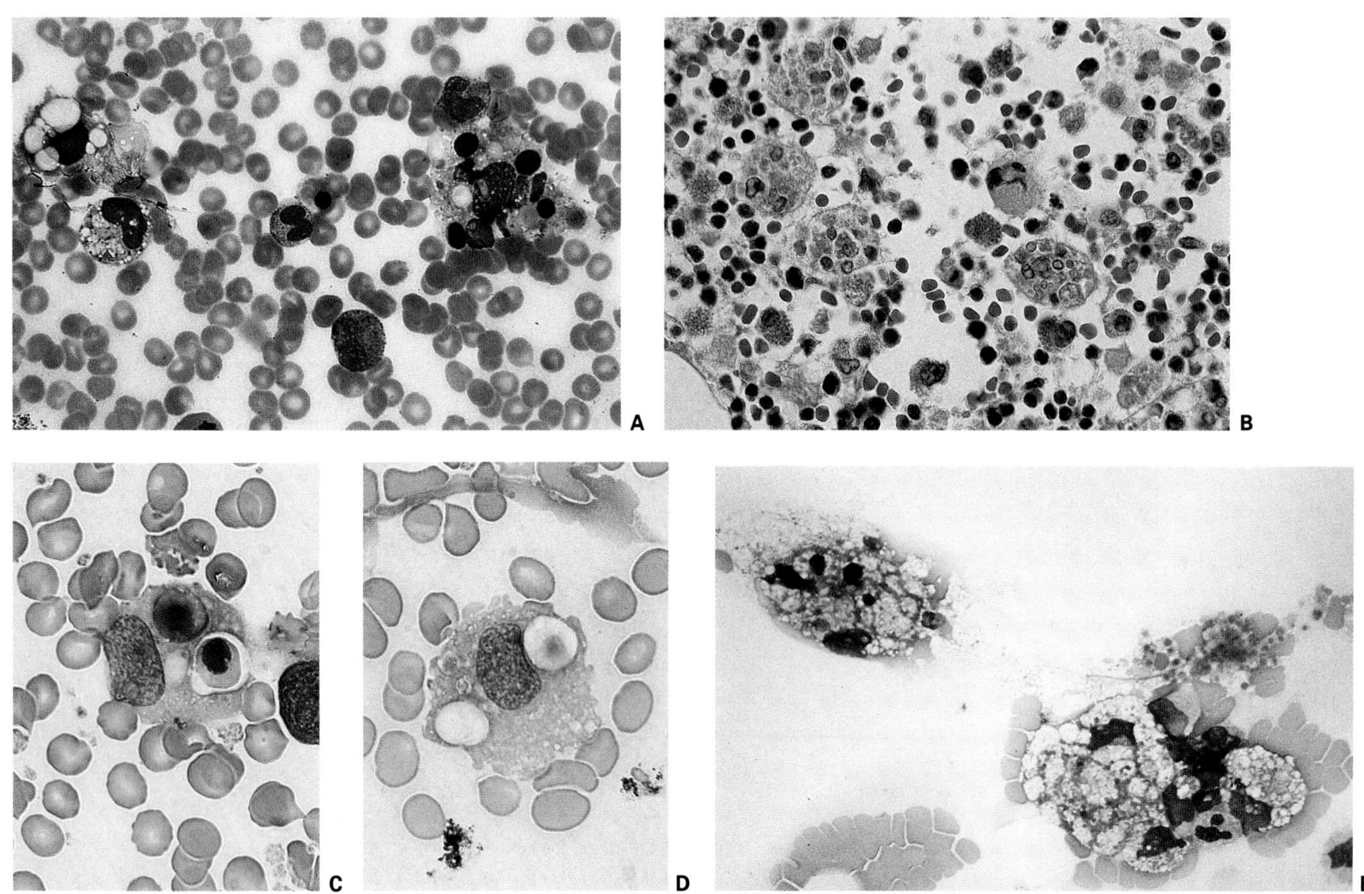

Fig. 7.16 Marrow, haemophagocytic syndromes, fatal, cause unidentified. **a,b** Probably infection-associated. **a** 3 months, **b** 11 months (vertebral marrow, autopsy, H & E). **c,d** 9-year-old girl who died 6 months after diagnosis; inclusions in **c** are an erythroblast and unidentified cell, and in **d**, 2 unidentified bodies, one possibly a digested erythrocyte. **e** 15-year-old boy who died 2 weeks after diagnosis; foaming is more prominent than phagocytosis of solid elements. **a,b** × 500; **c,d** × 750; **e** × 400. **c,d** Courtesy of Dr G Tauro. **e** Courtesy of Dr J Bell

REFERENCES

Ackerman B D 1964 Dysgammaglobulinemia: report of a case with a family history of a congenital gamma globulin disorder. Pediatrics 34: 211–219

Aggett P J, Cavanagh N P C, Matthew D J et al 1980 Shwachman's syndrome. A review of 21 cases. Archives of Disease in Childhood 55: 331–347

Alfaham M A, Ferguson S D, Sihra B, Davies J 1987 The idiopathic hypereosinophilic syndrome. Archives of Disease in Childhood 62: 601–613

Alter B P 1993 Fanconi's anaemia and its variability. British Journal of Haematology 85: 9–14

Ambruso D R, McCabe E R B, Anderson D et al 1985 Infectious and bleeding complications in patients with glycogenesis Ib. American Journal of Diseases of Children 139: 691–697

Anand A, Gray E S, Brown T et al 1987 Human parvovirus infection in pregnancy and hydrops fetalis. New England Journal of Medicine 316: 183–186

Bertotto A, Arcangeli C De F, Spinozzi F et al 1985 Acute infectious lymphocytosis: phenotype of the proliferating cell. Acta Paediatrica Scandinavica 74: 633–635

Bhat A M, Scanlon J W 1981 The pattern of eosinophilia in premature infants. A prospective study in premature infants using the absolute eosinophil count. Journal of Pediatrics 98: 612–616

Bishop C J, Moss D J, Ryan J M, Burrows S R 1985 T lymphocytes in infectious mononucleosis. II. Response in vitro to interleukin-2 and establishment of T-cell lines. Clinical and Experimental Immunology 60: 70–77

Björkstén B, Lundmark K M 1976 Recurrent bacterial infections in four siblings with neutropenia, eosinophilia, hyperimmunoglobulinemia A, and defective neutrophil chemotaxis. Journal of Infectious Diseases 133: 63–71

Blume R S, Wolff S M 1972 The Chediak-Higashi syndrome: studies in four patients and a review of the literature. Medicine 51: 247–280

Christensen R D, Rothstein G 1980 Exhaustion of mature marrow neutrophils in neonates with sepsis. Journal of Pediatrics 96: 316–318

Dacie J W, Lewis S M 1991 Practical haematology, 7th edn. Churchill Livingstone, Edinburgh

Dale D C, Hammond W P 1988 Cyclic neutropenia: a clinical review. Blood Reviews 2: 178–185

Ehrlich G D, Han T, Bettigole R et al 1988 Human T-lymphotropic virus type 1-associated benign transient immature T-cell lymphocytosis. American Journal of Hematology 27: 49–55

Epstein H D, Kruskall M S 1988 Spurious leukopenia due to in vitro granulocyte aggregation. American Journal of Clinical Pathology 89: 652–655

Fanning S F, Taylor K, Thong Y H 1994 Personal communication

Fleisher G R, Collins M, Fager S 1983 Limitations of available tests for diagnosis of infectious mononucleosis. Journal of Clinical Microbiology 17: 619–624

Gasparetto C, Smith C, Firpo M et al 1994 Dyshematopoiesis in combined immune deficiency with congenital neutropenia. American Journal of Hematology 45: 63–72

Geha R S, Akl K F 1976 Skin lesions, angioedema, eosinophilia and hypocomplementemia. Journal of Pediatrics 89: 724–727

Geha R S, Leung D Y M 1989 Hyper immunoglobulin E syndrome. Immunodeficiency Reviews 1: 155–172

Guibaud S, Plumet-Leger A, Frobert Y 1983 Transient neutrophil aggregation in a patient with infectious mononucleosis. American Journal of Clinical Pathology 80: 883–884

Gurbindo C, Seidman E G 1991 Gastrointestinal manifestations of immunodeficiency states. In: Walker W A, Durie P R, Hamilton J R, Walker-Smith J A, Watkins J B (eds) Pediatric gastrointestinal disease. B C Decker, Philadelphia, ch 27, part 7

Harmon D C, Weitzman S A, Stossel T P 1984 The severity of immune neutropenia correlates with the maturational specificity of antineutrophil antibodies. British Journal of Haematology 58: 209–215

Hernández A, Olivares F, Cantú J-M 1979 Autosomal recessive onychotrichodysplasia, chronic neutropenia and mild mental retardation. Delineation of the syndrome. Clinical Genetics 15: 147–152

Herring W B, Smith L G, Walker R I, Herion J C 1974 Hereditary neutrophilia. American Journal of Medicine 56: 729–734

Herrod H G, Wang W C, Sullivan J L 1985 Chronic T-cell lymphocytosis with neutropenia. Its association with Epstein-Barr virus infection. American Journal of Diseases of Children 139: 405–407

Heyderman R S, Morgan G, Levinsky R J, Strobel S 1991 Successful bone marrow transplantation and treatment of BCG infection in two patients with severe combined immunodeficiency. European Journal of Pediatrics 150: 477–480

Heyne K 1976 Konstitutionelle familiäre leukocytopenie mit partieller Pelger-anomalie und ossärer entwicklungsverzögerung. European Journal of Pediatrics 121: 191–201

Howard W A 1990 Pulmonary infiltrates with eosinophilia (Löffler syndrome). In: Chernick V, Kendig E L (eds) Disorders of the respiratory tract in children, 5th edn. W B Saunders, Philadelphia, ch 64

Hutchinson R J, Bunnell K, Thoene J G 1985 Suppression of granulopoietic progenitor cell proliferation by metabolites of the branched-chain amino acids. Journal of Pediatrics 106: 62–65

Jacobs P, Saxe N, Gordon W, Nelson M 1984 Dyskeratosis congenita. Haematologic, cytogenetic and dermatologic studies. Scandinavian Journal of Haematology 32: 461–468

Janka G E 1989 Familial hemophagocytic lymphohistiocytosis: diagnostic problems and differential diagnosis. Pediatric Hematology and Oncology 6: 219–225

Joyce R A, Boggs D R, Chervenick P A, Lalezari P 1980 Neutrophil kinetics in Felty's syndrome. American Journal of Medicine 69: 695–702

Kennedy C R, Singer H S 1988 Eosinophilia of the cerebrospinal fluid: late reaction to a silastic shunt. Developmental Medicine and Child Neurology 30: 378–390

Kirschner B S 1991 Miscellaneous intestinal inflammatory disorders. In: Walker W A, Durie P R, Hamilton J R, Walker-Smith J A, Watkins J B (eds) Pediatric gastrointestinal disease. B C Decker, Philadelphia, pp 630–631

Klaassen R J L, Vlekke A B J, Von Dem Borne A E G Kr 1991 Neutrophil-bound immunoglobulin in HIV infection is of autoantibody nature. British Journal of Haematology 77: 403–409

Kostmann R 1975 Infantile genetic agranulocytosis. A review with presentation of ten new cases. Acta Paediatrica Scandinavica 64: 362–368

Kozlowski C, Evans D I K 1991 Neutropenia associated with X-linked agammaglobulinaemia. Journal of Clinical Pathology 44: 388–390

Krilov L R, Jacobson M, Shende A 1987 Acute febrile neutrophilic dermatosis (Sweet's syndrome) presenting as facial cellulitis in a child with juvenile chronic myelogenous leukemia. Pediatric Infectious Disease 6: 77–79

Kuberski T 1979 Eosinophils in the cerebrospinal fluid. Annals of Internal Medicine 91: 70–75

Lancet Leader 1987 Neonatal lupus syndrome. Lancet 2: 489–490

Landolt R F 1945 Das Knockenmark bei Pertussis. Helvetica Paediatrica Acta 1: 153–163

Lensink D B, Barton A, Appelbaum F R, Hammond W P 1986 Cyclic neutropenia as a premalignant manifestation of acute lymphoblastic leukaemia. American Journal of Hematology 22: 9–16

Lightsey A L, Parmley R T, Marsh W L et al 1985 Severe congenital neutropenia with unique features of dysgranulopoiesis. American Journal of Hematology 18: 59–71

Lonsdale D, Deodhar S D, Mercer R D 1967 Familial

granulocytopenia and associated immunoglobulin abnormality. Report of three cases in young brothers. Journal of Pediatrics 71: 790–801

Lyall E G H, Lucas G F, Eden O B 1992 Autoimmune neutropenia of infancy. Journal of Clinical Pathology 45: 431–434

McClain K, Estrov Z, Chen H, Mahoney D H 1993 Chronic neutropenia of childhood: frequent association with parvovirus infection and correlations with bone marrow culture studies. British Journal of Haematology 85: 57–62

McCullough J, Press C, Clay M, Kline W 1988 Granulocyte serology. A clinical and laboratory guide. AACP Press, Chicago

McCune A B, Weston W L, Lee L A 1987 Maternal and fetal outcome in neonatal lupus erythematosus. Annals of Internal Medicine 106: 518–523

Malone M 1991 The histiocytoses of childhood. Histopathology 19: 105–119

Mamlok R J, Juneja H S, Elder F F B et al 1987 Neutropenia and defective chemotaxis associated with binuclear, tetraploid myeloid-monocytic leucocytes. Journal of Pediatrics 111: 555–558

Manroe B L, Weinberg A G, Rosenfeld C R, Browne R 1979 The neonatal blood count in health and disease. 1. Reference values for neutrophilic cells. Journal of Pediatrics 95: 89–98

Mentzer W C, Johnston R B, Baehner R L Nathan D G 1977 An unusual form of chronic neutropenia in a father and daughter with hypogammaglobulinaemia. British Journal of Haematology 36: 313–322

Miller M E, Oski F A, Harris M B 1971 Lazy-leucocyte syndrome. A new disorder of neutrophil function. Lancet 1: 665–669

Minchinton R M, McGrath K M 1987 Alloimmune neonatal neutropenia — a neglected diagnosis? Medical Journal of Australia 147: 139–141

Minchinton R M, Waters A H 1984 The occurrence and significance of neutrophil antibodies. British Journal of Haematology 56: 521–528

Minchinton R M, Waters A H 1985 Autoimmune thrombocytopenia and neutropenia after bone marrow transplantation. Blood 66: 752

Moore M A S 1991 Clinical implications of positive and negative hematopoietic stem cell regulators. Blood 78: 1–19

Morse S I, Barron B A 1970 Studies of the leucocytosis and lymphocytosis induced by Bordetella pertussis. III. The distribution of transfused lymphocytes in pertussis-treated and normal mice. Journal of Experimental Medicine 132: 663–672

Murray J A, Lilleyman J S 1983 T cell lymphocytosis with neutropenia. Archives of Disease in Childhood 58: 635–636

Naiman J L, Oski F A, Allen F H, Diamond L K 1964 Hereditary eosinophilia: report of a family and review of the literature. American Journal of Human Genetics 16: 195–203

Nathan C F 1987 Neutrophil activation on biological surfaces. Massive secretion of hydrogen peroxide in response to products of macrophages and lymphocytes. Journal of Clinical Investigation 80: 1550–1560

Norio R, Raitta C, Lindahl E 1984 Further delineation of the Cohen syndrome; report on chorioretinal dystrophy, leukopenia and consanguinity. Clinical Genetics 25: 1–14

Omenn G S 1965 Familial reticuloendotheliosis with eosinophilia. New England Journal of Medicine 273: 427–432

Parmley R T, Crist W M, Ragab A H et al 1980 Congenital dysgranulopoietic neutropenia: clinical, serologic, ultrastructural, and in vitro proliferative characteristics. Blood 56: 465–475

Parmley R T, Crist W M, Ragab A H et al 1981 Phagocytosis of neutrophils by marrow macrophages in childhood chronic benign neutropenia. Journal of Pediatrics 98: 207–212

Pattengale P K, Smith R W, Perlin E 1974 Atypical lymphocytes in acute infectious mononucleosis. Identification by multiple T and B lymphocyte markers. New England Journal of Medicine 291: 1145–1148

Pegels J G, Helmerhorst F M, van Leeuwen E F et al 1982 The Evans syndrome: characterization of the responsible autoantibodies. British Journal of Haematology 51: 445–450

Pinkerton P H, Robinson J B, Senn J S 1978 Lazy leucocyte syndrome — disorder of the granulocyte membrane? Journal of Clinical Pathology 31: 300–308

Plebani A, Cantù-Rajnoldi A, Collo G et al 1988 Myelokathexis associated with multiple congenital malformations: immunological study on phagocytic cells and lymphocytes. European Journal of Haematology 40: 12–17

Pui C-H, Wilimas J, Wang W 1980 Evans syndrome in childhood. Journal of Pediatrics 97: 754–758

Purtilo D T, DeFlorio D, Hutt L M et al 1977 Variable phenotypic expression of an X-linked recessive lymphoproliferative syndrome. New England Journal of Medicine 297: 1077–1081

Robinson L, Smith H 1966 Serological screening test for infectious mononucleosis using papain-treated sheep erythrocytes. Journal of Clinical Pathology 19: 339–342

Rodwell R L, Leslie A L, Tudehope D I 1988 Early diagnosis of neonatal sepsis using a hematologic scoring system. Journal of Pediatrics 112: 761–767

Rodwell R L, Leslie A L, Tudehope D I 1989 Evaluation of direct and buffy coat films of peripheral blood for the early detection of bacteraemia. Australian Paediatrics Journal 25: 83–85

Roper M, Parmley R T, Crist W M et al 1985 Severe congenital leukopenia (reticular dysgenesis). Immunologic and morphologic characterizations of leukocytes. American Journal of Diseases of Children 139: 832–835

Rosen R B, Kang S-J 1979 Congenital agranulocytosis terminating in acute myelomonocytic leukemia. Journal of Pediatrics 94: 406–408

Rosenberg L E, Fenton W A 1989 Disorders of propionate and methylmalonate metabolism. In: Scriver C R, Beaudet A L, Sly W S, Valle D (eds) The metabolic basis of inherited disease, 6th edn. McGraw-Hill, New York, ch 29

Ruco L P, Stoppacciaro A, Pezzella F et al 1985 The Omenn's syndrome: histological, immunochemical and ultrastructural evidence for a partial T cell deficiency evolving in an abnormal proliferation of T lymphocytes and S-100+/T-6+ Langerhans-like cells. Virchows Archiv (Pathological Anatomy) 407: 69–82

Schooley R T, Densen P, Harmon D et al 1984 Antineutrophil antibodies in infectious mononucleosis. American Journal of Medicine 76: 85–90

Schooley R T, Dolin R 1990 Epstein-Barr virus (infectious mononucleosis). In: Mandell G L, Douglas R G, Bennett J E (eds) Principles and practice of infectious diseases, 3rd edn. Churchill Livingstone, New York, ch 121

Shastri K A, Logue G L 1993 Autoimmune neutropenia. Blood 81: 1984–1995

Shepherd P C A, Corbett G M, Allan N C 1988 Neutropenia preceding acute lymphoblastic leukaemia. Journal of Clinical Pathology 41: 703–704

Slungaard A, Vercellotti G M, Tran T et al 1993 Eosinophil cationic granule proteins impair thrombomodulin function. A potent mechanism for thromboembolism in hypereosinophilic heart disease. Journal of Clinical Investigation 91: 1721–1730

Smith C H 1941 Infectious lymphocytosis. American Journal of Diseases of Children 62: 231–261

Smith H 1964 The prevalence and diagnostic significance of 'histiocytes' and phagocytic mononuclear cells in peripheral blood films. Medical Journal of Australia 2: 205–210

Smith H 1965 A morphological study of histiocytes and phagocytic mononuclear cells in human blood. MD Thesis, University of Melbourne

Smith H 1966 Leucocytes containing bacteria in plain blood films from patients with septicaemia. Australasian Annals of Medicine 15: 210–221

Smith H 1969 Leucocyte death in generalized virus infection. Australian Paediatrics Journal 5: 56–61

Stevens D L, Everett E D, Boxer L A, Landefeld R A 1979 Infectious mononucleosis with severe neutropenia and opsonic antineutrophil activity. Southern Medical Journal 72: 519–521

Stroncek D F 1993 Drug-induced immune neutropenia. Transfusion Medicine Reviews 7: 268–274

Stroncek D F, Vercellotti G M, Hammerschmidt D E et al 1992 Characterization of multiple quinine-dependent antibodies in a patient with episodic hemolytic uremic syndrome and immune agranulocytosis. Blood 80: 241–248

Suster S, Hilsenbeck S, Rywlin A M 1988 Reactive histiocytic hyperplasia with hemophagocytosis in hematopoietic organs: a reevaluation of the benign hemophagocytic proliferations. Human Pathology 19: 705–712

Sweetman L 1989 Branched chain organic acidurias. In: Scriver C R, Beaudet A L, Sly W S, Valle D (eds) The metabolic basis of inherited disease, 6th edn. McGraw-Hill, New York, ch 28

Tanaka Y, Hatano S, Nishi Y, Usui T 1980 Nutritional copper deficiency in a Japanese infant on formula. Journal of Pediatrics 96: 255–257

Van Nuys F 1907 An extraordinary blood. Presence of atypical phagocytic cells. Boston Medical and Surgical Journal 156: 390–391

Wagle S, Grauaug A, Kohan R, Evans S F 1994 C-reactive protein as a diagnostic tool of sepsis in very immature babies. Journal of Paediatrics and Child Health 30: 40–44

Weller P F, Bubley G J 1994 The idiopathic hypereosinophilic syndrome. Blood 83: 2759–2779

Weston B, Axtell R A, Todd R F et al 1991 Clinical and biologic effects of granulocyte colony stimulating factor in the treatment of myelokathexis. Journal of Pediatrics 118: 229–234

Wilson W G, Aylsworth A S, Folds J D, Whisnant J K 1978 Cartilage-hair hypoplasia (metaphyseal chondrodysplasia, type McKusick) with combined immune deficiency: variable expression and development of immunologic functions in sibs. Birth Defects 14, No 6A: 117–129

Yoda S, Morosawa H, Komiyama A, Akabane T 1980 Transient 'lazy-leukocyte' syndrome during infancy. American Journal of Diseases of Children 134: 467–469

Young G A R, Vincent P C 1980 Drug-induced agranulocytosis. Clinics in Haematology 9: 485–504

Yunis E J, Atchison R W, Michaels R H, DeCicco F A 1975 Adenovirus and ileocecal intussusception. Laboratory Investigation 33: 347–351

Zidar B L, Shadduck R K, Zeigler Z, Winkelstein A 1977 Observations on the anemia and neutropenia of human copper deficiency. American Journal of Hematology 3: 177–185

Zipursky A, Palko J, Milner R, Akenzua G I 1976 The hematology of bacterial infections in premature infants. Pediatrics 57: 839–853

Zuelzer W W 1964 "Myelokathexis" — a new form of chronic granulocytopenia. New England Journal of Medicine 270: 699–704

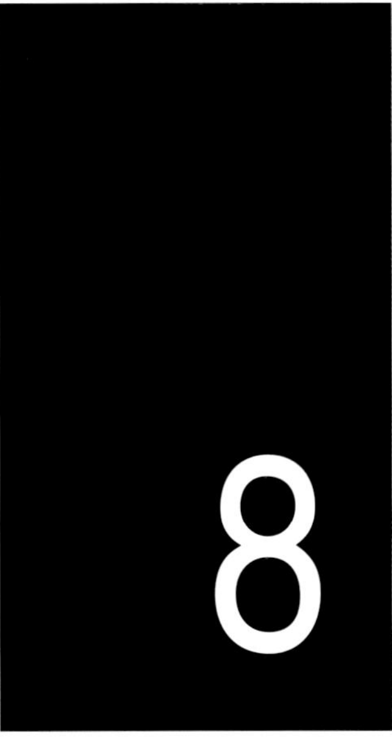

8 Disorders of haemostasis

Approach to diagnosis, value and limitations of a haemostatic screen and discussion of haemostatic defects where practicable within a framework of differential diagnosis of abnormal laboratory tests.

Abbreviations and notes

α_1AT: a_1 antitrypsin; α_2AP: α_2 antiplasmin; α_2M: α_2 macroglobulin; APTT: activated partial thromboplastin time; ATIII: antithrombin III; C_1EINH: C_1 esterase inhibitor; DAT: direct antiglobulin (Coombs) test; DDAVP: desamino-D-arginine-vasopressin; DIC: disseminated intravascular coagulation; F: (coagulation) factor; FDP: fibrinogen/fibrin degradation products; F VIII:C: the coagulant activity of the Factor VIII molecule measured in standard coagulation assays; F VIII:CAg: antigenic determinants on Factor VIII measured by immunoassay using human antibodies; Gp: glycoprotein; HCII: heparin cofactor II; hct: haematocrit; HMWK: high molecular weight kininogen (Fitzgerald, Flaujeac or Williams factor); HUS: haemolytic-uraemic syndrome; ITP: idiopathic thrombocytopenic purpura; LA: lupus anticoagulant/s; MPV: mean platelet volume; PAI: plasminogen activator inhibitor; PK: prekallikrein (Fletcher factor); PNH: paroxysmal nocturnal haemoglobinuria; PT: prothrombin time; PvWD: platelet type (pseudo) von Willebrand's disease; TAR: thrombocytopenia–absent radius; TCT: thrombin clotting time; tPA: tissue plasminogen activator; TTP: thrombotic thrombocytopenic purpura; TXA2: thromboxane; vWD: von Willebrand's disease; vWF: von Willebrand factor (ristocetin cofactor); vWF:Ag: antigenic determinants on vWF molecule measured by immunoassays using heterologous (usually rabbit) antibodies.

General references for haemostatic defects and their investigation: Colman (1993), Chanarin (1989).

Clinical features 274

The haemostatic screen 276

Peculiarities of haemostasis in infancy and childhood 278

Isolated prolongation of APTT 280

Isolated prolongation of PT 286

Prolongation of APTT + PT 286

Prolongation of TCT as only or primary abnormality 288

Incoagulable blood 290

Disseminated intravascular coagulation 290

Macrothrombotic states with little or no DIC 296

Thrombocytopenias 300
Megakaryocyte deficiency 300
Ineffective thrombopoiesis 302
Immune 304
Non-immune destruction 311
Hypersplenism 312
Dilution 312

Thrombocytopathies 312
Defects of adhesion to subendothelium 313
Defects of primary aggregation 314
Storage pool disease 314
Defects of platelet/plasma coagulation interaction 316
Other/multiple/unidentified 316

Clinical features

The clinical history and signs differentiate, with a high degree of probability, spontaneous from non-accidental bleeding and identify with some accuracy the broad nature of the defect.

- Recognition of bruising

Lesions to be distinguished from bruises include Mongolian blue spots, telangiectases (hereditary telangiectasia rarely manifests before puberty) and erythema nodosum.

- Significance of nature of bleeding

Platelet or small vessel disorder is suggested by: petechiae, ecchymoses, small haematomas, mucous membrane bleeding (e.g. epistaxis), short-lived bleeding after trauma. Exceptions to these generalizations are rare (Fig. 8.1).

Plasma coagulation defect is suggested by: large/deep haematomas, persistent oozing after trauma, haemarthrosis after minimal trauma. Absence of excessive bleeding after surgery or tooth extraction argues against significant haemostatic defect; however, a normal response to trauma in the neonate, e.g. at circumcision or heel puncture for blood taking, does not necessarily exclude a plasma coagulation defect such as haemophilia.

- Recognition of genuine bleeding disorder

Bleeding which is excessive for the degree of trauma is an important criterion. On the other hand, bleeding is a natural consequence of abnormal stress on the vasculature, e.g. prolonged coughing, vomiting or fitting (bleeding in distribution of superior vena cava), physical abuse and self-inflicted injury (almost invariably denied, limited to areas to which the child can personally get access). See Figure 8.2.

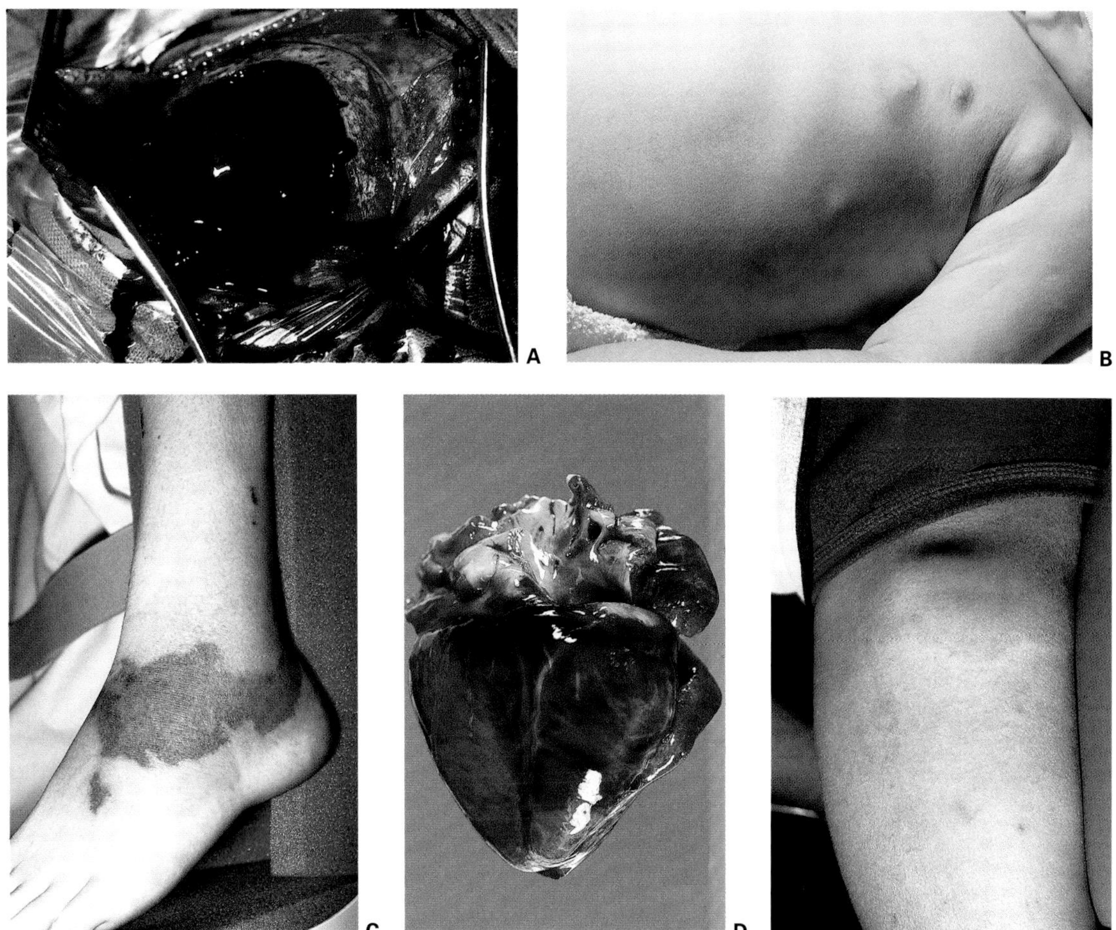

Fig. 8.1 Bleeding due to haemostatic defect. **a** F XIII deficiency. Extradural haematoma in a 19-day-old infant, oozing from umbilical cord from day 10. **b** Haematomas due to vitamin K deficiency from prolonged diarrhoea, severe combined immunodeficiency. **c** Snake bite which caused hypofibrinogenaemia (< 30 mg/dl, platelets normal, no fragmentation haemolysis). Fibrinogen rose spontaneously after about 36 h. An area of necrosis about 5 cm across became evident, which was grafted later. **d** Subepicardial haemorrhage, hypoprothrombinaemia of undetermined cause in a 22-day-old infant (delayed haemorrhagic disease of newborn). Vitamin K had been given at birth and the infant circumcised at 5 days without incident; breast-fed but the mother had not taken any medication. **e** Bubo-like haematoma in upper thigh of a 6-year-old boy with thrombocytopathy from fructose 1-6 diphosphatase deficiency.

The haemostatic screen

An effective screen should detect most defects but cannot be expected to identify rare or mild deficiencies.

A useful screen for haemostatic defect comprises:

- blood count and film (preferably unanticoagulated blood)
- prothrombin time
- activated partial thromboplastin time
- thrombin clotting time
- fibrinogen assay.

Table 8.1 Spurious results in the haemostatic screen

Result	Cause	Recognition	Correction
Low platelet count in automated counters	clotting in sample	visual inspection of sample	re-collect
	clumping in vitro of platelets	stained film	retake into citrate or heparin
	large platelets[1]	stained film	manual count
	platelet satellitism (EDTA samples)	stained film (Fig. 8.4)	retake into citrate or heparin
	EDTA-dependent platelet-agglutinating antibody[2]	stained film	manual count or use another anticoagulant
High platelet count in automated counters	extreme red cell fragmentation[3]	stained film	manual count
	leucocyte fragments[4]	stained film	manual count
	protein precipitation from overheating	stained film (Fig. 8.4) or phase-contrast	repeat at lower temp
Shortened PT, APTT	activation of clotting factors from difficulty in obtaining sample	results inappropriate for clinical state[5]	re-collect
	inadequate anticoagulation due to excess plasma	severe anaemia (hct < 0.2)	re-collect in appropriate volume of citrate[7]
Prolonged PT, APTT	delay in testing (> 4 h) (inactivation of V and VIII)	knowledge of time of sampling	re-collect
	excessive anticoagulation from plasma deficit	polycythaemia[6] (hct > 0.55)	re-collect in appropriate volume of citrate[7]
	excessive anticoagulation from plasma deficit	short sample	re-collect
	hypofibrinogenaemia	fibrinogen < 80 mg/dl	
	lipaemia	visual inspection	do manually
Prolonged TCT	faulty recognition by optical machines of poor quality/ transparent clot[8]	TCT inappropriate for clinical state	do manual TCT; factor assays except for fibrinogen normal
Low fibrinogen, incoagulable blood	clotting in sample	visual inspection of sample	re-collect
Low fibrinogen (automated)	lipaemia	visual inspection of sample	do manually
High fibrinogen (automated)	dysfunctional fibrinogen, aberrant kinetics of clotting	value inappropriate for clinical state	do manually
Failure to clot in clotting tests	heparin contamination	enquire of clinical staff	re-test after polybrene neutralization, or re-collect
Unexpected clotting of samples	hypercalcaemia from injected Ca	enquire of clinical staff; measure serum Ca	reduce Ca injections and re-test

[1] e.g. Bernard-Soulier
[2] Pegels et al 1982
[3] e.g. HUS, hereditary pyropoikilocytosis
[4] Extreme leucocytosis in leukaemia
[5] Genuine shortening rare, e.g. HUS
[6] Common causes: normal neonate and cyanotic congenital heart disease
[7] Volume of 3.8% citrate required (ml) = 1.85×10^{-3} x (100 – hct as %) $\times$ volume of blood
[8] Usually liver disease/jaundice

Unexpected results may be due to artefact (Table 8.1). This screen will not detect:

- Thrombocytopathies with normal platelet morphology

- Mild deficiency of coagulation factors

The minimum levels of coagulation factors required for normal PT and APTT vary with the factor and the reagents used within the range of approximately 25–50%. Minimum levels required for clinically normal haemostasis are given in Table 8.2.

- A proportion of cases of von Willebrand's disease

- A minority of lupus anticoagulants

- Factor XIII deficiency (Board et al 1993)

Clot solubility will detect severe deficiency. Clot solubility is also abnormal in dysfibrinogenaemia, but PT, APTT and TCT are usually abnormal as well. Precise quantitation of F XIII deficiency may be made by chromogenic assay, and subunits a and b may be measured immunochemically (subunit a carries site for fibrin stabilization).

a. Inherited (autosomal recessive). Deficiency usually severe. Subunits a + b deficient in some cases, only a in others. Bleeding is due to defective cross-linking of fibrin polymer. Characteristics are: bleeding from (neonatal) umbilical stump, delayed bleeding (24–36 h) after trauma, slow and poor wound healing with excessive scar formation (F XIII necessary for attachment of fibronectin to fibrin clot), intracranial bleeding (Fig. 8.1). Mothers of affected children have a high incidence of spontaneous miscarriage.
b. Acquired deficiency (impaired synthesis, excessive consumption, adsorption to fibrin) is mild and occurs in liver dysfunction, DIC, malignancy, inflammatory bowel disease, collagen disease and post surgery.
c. Inhibitors are rare, occurring as a response to replacement therapy in F XIII deficient patients, and after prolonged treatment with streptomycin or isoniazid.

- α_2 antiplasmin deficiency

Diagnosis is most conveniently made by immunologic assay. Whole blood clot lysis and euglobulin clot lysis times are shortened. Fibrinogen is usually normal. Inherited deficiency (autosomal recessive) is rare. Bleeding (hyperplasminaemia) is usually severe. Bleeding after trauma is characteristically delayed. Acquired deficiency is significant in the coagulopathy of AML M3 (p. 152).

Table 8.2 Minimum levels of coagulation factors required for clinically normal haemostasis

Factor	Minimum level required
Fibrinogen	50–80 mg/dl
II	0.3–0.4 IU/ml
V	0.10–0.15 U/ml
VII	0.3–0.4 IU/ml
VIII	0.3–0.4 IU/ml
IX	0.3–0.4 IU/ml
X	0.3–0.4 IU/ml
XI	approx 0.2 U/ml (variable)
XII[1]	0
XIII	0.01–0.02 U/ml
PK[1]	0
HMWK[1]	0

[1] Deficiency not associated with bleeding, because of diminution in drive to fibrinolysis

- Thrombotic states
- Small vessel dysfunction (Table 8.3, Fig. 8.2)

Bleeding is usually of 'platelet' type. In scurvy, however, haemophilia-type bleeding (subperiosteal and muscle) may occur in addition.

Table 8.3 Small vessel dysfunction which may be associated with bleeding tendency

Infection
Intraventricular haemorrhage of premature infants
Snake envenomation
Henoch-Schönlein purpura
Diabetes mellitus (retina especially)
Allergic vasculitis (food, drugs)
Hereditary haemorrhagic telangiectasia (telangiectases rare before puberty)
Steroid therapy, Cushing's disease
Scurvy
Osteogenesis imperfecta
Marfan's syndrome
Ehlers-Danlos syndrome
Pseudoxanthoma elasticum
Fabry's disease
Autoerythrocyte sensitization (Gardner-Diamond)
Fat embolism

Peculiarities of haemostasis in infancy and childhood

Coagulation

Peculiarities in normal infants and children are summarized in Tables 8.4–8.6 (coagulation components do not cross the placenta to any significant degree).

As a result of these peculiarities some inherited deficiencies cannot be diagnosed with confidence in infancy:

- mild F IX deficiency (F IX normally low)
- most cases of vWD (vWF normally high)
- heterozygous deficiency of inhibitors (C, S, ATIII normally low).

In sick infants values may be lower than for the healthy, and some values may take longer to reach adult levels (e.g. ATIII).

Table 8.4 Coagulation tests and factors in healthy premature and full-term[1] infants which differ from adult values

Test[2]	Premature, day 1	Full-term, day 1	Adult	Maturation time[3]
PT, s			12.4 (10.8–13.9)	
APTT, s	53.6 (27.5–79.4)	42.9 (31.3–54.5)	33.5 (26.6–40.3)	3 months
TCT, s			26.0 (19.7–30.3)	
Fibrinogen			278 (156–400)	
II	0.45 (0.20–0.77)	0.48 (0.26–0.70)	1.08 (0.70–1.46)	6 months
V		0.72 (0.36–1.08)	1.06 (0.62–1.50)	5 days
VII	0.67 (0.21–1.13)	0.66 (0.28–1.04)	1.05 (0.67–1.43)	5 days
VIII:C			0.99 (0.50–1.49)	
vWF:Ag	1.36 (0.78–2.10)	1.53 (0.19–2.87)	0.92 (0.50–1.58)	6 months
IX	0.35 (0.19–0.65)	0.53 (0.15–0.91)	1.09 (0.55–1.63)	6–9 months
X	0.41 (0.11–0.71)	0.40 (0.12–0.68)	1.06 (0.70–1.52)	6–9 months
XI	0.30 (0.08–0.52)	0.38 (0.10–0.66)	0.97 (0.67–1.27)	6 months
XII	0.38 (0.10–0.66)	0.53 (0.13–0.93)	1.08 (0.52–1.64)	6–9 months
PK	0.33 (0.09–0.57)	0.37 (0.05–0.69)	1.12 (0.62–1.62)	6–9 months
HMWK	0.49 (0.09–0.89)	0.54 (0.06–1.02)	0.92 (0.50–1.36)	5 days
XIIIa	0.70 (0.32–1.08)	0.79 (0.27–1.31)	1.05 (0.55–1.55)	5 days
XIII b	0.81 (0.35–1.27)	0.76 (0.30–1.22)	0.97 (0.57–1.37)	5 days
Plasminogen	1.70 (1.12–2.48)	1.95 (1.25–2.65)	3.36 (2.48–4.24)	6 months
D-dimer	may be ↑	may be ↑		days

Note: Values are the mean and range for 95% of population
Blanks are for values which are the same as in adults

[1] Premature = 30–36 weeks gestation; full-term = ≥ 37 weeks. All infants in these studies (Andrew et al 1987, 1988) had received vitamin K 1 mg intramuscular at birth

[2] Units of measurement: fibrinogen as mg/dl, all other coagulation factors in U or IU/ml

[3] Time taken for those values which in the full-term infant differ from the adult, to come within the adult range; this period is usually longer in prematures

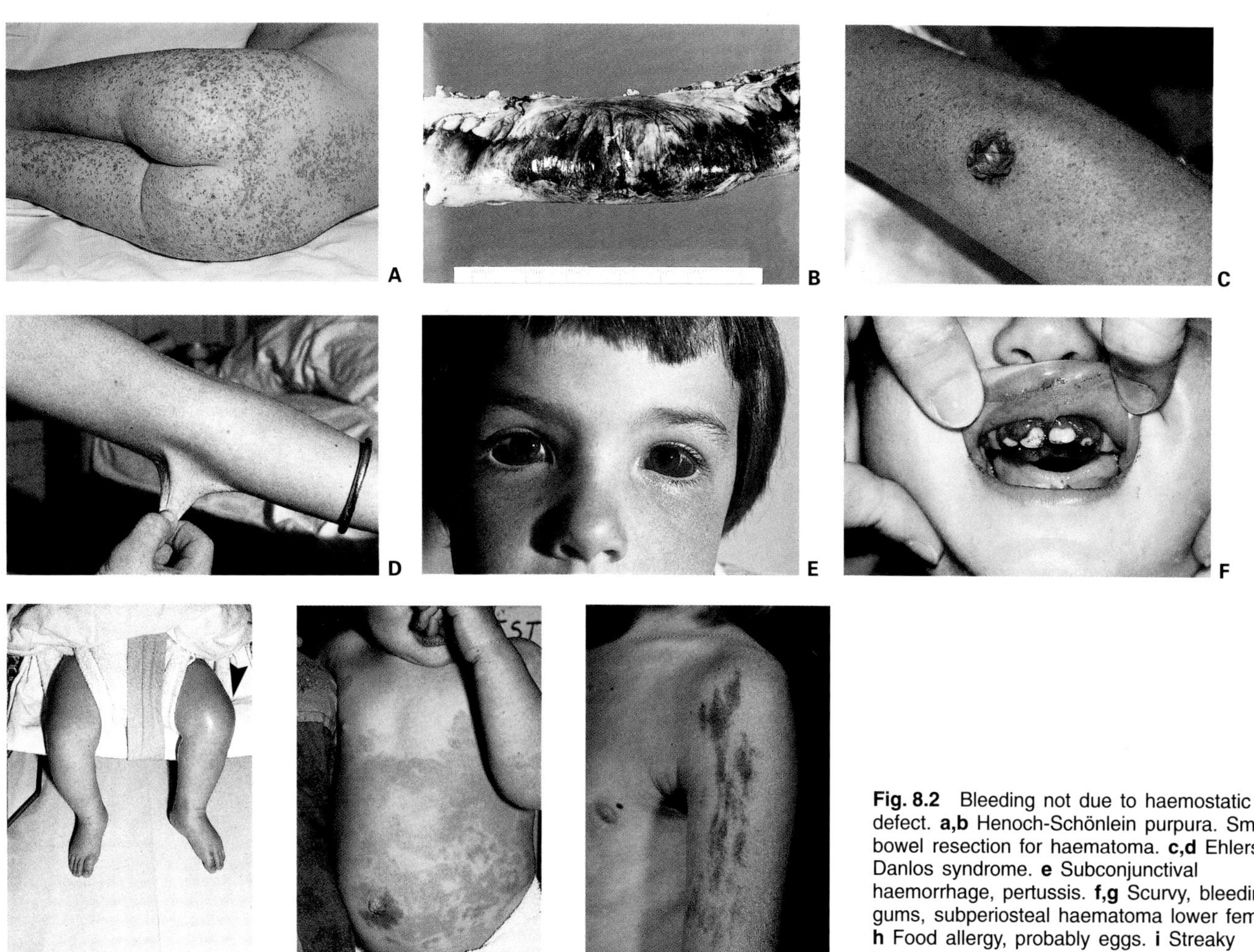

Fig. 8.2 Bleeding not due to haemostatic defect. **a,b** Henoch-Schönlein purpura. Small bowel resection for haematoma. **c,d** Ehlers-Danlos syndrome. **e** Subconjunctival haemorrhage, pertussis. **f,g** Scurvy, bleeding gums, subperiosteal haematoma lower femur. **h** Food allergy, probably eggs. **i** Streaky bruising in 7-year-old girl, diagnosed by exclusion as self-inflicted.

Table 8.5 Natural coagulation inhibitors in healthy premature and full-term[1] infants which differ from adult levels

Test[2]	Premature, day 1	Full-term, day 1	Adult	Maturation time[3]
ATIII	0.38 (0.14–0.62)	0.63 (0.39–0.87)	1.05 (0.79–1.31)	6 months
α_2M	1.19 (0.56–1.82)	1.39 (0.95–1.83)	0.86 (0.52–1.20)	still high at 6 months
α_2AP	0.78 (0.40–1.16)	0.85 (0.55–1.15)	1.02 (0.68–1.36)	5 days
C_1EINH	0.65 (0.31–0.99)	0.72 (0.36–1.00)	1.01 (0.71–1.31)	2 months, high till 6 months
HCII	0.32 (0.00–0.60)	0.43 (0.00–0.86)	0.96 (0.66–1.26)	4–6 months
Protein C	0.28 (0.12–0.44)	0.35 (0.17–0.53)	0.96 (0.64–1.28)	>6 months
Protein S total[4]	0.26 (0.14–0.38)	0.36 (0.12–0.60)	0.92 (0.60–1.24)	6–12 months

Note: Values are the mean and range for 95% of population

[1] Premature = 30–36 weeks gestation; full-term = ≥37 weeks. All infants in these studies (Andrew et al 1987, 1988) had received vitamin K 1 mg intramuscular at birth

[2] Units of measurement: ATIII and protein C as IU/ml, others as U/ml

[3] Time taken for those values which in the full-term infant differ from the adult, to come within the adult range; this period is usually longer in prematures

[4] Free protein S is present in relatively greater proportion than total S (54.2 vs 36.5% of adult in full-term infants), because of low levels of C_4 binding protein (Sthoeger et al 1989)

Platelets

Apart from minimal thrombocytopenia in some premature neonates, the count is the same in infancy as in childhood. Aggregation of neonatal platelets is normal with some reagents (ristocetin) but impaired with others (ADP, adrenalin, collagen); in spite of this the bleeding time is normal or even slightly shortened (Feusner 1980) due, it is thought, to the high hct and vWF levels of the neonate and diminished capacity to generate the platelet anti-aggregant, prostacyclin.

Isolated prolongation of APTT

Causes are listed in Table 8.7 and investigation summarized in Table 8.8. A schema of coagulation is given in Figure 8.3.

FACTOR VIII DEFICIENCY

Inherited (haemophilia A)

Grades of deficiency are: severe < 0.02 IU/ml, moderate 0.02–0.05 IU/ml, mild 0.05–0.50 IU/ml. Different members of the one kindred are affected to the same degree (cf vWD). Because VIII:C (like vWF) is an acute phase reactant, stress, fright, exercise, trauma and inflammation increase the level and may mask mild deficiency.

Gene defects include:

- rearrangement within intron 22 in almost half of severely affected patients (Goodeve et al 1994)
- point mutations in about 40%
- deletions in about 5%.

Inheritance is X-linked recessive but cannot be shown in about 25% of cases; the disorder in these is attributed to spontaneous mutation in the mother or a grandparent. Severe deficiency in phenotypic girls may be due to:

- extreme lyonization in carrier
- homozygous state from carrier mother and affected father (often consanguineous)
- homozygous state from spontaneous mutation in one X chromosome, the other from a carrier mother or affected father
- hemizygous state (Turner syndrome, XO)
- testicular feminization (XY in phenotypic female)
- Normandy variant of vWD (defective bonding of vWF to F VIII, autosomal recessive, Siguret et al 1994).

Table 8.6 Haemostatic components/tests in normal children which differ from those of adults[1]

	1–5 yr	6–10 yr	11–16 yr	Adult
Factors				
II	0.94 (0.71–1.16)	0.88 (0.67–1.07)	0.83 (0.61–1.04)	1.08 (0.70–1.46)
V		0.90 (0.63–1.16)	0.77 (0.55–0.99)	1.06 (0.62–1.50)
VII	0.82 (0.55–1.16)	0.85 (0.52–1.20)	0.83 (0.58–1.15)	1.05 (0.67–1.43)
IX	0.73 (0.47–1.04)	0.75 (0.63–0.89)	0.82 (0.59–1.22)	1.09 (0.55–1.63)
X	0.88 (0.58–1.16)	0.75 (0.55–1.01)	0.79 (0.50–1.17)	1.06 (0.70–1.52)
XI			0.74 (0.50–0.97)	0.97 (0.67–1.27)
XII			0.81 (0.34–1.37)	1.08 (0.52–1.64)
XIIIa	1.08 (0.72–1.43)	1.09 (0.65–1.51)		1.05 (0.55–1.55)
XIIIb	1.13 (0.69–1.56)	1.16 (0.77–1.54)		0.97 (0.57–1.37)
Inhibitors				
α_2M	1.69 (1.14–2.23)	1.69 (1.28–2.09)	1.56 (0.98–2.12)	0.86 (0.52–1.20)
C_1EINH	1.35 (0.85–1.83)			1.0 (0.71–1.31)
HCII	0.88 (0.48–1.28)	0.86 (0.40–1.32)	0.91 (0.53–1.29)	1.08 (0.66–1.26)
Protein C	0.66 (0.40–0.92)	0.69 (0.45–0.93)	0.83 (0.55–1.11)	0.96 (0.64–1.28)
Fibrinolytic				
Plasminogen			0.86 (0.68–1.03)	0.99 (0.77–1.22)
tPA, μg/ml	2.15 (1.0–4.5)	2.42 (1.0–5.0)	2.16 (1.0–4.0)	4.90 (1.40–8.40)
PAI		6.79 (2.0–12.0)	6.07 (2.0–10.0)	3.60 (0–11.0)
Bleeding time, min[2]	6 (2.5–10)	7 (2.5–13)	5 (3–8)	4 (1–7)

Values are the mean and limits for 95% of population
Units: U/ml or IU/ml unless otherwise shown
Blanks are for values which do not differ from the adult
[1] From Andrew et al 1992
[2] For uniformity all measurements, including adults, were done with a paediatric device (cut 3.5 mm long and 1 mm deep)

Table 8.7 Isolated prolongation of APTT

	Notes
F VIII:C deficiency	
Inherited	
Inhibitors	
von Willebrand's disease	
Inherited	APTT ↑ in about 1/3; (normal) high vWF in infancy masks deficiency
Acquired	
F IX deficiency	
Inherited	diagnosis of mild deficiency uncertain in infancy because F IX normally low
Acquired	
Lupus anticoagulant	APTT normal in minority
Heparin[1]	usually TCT also prolonged
Rare causes	
Deficiency of: F XI	
F XII, PK, HMWK	APTT usually > 70 s; no abnormal bleeding
F X	PT also usually prolonged
Passovoy defect	
Mild deficiency of several factors	
Origin obscure	
Post-viral thrombocytopenia	
Child abuse	

[1] Heparin-like glycosaminoglycans are released from damaged endothelium in septicaemia

Table 8.8 Investigation of isolated prolongation of APTT

Exclude heparin contamination if possibly relevant
Neutralize with polybrene
Remove with 'hepasorb' (Organon Teknika)
Reptilase time normal
Re-collect from vein distant to that cannulated
Mixing tests
No or only partial correction by normal plasma:
specific factor inhibitor
lupus anticoagulant
Correction by normal plasma:
factor deficiency
Specific factor assays
VIII
IX
XI
XII
HMWK
PK (or use long incubation, 10 min–1 h, of plasma + micronized silica)
Passovoy (no correction with Passovoy plasma)

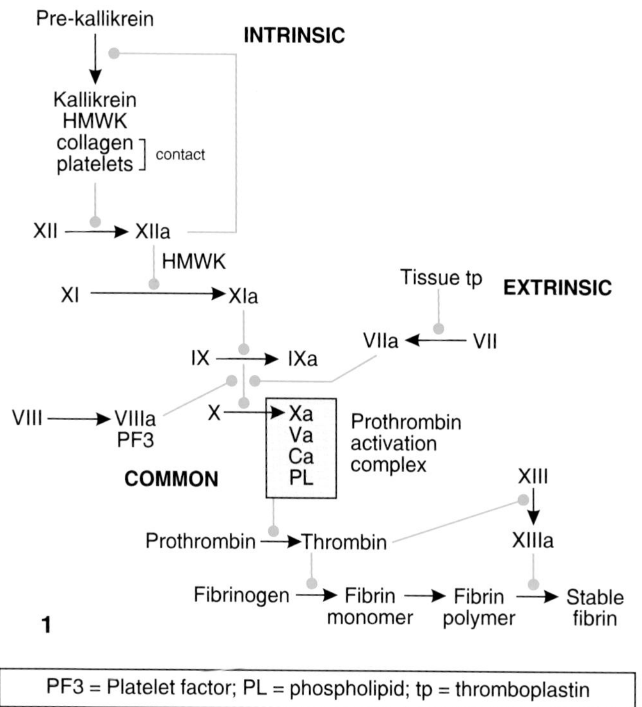

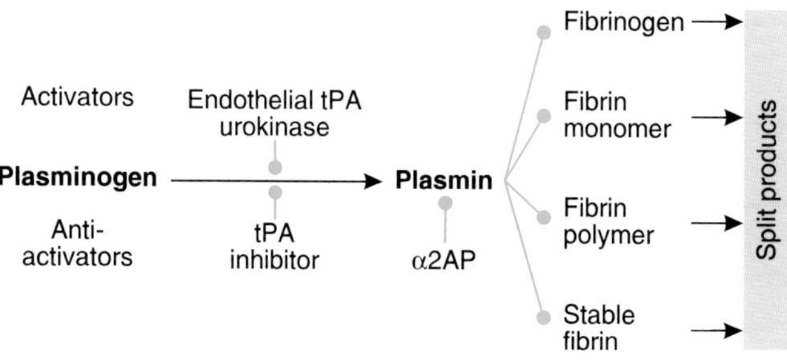

2

Fig. 8.3 The coagulation and fibrinolytic systems, simplified schema.

The carrier state in females may be detected by:

- F VIII:C levels
A reading < 0.5 IU/ml is presumptive evidence. Repeated testing may be needed to detect this. Testing is preferable after cessation of contraceptives and at end of menstrual cycle (contraceptives and oestrogen increase level).
- Excess of vWF over VIII:C (VIII:C 1/2–2/3 of antigen). Detects about 80% of carriers.
- Gene analysis for restriction fragment length polymorphisms or the gene defects above (Tuddenham 1994).

Inhibitors

Inhibitory activity is quantitated usually in Bethesda units — 1 unit = 50% destruction of F VIII:C after 2 hours incubation of a 1:1 mixture of patient and normal plasma; ≥ 5 units is regarded as 'strong'. Inhibitors are usually alloantibodies and almost always IgG.

Alloantibodies
These are generated in response to infused F VIII in up to 20% of patients with haemophilia, in those who are severely rather than mildly affected, and more often in those lacking the gene rearrangement within intron 22 (Goodeve et al 1994). These antibodies produce a progressive, log-linear destruction of F VIII:C to complete inactivation at antibody excess. Some patients show a large increase in antibody 4–7 days after F VIII infusion ('high responders'). Others show little or no increase ('low responders'). Weak inhibitors tend to disappear spontaneously. Spontaneous disappearance does not occur or is slow (years) in high responders and those with strong antibody, though there are exceptions (Leyva et al 1988). Examination for inhibitor should be made if response to F VIII infusion is less than expected, before surgery is contemplated, no matter how minor, and as a routine at least once a year.

Autoantibodies
A rare, de novo occurrence in SLE (lupus anticoagulant is more common and may be associated), rheumatoid arthritis, inflammatory bowel disease, skin disorders (erythema multiforme, dermatitis herpetiformis), drugs (penicillin, phenytoin) or without any obvious disease association (?viral myocarditis in a personal case). Unlike alloantibodies, autoantibodies produce early, rapid but incomplete destruction of F VIII:C, with a residuum of coagulation factor at antibody excess. They tend to disappear spontaneously over months to years.

VON WILLEBRAND'S DISEASE

Inherited

The commonest inherited disorder of coagulation. Due to quantitative or qualitative deficiency of vWF, which carries and protects F VIII:C, and binds platelets (at Gp Ib complex) to exposed subendothelial collagen at sites of vessel injury (Fig. 8.10). Because larger multimers of vWF are more effective in binding than the smaller, bleeding is more severe in deficiency of larger than of smaller multimers. vWF is produced by endothelial cells and megakaryocytes and stored in endothelial cells (Weibel-Palade bodies) and platelets (α granules).

Features of the main types are summarized in Tables 8.9–8.11.

Diagnosis, of less severe cases especially, remains a problem:

- Abnormal results for one or more routinely available screening procedure (bleeding time, F VIII:C, vWF, vWF:Ag) are obtained in only about 60% of patients (Miller et al 1979).
- Mild cases cannot be diagnosed in infancy because vWF is normally high for up to 6 months after birth.
- vWF, as an acute phase reactant, is increased by stress, fright, exercise, trauma, inflammation and oestrogen excess (mid-menstrual cycle).
- Except for the rare type III, test results may vary unpredictably over time and between members of the one kindred. Symptoms may improve spontaneously in late childhood or at puberty, lessening the pressure for investigation.
- The characteristically delayed and prolonged (2–4 days) normalization of tests (VIII:C, bleeding time) by infusion of vWF-containing material (e.g. cryoprecipitate, normal plasma), though reliable for diagnosis, is impractical.
- An expanding heterogeneity is being recognized (Ginsburg & Sadler 1993).
- Only type IIA, IIB and some type III have demonstrated gene defects.

Table 8.9 von Willebrand's disease

	I	II	III	Platelet type[1]
Defect	symmetric ↓ all multimers	large multimers absent — excessive avidity of abnormal vWF for n platelets[2,3]	severe ↓ or absence all multimers[4]	large multimers absent — excessive avidity for abnormal (GpIb) platelets[2]
Frequency	75%	20%	5%	< 1%
VIII:C	n to ↓	n to ↓	↓↓	n to ↓
vWF	usu ↓ (< VIII:C)	n to ↓	↓↓	n to ↓
vWF:Ag	n to ↓	n to ↓	↓↓	usu n
Bleeding time	n to ↑	n to ↑	↑	n to ↑
RIPA[5]	n to ↓	n to ↓	↓	n to ↓
Thrombocytopenia	no	often in IIb, chronic or inducible[6]	no	often, chronic or inducible[6], macroplatelets
Inheritance	AD	AD, some AR	AR or double heterozygous[7]	AD

[1] Pseudo von Willebrand's disease
[2] Coating renders platelets susceptible to aggregation and clearance (spontaneous or following further coating with vWF released by stress, DDAVP)
[3] Subtypes of II differ in multimer patterns of plasma and platelets
[4] Because of severity of deficiency, likely to have haemophilia-type bleeding, to present in infancy and to produce anti-vWF antibodies after infusion of vWF-containing plasmas
[5] Ristocetin-induced platelet aggregation at usual concentration (≥ 0.7 mg/ml); subnormal aggregation corrected by normal plasma or other source of vWF; aggregometry with other agents normal in all types
[6] Stress or DDAVP (release vWF from endothelium, megakaryocytes, platelets)
[7] One or both parents may be silent to testing
AD = autosomal dominant; AR = autosomal recessive; n = normal; usu = usually

Table 8.10 Type IIb vs platelet type vWD

	Agglutination by low concentration ristocetin (0.3–0.5 mg/ml[1]) of: Pt plasma + Pt platelets	n plasma + Pt platelets	Pt plasma + n platelets	Aggregation of Pt platelets by vWF[2]
IIb	↑, may be spontaneous[4]	normal[3]	↑	no aggregation
Platelet type	↑, may be spontaneous[4]	↑	normal[3]	aggregation

n = normal; Pt = patient
[1] Normal minimum required 0.7 mg/ml
[2] e.g. cryoprecipitate as source
[3] Normal response is absence of agglutination
[4] Excessive aggregation may also be noted in blood films

Table 8.11 Effect of DDAVP infusion (0.3 μg/kg) in vWD

	VIII:C	vWF	Bleeding time	Platelet count
I	↑	↑	↓	same
IIb[1]	same	may ↑	same (or ↑ if platelets ↓)	usu ↓
III[2]	same	same	same	same
Platelet type[1]				↓

[1] DDAVP contraindicated because of risk of induction or exacerbation of thrombocytopenia
[2] DDAVP ineffective because of severity of impairment of vWF production

Acquired

A rare occurrence in:

(i) Wilms tumour — vWD is due most likely to high levels of hyaluronic acid (Han et al 1987, Bracey et al 1987, see also Fig. 5.28). Haemostatic abnormalities disappear after effective treatment of the tumour.
(ii) Autoimmune disease, e.g. SLE, due to inhibition by IgG or IgA antibody (Sampson et al 1983).

Bleeding may be more severe than in the usual inherited vWD, because of greater reduction in vWF and F VIII:C (usually < 20%, often < 10%).

FACTOR IX DEFICIENCY

Inherited (haemophilia B, Christmas disease)

Frequency 10–20% that of haemophilia A. Diagnosis of mild disease may be uncertain for up to 6 months after birth because of physiologically low level of F IX (Table 8.4).

Inheritance as for F VIII deficiency. Severe deficiency may occur in phenotypic girls for the same reasons, though extreme lyonization appears to be more common than in F VIII deficiency.

Carriers tend to have lower levels of F IX and to be symptomatic more often than F VIII carriers. Gene analysis is important for detection of carrier state and for antenatal diagnosis; about half have point mutations and the rest, deletions (Giannelli et al 1991).

Acquired

(i) Inhibitors
The inhibitory effect is immediate and does not increase with further incubation (cf F VIII inhibitors). Most inhibitors occur in patients given F IX replacement, and are more likely in those with severe deficiency, those with dysfunctional variants and those with gene deletion rather than mutation; inhibitors are less frequent (about 3%) than F VIII inhibitors in haemophilia A. They may also occur without obvious cause or in association with Gaucher's disease or the disorders associated with F VIII inhibitors.

(ii) Loss
F IX may be lost in urine in nephrosis, together with F XII and ATIII; however, plasma F IX is rarely < 10%.

LUPUS ANTICOAGULANTS

Autoantibodies (usually IgG) which inhibit phospholipid-containing coagulants such as prothrombin converting complex (Fig. 8.3). Inhibitory effect is immediate and does not increase over time.

Detection (Exner et al 1991)

- APTT prolonged in most cases, normal in about 10%, perhaps because of excess of phospholipid in some test mixtures.
- No or incomplete correction on mixing with normal plasmas, but substantial correction in about 15%.
- Plasmas must be as platelet-poor as practicable to minimize phospholipid.
- The most sensitive method (containing minimum phospholipid) is kaolin clotting time of serial dilutions of patient + normal plasma.
- A more specific method (important when other inhibitors may be present) is the dilute Russell's viper venom time (venom directly activates F X), with correction of abnormal test by added phospholipid.

Co-occurrence with other haemostatic abnormalities (antiphospholipid syndrome) (Hughes et al 1989)

- Factor deficiencies, most commonly II, VIII

F II deficiency is due to rapid clearance of II-LA complex (LA binds at site away from phospholipid and F V binding sites). VIII deficiency is due to specific inhibitor (see below).

Suspect F II deficiency if PT is also prolonged. In the presence of LA, one-stage assays dependent on phospholipid may give spuriously low results (for all factors); assays approach true value with increasing dilution, due to enfeeblement of LA. Factor deficiency gives discordantly low assay for that factor; confirm by immunologic methods.

- Other inhibitors

In haemophiliacs LA from HIV infection may coexist with anti-F VIII from replacement therapy. Suspect inhibitors additional to LA if added phospholipid does not correct in the Russell's viper venom procedure. LA may coexist with anticardiolipin in autoimmune disease such as SLE (both are antiphospholipid but separable, McNeil et al 1989).

- Thrombocytopenia, platelet dysfunction, due to affinity of LA for platelet phospholipid.

Clinical effects
Usually no haemostatic disturbance, especially LA associated with viral infection or idiopathic. Bleeding, if present, is likely to be due to thrombocytopenia, platelet dysfunction or hypoprothrombinaemia. Thrombosis (inhibition of release of endothelial prostacyclin) is more likely than bleeding. Fetal loss is significant in pregnant women.

Causes
Viral infection (including HIV) is the most common association in childhood; APTT is usually only mildly prolonged, occasionally more so (to 120s); LA disappear within 6 months usually. Other associations include: SLE (about one third, may antedate overt clinical manifestations by months to years), rheumatoid disorder, remission induction of ALL, lymphoma and drugs (chlorpromazine, penicillin derivatives). In neonates LA may derive from mother by placental transfer.

HEPARIN (Table 8.8)

The use of heparin, e.g. for flushing of intravenous lines, may not be revealed to the laboratory, and ward staff may be unaware of its presence in a line. The TCT is usually prolonged as well as the APTT, but prolongation of APTT only is not uncommon from heparin in small doses. The effect of heparin lasts for up to 2–3 hours after an intravenous bolus and for up to 12 hours after a subcutaneous dose.

RARE CAUSES (see also Tables 8.7, 8.8)

- Factor XII deficiency

Inherited deficiency (Hageman trait) is usually severe and due to lack of synthesis of normal molecules or, rarely, dysfunctional variants. Inheritance autosomal recessive or rarely dominant. Deficiency may occur in nephrotic syndrome (loss in urine). Inhibitors of F XII (or other contact factors) are very rare (Lazarchick et al 1985).

- Factor XI deficiency (Colman et al 1994)

In inherited deficiency (haemophilia C, Rosenthal's syndrome), deficiency is usually mild to moderate and bleeding mild. Some homozygotes, however, have no bleeding, even after surgery. Inheritance is autosomal recessive with a high incidence among Ashkenazi Jews (about 3%). Because levels are normally low in the first months (Table 8.4), only severe deficiency (< 0.1 U/ml) is diagnosable in infancy. F XI may be lost in urine in nephrosis.

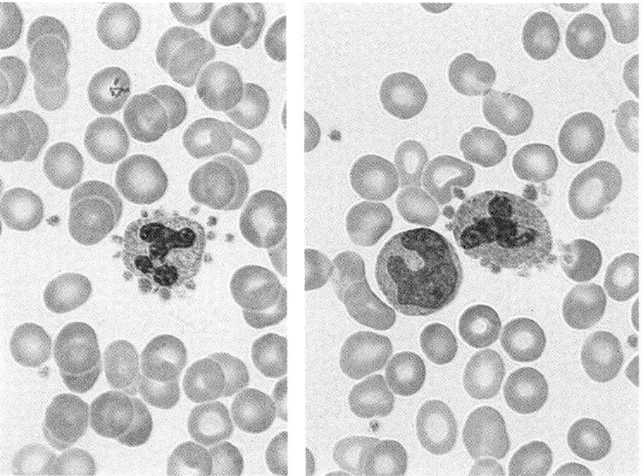

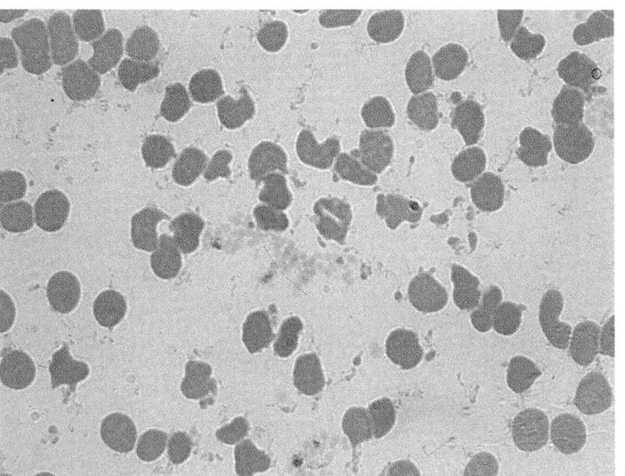

Fig. 8.4 Spurious platelet counts. **a** Low count due to platelet satellitism in a boy with (treated) neuroblastoma; monocyte not affected. **b** High count due to protein precipitation in blood inadvertently heated to 50°C (instead of 37°) to reverse cold agglutination of erythrocytes. × 750

- PK deficiency (Fletcher trait)

There is no abnormal bleeding, but rather a tendency to thromboembolism because of participation of PK in fibrinolysis (Fig. 8.4). Deficiency of HMWK may coexist (circulate as a complex). Autosomal recessive.

- HMWK deficiency (Fitzgerald, Flaujeac or Williams trait)

The APTT is not normalized by long incubation before addition of calcium (Fletcher trait is). Deficiency of PK may coexist (see above). Inheritance autosomal recessive.

- Isolated deficiency of Factor X

In occasional cases only the APTT is prolonged. Usually both APTT and PT are prolonged (see below).

- Passovoy defect

Mild prolongation of APTT of obscure origin, associated with significant bleeding tendency, autosomal dominant. May not be rare (Jackson et al 1981).

- Mild deficiency of multiple coagulation factors

The APTT (and PT) may be prolonged by summation of mild deficiency of several factors (in a personal case, F XI + XII in neuraminidase-induced HUS). See also Burns et al 1993.

PROLONGED APTT OF OBSCURE ORIGIN

- Transient (< 1 week) prolongation by a few seconds is occasionally seen in children with post-viral thrombocytopenia (? virus-induced LA).
- Transient prolongation also occurs occasionally in physically abused children (? virus-induced LA, mild liver hypoxia, dietary deficiency of vitamin K); brain damage in abused children may cause DIC (Fig. 8.5c).

Isolated prolongation of PT

ISOLATED FACTOR VII DEFICIENCY

Russell's viper venom time (direct activation of F X) is normal. Diagnosis requires factor assay.

Inherited

In symptomatic patients PT is usually grossly prolonged (> 50 s), with factor levels < 0.01–0.20 U/ml. Often first manifests in infancy as bleeding from umbilical cord, cephalhaematoma or intracranial haemorrhage. Inheritance autosomal recessive; heterozygotes have about half normal values. Most deficiencies are due to underproduction of normal molecules. May be associated with F X deficiency and with hereditary disorders of bilirubin metabolism (Dubin-Johnson, Rotor syndromes with predominantly conjugated hyperbilirubinaemia, Gilbert syndrome with predominantly unconjugated hyperbilirubinaemia). Mild deficiency has been observed in homocystinuria.

Acquired

In prothrombin complex deficiency (II, VII, IX, X) only the PT may be abnormal for the first 2–3 days before the APTT also prolongs (F VII earliest affected and has shortest half life). In mild prothrombin complex deficiency also, only the PT may be prolonged (APTT insensitive to mild deficiency of II, IX, X). Antibodies are very rare.

Prolongation of both PT and APTT
(Table 8.12)

DEFICIENCY OF PROTHROMBIN COMPLEX (II, VII, IX, X) (Table 8.13, Fig. 8.1)

The commonest cause of prolonged PT + APTT. PT is usually prolonged to a greater degree than APTT, and only the PT may be abnormal in the first 2–3 days of deficiency and in mild deficiencies (see above).

Confirmation of diagnosis may be made by:

(i) Echis time (venom from *Echis carinatus*; directly activates F II, carboxylated or not). Echis time is normal in vitamin K deficiency and remains prolonged in F II deficiency.
(ii) Assay of specific factors.
(iii) Partial or complete correction of results within 12 hours after a dose of vitamin K_1 occurs in vitamin K deficiency but not in factor deficiency.

Acquired

Haemorrhagic disease of the newborn, an exaggeration of the mild deficiency of II, VII, IX and X of the normal neonate (Table 8.4), has become rare since the routine use of vitamin K prophylaxis at birth. Contributing factors are listed in Table 8.13, but severe deficiency may occur without obvious potentiating factors.

Delayed haemorrhagic disease of the newborn is an uncommon occurrence 1–3 months after birth. The cause/s may be obscure (Fig. 8.1). It may occur even when vitamin K prophylaxis has been given at birth, and is more likely in breast-fed than formula-fed infants. In some cases vitamin K deficiency (e.g. biliary atresia, cystic fibrosis, non-specific diarrhoea) or liver damage (e.g. hepatitis) contribute.

Hereditary

Very rare. In most cases the molecules are dysfunctional. High dose vitamin K may produce partial response. Hereditary deficiency may be associated with warfarin-type embryopathy, both perhaps due to under-carboxylation of glutamyl residues of proteins (Pauli et al 1987). Deficiency of

Table 8.12 Prolongation of PT + APTT

Deficiency of II, VII, IX, X (Table 8.13)
Lupus anticoagulant[1]
Massive transfusion of stored blood (deficient in VIII:C,V)
Rare
Combined deficiency V + VIII
Isolated deficiency:
II
V
X
Citrate excess (Table 8.1)
Hypofibrinogenaemia < 80 mg/dl

[1] In those (a minority) with F II deficiency as well

Table 8.13 Deficiency of factors II, VII, IX and X

Acquired	
(breast feeding accentuates because of low content of vitamin K in human milk[1])	
Vitamin K deficiency	
Decreased intake	omission of vitamin K prophylaxis at birth[2]
	low intake of milk in first days of life[2]
	prolonged anorexia
	prolonged unsupplemented parenteral feeding
	deficiency of vitamin K-producing gut bacteria:
	physiologic (neonate)[2]
	prolonged antibiotics (especially cephalosporins) given to child or nursing mother
Malabsorption	biliary obstruction
	bowel disease — coeliac disease, inflammatory bowel disease
	cystic fibrosis
Impaired liver function	physiologic (neonate)
	vitamin K antagonism: coumarins given to child[3] or nursing mother
	other drugs given to mother which may affect vitamin K stores or function in neonate:
	anticonvulsants
	rifampicin
	isoniazid
	structural damage
	fulminant hepatic destruction
	cirrhosis — biliary atresia, metabolic disorders, e.g. α_1 antitrypsin deficiency
Inherited	
Origin obscure	delayed haemorrhagic disease of newborn
	child abuse

[1] There is little placental transfer of vitamin K
[2] Contribute to haemorrhagic disease of newborn
[3] Or poisoning with coumarin-containing rodenticides

vitamin K-dependent anticoagulants (proteins C, S) may accompany factor deficiencies (Brenner et al 1990).

Obscure origin

A transient (< 1 week) mild prolongation of values (by a few seconds) in some children who have been physically abused has been attributed to liver hypoxia and/or vitamin K deficiency due to inadequate diet.

CITRATE EXCESS

Usually the APTT is prolonged to a greater degree than the PT. See also Table 8.1.

RARE CAUSES

Combined deficiency of V, VIII

This rare defect is the commonest of the inherited combinations. In most congenital cases V and VIII are reduced to the same degree (< 0.10 U/ml), suggesting an effect of a single gene (autosomal recessive). Somatic defects are often associated (mental retardation, syndactyly, hypogonadism). Some cases are attributed to over-degradation of V and VIII by activated protein C due to autosomal dominant deficiency of protein C inhibitor.

Acquired deficiency is most commonly due to massive transfusion of stored blood. A mild decrease in F V, VIII and fibrinogen in some cases of essential thrombocythaemia and polycythaemia vera is attributed to hypercoagulable state.

Isolated deficiency of F II

Most commonly acquired in (occasional) cases of LA (p. 284). Inherited deficiency is autosomal recessive.

Isolated deficiency of F V

The Russell's viper venom time is prolonged (direct activation of F X). Bleeding is likely at levels < 0.10 U/ml. Mild platelet dysfunction occurs in about one third of patients with inherited deficiency. Inheritance in most is autosomal recessive (rare cases autosomal dominant). Inhibitors occur in some patients with genetic deficiency and in rare patients with malignancy or inflammatory disorders. Inhibitors usually disappear spontaneously within 6 weeks.

Isolated deficiency of F X (Stuart factor)

The Russell's viper venom time is prolonged. In inherited cases, F X deficiency may be associated with F VII deficiency or with carotid body tumour (F X not increased by removal). Autosomal recessive. Acquired deficiency of only F X occurs in rare cases of malignancy, exposure to fungicides and without obvious cause.

Prolongation of TCT as the only or primary abnormality (Tables 8.14–8.16)

Prolongation of TCT occurs when functional fibrinogen is < 100 mg/dl or when there is interference with fibrinogen–fibrin conversion (Table 8.14). Automated optical methods for TCT may give spuriously prolonged values (Table 8.1).

FIBRINOGEN DEFICIENCY (Table 8.14)

- Impaired production

Congenital afibrinogenaemia (< 5 mg/dl) is more common than congenital hypofibrinogenaemia (50–150 mg/dl). Hypofibrinogenaemia is probably the heterozygous state. However, parents of children with afibrinogenaemia usually have normal levels. Platelet function may be impaired because of deficiency of fibrinogen on the platelet surface (p. 314).

Hypofibrinogenaemia due to decreased production is a late occurrence in severe liver disease. A mild reduction (120–160 mg/dl) of unknown cause occurs in some cases of anorexia nervosa (no or minimal liver dysfunction); values return to normal over some weeks as clinical state improves.

- Hyperfibrin(ogen)olysis

Direct assessment of fibrinolysis by measurement of plasmin concentration is impractical because of its short half life; accordingly, recognition of fibrinolysis is made on a combination of indirect indicators (Table 8.15).

Primary fibrinolysis is rare in childhood but the effects are usually more striking than those of secondary fibrinolysis.

- Other causes

Moderate to severe hypofibrinogenaemia occurs in some patients receiving sodium valproate (cause obscure) or L-asparaginase (impairment of production + destruction by circulating trypsin from drug-induced pancreatitis).

Antibodies to fibrinogen are very rare. The reptilase time (Table 8.16) is prolonged as well as TCT. Fibrinogen concentration is usually normal or increased; cryofibrinogen is demonstrable in some cases. Antibodies are usually IgG and occur most commonly in patients with congenital afibrinogenaemia given replacement products. De novo occurrence has been noted in ulcerative colitis with liver disease.

DYSFIBRINOGENAEMIA (Table 8.16)

Diagnostic features include:

- small, friable clot with excessive red cell dropout; F XIII deficiency screen also abnormal
- excess of total over clottable fibrinogen; total assessed as antigen or by physico-chemical methods (heat precipitation, turbidimetry; these also measure FDP)
- PT, APTT as well as TCT prolonged, reptilase time prolonged
- TCT corrected by toluidine blue
- further characterization by immunoelectrophoresis and purification of fibrinogen.

Dysfibrinogenaemia is most commonly associated with liver disease (cirrhosis, hepatoma, secondary malignancy, tyrosinaemia) or pseudotumour cerebri (benign intracranial hypertension). Abnormal fibrinogen in liver disease has some resemblances to fetal fibrinogen (especially increased sialic acid content) and is not associated with haemorrhage, thrombosis or defective wound healing.

Congenital dysfibrinogenaemias are defects of cleavage of fibrinopeptides by thrombin, or of polymerization of fibrin monomer or of stabilization of fibrin polymer. Autosomal dominant. Most individuals are heterozygous and asymptomatic. Homozygotes and some heterozygotes have abnormal bleeding, and in some types, thrombosis (p. 298) or poor wound healing.

INHIBITION OF FIBRINOGEN–FIBRIN CONVERSION

Interference may be caused by heparin or FDP (Table 8.16).

FDP interfere with fibrin monomer polymerization. Increase is most conveniently shown as D-dimer (from lysis of cross-linked fibrin; test applicable to serum, plasma or whole blood, containing heparin or not). Increase is a result of fibrinolysis, either primary or secondary to coagulation within or outside the vasculature (large haematomas). Mild increase is normal in the first week of life (usually insufficient to prolong the TCT). An increase of uncertain origin may occur in nephrotic syndrome (fibrinogen normal).

Table 8.14 Prolongation of TCT as the only or primary abnormality

	Mechanism/notes
Fibrinogen deficiency	
Impaired production	
Hereditary	
Acquired	
Liver disease	
Anorexia nervosa[1]	mechanism obscure
Increased utilization	
Intravascular coagulation[2]	
Fibrin(ogen)olysis	
Secondary	
Intravascular coagulation[2]	
Primary	
Liver cirrhosis	↓ synthesis of α_2 antiplasmin
Trauma, esp bone	release of tPA
Envenomation	fibrinolysis primary (Fig. 8.1) or secondary to intravascular coagulation
Extreme fear	release of tPA from endothelium
Therapeutic	
Strepto/urokinase	
Hereditary	
↓ α_2 antiplasmin	fibrinogen usually normal
↑ tPA	fibrinogen usually normal
↓ PAI 1[3]	
Other	
Sodium valproate, L-asparaginase, antibiotics	
Dysfibrinogenaemia[4]	
Acquired	
Hereditary	
Inhibition of fibrinogen–fibrin conversion	
Heparin[5]	
FDP	
Dysproteinaemia	
Origin obscure	
Carbenicillin	
Hypoalbuminaemia (< 2 g/l)[6]	

[1] Fibrinogen deficiency usually not severe enough to prolong TCT
[2] With deficiency of other factors
[3] Lee et al 1993
[4] PT and APTT also prolonged and F XIII deficiency screen abnormal
[5] APTT also usually prolonged
[6] Correctable in vitro by adding albumin

Table 8.15 Evidence for fibrinolysis[1]

- Poor quality clot[2]
- Brisk clot lysis[2]
- Shortened euglobulin lysis time[2]
- ↑ FDP
- Hypofibrinogenaemia (inconstant, fibrinogen may be normal)
- Minimal or no thrombocytopenia[3]
- ↑ plasminogen
- tPA: release from endothelium by venous occlusion for 10 minutes, DDAVP infusion or exercise; measure either directly (antigen, function) or by shortening of euglobulin lysis time
- ↓ F V,VIII (destroyed by plasmin)
- Fibrin monomer normal[3,4]

[1] Features of primary ('pure') fibrinolysis; in secondary fibrinolysis (intravascular coagulation) deficiency of other coagulation factors and thrombocytopenia added
[2] Abnormal also in hypofibrinogenaemia and F XIII deficiency
[3] Features of value in differentiation from DIC
[4] Satisfactory, rapid method not available

Table 8.16 Investigation of prolonged TCT

	Hypofibrinogenaemia	Dysfibrinogenaemia	Heparin[1]	FDP
Fibrinogen	↓	total normal; clottable ↓	normal	variable
Added normal plasma	C	C	NC	NC
Reptilase[2]	NC	NC	C	NC
Toluidine blue	NC	C (in most)	C	NC
Polybrene	NC	NC	C	variable

[1] Usually APTT also prolonged
[2] Cleaves fibrinogen on a chain to liberate only fibrinopeptide A; not inhibited by heparin
C = corrected; NC = not corrected

Incoagulable blood

Before concluding that blood is truly incoagulable, artefact (over-anticoagulation) should be excluded, as well as poor, friable clot formation. The most likely causes in childhood are given in Table 8.17.

Disseminated intravascular coagulation (DIC)

DIAGNOSIS

There is no single, specific, invariably positive and readily applicable diagnostic test. Of procedures in Table 8.18, the most specific are those for D-dimer, fibrin monomer and fibrinopeptides A + B. Circulating thrombin is specific if entry into the circulation from extravascular haematomas can be excluded.

Figures for frequency in Table 8.18 are averages for a heterogeneous collection of disorders. Frequency, however, varies from one disorder to another as well as from case to case with the same disease, for example abnormality is more frequent and more severe in purpura fulminans than in septicaemia, and there is little if any systemic haemostatic disturbance in renal autograft rejection.

Utilization in thrombosis may not be the only cause of haemostatic depletion in DIC — for example, thrombin may aggregate platelets to contribute to thrombocytopenia, cleavage by thrombin and plasmin contributes to fibrinogen deficiency, destruction by plasmin and thrombin-activated protein C contributes to deficiency of V and VIII, and activation by thrombin contributes to F XIII deficiency.

Table 8.17 Genuinely incoagulable blood in childhood

Congenital afibrinogenaemia
Dysfibrinogenaemia
Severe intravascular coagulation or defibrinogenation
Envenomation
Cardiac arrest
Purpura fulminans

DIFFERENTIAL DIAGNOSIS OF DIC

- Liver disease

Differentiation of intravascular coagulation from the complex (and often opposing) haemostatic changes in liver disease (Table 8.19) cannot be made with certainty on laboratory features — similar changes occur in both and the two may coexist. In general, intravascular coagulation is not a dominating component in liver disease, especially if chronic. A trial of heparin is useful for differentiation but has unacceptable risks. The possibility of mimicry of DIC by acute liver disease is also to be considered; fulminant viral hepatitis, for example, may cause hypofibrinogenaemia (impaired synthesis) and thrombocytopenia (viral or immune destruction).

- Primary fibrinolysis

See Table 8.15.

- Extravascular coagulation

Utilization of haemostatic components within a haematoma, together with leakage of thrombin into the circulation may mimic DIC. Haemostatic changes, however, are unlikely unless the haematoma is clinically obvious (e.g. cephalhaematoma in newborns) and are usually mild, with increase in FDP (or thrombin if measured) as the only abnormal finding. However, plasma F VIII:C may be depressed by pseudotumour in haemophilia, rising after removal of the mass.

CONDITIONS ASSOCIATED WITH DIC IN CHILDHOOD

An outline classification of causes by mechanism or presumed mechanism is given in Table 8.20.

Table 8.18 Evidence for DIC

	Frequency, %[1]
Circulating fibrin monomer[2]	66
Depletion of: platelets[3]	95
II	68
V[3]	58
I[3]	57
VIII[3]	16
X	
XIII	
ATIII	75
protein C, S	
HCII	
Increase in FDP[4]	76
Fragmentation haemolysis	70
Increased: TCT ($\downarrow$ I, $\uparrow$ FDP)	67
PT + APTT ($\downarrow$ factors)	56
Research procedures	
Circulating thrombin (prothrombin fragments F 1 + 2 are an indirect estimate)	
Fibrinopeptides A + B	
Fibrin monomer by precise techniques, e.g. monoclonal antibodies	

[1] From Weiss 1988
[2] Ethanol gelation/protamine paracoagulation; neither is specific (positive also with larger breakdown fragments e.g. X,Y)
[3] Acute phase reactants whose values may be above normal at onset, but which, as DIC develops, will fall, though not necessarily to below normal
[4] FDP sensitive but not specific (fragments D, E from lysis of fibrinogen and uncross-linked fibrin). D-dimer less sensitive but more specific (D-dimeric units from lysis of cross-linked fibrin)

Table 8.19 Abnormal haemostasis in liver disease

	Effect
Impaired synthesis of factors	$\downarrow$ I, II, VII[1], IX, X, V
Impaired synthesis of inhibitors	$\downarrow$ ATIII, protein C, S enhance intravascular coagulation, $\rightarrow$ $\downarrow$ I, II, V, VIII, X; $\uparrow$ FDP; thrombocytopenia
	$\downarrow$ α_2 antiplasmin $\rightarrow$ hyperfibrinolysis (Table 8.15)
Impaired synthesis of C4 binding protein	$\uparrow$ free protein S
Impaired clearance	of tPA and plasmin $\rightarrow$ hyperfibrinolysis
	of FDP $\rightarrow$ $\uparrow$ FDP
Perverted synthesis	dysfibrinogenaemia
Hypersplenism (chronic liver disease)	thrombocytopenia
Deficiency of platelet dense bodies	thrombocytopathy

[1] Normal values for VII in DIC useful in distinction from liver disease

Table 8.20 DIC in childhood[1]

Endothelial damage (activation of intrinsic pathway)	
Organisms or their endotoxins	infection HUS, TTP
Antigen/antibody complexes	renal autograft rejection anaphylaxis
Hypoxia[2]/acidosis	shock, hypotension hypoxia hypothermia cardiac arrest immersion heat stroke status epilepticus
Haemangioma	
Deficiency of inhibitors (Protein C, S)	purpura fulminans
Release of thromboplastins into circulation (activation of extrinsic pathway)	
Neoplasm[3] — AML M3[4], M5, disseminated neuroblastoma, tumour lysis syndrome	
Tissue death — trauma, head injury, burns, necrotizing enterocolitis, dead twin fetus	
Maternal disease and intravascular coagulation in neonate	
Envenomation	
Blood cell destruction — incompatible blood transfusion, erythroblastosis fetalis	
Amniotic fluid inhalation	
Fat embolism	
Other or unknown mechanisms	
Kawasaki disease	
Cyanotic congenital heart disease	
Administration of prothrombin complex concentrates[5]	
Liver disease (Table 8.19)	
Juvenile rheumatoid arthritis[6]	

[1] Process affecting predominantly the microvasculature. In some disorders intravascular coagulation is most severe in or confined to one organ, e.g. kidney in HUS and renal autograft rejection
[2] Hypoxia is of especial significance in the neonate (Favara et al 1974)
[3] Irritation of endothelium by tumour deposits may contribute to thrombosis
[4] Decrease in α_2 antiplasmin is probably more significant than DIC in the bleeding tendency
[5] Especially in those with liver disease (impaired clearance of F IXa, Xa, decreased synthesis of ATIII)
[6] Disease itself or treatment (gold, indomethacin, ibuprofen, Silverman et al 1983)

Bacterial infection

Septicaemia

DIC is common in hypotensive septicaemia (Fig. 8.5) but is not necessarily the only cause of haemostatic changes; liver damage from hypotension or infection depletes coagulation factors, and heparin-like glycosaminoglycans released into the circulation from damaged endothelium contribute to increase in the APTT. Fragmentation haemolysis is infrequent. Organisms most commonly implicated are Gram-negative rods, meningococcus, pneumococcus, *H. influenzae* and β haemolytic streptococci. Mechanism/s for disturbing the normally antithrombic properties of the endothelial surface are not clear (Heyderman 1993). Isolated thrombocytopenia in bacterial infection is considered on page 307.

Haemolytic-uraemic syndrome

Major characteristics are fragmentation haemolysis (p. 80), renal failure and thrombocytopenia, due to thrombosis, which for unknown reasons is confined to or most severe in the kidneys. Thrombi consist mainly of platelets, with a variable component of fibrin and vWF multimers (Fig. 8.5, Kaplan B S et al 1992, Moake 1994). The relatively minor nature of the haemostatic changes, apart from thrombocytopenia (Table 8.21) is a reflection of this process.

In the most common (diarrhoea-associated) form, platelet aggregation is attributed to binding to their glycoprotein receptors of unusually large vWF multimers released from endothelium by exotoxins (especially verotoxin) absorbed from bacteria in the bowel (usually *E. coli* or *S. dysenteriae*). A relation between neutrophil count and severity of renal damage is attributed to release from neutrophils of components (e.g. platelet-activating factor, cathepsin) that damage endothelium or activate platelets. In pneumococcus-associated HUS, endothelial damage is due to neuraminidase produced by the organism, cryptantigen exposure occurring in the kidney and other tissues (p. 74). HUS may occasionally be associated with upper respiratory infection, diphtheria-pertussis-tetanus inoculation or viral vaccination. Most patients with infection-associated HUS are under 4 years of age.

An HUS-like disorder may occur in patients receiving metronidazole, mitomycin, cisplatin or cyclosporin (usually not until weeks or months after exposure) and as an immune reaction to quinine (activation and adhesion of neutrophils to endothelium, Stroncek et al 1992).

The relation between HUS and TTP is considered on page 80.

Purpura fulminans

See below.

Viral infection

Severe viraemias may be associated with DIC, e.g. haemorrhagic varicella, rubella, rubeola, influenza and dengue, Korean haemorrhagic fever and Rocky Mountain spotted fever. However, bleeding into skin lesions may not necessarily be due to DIC but to a combination of isolated thrombocytopenia and vasculitis. Viraemias in the neonate or in utero are especially likely to be associated with DIC, e.g. herpes simplex, CMV, mumps and rubella; the normal deficiency at this age of natural inhibitors (Table 8.5) and impaired capacity for reticuloendothelial clearance of activated coagulation factors may facilitate thrombosis. Liver damage from virus may accentuate coagulation factor deficiencies.

Purpura fulminans, which is most commonly associated with viral infection, is considered below.

The commonest haemostatic abnormality in viral infection, isolated thrombocytopenia, is not due to DIC (see p. 306).

Other infections

An element of DIC is not infrequent in severe falciparum malaria.

Haemangioma

Haemangiomas may consume haemostatic components to cause a generalized bleeding tendency (Kasabach-Merritt syndrome). Fragmentation haemolysis however is infrequent. Consumption of components is attributed to fibrin-platelet thrombosis in the haemangioma but histologic evidence of this may be slight (Fig. 8.6). Though the lesion is congenital, haemostatic deficiency may not manifest till some years after birth. In some cases haemostatic depletion occurs only when the haemangioma is infected.

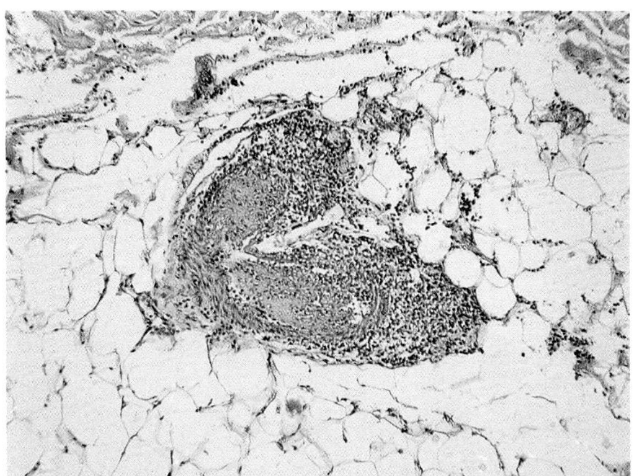

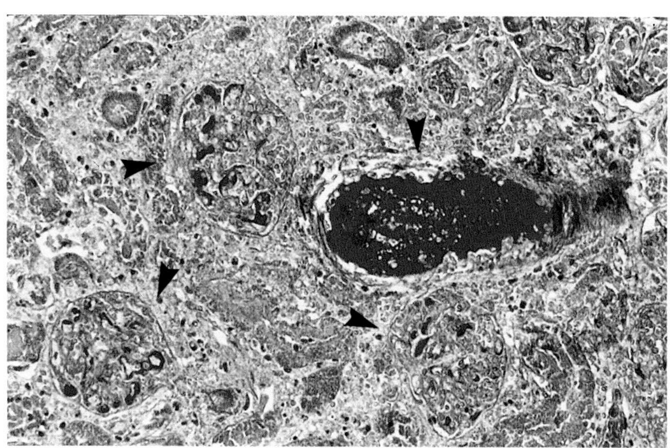

Fig. 8.5 Intravascular coagulation. **a** Subcutaneous vessel, meningococcal septicaemia. H & E × 130. **b** Kidney, HUS, fibrin thrombus (red) in arteriole and glomerular capillaries (arrows). Acid picro-Mallory × 160. **c** DIC due to brain damage (child abuse) in a 19-day-old infant. Arrows show, clockwise from 12 o'clock, hyperdense area (haemorrhage), gap between skull and brain (subdural fluid) and large hypodense area (infarction). Plasma fibrinogen 114 mg/dl, D-dimer titre 1/128, platelet count normal. Prolongation of PT (33 s, n < 17) and APTT (80 s, n < 41) was regarded as a spurious effect of hypofibrinogenaemia.

Table 8.21 Haemostatic abnormalities in HUS[1]

	Frequency
Thrombocytopenia (usually severe, to 30 × 10^9/l) or falling count	85%
APTT shortened by a few seconds ('Hypercoagulable state' from ↑ I, V, VIII, IX, XI)	1/3
D-dimer ↑	80%
Consumption of factors (I, V, VIII)	5%
ATIII ↓	occasional

[1] Adapted in part from Kaplan B S et al 1992

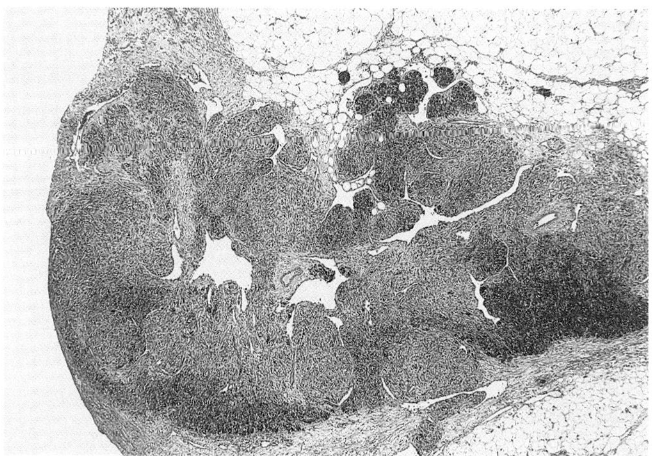

Fig. 8.6 Haemangioendothelioma of upper arm in a 5-month-old girl associated with haemostatic depletion. No thrombus discernible. Coagulation factor deficiencies corrected in about 2 weeks, and thrombocytopenia in 10 weeks. H & E × 30

While most haemangiomas associated with haemostatic depletion are large and external, some are small or internal, e.g. disseminated haemangiomatosis of bones and spleen (cure by splenectomy, Dadash-Zadeh et al 1976), haemangioma of placenta (chorangioma) producing DIC and fragmentation haemolysis in the neonate (Bauer et al 1978) and disseminated lymphangiomatosis (Dietz & Stuart 1977).

Deficiency of natural inhibitors of coagulation

DIC is characteristic of purpura fulminans associated with severe deficiency of proteins C and S.

Patches of haemorrhagic ischaemia and necrosis appear in the skin, often evolving to painful bullae (Fig. 8.7), with a high risk of gangrene of digits or whole limbs if effective treatment is not given within 2 days of onset. Thrombosis of small and large vessels occurs, usually associated with clear evidence of DIC; thrombocytopenia and hypofibrinogenaemia are usual, but fragmentation haemolysis is infrequent. ATIII and proteins C and S are mildly to moderately reduced secondary to consumption (C or S severely reduced in homozygous deficiency).

Protein C deficiency
Inherited deficiency may be heterozygous (approx half normal values) or (rare) homozygous (< 5% of normal). Thrombosis is unusual in heterozygotes before adolescence, though occurring occasionally in the neonate. Hypothalamic failure is prominent in some cases (Schmitt et al 1992). Skin necrosis after administration of coumarins is also a risk in heterozygotes; because of its short half life there is a lag between drop in protein C and drop in other vitamin K-dependent factors (II, VII, IX, X), during which thromboembolism is a risk. Inheritance autosomal dominant.

Homozygotes present usually in the neonatal period as purpura fulminans, though presentation may occasionally be delayed until early adulthood (Melissari & Kakkar 1989). The heterozygous parents of these children do not, for unexplained reasons, have the thrombotic proclivity of other heterozygotes. Deficiency is rarely part of a broad deficiency of vitamin K-dependent proteins (C, S, II, VII, IX, X, Brenner et al 1990).

Acquired deficiency is mild to moderate and is a result of impaired synthesis (liver disease, coumarins), loss in urine (nephrosis) or consumption (intravascular coagulation of any aetiology); deficiency also occurs, for obscure reasons, in renal failure (increases after dialysis).

Protein S deficiency
The significant component is the free protein, as the bound fraction (to C4B binding protein) is unavailable as cofactor for protein C.

Inherited deficiency is usually heterozygous, with approximately half normal values. About half of these individuals have recurrent thrombosis, presenting usually in adult life, but occasionally in childhood (Mannucci et al 1986). Protein S deficiency does not predispose to skin necrosis after warfarin; S has a longer half life than C and reduces simultaneously with other vitamin K-dependent factors after treatment. Homozygous deficiency may present in the neonate as purpura fulminans (Mahasandana et al 1990). Deficiency is rarely part of a broad deficiency of vitamin K-dependent proteins (see above).

Acquired deficiency of mild to moderate degree occurs in liver disease and intravascular coagulation of any cause. Severe deficiency due to autoantibody (with rapid clearance of S-antibody complex) occurs in the thromboembolic disorder of the recovery phase of (rare cases of) varicella. Some of these cases have typical purpura fulminans (Levin M 1994, personal communication), others do not (D'Angelo et al 1993). The antibody is potent; replacement with plasma restores coagulation components except protein S, which takes up to 8 weeks to return to normal as antibody wanes.

Purpura fulminans may be due to other mechanisms (e.g. lupus anticoagulant, p. 285), and in some cases, e.g. those associated with bacterial infection such as meningococcus and streptococcus, the mechanism is obscure.

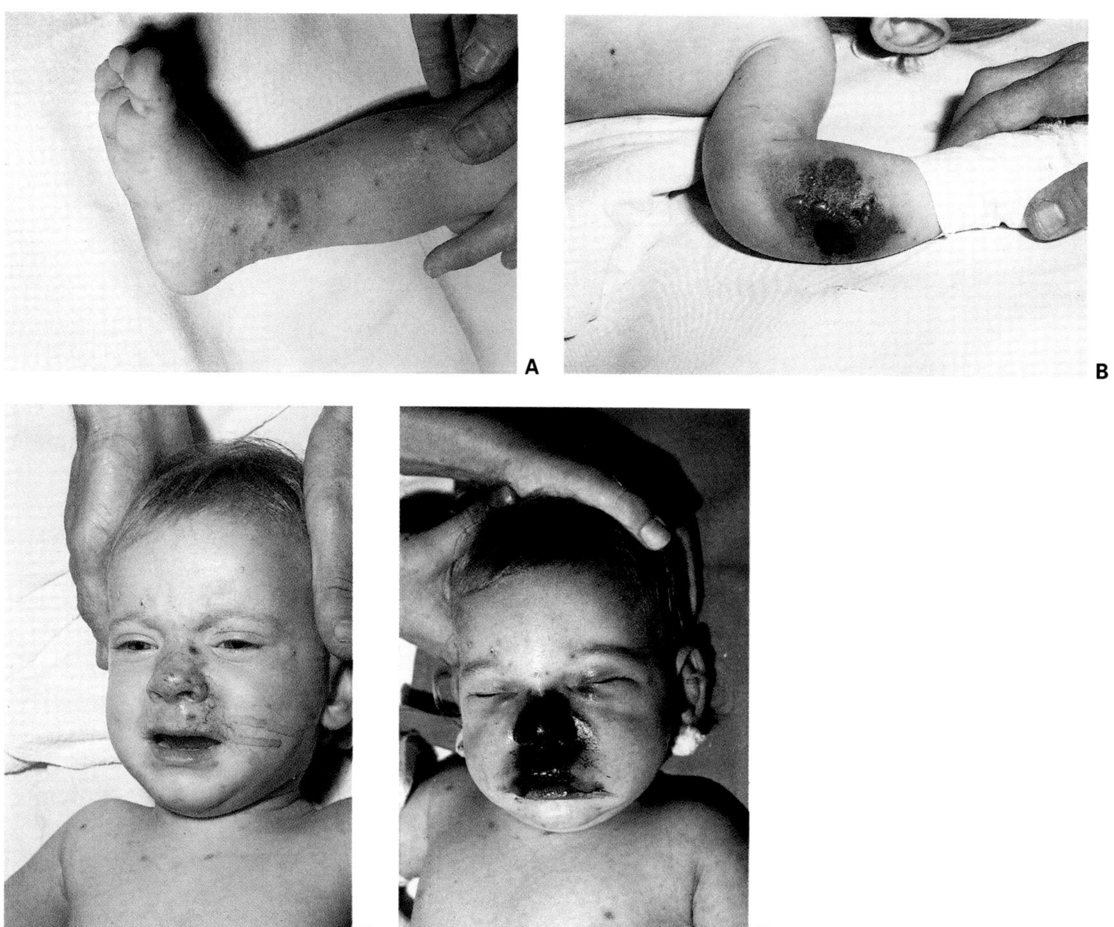

Fig. 8.7 Purpura fulminans in a 17-month-old girl convalescing from varicella. **a–c** (taken at same time): early lesions. **d** (next day): established necrosis. Protein C normal, protein S < 0.06 U/ml. A satisfactory arrest and resolution were achieved with low molecular weight dextran and steroid. Copyright The Medical Journal of Australia 1967; 2: 685–687. Reproduced with permission

Malignancy

In malignancy haemostatic deficiencies are usually due to causes other than DIC, e.g. thrombocytopenia from marrow infiltration, and coagulation factor deficiencies from liver infiltration or deficient intake or absorption of vitamin K. Convincing evidence of intravascular coagulation is however noted in some malignancies (Table 8.20), though fragmentation haemolysis is uncommon.

Trauma, burns

Coagulation tests are more consistently abnormal than the platelet count. In head injury, depletion of factors occurs in some cases (Fig. 8.5c) and shortening of APTT and TCT from activation of factors in others.

Maternal disease and intravascular coagulation in the neonate

Thrombosis in the neonate may be associated with abruptio placentae, severe maternal eclampsia (placental passage of thromboplastin, fetal hypoxia) and maternal diabetes mellitus (attributed to diminished capacity of endothelium to synthesize prostacyclin, Stuart et al 1985).

Envenomation

There is great variation in rate of development, severity and chronicity of haemostatic disturbance in snake and spider envenomation, with variable defibrinogenation/DIC, thrombocytopenia and haemolysis of fragmentation, normocytic, or spherocytic type. Venoms may act directly on fibrinogen (Fig. 8.1) or activate factors X or II. Although haemostatic abnormalities may be severe (e.g. incoagulable blood), bleeding may be surprisingly mild and is more likely if thrombocytopenia (platelet aggregation) accompanies hypofibrinogenaemia.

Blood cell destruction

Some types of blood cell destruction are associated with (usually mild) DIC, attributed to release of thromboplastins by direct damage or complement activation: incompatible blood transfusion, severe Rh disease of newborn, sickle cell crisis, paroxysmal nocturnal haemoglobinuria and extracorporeal bypass cardiac surgery (damage to platelets and erythrocytes).

Amniotic fluid inhalation

A persistent pulmonary hypertension in neonates associated with pulmonary microthrombi is attributed to the thromboplastic effect of amniotic fluid inhaled at birth (Levin et al 1983).

Cyanotic congenital heart disease (Maurer 1972, Waldman et al 1975)

Mild haemostatic abnormalities are common and associated with bleeding during and after surgery, haematuria, or less often thrombosis:

- thrombocytopenia in up to half of patients, especially if > 3 years old, and hct is > 0.6 and Hb > 16.0 g/dl; platelet survival is diminished
- thrombocytopathy (bleeding time, aggregations) in up to 40% of patients
- hyperfibrinolysis commonly accompanies thrombocytopenia
- increase in FDP
- deficiency of isolated coagulation factors (I, II, V, VII, VIII), not due to liver dysfunction
- during surgery, dilution of coagulation factors in the bypass system and inadequate neutralization of heparin by protamine
- artefactual prolongation of PT + APTT from citrate excess in polycythaemia (plasma lack, Table 8.1) is to be excluded.

The pathogenesis of the abnormalities is obscure. Low-grade intravascular coagulation from hyperviscosity is possible but unlikely; liver hypoxia may be a component.

Haemostatic abnormalities are infrequent in acyanotic disease and include loss of large vWF multimers, mild deficit in platelet function and mild F XII deficiency (Gill et al 1986).

Macrothrombotic states with little or no DIC (Table 8.22)

As a rough generalization, macroscopic thrombosis, because it is usually not widespread, is less likely to be associated with DIC than microvascular thrombosis. The distinction, however, is unrealistic or unsharp for some disorders; for example, in purpura fulminans, small and large vessels may be affected, and in protein C/S deficiency widespread thrombosis with DIC is common in the homozygote and rare in the heterozygote.

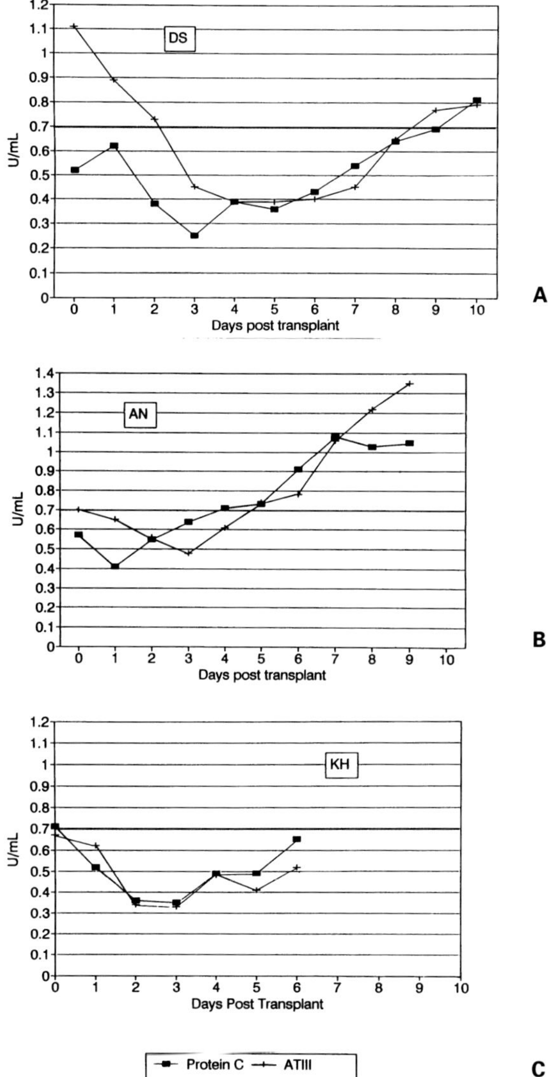

Fig. 8.8 Plasma levels of coagulation inhibitors in relation to thrombosis of hepatic artery post liver transplant. **a** Transplant of child liver, thrombosis recognized on day 5. **b** Transplant of child liver, no thrombosis. **c** Transplant of cut-down adult liver, no thrombosis.

Table 8.22 Macroscopic thrombosis in childhood with little or no DIC[1]

Endothelial damage	
Mechanical or other irritation	catheters
	cardiac valve prosthesis
	disseminated malignancy
	vasculitis (polyarteritis, Wegener's, Kawasaki)
	myocardial infarction
	endocardial fibroelastosis
Stasis	immobilization of limb
Other	lupus anticoagulant[2]
	hypereosinophilic syndrome
	homocystinuria
	PNH
Hypercoagulable state	
Hyperviscosity	erythrocytosis (cyanotic congenital heart disease, dehydrated infant, polycythaemia vera)
	sickle cell disease
	thrombocytosis (essential thrombocythaemia, infantile cortical hyperostosis[3])
	hyperleucocytosis (leukaemia)
Inhibitor deficiency	ATIII
	protein C
	protein S
Resistance to inhibitors	mutant F V
Defective fibrinolysis	inherited dysfibrinogenaemias (some types)
	plasminogen deficiency
	tPA deficiency
	F XII deficiency
Coagulants	prothrombin complex concentrate
	ϵ-aminocaproic acid
	tranexamic acid
Platelet hyperreactivity	diabetes mellitus
	nephrotic syndrome
	Kawasaki disease
	cyclosporin
	hyperlipoproteinaemia
Origin obscure	neonatal thrombosis (many cases)

[1] Mechanism for thrombosis in some disorders uncertain. More than 1 mechanism operates in some disorders
[2] Crosses placenta if IgG
[3] Pickering & Cuddigan 1969. Other causes of secondary thrombocytosis do not appear to predispose to thrombosis

As a general guide, endothelial damage predisposes to either venous or arterial thrombosis, and hypercoagulable states to venous thrombosis. A predisposing cause should be sought if:

- no clinically identifiable cause can be found
- there is a family history of thrombosis
- thrombosis is recurrent.

Homocystinuria (cystathione synthetase deficiency)

A syndrome of mental retardation, ectopia lentis, skeletal deformity, progressive cardiovascular disease and thromboembolism (myocardial, cerebral, renal, pulmonary). Thrombosis is attributed to endothelial damage from high plasma homocystine, but diminished ATIII and F VII (impaired synthesis) may contribute (Palareti et al 1986).

ATIII deficiency

Inherited deficiency is heterozygous (autosomal dominant), with values about half normal. Homozygous deficiency is probably incompatible with life. Thromboembolism is unlikely before 20 years and may be spontaneous or follow trauma, surgery or acute illness. Deficiency may however manifest in the neonate (Brenner et al 1988). Thrombosis in the neonate is unlikely to be due to ATIII deficiency unless levels are well below (< 0.3 U/ml) the normal for the neonate (Table 8.5).

Acquired deficiency occurs in:

- liver disease (impaired synthesis); other factors contributing to thrombosis include impaired synthesis of protein C and plasminogen, administration of prothrombin complex concentrates, and (post liver transplant) small size of hepatic/portal vessels (if donor a child, Fig. 8.8, Harper et al 1988)
- nephrotic syndrome (loss in urine); loss of protein C and plasminogen in urine and platelet hyperreactivity (below) contribute to thrombotic tendency
- L-asparaginase (Mitchell et al 1994); alteration in multimeric structure of vWF may contribute to thrombosis (Pui et al 1985)
- DIC, as part of the consumption process.

Protein C, S deficiency

See page 294.

Resistance to inhibitors

A heterozygous or homozygous point mutation in the F V gene which renders F V resistant to activated protein C (APC resistance) is the commonest cause of inherited predisposition to venous thrombosis (Bertina et al 1994).

Defective fibrinolysis

Thrombosis is usually not manifest before adolescence and may be precipitated by trauma. Most cases have autosomal dominant inheritance.

In the inherited dysfibrinogenaemias, thrombosis occurs in that minority in which there is suboptimal interaction of the abnormal fibrin with the plasminogen system. See also page 288.

Plasminogen deficiency may be inherited or, more commonly, acquired: in liver disease from impaired synthesis and in nephrosis from loss in urine. Deficiencies of ATIII and protein C are usually associated.

TPA deficiency may result from subnormal production/release from endothelial cells (Table 8.15) or from hereditary high levels of PAI.

Heterozygous or homozygous F XII deficiency is associated with thromboembolism attributed to diminished activation of the fibrinolytic system.

Platelet hyperreactivity

Characterized by exaggerated aggregability in response to a variety of agonists, due, in part at least, to enhanced synthesis of TXA2 from arachidonic acid.

In diabetes mellitus platelet hyperreactivity may be noted early in the disease (Kobbah et al 1985) and persist despite adequate control of blood sugar (Jackson et al 1984).

In nephrosis, hyperreactivity is attributed to greater availability of arachidonic acid, less of which is bound to the depleted serum albumin (Jackson et al 1982). Other factors contributing to thrombosis include loss in urine of ATIII, protein C and plasminogen.

In Kawasaki disease hyperreactivity is due to increased TXA2 synthesis. Increase in β thromboglobulin, another index of platelet activation, may identify those at risk for coronary artery aneurysm and thrombosis (Burns et al 1984). Hyperreactivity may persist for up to 9 months. Also possibly contributing to thrombosis is an increase in acute phase reactants such as VIII:C, fibrinogen and platelets.

Thrombosis in patients receiving cyclosporin is attributed to platelet hyperaggregability (Grace et al 1987). Other factors may contribute, e.g. after liver transplantation, reduction in ATIII, protein C and plasminogen (Fig. 8.8).

Platelet hyperreactivity has been noted in hyperlipoproteinaemia (Tremoli et al 1984).

Thrombosis of obscure origin

Thrombosis in the neonate may be a consequence of catheter placement, hypoxia (Favara et al 1974), myocardial infarction (Fig. 8.9) or maternal disease (p. 296), and is more frequent in infants who are sick or of low birth weight and in those receiving hyperosmolar solutions.

In a significant proportion however a satisfactory explanation is not found (Fig. 8.9). Factors thought to predispose the neonate to thrombosis include diminished capacity for clearance of activated coagulation factors and naturally low level of inhibitors (Table 8.5).

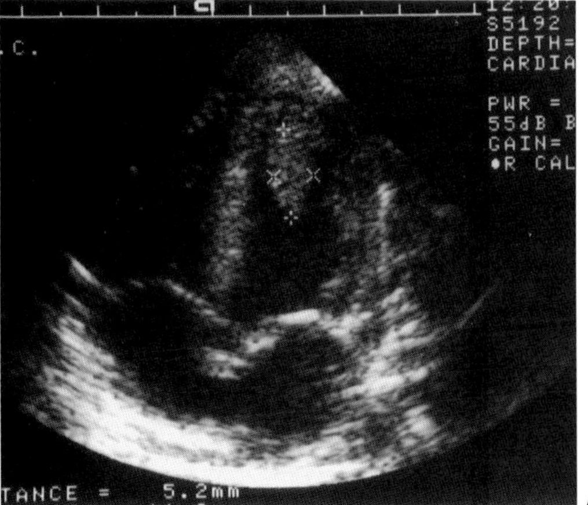

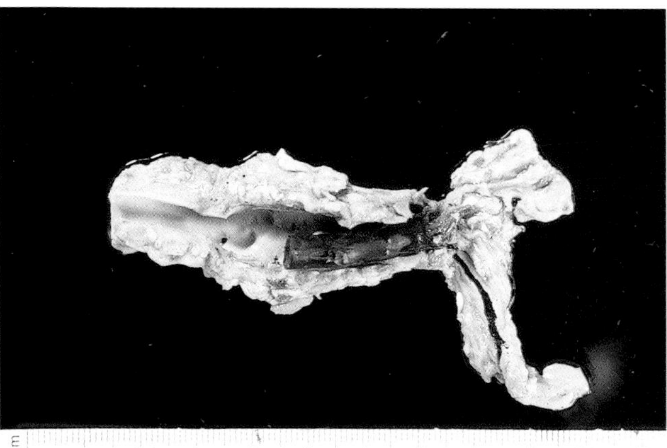

B

Fig. 8.9 Macroscopic thrombosis/embolus in the neonate. **a** Echocardiogram of a 2-week-old infant, showing thrombus in left ventricle (asterisks) attributed to myocardial damage from birth asphyxia. The infant presented with blanching of both legs due to embolus at the aorto iliac bifurcation. **b** Aorto-iliac thrombosis of unknown cause associated with thrombocytopenia (to 8×10^9/l) in a 15-day-old infant. Thrombosis also affected portal and left renal veins. The infant was well until onset of cyanosis and fever on 5th day.

Thrombocytopenias of childhood

An outline classification by mechanism is given in Table 8.23 and an outline of investigation in Table 8.24. Artefacts to be considered include:

- Spurious thrombocytopenia, usually due to clotting in sample (Table 8.1).
- Spurious megakaryocyte deficiency in marrow aspirates from neonates. More than one sample (or trephine biopsy) may be required for correct assessment.

THROMBOCYTOPENIAS DUE TO MEGAKARYOCYTE DEFICIENCY

a. Megakaryocyte numbers diminished, with pancytopenia

'Acquired amegakaryocytic' thrombocytopenia
Excessively rare in childhood (Scarlett et al 1992). Diagnosis requires exclusion of other disorders in Table 8.25, especially Fanconi anaemia. In addition to virtual absence of megakaryocytes, the erythron is dyspoietic (macrocytosis) and hyperplastic. Thrombocytopenia is severe, with mild to moderate anaemia and leucopenia. Precursor cells for each lineage are deficient in marrow. Chromosomal fragility (p. 48) is not excessive. About 20% evolve to frank aplasia of marrow.

Other causes
These are considered in appropriate chapters.

b. Megakaryocyte numbers diminished, with isolated thrombocytopenia

Fetal infection
Megakaryocyte deficiency tends to be most severe in viral infections, may be associated with haemophagocytosis and is due to damage by the organism directly or by antigen/antibody complexes.

Thrombocytopenia is usually not severe, usually does not persist for more than 6 weeks after birth, and may be associated with leucoerythroblastic anaemia (erythroblasts and immature granulocytes in blood film).

Fanconi syndrome
The usual presentation is pancytopenia at 5–10 years of age. Occasionally, however, isolated thrombocytopenia antedates other cytopenias (this may first manifest shortly after birth). See page 48.

TAR syndrome (Hall 1987, Fig. 8.11)

Major characteristics
- severe thrombocytopenia at (and before) birth; may be worsened by stress, infection or surgery
- bilateral absence of radius (radial deviation of wrists, flexion of elbows)
- megakaryocytes absent or virtually absent in marrow; the few remaining are small, immature, vacuolated and agranular (presumed signs of poor function)
- platelet antibodies not demonstrable.

Other features
- Gradual improvement in platelet count, especially after the first year, is usual; count may reach almost normal by adulthood; platelets deficient in dense bodies (storage pool deficiency), with shortened survival.
- A transient CML-like myeloproliferation of unknown nature occurs in 60–70% of cases in the first year, with leucocyte counts up to about $140 \times 10^9/l$, a small percentage of blast cells, and (in about half) mild eosinophilia. NAP is normal to increased. Enlargement of liver, spleen and lymph nodes may occur.
- Limb bones additional to radii may be absent or dysplastic.
- Congenital heart disease (Fallot's tetralogy, atrial septal defect) in some cases.
- No propensity to aplastic anaemia or leukaemia.
- Autosomal recessive.

Table 8.23 Isolated thrombocytopenia in childhood: outline

Impaired production[1]
Ineffective thrombopoiesis[1]
Excess destruction
Immune
Non-immune: extrinsic
intrinsic (faulty platelets)
Excess utilization[1]
DIC
Macroscopic thrombosis
Redistribution
Hypersplenism[1]
Dilution
Massive transfusion of stored blood[2]

[1] Usually with other cytopenias
[2] > 1 blood volume in < 24 h

Table 8.24 Isolated thrombocytopenia in childhood: investigation

Associated clinical features, e.g.
Eczema
Renal disease
Deafness
Familial occurrence
Platelet morphology
Light microscopy
Electron microscopy
Marrow megakaryocytes (aspirate + trephine biopsy)
Number
Morphology
Platelet function if suspect thrombocytopathy (bleeding tendency excessive for platelet count)
Platelet antibodies
As indicated
Platelet glycoproteins
Tests for autoimmune disease
Direct antiglobulin test
Cardiolipin antibodies
Tests for vWD
Platelet survival

Table 8.25 Thrombocytopenia with diminished megakaryocytes

With other cytopenias
Marrow hypoplasia
Leukaemia
Myelodysplasia
Gaucher's disease[1]
'Acquired amegakaryocytic' thrombocytopenia
Isolated thrombocytopenia
Fetal: infection (rubella, CMV, toxoplasmosis, syphilis)
drugs (? thiazides)
Immune[2]
Fanconi syndrome, before global aplasia
TAR syndrome
Other congenital syndromes, e.g. trisomy 18, phocomelia
Congenital amegakaryocytic thrombocytopenia

[1] Hypersplenism contributes to thrombocytopenia
[2] In occasional cases of immune thrombocytopenia destruction of megakaryocytes contributes to thrombocytopenia

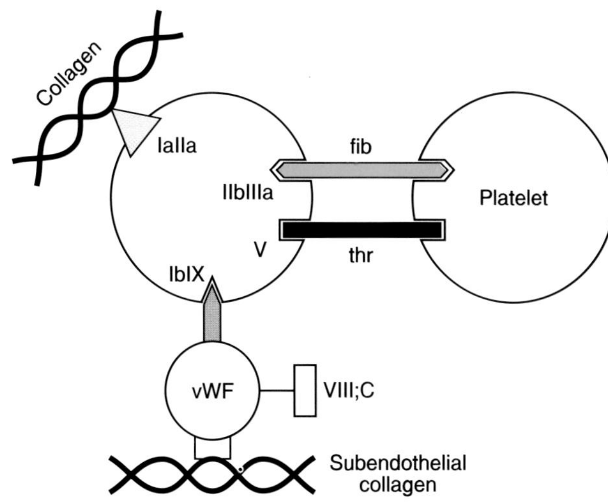

Fig. 8.10 Some aspects of platelet function, simplified schema. fib = fibrinogen; thr = thrombin.

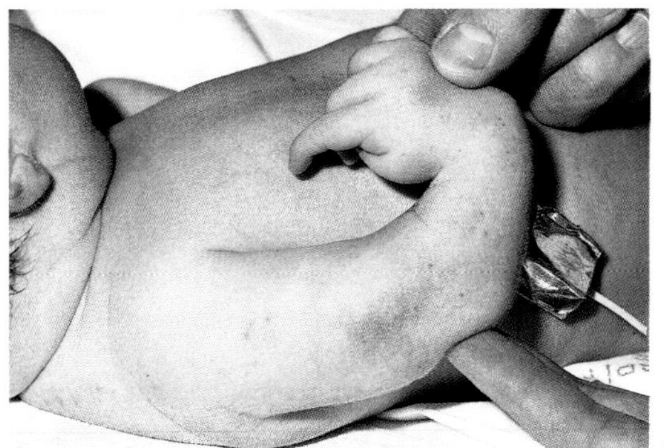

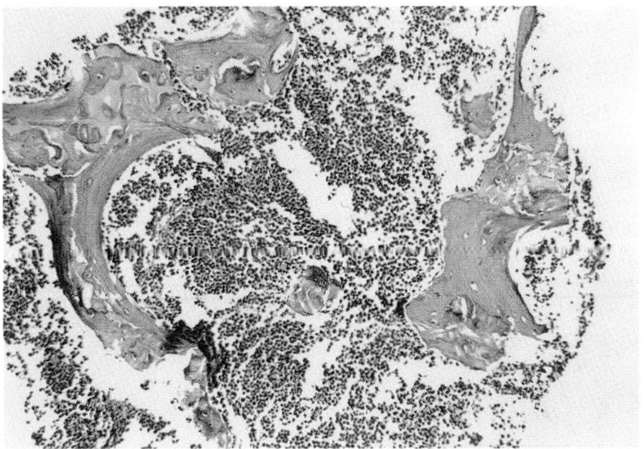

Fig. 8.11 TAR syndrome. **a** Radial deviation of wrist, age 6 days. **b** Marrow (autopsy, 5 weeks) showing absence of megakaryocytes. H & E × 60

Differential diagnosis

a. Fanconi syndrome (p. 48)

- absence of both radii with preservation of fingers and thumbs does not occur
- thrombocytopenia rarely isolated
- marrow deficient in all cell lines rather than megakaryocytes only
- chromosomal fragility increased.

b. CML adult type (p. 176)

- no association with absent radii
- leucocyte counts often $> 140 \times 10^9/l$
- NAP usually decreased
- karyotype abnormal.

Other congenital syndromes

Thrombocytopenia with deficiency or absence of megakaryocytes in marrow may be associated rarely with trisomy 18, phocomelia (truncation of limbs with variable preservation of hands and feet) and other syndromes. Myeloid leukaemoid reactions may be noted, similar to but milder than those in TAR (above). In some cases thrombocytopenia tends to improve with age (Dignan et al 1967, Rabinowitz et al 1967, Cherstvoy et al 1980, Gardner et al 1983).

Congenital amegakaryocytic thrombocytopenia (Freedman & Estrov 1990)

This rare syndrome has similarities to acquired amegakaryocytic thrombocytopenia (p. 300). Severe deficiency of megakaryocytes, attributed to stem cell defect, occurs without associated physical defects; chromosome fragility is normal. At first there are no other haematologic abnormalities, but about 80% evolve, at a median age of about 3 years, to aplastic anaemia.

THROMBOCYTOPENIAS DUE TO INEFFECTIVE THROMBOPOIESIS (Table 8.26)

Diagnosis requires demonstration of adequate numbers of megakaryocytes in marrow together with normal or only mildly shortened survival of blood platelets.

May-Hegglin anomaly (Hamilton et al 1980)

A syndrome of large platelets (Fig. 8.12) and Döhle-like bodies in granulocytes (Fig. 6.10). Unusually small platelets also occur. Internal platelet structure is normal by light microscopy. Thrombocytopenia, usually mild, occurs in about half of patients and is attributed to defective fragmentation of megakaryocytes. The bleeding time is prolonged for the platelet count but survival and in vitro tests of platelet function are normal. Inheritance autosomal dominant. For differential diagnosis (from Fechtner and Sebastian anomalies) see Table 8.29 and page 216.

Bernard-Soulier syndrome

See page 313.

Table 8.26 Thrombocytopenias due to ineffective thrombopoiesis

Thrombocytopenias due to ineffective thrombopoiesis
Impaired megakaryocyte maturation
May-Hegglin
Bernard-Soulier[1]
Wiskott-Aldrich
Greaves
Thrombopoietin deficiency[2]
Megaloblastic anaemias (Ch. 2)
Other
Intramedullary death of platelets
Myeloproliferative disease
Impaired egress of platelets from marrow
Najean-Lecompte

[1] Shortened survival of platelets contributes to thrombocytopenia
[2] Existence as a genuine anomaly uncertain

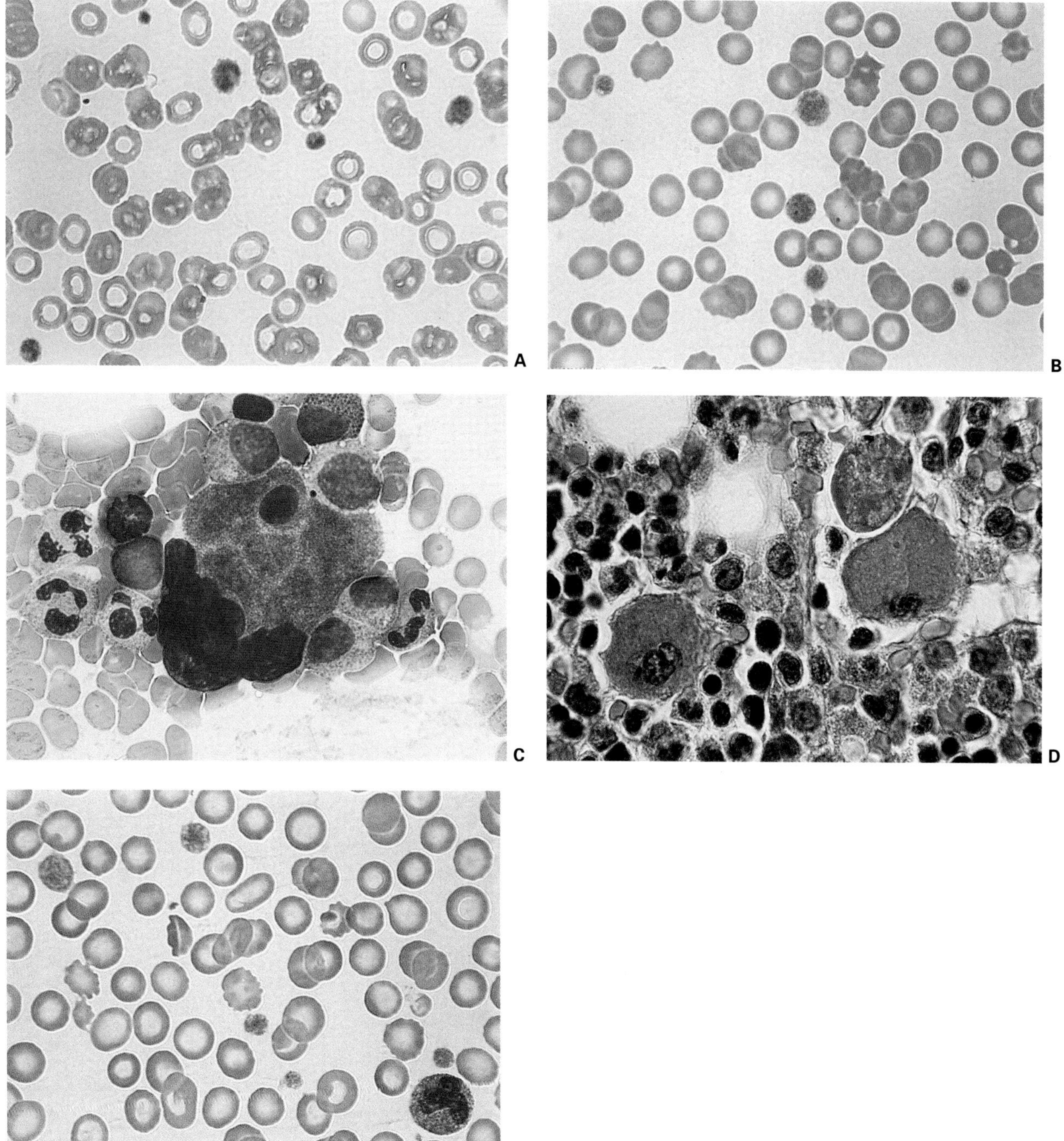

Fig. 8.12 Macroplatelet disorders. **a** May-Hegglin anomaly. **b** Inherited Bernard-Soulier syndrome. **c,d** Unidentified macrothrombocytopenia with degenerate megakaryocytes, platelet glycoproteins normal. Aspirate (**c**) shows megakaryocyte with lumpy cytoplasm; trephine biopsy (**d**) shows 2 of 3 megakaryocytes degenerate, one with single small peripheral nucleus, one anuclear. **e** As a transient (weeks) phenomenon in a 7-week-old infant with staphylococcal pneumonia and adenosine deaminase deficiency. **c,d** Courtesy of Dr K Taylor

Wiskott-Aldrich syndrome (WAS) (Ochs et al 1980)
An X-linked combination of:

- Thrombocytopenia

Severe, present from (and before) birth. Platelets are small (Fig. 8.13) and stain poorly with PAS (subnormal glycogen). Platelet survival is near normal if immunization by platelet transfusions has not occurred. The major component in thrombocytopenia is ineffective thrombopoiesis; megakaryocyte numbers are normal to increased and nuclei may show fragmentation and other signs of damage.

- Eczema

Appears usually by 3 months.

- Immunodeficiency

Symptoms begin after about 6 months. Inability to produce antibody to polysaccharide antigens manifests as susceptibility to pyogenic, polysaccharide-encapsulated bacteria, especially pneumococcus, meningococcus and *H. influenzae*. Patients are susceptible also to viruses, especially herpes and warts, as well as pneumocystis. Serum IgM and ABO isoagglutinins (IgM) are diminished or absent. Increases occur in IgA, IgE (usually considerable) and often IgG. Ig levels may be normal in the first 2 years. Lymphocytes lack the 115 kD surface sialophorin.

Other features
Lymphopenia and eosinophilia are common. Lymphopenia however is usually not evident till about 6 years. A Coombs-positive haemolysis occurs in some cases and may be transient. Lymphoid malignancy, especially of the central nervous system, is a risk.

Partial forms of WAS may occur (Weiden & Blaese 1972). The relation between WAS and other X-linked thrombocytopenias (Table 8.29) is uncertain.

Greaves syndrome (Greaves et al 1987)
Congenital thrombocytopenia (to $51 \times 10^9/l$) with plentiful but abnormal megakaryocytes in marrow. MPV normal but platelets abnormal in size (small and large), ultrastructure and aggregability (ADP, adrenalin, collagen). Arachidonic acid mobilization is defective. Megakaryocyte abnormalities include nuclear/cytoplasmic asynchrony, cytoplasmic inclusions of nuclear material and shift to higher nuclear ploidy. Thrombocytopenia is attributed to defective fragmentation of megakaryocyte cytoplasm. Autosomal dominant.

Thrombopoietin deficiency
Rare cases of congenital thrombocytopenia responsive to infusions of whole plasma have been attributed to deficiency of a thrombopoietin (Schulman et al 1960). Marrow megakaryocytes are adequate in number but of immature appearance. This interpretation however is uncertain — Schulman's patient was diagnosed at the age of 31 years as chronic relapsing thrombotic thrombocytopenic purpura (Moake et al 1982).

Other megakaryocyte anomalies
See Figure 8.12c,d.

Myeloproliferative disease
Faulty quality of megakaryocytes/platelets may be surmised from excessive phagocytosis by marrow macrophages (Fig. 5.18).

Impaired egress of platelets from marrow (Najean & Lecompte 1990)
Megakaryocytes are normal in number and morphology (light and electron microscopy). Platelet survival is normal (autologous and homologous). Thrombocytopenia is moderate to severe (to $10 \times 10^9/l$), with a tendency to uniformity among family members (autosomal dominant). Platelets are large (MPV 10–18 fl) but of normal function, and there is no excess of platelet-bound IgG. Bleeding tendency is mild or absent. There may be a propensity to AML (3 of 54 cases).

Distinction from immune thrombocytopenia is important as presently available treatments, including splenectomy, are ineffective.

IMMUNE THROMBOCYTOPENIAS (Table 8.27)

The commonest isolated thrombocytopenias of childhood. Antibody and/or complement-coated platelets are removed by reticuloendothelial macrophages, especially in spleen (Fig. 8.14) and, in severe cases, liver also. Thrombocytopenia is usually severe ($< 50 \times 10^9/l$) but in ITP and SLE counts tend to be higher than in other disorders. Usually some platelets in blood films are large (young active platelets).

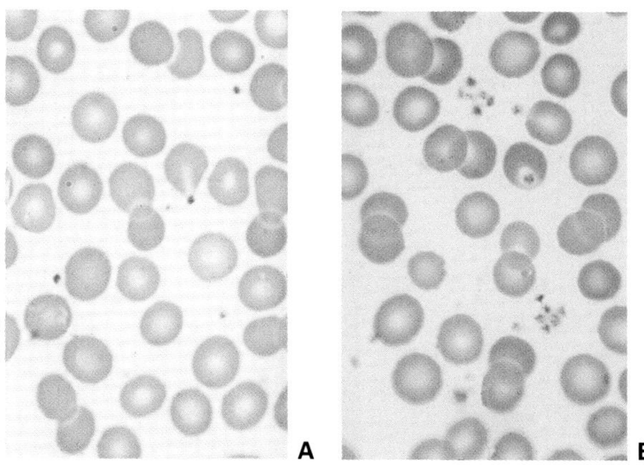

Fig. 8.13 Wiskott-Aldrich syndrome — small, sparse platelets (**a**) vs normal platelets (**b**). × 750

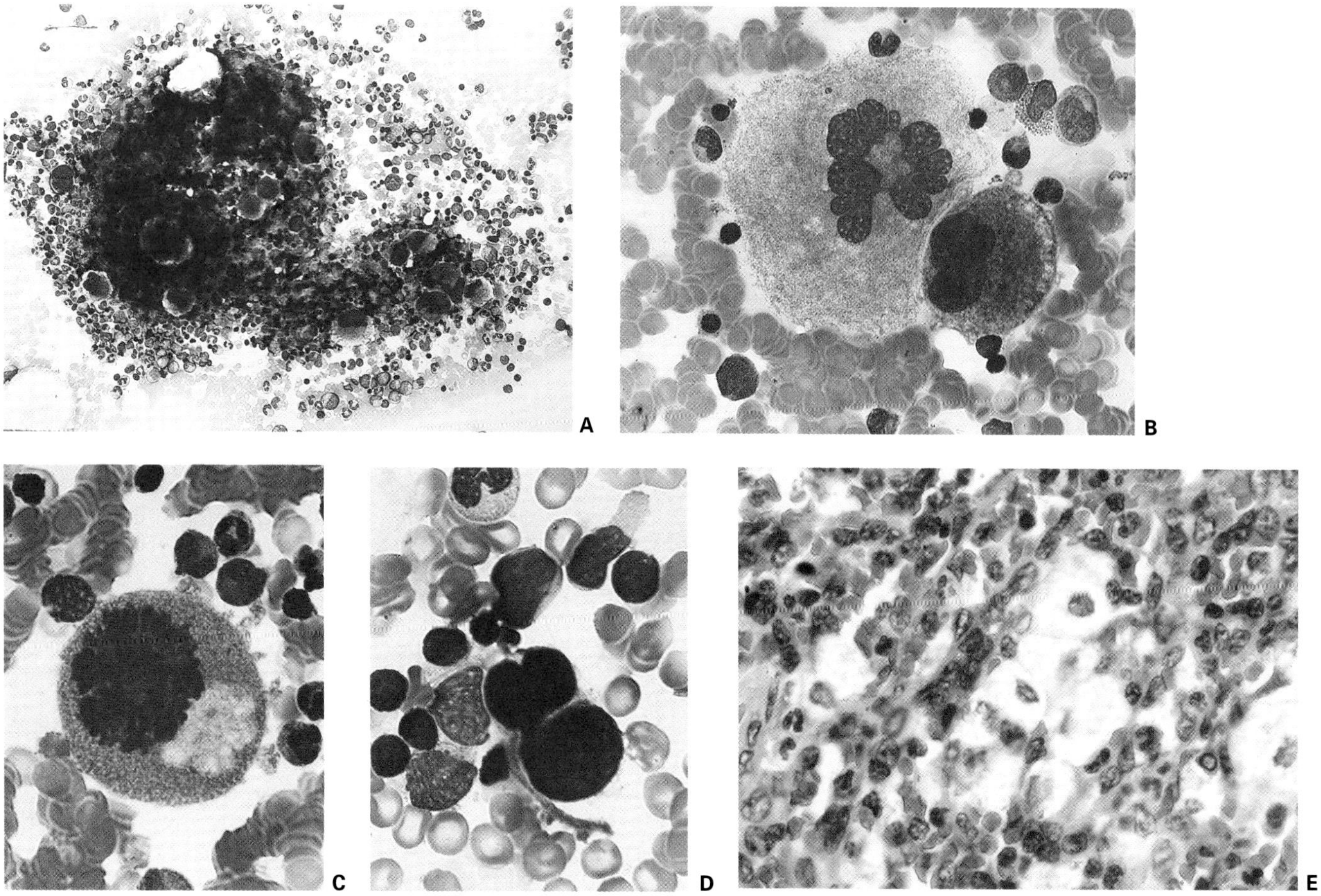

Fig. 8.14 Autoimmune thrombocytopenias. **a–d** Megakaryocytes in marrow, post-viral thrombocytopenia. Cells in abundance (**a**), mature and immature forms (**b**), mitosis (**c**), cell death (**d**). **e** Spleen, chronic immune thrombocytopenia, showing groups of macrophages, a site of platelet destruction. **a** × 120; **b** × 500; **c,d** × 750; **e** × 600

Megakaryocytes in marrow (Fig. 8.14) are normal to increased in number, often with some shift to the left. Dead megakaryocytes may rarely be noted. Megakaryocytes are occasionally severely depleted as a result of destruction by antibody (Bizzaro & Dianese 1988).

Foamy macrophages, presumably a result of platelet phagocytosis and destruction, may be noted in small numbers, and are more prominent in patients on steroids. Plasma acid phosphatase may be increased due to platelet destruction.

Table 8.27 Thrombocytopenias in childhood due to excess destruction: immune

Autoimmune
- Post-viral[1]
- Other infections
- Idiopathic
- Autoimmune disease or component of disease
  - SLE[2]
  - Antiphospholipid syndrome
  - Rheumatoid arthritis[3]
  - Evans syndrome
  - Hodgkin's disease[4]
  - Non-Hodgkin lymphoma[4]
  - Hyperthyroidism
  - Ulcerative colitis
  - Solid tumours
- Drug-immune (Table 8.30)[5]
- Acquired passively from mother
  - ITP
  - Gestational thrombocytopenia
  - SLE
  - Drugs/food additives (e.g. quinidine)

Alloimmune
- Fetomaternal incompatibility
- Platelet refractoriness
- Transplantation of fetal thymus, marrow

[1] May not be true autoimmune — in at least some cases, platelet antibody cross-reacts with viral antigens
[2] Thrombocytopenia may precede overt disease by years
[3] Thrombocytopenia rare (Sherry & Kredich 1985); thrombocytosis more characteristic
[4] Thrombocytopenia may precede overt disease by months and may presage relapse
[5] True autoimmune in only few cases

Post-viral thrombocytopenia

The commonest thrombocytopenia of childhood beyond the neonatal period.

Major characteristics

● Onset in phase of recovery (1–6 weeks, initiation of antibody production) from viral infection. This may be of specific type (varicella, rubella, rubeola, mumps, infectious mononucleosis, hepatitis, HIV, CMV), or more commonly a nondescript, especially respiratory or gastrointestinal infection. In HIV infection, thrombocytopenia may antedate or follow onset of characteristic symptoms. Antiviral vaccination may also be followed by thrombocytopenia. The propensity to thrombocytopenia may be greater for rubella than for other viral illnesses. Familial occurrence is rare.

Viral infections are so common in childhood that a causal connection with thrombocytopenia in an individual case may be unconvincing. Nevertheless, a history of recent viral illness or viral vaccination justifies a diagnosis of post-viral thrombocytopenia and optimism for recovery.

● Thrombocytopenia characteristically is sudden in onset (< 2 weeks, usually days) and is due to antigen/antibody complexes attaching to the surface (see below). By contrast, thrombocytopenia at the height of viral illness is likely to be due to destruction by virus itself or consumption in a process of DIC.

● Minimal changes in blood and marrow apart from thrombocytopenia (see below).

Other characteristics

1. Blood

● Thrombocytopenia

Usually severe (< 50 and often < 20×10^9/l). Measurement of bleeding time at this stage is not useful and not recommended. MPV is usually increased (young, active platelets).

● Leucocytes

Reactive lymphocytes are present in variable numbers, depending on the nature of the viral infection (Tables 7.14, 7.15) and the relation in time to the infection. Toxic change in neutrophils is usually mild, in keeping with viral infection. Occasionally, immune neutropenia accompanies thrombocytopenia. A mild eosinophilia (< 1.0×10^9/l) is frequent.

• Erythrocytes
Anaemia occurs in a minority (about 20%), usually in proportion to blood loss. Occasionally erythrocytes also are a target for antibody: if IgM, without morphologic changes (the usual), or with variable agglutination, spherocytosis and positive Coombs test; if IgG, usually more severe changes (p. 74).

• Platelet antibody
IgM and/or IgG autoantibodies to platelet glycoproteins are detectable in most cases. The transient course of most post-viral thrombocytopenias correlates with the high incidence of IgM antibody (Winiarski 1989). Antibodies to Gp Ib, IIb and IIIa are the most commonly identified by Western immunoblot. Antibody may not be true autoantibody — in some cases at least, platelet antibodies cross-react with viral antigens (Wright et al 1994).

Examination for platelet antibody has little impact at present on diagnosis and management and in any case is usually not feasible in severe thrombocytopenia. However, a sensitive method such as platelet immunofluorescence by flow cytometry gives useful information if some platelets can be harvested. There is no correlation between quantity of platelet-associated Ig and severity of thrombocytopenia. Free antibody and platelet-associated Ig may persist for a short time after recovery of platelet count, spontaneously or post-splenectomy ('compensated' platelet destruction).

Muffling of Gp by antibody may affect platelet function; bleeding time may be excessive for the thrombocytopenia (testing not recommended in severe thrombocytopenia), aggregations may be defective (whole blood more reliable than conventional aggregometry if count $< 100 \times 10^9/l$), and bleeding may be exacerbated.

Measurement of survival and organ uptake of labelled platelets does not predict the possible effect of splenectomy on count.

• Other autoantibodies
Thyroid or parietal cell autoantibodies occur in a small proportion (< 1%) of cases (Walker & Walker 1984, Reid M 1993, personal communication). The frequency of thyroid antibodies is no greater than in a random population of similar age, but parietal cell antibody in children without intrinsic factor antibody or abnormality of plasma B_{12} or Hb level is unusual.

• Coagulation factor abnormalities
A mild, temporary prolongation of APTT, due to viral-induced lupus anticoagulant (p. 285), occurs occasionally.

2. Marrow
Because of the virtual certainty that isolated thrombocytopenia following viral infection in an otherwise healthy child is post-viral, some paediatricians may not request marrow examination for confirmation. However, marrow examination is recommended to exclude the rare possibility of thrombocytopenia as the only blood manifestation of leukaemia or marrow aplasia, and especially if steroid treatment is contemplated (which may efface evidence of leukaemia).

Changes which may be noted additional to those mentioned (p. 306) include:

- reactive lymphocytes, as an indication of viral infection, but in notably fewer numbers than in blood
- eosinophils often at upper normal or slightly increased
- except for distinctive inclusion-containing giant cells in some cases of CMV (Fig. 5.9), marrow changes are not specific for viral infection.

3. Natural history
Incidence of cerebral haemorrhage is < 1%. There is no correlation between severity of thrombocytopenia and long-term outlook for recovery (Table 8.28). Recurrence is rare. Failure of the platelet count to exceed $300 \times 10^9/l$ after 2 weeks is a predictor of failure of splenectomy (Walker & Walker 1984).

Immune thrombocytopenia in non-viral infections

Ig coating of platelets is a more frequent cause of thrombocytopenia in bacterial infection than DIC (Kelton et al 1979). Thrombocytopenia tends to be of shorter duration (< 2 weeks) than viral-immune thrombocytopenia. An immune component is likely also in the thrombocytopenia of malaria (Kelton et al 1983).

Idiopathic thrombocytopenic purpura (ITP)

In childhood about one third as common as post-viral thrombocytopenia.

Major characteristics

- isolated thrombocytopenia without obvious cause or antecedent, and especially no clear history of preceding infection
- minimal changes in blood and marrow apart from thrombocytopenia
- exclusion of other causes of isolated thrombocytopenia (see differential diagnosis).

Other characteristics

Platelet-bound Ig is detectable in about three quarters of patients, specificity in most to the GpIIb–IIIa complex, less often Ib, occasionally both (McMillan et al 1987). As in post-viral thrombocytopenia, attached antibody may affect platelet function. Measurement of platelet survival and organ uptake of labelled platelets does not predict the effect of splenectomy on count.

Differential diagnosis

Isolated thrombocytopenias which may be misidentified as ITP include:

- post-viral thrombocytopenia (Table 8.28), including chronic viraemias such as HIV infection
- autoimmune disease, e.g. SLE
- familial/inherited thrombocytopenias.

Hereditary thrombocytopenias which are, or appear to be, separate disorders are summarized in Table 8.29 (most are considered again elsewhere in this chapter). The most important which might be confused with ITP are: Wiskott-Aldrich syndrome (or 'partial' forms of this), May-Hegglin anomaly, type IIb and platelet-type vWD and Najean-Lecompte thrombocytopenia.

Natural history

The outlook for recovery is not as optimistic as for post-viral thrombocytopenia (Table 8.28). Failure of platelet count to exceed $300 \times 10^9/l$ after 2 weeks is a predictor of failure of splenectomy (Walker & Walker 1984). Isolated thrombocytopenia may be a prodrome (up to several years) of autoimmune disease such as SLE or acquired haemolytic anaemia.

Thrombocytopenia in autoimmune disease or as an autoimmune component of a disease

Thrombocytopenia occurs in up to 15% of patients with SLE and may antedate (years) overt expression (possibility of misdiagnosis as ITP). Lupus-type anticoagulant may coexist as part of the antiphospholipid syndrome (Hughes et al 1989). The Coombs test may be positive in the absence of anaemia or morphologic change in erythrocytes such as spherocytosis.

Autoimmune haemolysis and/or neutropenia may be associated with thrombocytopenia in:

- viral infection (p. 75)
- SLE, rheumatoid arthritis
- other, uncharacterized immune disease, e.g. a syndrome of eczema, alopecia and benign lymphoid hyperplasia (Miller & Beardsley 1983)
- Evans syndrome (no evidence of associated disease, Pui et al 1980).

The antibodies to the various cell lines are different. Cytopenias may antedate tissue manifestations of the disorder.

Table 8.28 Post-viral vs idiopathic thrombocytopenia in childhood

	Post-viral	Idiopathic
Age	peak 2–4 yrs	most > 5 yrs, no peak
Sex incidence	about equal	girls > boys
Onset	rapid, < 2 weeks	slow, > 2 weeks
Preceding viral infection	symptomatic, in about 80%	infrequent[1]
Splenomegaly	about 10%	unusual
Evidence of infection in blood, marrow films	often	no
Spontaneous recovery[2]	90%	36%
Speed of recovery[2]		
< 3 months	75%[3]	20%
> 1 year	10%[4]	80%[4]

[1] Chronic viraemia, e.g. HIV, to be considered
[2] From Walker & Walker 1984
[3] Thrombocytopenia at height of virus infection (direct viral destruction, DIC) usually lasts < 2 weeks
[4] Rare cases take > 4 yrs to recover (Tait & Evans 1993)

Table 8.29 Familial thrombocytopenias with adequate megakaryocytes in marrow

	Platelets, light microscopy	Thrombocytopathy	Other features	References[1]
Autosomal dominant				
Carrington	n	0	myopathy	Carrington 1989
Danielsson	large	+	0	Danielsson 1980
Dowton	n	+	tendency to malignancy, esp haemopoietic	Dowton 1985
Epstein	large	+	nephritis, neural deafness	Epstein 1972
Fechtner	large	0	nephritis, deafness, cataracts, granulocyte inclusions	Peterson 1985
grey platelet	large, pale, grey	+	tendency to myelofibrosis	Berndt 1983a
Greaves	large + small	+	0	Greaves 1987
May-Hegglin	large	+/–	granulocyte inclusions	Hamilton 1980
'Montreal'	large, spontaneous aggregation	+	0	Lacombe 1963
Najean-Lecompte	large	0	tendency to AML	Najean 1990
Sebastian	large	0	as for Fechtner but no clinical disorder	Greinacher 1990
Stormorken	large	+	small pupils, muscle fatigue, migraine, dyslexia, asplenia, ichthyosis	Stormorken 1985
'Swiss-cheese'[2]	large	+	0	Smith 1973
vWD, IIb and platelet types	n to large	+	0	Weiss 1982
Autosomal recessive				
Bernard-Soulier	large	+	0	Berndt 1983b
Chediak-Higashi[3]	large granules in some platelets	+	giant granulation in leucocytes and other cells, albinism, infections	Apitz-Castro 1985
Organic acidaemias	n		variable neutropenia and anaemia; acidosis	Sweetman 1989
X-linked recessive				
Chiaro	n		0	Chiaro 1972
Gutenberger	n	0	nephritis, ↑ serum IgA	Gutenberger 1970
Thompson	n	+	β thal minor	Thompson 1977
Wiskott-Aldrich	small	+/–	eczema, infections	Ochs 1980
Inheritance obscure				
Antiphospholipid syndrome	n		autoimmune disease, lupus anticoagulant	Hughes 1989
Mediterranean	large	0	stomatocytosis, abdominal pain	Ducrou 1969, von Behrens 1975
Stewart	large	+/–	stomatocytosis, ↑ cholesterol, xanthomas	Stewart 1987

n = normal; +/– = minimal or disputed; gaps = insufficient information
[1] Only first author given
[2] Because of vacuolated ultrastructure
[3] Thrombocytopenia more severe in accelerated, lymphoma-like phase

Drug-immune thrombocytopenia (Table 8.30)

Drug-immune effect is a rare or rarely provable cause of thrombocytopenia in childhood. Antibodies are of 2 kinds, both of which may be produced by the same drug (Mueller-Eckhardt & Salama 1990):

- Drug-dependent antibodies are a response to an antigen which is a combination of drug and membrane components. Cytopenias result from complement-mediated intravascular destruction and are acute and severe.
- Drug-independent antibodies are true autoantibodies stimulated by drug-induced alteration of membrane. Cytopenias are a result of extravascular destruction and are milder and more protracted than those from drug-dependent antibodies.

Rarely, immune neutropenia and/or haemolysis accompany thrombocytopenia.

Requirements for diagnosis include: (i) demonstration of plentiful megakaryocytes in marrow; (ii) exclusion of other causes of thrombocytopenia; (iii) recovery of platelet count after withdrawal of drug (usually within 3 days, occasionally weeks, rarely months because of slow excretion, e.g. gold).

The most useful in vitro tests are:

- for quinine/quinidine, drug-enhanced deposition of patient Ig on to normal platelets, assessed by immunofluorescence
- for heparin, drug-induced aggregation of normal platelets in patient plasma, with neutralization by protamine and omission of heparin as controls; serotonin release from platelets is more sensitive and specific than aggregation (Chong & Gallus 1993).

Heparin-induced thrombocytopenia occurs in < 5% of those treated and may occur with only small doses, for example of the order used for flushing intravenous lines. A mild, transient thrombocytopenia occurring within a few days (type 1) is due to direct toxic or aggregating effect and recovers spontaneously, even if heparin is continued. More severe and persistent (immune) thrombocytopenia (type 2) occurs after 5–14 days (< 24 hours if previously exposed) and may be associated, though rarely in children, with arterial thrombosis (platelet aggregation, damage to endothelium by reaction of the antibody with heparin bound to or synthesized by endothelium).

Thrombocytopenia in neonate due to antibody passively acquired from mother

Although any IgG autoimmune thrombocytopenia in the mother may cause thrombocytopenia in the newborn, this occurs with significant frequency in few disorders (Table 8.27).

- ITP

Thrombocytopenia may occur in the newborn whether the mother's ITP is active or in remission (e.g. post-splenectomy). Thrombocytopenia ($< 150 \times 10^9/l$) occurs in 15–65% (McCrae et al 1992), and severe thrombocytopenia ($< 50 \times 10^9/l$, with risk of intracranial bleeding from spontaneous vaginal delivery) in approximately 9% (Burrows & Kelton 1993). Recovery is usual within 3–4 weeks. Rarely, thrombocytopenia in the neonate antedates overt manifestation of thrombocytopenia in the mother.

- Gestational thrombocytopenia (incidental thrombocytopenia of pregnancy) (Aster 1990)

In contrast to the situation in ITP, thrombocytopenia in infants of mothers whose thrombocytopenia is noted first in pregnancy is infrequent (about 4%) and mild. Platelet-binding IgG is found in serum of approximately 60% of these mothers but it is not known if this is autoantibody (Gp specific, true ITP) or alloantibody against HLA antigens (common in pregnant women). Non-immune platelet consumption is another possibility.

- SLE

Transient haemolytic anaemia/thrombocytopenia/leucopenia occurs in about 15% of newborns but is seldom of clinical importance (Hardy et al 1979).

Fetomaternal incompatibility (Kaplan C et al 1992)

The fetus inherits a platelet antigen from the father to which the mother reacts with IgG antibody. In Caucasians antigen is usually (about 3/4) Pl^{A1}(HPA-1a), the mother belonging to the 3% of the population who are negative; rarer antigens are Pl^{A2} (HPA-1b), Bak (HPA-3a,b) or antigens which are not specific to platelets, e.g. HLA. However, only a minority (< 10%) of pregnancies with the potential for sensitization result in fetal thrombocytopenia. Antibody is demonstrable in most but not all cases. The most practical approach is to react maternal serum with paternal platelets (infant platelets too sparse in acute stage). Because antibody may be slow to appear, repeat examination is recommended at 1–2 months if results at birth are negative or equivocal. There is a strong association with HLA DR3 phenotype in the mother (Flug et al 1994). Maternal platelet count is normal (cf ITP).

Thrombocytopenia originates before birth and fetal blood may be tested in the 2nd or 3rd trimester. Thrombocytopenia is usually severe, and mortality (cerebral haemorrhage) is higher (approx 5–10%, highest at birth) than for immune thrombocytopenia in childhood (< 1%). Counts become normal usually within 6 weeks. Neonatal thrombocytopenia in preceding siblings is common (about half the families, sensitization established in first pregnancy), succeeding infants being equally or more severely affected.

Refractoriness to platelet transfusion

Antigens responsible are usually class 1 HLA (contaminating leucocytes being the most important stimulus), less often platelet-specific or ABO (Schiffer 1991). In children requiring platelet support, infection, with or without DIC, may diminish the effectiveness of platelet transfusions.

NON-IMMUNE DESTRUCTION OF PLATELETS (Table 8.31)

- Infection

Thrombocytopenia for which an immune mechanism cannot be demonstrated is attributed to direct damage (organism itself or exotoxins) or consumption in DIC. This thrombocytopenia lasts for usually < 2 weeks (cf post-viral thrombocytopenia, Table 8.28).

- Congenital heart disease

Thrombocytopenia is common in cyanotic disease (p. 296). Surgically corrected defects and, less often, uncorrected calcified valve disease may be associated with thrombocytopenia and fragmentation haemolysis ('Waring blender' syndrome, Maurer 1972).

- Uraemia

Thrombocytopenia (usually mild–moderate) and platelet dysfunction (e.g. impaired ristocetin aggregation) are common. Reduction in concentration of the largest vWF multimers appears to be a significant factor (Gralnick et al 1988).

Table 8.30 Drugs and other chemicals used in childhood which may cause immune thrombocytopenia

Connection accepted
Sodium valproate
Quinine
Quinidine
Sulphonamides
Trimethoprim
Interferon
Heparin[1]
Gold
Connection suspected
Analgesics
Aspirin
Paracetamol
Anticonvulsants
Diphenylhydantoin
Carbamazepine
Antibiotics
Rifampicin
Ampicillin
Other
Acetazolamide
Chlorothiazide
Cimetidine
Chloroquine
Insecticides

[1] May also damage platelets directly

Table 8.31 Isolated thrombocytopenias in childhood: non-immune platelet damage[1]

Intrinsic platelet defect
Inherited thrombocytopathies (Table 8.29)
Extrinsic
Infection
Drugs
Cytotoxics[2]
Heparin[3]
Antilymphocyte/thymocyte globulin
Amphotericin B
Steroids
Intralipid (high dosage)[4]
Thiazides
Cyanotic congenital heart disease
Surgical heart repair[5]
Uraemia[6]
vWD (IIb type)
Organic acidaemias[7]
Isovaleric
Methylmalonic
Propionic
Phototherapy[8]

[1] Direct damage or non-immune coating to enhance aggregation/thrombosis
[2] Thrombocytopenia due more often to marrow damage than toxicity to platelets
[3] May also cause immune thrombocytopenia
[4] Lipson et al 1974
[5] Usually with fragmentation haemolysis
[6] Usually with anaemia
[7] Often with neutropenia, occasionally pancytopenia
[8] Maurer et al 1976

HYPERSPLENISM

Thrombocytopenia is unlikely unless the spleen is palpably enlarged, is usually not severe (> 50×10^9/l), and is usually part of pancytopenia. The marrow is normal, or hyperplastic for all cell lines. Platelet survival is normal or slightly diminished. Causes include portal hypertension, storage disorder (e.g. Gaucher, Niemann-Pick), infiltration (Letterer-Siwe disease, non-Langerhans histiocytosis, lymphoma) and SLE.

DILUTIONAL THROMBOCYTOPENIA

Thrombocytopenia is usually not severe but may be more severe than anticipated from the degree of dilution, and lasts up to 1 week.

Disorders of platelet function (thrombocytopathies)

An expanding heterogeneity (Hutton & Ludlam 1989) continues to be recognized. Identification is important because, although in general spontaneous bleeding is mild, bleeding may be troublesome with trauma or surgery.

Major features:

- Bleeding time excessive for platelet count (by > 5 min)

An appropriate bleeding time for a particular platelet count between 10 and 100×10^9/l may be calculated from the Harker-Slichter (1972) formula:

$$\text{bleeding time (min)} = 30.5 - \frac{\text{platelet count } (10^9/\text{l})}{3.85}$$

A normal bleeding time does not exclude platelet dysfunction.

- Defect in function demonstrable by in vitro testing
- History of easy bruisability with no evidence of plasma coagulation or vessel defect.

An outline classification is given in Table 8.32, a suggested schema for investigation in Table 8.33, information to be gained from simple investigations in Table 8.34, and aggregability characteristics of those disorders in which they are of diagnostic value in Table 8.35.

Table 8.32 Thrombocytopathies: outline

Adhesion to subendothelium
  vWD
  Bernard-Soulier
  Gpla deficiency
Primary aggregation
  Glanzmann
  Afibrinogenaemia
Storage pool disease (Table 8.36)
  Storage pool deficiency
  Release defect
Platelet/plasma coagulation interaction
  F V deficiency
Other/multiple/unidentified mechanisms
  Hereditary
    Most thrombocytopathies in Table 8.29
    Inherited connective tissue disorder[1]
      Osteogenesis imperfecta
      Ehlers-Danlos
      Marfan
    Inherited disorders of carbohydrate metabolism[2]
      Glucose-6-phosphatase (glycogen storage disease type I)
      Fructose-1-6-diphosphatase (Fig. 8.1)
  Acquired[3]
    Uraemia
    Liver cirrhosis
    Drugs (Tables 8.31, 8.38)
    Congenital heart disease
    Essential thrombocythaemia
    Antiphospholipid syndrome
    Extracorporeal circulation

[1] The (mild) bleeding tendency is due more to the connective tissue abnormality than to thrombocytopathy
[2] Inadequate synthesis of storage nucleotides secondary to chronic hypoglycaemia
[3] Bleeding due more to thrombocytopenia/coagulation factor deficiency than to thrombocytopathy

Table 8.33 Suspected thrombocytopathy: lab investigation

Blood count, film
Bleeding time
Plasma coagulation for vWD
Platelet aggregation
  ADP
  Collagen
  Arachidonate
  Ristocetin
Platelet glycoproteins
Dense body adequacy
  Fluorescence microscopy of mepacrine-treated platelets
  Electron microscopy
  5HT uptake and secretion
  Content of adenine nucleotides
α granule adequacy
  Electron microscopy
  β thromboglobulin, PF4
Arachidonate metabolism
  Screening procedures (Table 8.37)
Calcium mobilization
  Aggregation by cation-ionophore A23187 as screen

DEFECTS OF ADHESION TO SUBENDOTHELIUM

von Willebrand's disease

Except for the platelet type, platelet abnormality is secondary to deficiency of plasma vWF. Thrombocytopenia, either continuous or intermittent, may occur in the IIb and platelet types (Table 8.9).

Bernard-Soulier syndrome (BSS) (Berndt et al 1983b)
Platelets lack GpIb–IX and GpV, resulting in deficient binding by vWF of platelets to subendothelium at sites of injury. This grouping is also the binding site for quinine/quinidine-dependent antibodies (GpV) and is the site of the antigen Pl^{A1} (HPA-Ia).

Platelets are large (Fig. 8.12), up to the size of lymphocytes, and in some, the granules are clustered in the centre (pseudonucleus). Thrombocytopenia is moderate (50–100 × 10^9/l), with machine counts usually spuriously low because large platelets are counted as erythrocytes. Thrombocytopenia is due to impaired production (megakaryocyte numbers normal) and reduced survival.

Aggregation with ristocetin is defective because of requirement for vWF in binding (Table 8.35). Whole blood is preferred to conventional aggregometry (loss of larger platelets with erythrocytes in preparation of platelet concentrate). Diagnosis may be confirmed by examination for Gp using monoclonal antibodies in a fluorescence procedure.

Table 8.34 Thrombocytopathies with abnormal light microscopic morphology

	Platelet morphology	Platelet count	Inheritance	Other
Bernard-Soulier	large	↓	AR	
Chediak-Higashi	giant granules in some platelets	↓ in accelerated phase	AR	giant granules in granulocytes, lymphocytes
Grey platelet	large, pale, grey	↓	AD	
Greaves	large	↓	AD	
May-Hegglin	large + small	n to ↓	AD	Döhle-like bodies in granulocytes
Stormorken	minority large	occasionally mild transient ↓	AD	↓ adrenalin aggregation
'Swiss-cheese'	large	↓	AD	
vWD, IIb and platelet types	may be large	may be ↓	AD	
Wiskott-Aldrich[1]	small	↓↓	XLR	

[1] Existence of thrombocytopathy disputed
AD = autosomal dominant; AR = autosomal recessive; XLR = X-linked recessive

Table 8.35 Platelet aggregability in thrombocytopathies

	ADP 2 μmol/l	Collagen 1 μmol/l	Arachidonate 1 μmol/l	Ristocetin, 0.4	mg/ml 1.25
Normal	1° + 2°	2° after lag	monophasic, no lag	0	1° + 2°
Bernard-Soulier	n	n	n	0	0[1]
Glanzmann	0	0	0	0	1°
Grey platelet	n	v	n	0	1° + 2°
May-Hegglin	n	n			1° + 2°
Storage pool deficiency[2]	1°	↓	n to ↓	0	1°
TXA2 synthesis defect[2]	1°	0	0	0	1° + 2°
vWD	n	n	n	+[3]	n to ↓[4]

1° = primary wave; 2° = secondary wave; n = normal; v = variable
[1] Not normalized by addition of vWF
[2] Aggregation with thrombin subnormal in storage pool deficiency, normal in TXA2 deficiency; it may be difficult however to find a concentration of thrombin which does not clot samples
[3] IIb and platelet types only
[4] Normalized in IIb by added vWF

Bleeding is variable and may be pronounced. Symptoms start in infancy or early childhood and tend to improve with age.

Heterozygotes may show occasional large platelets, but platelet count, bleeding time and ristocetin aggregation are normal, and Gp quantitation is required for identification.

Differential diagnosis:

- other inherited large-platelet syndromes (Table 8.29)
- acquired BSS in myelodysplastic disease such as monosomy 7 MPD (Fig. 5.18)
- reactive conditions with large, young active platelets (Fig. 8.12).

GpIa deficiency
This rare defect results in failure of aggregation specifically to collagen (GpIa–IIa contains a binding site for collagen). Platelet count and morphology are normal (Nieuwenhuis et al 1985).

DEFECTS OF PRIMARY AGGREGATION

Glanzmann's thrombasthenia
A deficiency of the IIb–IIIa Gp complex, which binds fibrinogen essential for platelet–platelet aggregation (Fig. 8.10).

Platelets aggregate in response to ristocetin (binds vWF to GpIb) but not other agents (Table 8.35, Fig. 8.15). Diagnosis may be confirmed by assessing the binding of specific Gp monoclonal antibodies. Gp is undetectable or, in some patients, about 15% of normal. Platelet morphology and count are normal, though aggregates may not be seen in films when they might be expected (unanticoagulated blood films). Clot retraction is absent or severely diminished.

Specific platelet antigens Pl^{A1}, Pl^{A2} (HPA-1a,b), Bak^{a} and Bak^{b} (HPA-3a,b) are located in this Gp complex. Glanzmann patients who are completely lacking in GpIIb–IIIa are at risk of producing IgG anti-Pl^{A1} if given Pl^{A1} positive platelets (98% of normal population).

Bleeding may be severe but tends to diminish with age. Inheritance is autosomal recessive; heterozygotes have 50–60% normal Gp but normal platelet aggregations and no abnormal bleeding.

Afibrinogenaemia
Some patients with inherited afibrinogenaemia or hypofibrinogenaemia have prolonged bleeding time, impaired aggregations (ADP, collagen, but normal with ristocetin) and mild thrombocytopenia.

STORAGE POOL DISEASE

Storage pool disease is common, but bleeding is usually mild. Deficient discharge of agonists, especially ADP, is due to either deficiency of granule-stored components (storage pool deficiency) or defect in release (release defects). In many the precise defect is not identified.

Storage pool deficiency (Table 8.36)

Deficiency of dense bodies
Major characteristics:

— Deficiency or defect of dense bodies as such (electron microscopy, fluorescence microscopy of mepacrine-treated platelets).
— Deficiency of components normally stored in dense granules (ADP, ATP, 5HT, calcium), assessed most simply by thrombin-stimulated release of ATP.
— Impaired aggregations (Table 8.35). A single set of aggregations however is normal in up to one quarter of patients (Nieuwenhuis et al 1987).

Grey platelet syndrome (Berndt et al 1983a)
Platelets are large, poorly granulated and pale staining (Fig. 8.16). Moderate thrombocytopenia is usual. Deficiency (α granules) can be identified by electron microscopy (platelets vacuolated with normal to increased number of dense bodies), or by quantitation of α granule components such as β thromboglobulin, platelet-derived growth factor, thrombospondin and platelet factor 4. These may be increased in serum (i.e. granule defect is in packaging of components and not synthesis). Megakaryocytes are plentiful but poorly granular.

Bleeding tendency is mild. Inheritance is autosomal dominant. Myelofibrosis is frequent, due to leakage of platelet-derived growth factor and platelet factor 4 from α granules of megakaryocytes.

Similar appearances may rarely be due to artefact (Fig. 8.16).

Release defects

Most are due to defective TXA2 generation/effect (TXA2 is the most potent natural stimulant of platelet aggregation and release reactions); synthesis may be deficient, or effectiveness impaired by receptor malfunction or defect in intracellular calcium mobilization (Fig. 8.17).

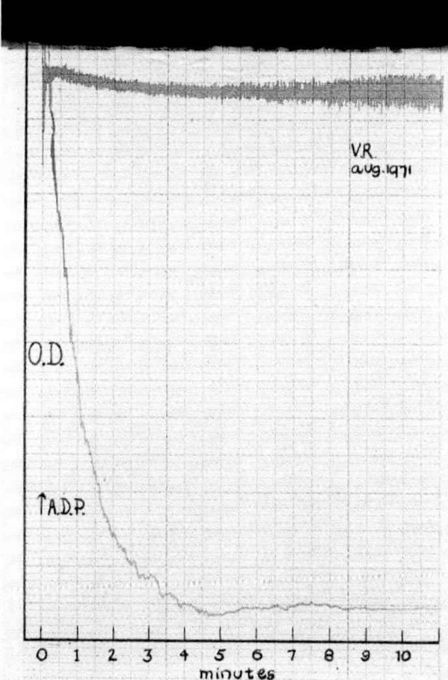

Fig. 8.15 Glanzmann's thrombasthenia: absence of platelet aggregation with ADP in patient (VR) vs normal.

Table 8.36 Thrombocytopathies: storage pool disease[1]

Storage pool deficiency
Dense bodies
Inherited
Isolated[2]
Part of syndrome
TAR
Hermansky-Pudlak
Chediak-Higashi
Niemann-Pick B
Acquired
AML or harbinger (years) of AML
HUS, TTP
Cardiopulmonary bypass
Burns
Liver disease
Autoimmune disease
α granules
Grey platelet
Release defect
TXA2 synthesis/receptor (Table 8.37)
Calcium mobilization
Other

[1] In disorders with thrombocytopenia, bleeding may be due more to this than to dense body deficiency
[2] Autosomal dominant, Ingerman et al 1978

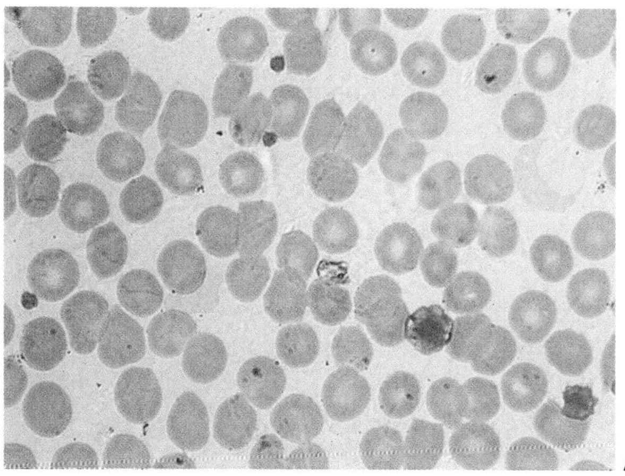

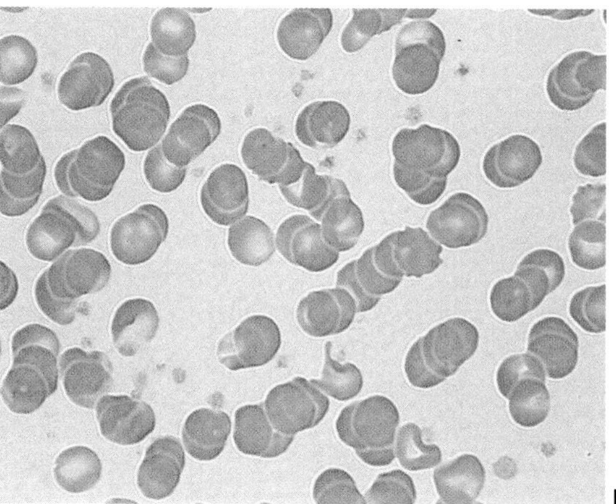

Fig. 8.16 Grey platelet (**a**) and transient grey platelet-like disorder (**b**). The cause of the hypogranulation in **b** was not determined; 11-year-old boy with eczema, morphology normal 2 days later.

Release defects may be distinguished from storage pool deficiency by thrombin-induced aggregation of platelets (Table 8.35) or thrombin-induced release of granule components, most conveniently ATP as a measure also of constituents released with it, such as ADP. A normal bleeding time in these defects may be strikingly prolonged by aspirin ingestion (not specific). Bleeding tendency is usually absent or mild.

Preliminary identification of the precise defect may be made from the pattern of aggregations with a variety of agonists (Tables 8.33, 8.35, 8.37).

Impaired release of arachidonic acid
A deficiency/defect in phospholipases which release arachidonic acid from membrane phospholipids. Platelet count and morphology are normal in some families (Rao et al 1984), macrothrombocytopenia occurs in others (Greaves et al 1987). Inheritance is autosomal dominant when demonstrable.

Cyclo-oxygenase deficiency ('aspirin-like' defect)
Deficiency is most commonly due to drugs. Aspirin causes irreversible enzyme acetylation. Since the enzyme is synthesized in megakaryocytes but not platelets, the effect lasts for the lifetime of the platelet (about 10 days). Mild increase in bleeding time and abnormal aggregations are evident within 2 hours of ingestion. Indomethacin, phenylbutazone and sulphinpyrazone cause a weaker and more transient inhibition. Enzyme deficiency is rarely inherited (Horellou et al 1983).

Drugs may induce platelet dysfunction by mechanisms other than cyclo-oxygenase inhibition (Table 8.38). The platelet dysfunction induced by dextrans may arrest some thrombotic states (Fig. 8.6).

Defective calcium mobilization
Some of these defects are associated with attention deficit-hyperactivity disorder (Koike et al 1984, Lages & Weiss 1988b).

Other release defects
Mild bleeding tendency may be associated with defect in exposure of the fibrinogen-binding site (GpIIb–IIIa, essential for the aggregation preceding secretion, Lages & Weiss 1988a). Absence of adrenalin-induced aggregability is described in a kindred (Stormorken et al 1983); the significance of this is uncertain — response to adrenalin is variable in normal persons and diminished response is usually ignored if this is the only abnormality.

DEFECTS OF PLATELET/PLASMA COAGULATION INTERACTION

Mild prolongation of bleeding time and mild thrombocytopenia (but normal aggregations) occur in about one third of patients with congenital isolated F V deficiency (lack of F V on platelet surface).

THROMBOCYTOPATHIES DUE TO OTHER/ MULTIPLE/UNIDENTIFIED MECHANISMS

(Table 8.32)

- Renal failure (Remuzzi 1988)

Thrombocytopathy is an important cause of bleeding. Significant causes include:

- — unidentified dialysable components in plasma (platelet function improved by dialysis)
- — erythropenia per se (platelet function improved by increasing Hb by transfusion or erythropoietin)
- — deficiency of largest vWF multimers in plasma, with platelet vWF also reduced (Gralnick et al 1988).

Thrombocytopenia is an additional cause of bleeding in renal disease, especially HUS.

- Others

Other thrombocytopathies listed in Table 8.32 are discussed elsewhere.

Table 8.37 Defects of TXA2 synthesis/receptor

	Platelet aggregation with: Arachidonic acid	Prostaglandin G2	U46619[1]
Impaired arachidonic acid release	n	n	n
Cyclo-oxygenase deficiency ('aspirin-like' defect)	↓	n	n
TXA2 synthetase deficiency[2]	↓	↓	n
TXA2 receptor defect[3]	↓	↓	↓

[1] TXA2 agonist
[2] Defreyn et al 1981
[3] Wu et al 1981

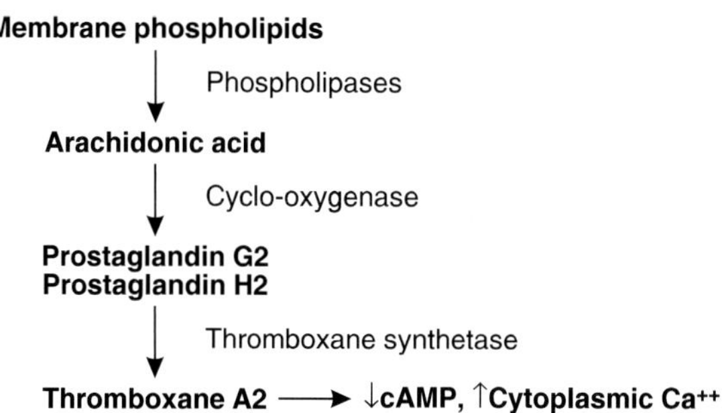

Fig. 8.17 Arachidonic acid metabolism in platelets, simplified schema.

Table 8.38 Drugs and chemicals used in paediatrics which may affect platelet function[1]

Cyclo-oxygenase inhibitors
- Aspirin
- Indomethacin
- Phenylbutazone
- Sulphinpyrazone

Other or unknown mechanisms
- Dipyridamole[2]
- Aminophylline
- Antihistamines
- Phenothiazines
- Tricyclic antidepressants
- Sodium valproate
- Carbenicillin, high dose[3]
- Cephalosporins, high dose[3]
- Radiographic contrast agents
- Heparin
- β blockers
- Dextrans[4]
- Phototherapy
- Foods — onions, garlic, peppers, ginger, alcohol[5]

[1] Mode of action not known for many drugs
[2] Phosphodiesterase inhibition, increase in platelet cAMP
[3] Platelet coating reduces binding by agonists (Shattil et al 1980)
[4] Evans & Gordon 1974
[5] Hutton & Ludlam 1989

REFERENCES

Andrew M, Paes B, Milner et al 1987 Development of the human coagulation system in the full-term infant. Blood 70: 165–172

Andrew M, Paes B, Milner R et al 1988 Development of the human coagulation system in the healthy premature infant. Blood 72: 1651–1657

Andrew M, Vegh P, Johnston M et al 1992 Maturation of the hemostatic system during childhood. Blood 80: 1998–2005

Apitz-Castro R, Cruz M R, Ledezma E et al 1985 The storage pool deficiency in platelets from humans with the Chédiak-Higashi syndrome: study of six patients. British Journal of Haematology 59: 471–483

Aster R H 1990 "Gestational thrombocytopenia". A plea for conservative management. New England Journal of Medicine 323: 264–266

Bauer C R, Fojaco R M, Bancalari E, Fernandez-Rocha L 1978 Microangiopathic hemolytic anemia and thrombocytopenia in a neonate associated with a large placental chorioangioma. Pediatrics 62: 574–577

Berndt M C, Castaldi P A, Gordon S et al 1983a Morphological and biochemical confirmation of gray platelet syndrome in two siblings. Australian and New Zealand Journal of Medicine 13: 387–390

Berndt M C, Gregory C, Chong B H et al 1983b Additional glycoprotein defects in Bernard-Soulier's syndrome: confirmation of genetic basis by parental analysis. Blood 62: 800–807

Bertina R M, Koeleman B P C, Koster T et al 1994 Mutation in blood coagulation factor V associated with resistance to activated protein C. Nature 369: 64–67

Bizzaro N, Dianese G 1988 Neonatal alloimmune amegakaryocytosis. Case report. Vox Sanguinis 54: 112–114

Board P G, Losowsky M S, Miloszewski K J A 1993 Factor XIII: inherited and acquired deficiency. Blood Reviews 7: 229–242

Bracey A W, Wu A H B, Aceves J et al 1987 Platelet dysfunction associated with Wilms tumor and hyaluronic acid. American Journal of Hematology 24: 247–257

Brenner B, Fishman A, Goldsher D et al 1988 Cerebral thrombosis in a new born with a congenital deficiency of antithrombin III. American Journal of Hematology 27: 209–211

Brenner B, Tavori S, Zivelin A et al 1990 Hereditary deficiency of all vitamin K-deficient procoagulants and anticoagulants. British Journal of Haematology 75: 537–542

Burns E R, Goldberg S N, Wenz B 1993 Paradox effect of multiple mild coagulation factor deficiencies on the prothrombin time and activated partial thromboplastin time. American Journal of Clinical Pathology 100: 94–98

Burns J C, Glode M P, Clarke S H et al 1984 Coagulopathy and platelet activation in Kawasaki syndrome: identification of patients at high risk for development of coronary artery aneurysms. Journal of Pediatrics 105: 206–211

Burrows R F, Kelton J G 1993 Fetal thrombocytopenia and its relation to maternal thrombocytopenia. New England Journal of Medicine 329: 1463–1466

Carrington P A, Evans D I K, Cumming W J K et al 1989 Familial thrombocytopenia and myopathy. Clinical and Laboratory Haematology 11: 323–329

Chanarin I (ed) 1989 Laboratory haematology. An account of laboratory techniques. Churchill Livingstone, Edinburgh

Cherstvoy E, Lazjuk G, Lurie I et al 1980 Syndrome of multiple congenital malformations including phocomelia, thrombocytopenia, encephalocele, and urogenital abnormalities. Lancet ii: 485

Chiaro J J, Dharmkrong-at A, Bloom G E 1972 X-linked thrombocytopenic purpura. I. Clinical and genetic studies of a kindred. American Journal of Diseases of Children 123: 565–568

Chong B H, Gallus A S 1993 Diagnosis of heparin-induced thrombocytopenia. Royal College of Pathologists of Australasia, Broadsheet No 31

Colman R W 1993 Hemostasis and thrombosis: basic principles and clinical practice, 3rd edn. Lippincott, Philadelphia

Colman R W, Rao A K, Rubin R N 1994 Factor XI deficiency and hemostasis. American Journal of Hematology 45: 73–78

Dadash-Zadeh M, Czapek E E, Schwartz A D 1976 Skeletal and splenic hemangiomatosis with consumption coagulopathy: response to splenectomy. Pediatrics 57: 803–806

D'Angelo A, Valle P D, Crippa L et al 1993 Brief report: autoimmune protein S deficiency in a boy with severe thromboembolic disease. New England Journal of Medicine 328: 1753–1757

Danielsson L, Jelf E, Lundkvist L 1980 A new family with inherited thrombocytopenia. Scandinavian Journal of Haematology 24: 427–429

Defreyn G, Machin J J, Carreras L O et al 1981 Familial bleeding tendency with partial platelet thromboxane synthetase deficiency: reorientation of cyclic endoperoxide metabolism. British Journal of Haematology 49: 29–41

Dietz W H, Stuart M J 1977 Splenic consumptive coagulopathy in a patient with disseminated lymphangiomatosis. Journal of Pediatrics 90: 421–423

Dignan P St J, Mauer A M, Fantz C 1967 Phocomelia with congenital hypoplastic thrombocytopenia and myeloid leukemoid reactions. Journal of Pediatrics 70: 561–573

Dowton S B, Beardsley D, Jamison D et al 1985 Studies of a familial platelet disorder. Blood 65: 557–563

Ducrou W, Kimber R J 1969 Stomatocytes, haemolytic anaemia and abdominal pain in Mediterranean migrants. Some examples of a new syndrome? Medical Journal of Australia 2: 1087–1091

Epstein C J, Sahud M A, Piel C F et al 1972 Hereditary macrothrombocytopathia, nephritis and deafness. American Journal of Medicine 52: 299–310

Evans R J, Gordon J L 1974 Mechanism of the antithrombotic action of dextran. New England Journal of Medicine 290: 748

Exner T, Triplett D A, Taberner D, Machin S J 1991 Guidelines for testing and revised criteria for lupus anticoagulants. SSC subcommittee for the standardization of lupus anticoagulants. Thrombosis and Haemostasis 65: 320–322

Favara B E, Franciosi R A, Butterfield J 1974 Disseminated intravascular and cardiac thrombosis of the neonate. American Journal of Diseases of Children 127: 197–204

Feusner J H 1980 Normal and abnormal bleeding times in neonates and young children utilizing a fully standardized template technic. American Journal of Clinical Pathology 74: 73–77

Flug F, Karpatkin M, Karpatkin S 1994 Should all pregnant women be tested for their platelet PLA (Zw, HPA-1) phenotype? British Journal of Haematology 86: 1–5

Freedman M H, Estrov Z 1990 Congenital amegakaryocytic thrombocytopenia: an intrinsic hematopoietic stem cell defect. American Journal of Pediatric Hematology/Oncology 12: 225–230

Gardner R J M, Morrison P S, Abbott G D 1983 A syndrome of congenital thrombocytopenia with multiple malformations and neurologic dysfunction. Journal of Pediatrics 102: 600–602

Giannelli F, Green P M, High K A et al 1991 Haemophilia B: database of point mutations and short additions and deletions, 2nd edn. Nucleic Acids Research 19: 2193–2219

Gill J C, Wilson A D, Endres-Brooks J, Montgomery R R 1986 Loss of the largest von Willebrand factor multimers from the plasma of patients with congenital cardiac defects. Blood 67: 758–761

Ginsburg D, Sadler J E 1993 Von Willebrand disease: a database of point mutations, insertions, and deletions. Thrombosis and Haemostasis 69: 177–184

Goodeve A C, Preston F E, Peake I R 1994 Factor VIII gene rearrangements in patients with severe haemophilia A. Lancet 343: 329–330

Grace A A, Barradas M A, Mikhailidis D P et al 1987 Cyclosporine A enhances platelet aggregation. Kidney International 32: 889–895

Gralnick H R, McKeown L P, Williams S B et al 1988 Plasma and platelet von Willebrand factor defects in uremia. American Journal of Medicine 85: 806–810

Greaves M, Pickering C, Martin J et al 1987 A new familial 'giant platelet syndrome' with structural, metabolic and functional abnormalities of platelets due to a primary megakaryocyte defect. British Journal of Haematology 65: 429–435

Greinacher A, Mueller-Eckhardt C 1990 Hereditary types of thrombocytopenia with giant platelets and inclusion bodies in the leucocytes. Blut 60: 53–60

Gutenberger J, Trygstad C W, Stiehm E R et al 1970 Familial thrombocytopenia, elevated serum IgA levels and renal disease. American Journal of Medicine 49: 729–741

Hall J G 1987 Thrombocytopenia and absent radius (TAR) syndrome. Journal of Medical Genetics 24: 79–83

Hamilton R W, Shaikh B S, Ottie J N et al 1980 Platelet function, ultrastructure and survival in the May-Hegglin anomaly. American Journal of Clinical Pathology 74: 663–668

Han P, Lou J, Wong H B 1987 Wilms' tumour with acquired von Willebrand's disease. Australian Paediatric Journal 23: 253–255

Hardy J D, Solomon S, Banwell G S et al 1979 Congenital complete heart block in the newborn associated with maternal systemic lupus erythematosus and other connective tissue disorders. Archives of Disease in Childhood 54: 7–13

Harker L A, Slichter S J 1972 The bleeding time as a screening test for evaluation of platelet function. New England Journal of Medicine 287: 155–159

Harper P L, Luddington R J, Carrell R W et al 1988 Protein C deficiency and portal thrombosis in liver transplantation in children. Lancet ii: 924–927

Heyderman R S 1993 Sepsis and intravascular thrombosis. Archives of Disease in Childhood 68: 621–625

Horellou M H, Lecompte T, Lecrubier C et al 1983 Familial and constitutional bleeding disorder due to platelet cyclo-oxygenase deficiency. American Journal of Hematology 14: 1–9

Hughes G R V, Asherson R A, Khamashta M A 1989 Antiphospholipid syndrome: linking many specialties. Annals of the Rheumatic Diseases 48: 355–356

Hutton R A, Ludlam C A 1989 Platelet function testing. Journal of Clinical Pathology 42: 858–864

Ingerman C M, Smith J B, Shapiro S et al 1978 Hereditary abnormality of platelet aggregation attributable to nucleotide storage pool deficiency. Blood 52: 332–344

Jackson C A, Greaves M, Patterson A D et al 1982 Relationship between platelet aggregation, thromboxane synthesis and albumin concentration in nephrotic syndrome. British Journal of Haematology 52: 69–77

Jackson C A, Greaves M, Boulton A J M et al 1984 Near-normal glycaemic control does not correct abnormal platelet reactivity in diabetes mellitus. Clinical Science 67: 551–555

Jackson J M, Marshall L R, Herrmann R P 1981 Passovoy factor deficiency in five Western Australian kindreds. Pathology 13: 517–524

Kaplan B S, Levin M, De Chadarevian J-P 1992 The hemolytic-uremic syndrome. In: Edelman C M (ed) Pediatric kidney disease, 2nd edn. Little Brown, Boston, ch 60

Kaplan C, Morel-Kopp M-C, Clemenceau S et al 1992 Fetal and neonatal alloimmune thrombocytopenia: current trends in diagnosis and therapy. Transfusion Medicine 2: 265–271

Kelton J G, Neame P B, Gauldie J, Hirsh J 1979 Elevated platelet-associated IgG in the thrombocytopenia of septicemia. New England Journal of Medicine 300: 760–764

Kelton J G, Keystone J, Moore J et al 1983 Immune-mediated thrombocytopenia of malaria. Journal of Clinical Investigation 71: 832–836

Kobbah M, Ewald U, Tuvemo T 1985 Platelet aggregation during the first year of diabetes in childhood. Acta Paediatrica Scandinavica (suppl) 320: 50–55

Koike K, Rao A K, Holmsen H, Meuller P S 1984 Platelet secretion defect in patients with the attention deficit disorder and easy bruising. Blood 63: 427–433

Lacombe M, D'angelo G 1963 Etudes sur une thrombopathie familiale. Nouvelle Revue Francaise d'Hematologie 2: 611–614

Lages B, Weiss H J 1988a Heterogeneous defects of platelet secretion and responses to weak agonists in patients with bleeding disorders. British Journal of Haematology 68: 53–62

Lages B, Weiss H J 1988b Impairment of phosphatidylinositol metabolism in a patient with bleeding disorder associated with defects of initial platelet responses. Thrombosis and Haemostasis 59: 175–179

Lazarchick J, Dainer P M, Teaford M J, Oswald M W 1985 An unusual circulating anticoagulant in an asymptomatic child. American Journal of Pediatric Hematology/Oncology 7: 199–202

Lee M H, Vosburgh E, Anderson K, McDonagh J 1993 Deficiency of plasma plasminogen activator inhibitor I results in hyperfibrinolytic bleeding. Blood 81: 2357–2362

Levin D L, Weinberg A G, Perkin R M 1983 Pulmonary microthrombi syndrome in newborn infants with unresponsive persistent pulmonary hypertension. Journal of Pediatrics 102: 299–303

Leyva W H, Knutsen A P, Joist H 1988 Disappearance of a high response factor VIII inhibitor in a hemophiliac with AIDS. American Journal of Clinical Pathology 89: 414–418

Lipson A H, Pritchard J, Thomas G 1974 Thrombocytopenia after intralipid infusion in a neonate. Lancet ii: 1462–1463

McCrae K R, Samuels P, Schreiber A D 1992 Pregnancy-associated thrombocytopenia: pathogenesis and management. Blood 80: 2697–2714

McMillan R, Tani P, Millard F et al 1987 Platelet-associated plasma anti-glycoprotein autoantibodies in chronic ITP. Blood 70: 1040–1045

McNeil H P, Chesterman C N, Krilis S A 1989 Anticardiolipin antibodies and lupus anticoagulants comprise separate antibody subgroups with different phospholipid binding characteristics. British Journal of Haematology 73: 506–513

Mahasandana C, Suvatte V, Chuansumrit A et al 1990 Homozygous protein S deficiency in an infant with purpura fulminans. Journal of Pediatrics 117: 750–753

Mannucci P M, Tripodi A, Bertina R M 1986 Protein S deficiency associated with "juvenile" arterial and venous thromboses. Thrombosis and Haemostasis 55: 440

Maurer H M 1972 Hematologic effects of cardiac disease. Pediatric Clinics of North America 19: 1083–1093

Maurer H M, Fratkin M, McWilliams N B et al 1976 Effects of phototherapy on platelet counts in low-birthweight infants and on platelet production and life span in rabbits. Pediatrics 57: 506–512

Melissari E, Kakkar V V 1989 Congenital severe protein C deficiency in adults. British Journal of Haematology 72: 222–228

Miller B A, Beardsley D S 1983 Autoimmune pancytopenia of childhood associated with multisystem disease manifestations. Journal of Pediatrics 103: 877–881

Miller C H, Graham J B, Goldin L R, Elston R C 1979 Genetics of classic von Willebrand's disease. I. Phenotypic variation within families. Blood 54: 117–136

Mitchell L, Hoogendoorn H, Giles A R et al 1994 Increased endogenous thrombin generation in children with acute lymphoblastic leukemia: risk of thrombotic complications in L'asparaginase-induced antithrombin III deficiency. Blood 83: 386–391

Moake J L 1994 Haemolytic-uraemic syndrome: basic science. Lancet 343: 393–397

Moake J L, Rudy C K, Troll J H et al 1982 Unusually large plasma factor VIII:von Willebrand factor multimers in chronic relapsing thrombotic thrombocytopenic purpura. New England Journal of Medicine 307: 1432–1435

Mueller-Eckhardt C, Salama A 1990 Drug-induced cytopenias: a unifying pathogenetic concept with special emphasis on the role of drug metabolites. Transfusion Medicine Reviews 4: 69–77

Najean Y, Lecompte T 1990 Genetic thrombocytopenia with autosomal dominant transmission: a review of 54 cases. British Journal of Haematology 74: 203–208

Nieuwenhuis H K, Akkerman J-W N, Houdijk W P M, Sixma J J

1985 Human blood platelets showing no response to collagen fail to express surface glycoprotein I. Nature 318: 470–472
Nieuwenhuis H K, Akkerman J-W N, Sixma J J 1987 Patients with a prolonged bleeding time and normal aggregation tests may have storage pool deficiency: studies on one hundred and six patients. Blood 70: 620–623
Ochs H D, Slichter S J, Harker L A et al 1980 The Wiskott-Aldrich syndrome: studies of lymphocytes, granulocytes and platelets. Blood 55: 243–252
Palareti G, Salardi S, Piazzi S et al 1986 Blood coagulation changes in homocystinuria: effects of pyridoxine and other specific therapy. Journal of Pediatrics 109: 1001–1006
Pauli R M, Lian J B, Mosher D F, Suttie J W 1987 Association of congenital deficiency of multiple vitamin K-dependent coagulation factors and the phenotype of warfarin embryopathy: clues to the mechanism of teratogenicity of coumarin derivatives. American Journal of Human Genetics 41: 566–583
Pegels J G, Bruynes E C E, Engelfriet C P, von dem Borne A E G Kr 1982 Pseudothrombocytopenia: an immunologic study on platelet antibodies dependent on ethylene diamine tetra-acetate. Blood 59: 157–161
Peterson L C, Rao K V, Corsson J T, White J G 1985 Fechtner syndrome — a variant of Alport's syndrome with leucocyte inclusions and macrothrombocytopenia. Blood 65: 397–406
Pickering D, Cuddigan B 1969 Infantile cortical hyperostosis associated with thrombocythaemia. Lancet ii: 464–465
Pui C-H, Wilimas J, Wang W 1980 Evans syndrome in childhood. Journal of Pediatrics 97: 754–758
Pui C-H, Chesney C M, Weed J, Jackson C W 1985 Altered non Willebrand factor molecule in children with thrombosis following asparaginase-prednisone-vincristine therapy for leukemia. Journal of Clinical Oncology 3: 1266–1272
Rabinowitz J G, Moseley J E, Mitty H A, Hirschhorn K 1967 Trisomy 18, esophageal atresia, anomalies of the radius and congenital hypoplastic thrombocytopenia. Radiology 89: 488–491
Rao A K, Koike K, Willis J et al 1984 Platelet secretion defect associated with impaired liberation of arachidonic acid and normal myosin light chain phosphorylation. Blood 64: 914–921
Remuzzi G 1988 Bleeding in renal failure. Lancet i: 1205–1208
Sampson B M, Greaves M, Malia R G, Preston F E 1983 Acquired von Willebrand's disease: demonstration of a circulating inhibitor to the factor VIII complex in four cases. British Journal of Haematology 54: 233–244
Scarlett J D, Williams N T, McKellar W J D 1992 Acquired amegakaryocytic thrombocytopaenia in a child. Journal of Paediatrics and Child Health 28: 263–266
Schiffer C A 1991 Prevention of alloimmunization against platelets. Blood 77: 1–4
Schmitt S, Auberger K, Fendel T, Kiess W 1992 Hypothalamic failure as a sequela of heterozygous protein C deficiency? European Journal of Pediatrics 151: 428–431
Schulman I, Pierce M, Lukens A, Currimbhoy Z 1960 Studies in thrombopoiesis. I. A factor in normal human plasma required for platelet production; chronic thrombocytopenia due to its deficiency. Blood 16: 943–957
Shattil S J, Bennett J S, McDonough M, Turnbull J 1980 Carbenicillin and penicillin G inhibit platelet production in vitro by impairing the interaction of agonists with the platelet surface. Journal of Clinical Investigation 65: 329–337
Sherry D D, Kredich D W 1985 Transient thrombocytopenia in systemic onset juvenile rheumatoid arthritis. Pediatrics 76: 600–603
Siguret V, Lavergne J-M, Chérel G et al 1994 A novel case of compound heterozygosity with "Normandy"/type I von Willebrand disease (vWD). Direct demonstration of the segregation of one allele with a defective expression at the mRNA level causing type I vWD. Human Genetics 93: 95–102
Silverman E D, Miller III J J, Bernstein B, Shafai J 1983 Consumption coagulopathy associated with systemic juvenile rheumatoid arthritis. Journal of Pediatrics 103: 872–876
Smith T P, Dodds W J, Tartaglia A P 1973 Thrombasthenic-thrombopathic thrombocytopenia with giant, "Swiss-cheese" platelets. A case report. Annals of Internal Medicine 79: 829–834
Stewart G W, O'Brien H, Morris S A et al 1987 Stomatocytosis, abnormal platelets and pseudo-homozygous hypercholesterolaemia. European Journal of Haematology 38: 376–380
Sthoeger D, Nardi M, Karpatkin M 1989 Protein S in the first year of life. British Journal of Haematology 72: 424–428
Stormorken H, Gogstad G, Solum N O 1983 A new bleeding disorder: lack of platelet aggregatory response to adrenalin and lack of secondary aggregation to ADP and platelet activating factor (PAF). Thrombosis Research 29: 391–402
Stormorken H, Sjaastad O, Langslet A et al 1985 A new syndrome: thrombocytopathia, muscle fatigue, asplenia, miosis, migraine, dyslexia and ichthyosis. Clinical Genetics 28: 367–374
Stroncek D F, Vercellotti G M, Hammerschmidt D E et al 1992 Characterization of multiple quinine-dependent antibodies in a patient with episodic hemolytic uremic syndrome and immune agranulocytosis. Blood 80: 241–248
Stuart M J, Sunderji S G, Walenga R W, Setty B N Y 1985 Abnormalities in vascular arachidonic acid metabolism in the infant of the diabetic mother. British Medical Journal 290: 1700–1702
Sweetman L 1989 Branched chain organic acidurias. In: Scriver C R, Beaudet A L, Sly W S, Valle D (eds) The metabolic basis of inherited disease, 6th edn. McGraw-Hill, New York, ch 28
Tait R C, Evans D I K 1993 Late spontaneous recovery of chronic thrombocytopenia. Archives of Disease in Childhood 68: 680–681
Thompson A R, Wood W G, Stamatoyannopoulos G 1977 X-linked syndrome of platelet dysfunction, thrombocytopenia, and imbalanced globin chain synthesis with hemolysis. Blood 50: 303–316
Tremoli E, Maderna P, Colli S et al 1984 Increased platelet sensitivity and thromboxane B2 formation in type II hyperlipoproteinaemic patients. European Journal of Clinical Investigation 14: 329–333
Tuddenham E G D 1994 Flip tip inversion and haemophilia A. Lancet 343: 307–308
von Behrens W E 1975 Mediterranean macrothrombocytopenia. Blood 46: 199–208
Waldman J D, Czapek E E, Paul M H et al 1975 Shortened platelet survival in cyanotic heart disease. Journal of Pediatrics 87: 77–79
Walker R W, Walker W 1984 Idiopathic thrombocytopenia, initial illness and long term follow up. Archives of Disease in Childhood 59: 316–322
Weiden P L, Blaese R M 1972 Hereditary thrombocytopenia: relation to Wiskott-Aldrich syndrome with special reference to splenectomy. Journal of Pediatrics 80: 226–234
Weiss A E 1988 Acquired coagulation disorders. In: Corriveau D M, Fritsma G A (eds) Hemostasis and thrombosis in the clinical laboratory. JB Lippincott, Philadelphia, p 196
Weiss H J, Meyer D, Rabinowitz R et al 1982 Pseudo-von Willebrand's disease. An intrinsic platelet defect with aggregation by unmodified human factor VIII/von Willebrand factor and enhanced adsorption of its high-molecular-weight multimers. New England Journal of Medicine 306: 326–333
Winiarski J 1989 IgG and IgM antibodies to platelet membrane glycoprotein antigens in acute childhood idiopathic thrombocytopenic purpura. British Journal of Haematology 73: 88–92
Wright J F, Blanchette V S, Freedman J 1994 Virus-reactive antibodies cross-react with autologous platelets in a patient with varicella zoster virus (VZV)-associated acute idiopathic thrombocytopenic purpura (ITP). Blood 84, No 10 (suppl 1): 185a (abstract)
Wu K K, Le Breton G C, Tai H-H, Chen Y-C 1981 Abnormal platelet response to thromboxane A2. Journal of Clinical Investigation 67: 1801–1804

Index

Page numbers refer to text and/or tables (T)
Page numbers in bold refer to figures
Only some drugs are indexed individually; for others *see* under Drugs

abetalipoproteinaemia
and acanthocytosis, 88
ABH antigens
normal development, 6
ABO incompatibility, immune haemolysis
blood transfusion, 72
bone marrow transplant, 72
fetomaternal, 71
liver transplant, 72
abuse, child
see **child abuse**
acanthocytosis, 86, **87**, **89**
Hallervordern-Spatz disease, 86, **87**
hypobetalipoproteinaemia, 88, **15**, **89**
hypothyroidism 88, **89**
obscure origin 88, **89**
transfused damaged cells, **89**
with:
hereditary elliptocytosis, **77**
hereditary spherocytosis, 66, **67**
acidified glycerol lysis
in hereditary spherocytosis, 68
acid phosphatase cytochemistry
ALL, 126, **125**
neuroblastoma, **185–187**
***Acinetobacter* septicaemia**
bacteria in leucocytes, **262**
differential diagnosis, 260, **263**
actin filaments
inclusions of, in leucocytes, 220
activated partial thromboplastin time
normal, 278
prolonged
artefact, 276
causes, 280
investigation, 281
obscure origin, 286
+prolonged PT
artefact, 276, **293**
causes, 287
shortened
artefact, 276
haemolytic-uraemic syndrome, 293
activated protein C (APC) resistance
and thrombosis, 298
acute lymphoblastic leukaemia, ch 4, 113ff.
acid phosphatase cytochemistry, 126, **125**
AML M5 as relapse after, **161**
ANAE cytochemistry 124, **125**
anaemia, erythrocyte changes, 133, **131**
ANBE cytochemistry, 126
antigen expression, asynchrony of, 116
antinuclear antibody, 132
aplasia of marrow preceding, 134, **135**
apoptosis
of leukaemic cells, 130, **131**
of multinucleate cells, 132, **133**
azurophil granulation, 120, **121**
B cell, 116, **117**, **119**
β glucuronidase cytochemistry, 126, **127**
bilineage/biphenotypic, 116, **117**
blood changes, 133
bone marrow
aplasia/hypoplasia preceding, 134, **135**
necrosis, 128, **129**
Burkitt-like, **119**
chloroacetate esterase cytochemistry, 126
chromatin, altered, 122, **122**
CML adult type as relapse after, **171**
coagulation abnormalities, 133
common immunophenotype, 116
cyclic neutropenia preceding, 240
cytochemistry
see this section, individual tests
cytogenetics, 126, **128**
cytopenias preceding, 134, **135**
demarcations, intranuclear, 124, **124**
diagnosis, criteria, 114
differential diagnosis
benign lymphoblastosis 136, **137**
Hodgkin's disease, **140**
non-haemopoietic malignancy, 138, 188

acute lymphoblastic leukaemia (*contd*)
differential diagnosis (*contd*)
non-Hodgkin lymphoma, 138, **139**
non-lymphocytic leukaemias, 136
normal marrow, immature lymphocytes, 10, **11**
disseminated intravascular coagulation, 133
DNA content, 128, **128**
early precursor B, 116
eosinophilia, 132, **133**
erythroblastopenia preceding, 134
erythrophagocytosis, **123**
FAB classification 118, **119**
fetal
marker in leukaemic cells, 124, **124**
origins of childhood malignancy, 124
Gaucher-like cells 132, **133**
gene rearrangements, 128
haemostasis, abnormalities, 133
'hand-mirror' variant 118, **119**
vs Hodgkin's disease, **140**
hypereosinophilic syndrome, 132, 256
Ig gene rearrangements, 128
immunophenotype, 116
L1, L2, L3, 118, **119**
lineage switch at relapse, 134, **117**, **161**, **171**
lupus anticoagulant, 285
minimal residual disease, detection, 134
morphologic types, 118, **119**
multinucleate cells, apoptotic, 132, **133**
myelofibrosis, 130, **131**
myeloid leukaemia secondary to, 134, **117**, **161**, **171**
myeloperoxidase cytochemistry, 114
neutropenia preceding, 240, 247
nucleus
demarcations in, 124, **124**
part degeneration, 122, **122**
oil red O cytochemistry, 126, **127**
PAS cytochemistry, 124, **125**
Ph chromosome, 127, **171**
phagocytosis by lymphoblasts, **123**
pre-B, 116
preceded by
bone marrow hypoplasia, 134, **135**
neutropenia, 240, 247
relapse
as AML M5, **161**
as CML adult type, **171**
diagnosis, 134
residual disease, detection, 134
secondary leukaemia, 134, **117**, **161**, **171**
sea-blue histiocytes, 232, **233**
smudge cells, **131**
splenic hypofunction, 133
sudan black positive, 124, **117**
T cell, 116
T receptor gene rearrangements, 128
thrombocytopenia, 133
tumour lysis, 131, **131**
vacuolation, 120, **119**, **127**
virus-like particles, 122, **123**
acute myeloid leukaemia (AML), ch 5, 143ff.
AML M0, 144
AML M1, 144, **145**
AML M2, 146, **147**, **149**, **151**
ANAE positive, **147**
Chediak-Higashi-like granulation, 148, 150, **149**
granulocyte dysplasia/M2 variants
Baso, 150, **149**, **151**
Eo, 148, **149**
mast cell, **149**
neutrophil, 146, **147**, **149**, **151**
lineage switch at relapse, M2 Neut→M2Baso, **151**
AML M3, 152, **153**, **155**
differential diagnosis, 156, **157**
microgranular, 154, **155**
variants, 154, **153**, **155**
AML M4, 156, **159**
differential diagnosis, 158, **157**
M4 Baso, 158
M4Eo, 158, **159**
AML M5, 160, **160**, **161**
adenovirus in, 160, **160**
ANAE negative, 160, **161**
congenital, 162, **161**
haemophagocytic variant, 162, **161**
as relapse after ALL, **161**
AML M6, 162, **163**, **165**
AML M7, 166, **167**
differential diagnosis, 168, **169**
myelofibrosis, 166, **167**
differential diagnosis, summary, 144
disseminated intravascular coagulation, 291
FAB classification, general remarks, 144
secondary to ALL, 134, **117**, **161**
with Sweet's syndrome, 248
thrombocytopathy in, 315
adenosine deaminase, 97
deficiency
severe combined immunodeficiency, 254
overproduction
Diamond-Blackfan anaemia, 53
with stomatocytosis, 96
adenovirus
atypical lymphocytes, 252, **137**
benign lymphoblastosis, **137**
in:
AML M5, 160, **160**
intussusception, 252(T7.14)
adrenalin unresponsiveness (platelet), 313(T8.34), 316
***Aerococcus* sp. septicaemia**
bacteria in leucocytes, **261**
differential diagnosis, 260, **263**
afibrinogenaemia, 288
platelet dysfunction in, 314
Albers-Schönberg disease (osteopetrosis)
leuco-erythroblastic anaemia, 56, **57**
Alder anomaly, 214
infantile free sialic acid storage disease, **215**
Maroteaux-Lamy MPS, **215**
alkaline phosphatase, neutrophil
in:
CML adult type, 173
infection, 257
juvenile chronic myeloid leukaemia, 173
allergy
eosinophilia in, 255
food, vasculitis in, **279**
plastic tubing, **257**
alloimmune haemolysis, 70, 98, **73**, **99**
ABO fetomaternal, 71
incompatible transfusion, 72
non-ABO fetomaternal, 72, **73**
of obscure origin, 70, **73**
organ transplantation, 72
Rh fetomaternal, 72, 98, **99**
disseminated intravascular coagulation, 296
erythroblastopenia, 56
alloimmune neutropenia
neonatal, 244, **243**
from transfusion, 245
alloimmune thrombocytopenia, 306
fetomaternal, 310
after platelet transfusions, 311
alpha-2 antiplasmin
deficiency, and bleeding
AML M3, 152
inherited, 277
normal values, 279
alpha-2 macroglobulin
normal values, 279
alpha globin chains of Hb
inclusions, congenital dyserythropoiesis type I, **40**
synthesis, 6
amegakaryocytic thrombocytopenia
acquired, 52
inherited
congenital, preceding marrow aplasia, 50, 302
Fanconi syndrome
see **Fanconi's anaemia**
phocomelia, 302
thrombocytopenia-absent radius, 300, **301**
trisomy 18, 302
spurious megakaryocytic deficiency, 300
amniotic fluid inhalation
disseminated intravascular coagulation, 291
pulmonary hypertension, 296
ANAE cytochemistry
ALL, 124, **125**
AML
M2, ANAE positive variant, **147**
M3, ANAE positive variant, **155**
M5, **160**
ANAE negative variants, **161**
M7, 166
malignant histiocytosis, **198**
anaemia
aplastic
see **aplastic/hypoplastic anaemia**
of chronic disease
see **chronic disease**
haemolytic
see **haemolysis**
in infection, 98
macrocytic
see **macrocytosis/macrocytic anaemias**
microcytic
see **microcytosis/microcytic anaemias**
normocytic
see **normocytic anaemias**
of prematurity, 64
ANBE cytochemistry
ALL, 126
AML M7, 166
Angiostrongylus cantonensis
eosinophilia, 255(T7.19)
ankyrin, 66
in hereditary spherocytosis, 66
anorexia nervosa
acanthocytosis, 88
bone marrow hypoplasia, 52
hypofibrinogenaemia, 288
anti-A, B isoagglutinins
immune haemolysis from I/V anti A/B/D, 75
normal development, 6
in Wiskott-Aldrich syndrome, 305
anticardiolipin
with lupus anticoagulant, 284
anticonvulsants
atypical lymphocytes (phenytoin sensitivity), 252
bone marrow aplasia, 47
eosinophilia, 256

immune
neutropenia, 247
thrombocytopenia, 311
macrocytosis, 57
anti-D
immune haemolysis from I/V anti A/B/D, 75
antigens
erythrocytic
ABH, normal development, 6
i, I in
congenital dyserythropoietic anaemias, 42
Diamond-Blackfan anaemia, 53
Fanconi's anaemia, 48
juvenile chronic myeloid leukaemia, 173
normal values, 6
antiglobulin (Coombs) test, direct
alloimmune haemolysis, 70
autoimmune haemolysis, 72ff., **73**
positive, causes of, 71
unexplained positive, 76
antinuclear antibody
in ALL, 132
antiphospholipid syndrome
lupus anticoagulant/F II deficiency/platelet damage, 284
anti-Pr
autoimmune haemolysis, 75, **73**
antithrombin III
deficiency and thrombosis, 298
post liver transplant, **297**
normal values, 279
aplasia, pure red cell
see **erythroblastopenia**
aplastic/hypoplastic anaemia, 44ff.
acquired, 47
anorexia nervosa, 52
drugs, 46, **43**
graft vs host disease, 50
infection, 46, **45**
monosomy 7 MPD, 174, **177**
neonatal, maternal SLE, 52
PNH, 50
preceded by acquired amegakaryocytic thrombocytopenia, 52
preceding ALL, 134, **135**
SLE, 52
thymoma, 52
inherited, 48
ataxia-pancytopenia-monosomy 7, 51
chronic mucocutaneous candidiasis, 52
Dubowitz syndrome, 51
dyskeratosis congenita, 48, **49**
Fanconi's anaemia, 48, **49**
Pearson's syndrome, 216, **217**
preceded by congenital amegakaryocytic thrombocytopenia, 50, 302
rare defects, 51
Sekel syndrome, 51
Shwachman's syndrome, 50
WT syndrome, 51
obscure nature
atypical cystic fibrosis, 50, **49**
defective cellular uptake of folate, 50
apoptosis
atypical lymphocytes, infectious mononucleosis, **253**
leukaemic cells, ALL, 130, **131**
lymphocytes, viral infection, 264, **264**
neutrophils, infection, SLE, 264, **264**, **265**
multinucleate cells, ALL, 132, **133**
appendicitis
vs non-surgical abdominal pain, haematology of, 248, 249
arachidonic acid, **317**
impaired release, platelet dysfunction in, 316, 317
artefact
acanthocytosis, 88
coagulation tests, 276, **293**
crenation, 90
leucopenia, 240
macrocytosis, 32
neutropenia, 240
neutrophilia, 248
platelet count, 276, **285**
spherocytosis, 64
stomatocytosis, 94
target cells, 82
ascorbic acid
see **vitamin C**
Askin tumour
in bone marrow, 192, **192**
L-asparaginase
hypofibrinogenaemia, 288
thrombosis, 298
aspartylglycosaminuria, 202(T6.2), 205, 206
aspirin
eosinophilia, 256
immune thrombocytopenia, 311
platelet dysfunction, cyclo-oxygenase deficiency, 316, 317
asplenia
see **spleen absence/atrophy**
asthma
eosinopenia, lymphopenia from steroids, 257
eosinophilia, 255
ataxia-pancytopenia-monosomy 7
marrow aplasia, 51
ataxia telangiectasia
and lymphopenia, 254
ATP
depletion and haemolysis, 102
atransferrinaemia
congenital, 18
attention deficit disorder
platelet calcium, defective mobilization of, 316
atypical (reactive) lymphocytes
see **lymphocytes**
Auer rods
in AML, **147**, **153**, **159**, **163**
Austin type metachromatic leucodystrophy (multiple sulphatase deficiency, mucosulphatidosis), 209, 212
deficient eosinophil granulation, 219
autoagglutination
erythrocytes, immune haemolysis, 74, **73**
leucocytes, mycoplasma infection, **73**
autoerythrocyte sensitization (Gardner-Diamond)
bleeding in, 278
autohaemolysis test
in:
enzyme deficiencies, 106
hereditary spherocytosis, 68
autoimmune haemolysis, 72ff., **73**
associated diseases, 75
Donath-Landsteiner, 74
drugs, 76
unexplained, 76
autoimmune neutropenia, 245
bone marrow transplant, 246
drugs, 246
Evans syndrome, 246
Felty's syndrome, 246
of infancy (chronic benign), 245
neonatal lupus (maternal SLE), 246
SLE, 246
virus infection, 246
autoimmune protein S deficiency, 294
autoimmune thrombocytopenia, 306
in autoimmune disease (SLE, other), 308
with autoimmune haemolysis/neutropenia, 308
bacterial infection, 307
drug autoimmune, 310
Evans syndrome, 75 (T3.10), 246
ITP, 308
maternal, and neonatal thrombocytopenia, 310
post-viral, 306, **305**
with:
autoimmune haemolysis, 307
parietal cell, thyroid autoantibodies, 307
vs ITP, 308
azurophil granulation
in:
leukaemic lymphoblasts, 120, **121**
normal lymphocytes, **263**

Babesia
haemolysis, 65
bacteria in leucocytes, septicaemia, 260, **261**, **262**
differential diagnosis, 260, **263**
see also individual bacteria
Bartonella
haemolysis, 65
Bart's haemoglobin, **31**
normal values, 6
in thalassaemias, 25, 26, **25**, **27**
basophilic stippling, erythrocyte, 97
lead poisoning, **21**
pyrimidine 5′ nucleotidase deficiency, 97
basophils
aberrant, AML, **149**, **151**
absence, acquired, 218
Alder anomaly, **215**
Charcot-Leyden crystals in, AML, 150, **151**
grey-staining inclusions, 220, **221**
normal, granules vs cocci, 260, **263**
Batten's disease (neuronal lipofuscinosis)
infantile (Hagberg-Santavuori)
granular osmiophilic deposits, lymphocytes, 204
juvenile (Spielmeyer-Vogt), 204, 205
lymphocyte vacuolation, 202, **203**
late infantile (Bielschowsky-Jansky), 204
curvilinear bodies, lymphocytes, **205**
B cell ALL, 116, **117**, **119**
B cell lymphoma, **139**
vs ALL, 138
benign intracranial hypertension
and dysfibrinogenaemia, 288
Bernard-Soulier syndrome
acquired, monosomy 7 MPD, 174, **175**
inherited, 313, **303**
β glucuronidase cytochemistry
ALL, 126, **127**
AML, **145**, **161**
neuroblastoma, 184, **187**
Bielschowsky-Jansky disease, 204
curvilinear bodies, lymphocytes, **205**
bilineage/biphenotypic ALL, 116
as lineage switch from ALL, **117**
bilirubin
in monocytes, **225**
Birbeck bodies
Langerhans cells, 194

bite cells, 86, **87**
bleeding
clinical evaluation, 274
haemostatic screen for, 276
from raised intravascular pressure, 274, **279**
self-inflicted, 274, **279**
bleeding time
aspirin prolongation of, platelet-release defects, 316
normal, 280
in:
platelet dysfunction, 312
thrombocytopenia, 312
blister cells (eccentrocytes, hemighosts), 92
favism, **93**
idiopathic neonatal Heinz body haemolysis, **85**
blood group incompatibility
see **incompatibility**
blood loss
iron deficiency anaemia, 16, 17, **15**
normocytic anaemia, 62, **63**
blood transfusion
see **transfusion**
bone marrow
aplasia/hypoplasia
see **aplastic/hypoplastic anaemia**
failure, 65
see also specific disorders
necrosis, ALL, 128, **129**
normal
cell composition, 10, **11**
cellularity, **11**
fibrils, **187**
immature lymphocytes/lymphoblasts, 10, **11**
iron, 11
osteoblasts, **185**
rosettes, **186**
transplantation, and
alloimmune
haemolysis, ABO incompatibility, 72
thrombocytopenia, 306
autoimmune neutropenia, 246
graft-vs-host disease, 47
botryoid nuclei
heat stroke, 224
brain damage
causing DIC, 286, **293**
brucellosis
atypical lymphocytes, 252
neutropenia, 241
Buckley's syndrome
and eosinophilia, 255, 256
Budd-Chiari syndrome
in PNH, 52
Buhot plasma cells, 212, **213**
burns
disseminated intravascular coagulation, 296
lymphopenia, 254
neutropenia, 240
spherocytosis, 68, **69**
thrombocytopathy, 315

C1 esterase inhibitor
normal values, 279
Cabot rings
AML M6, **163**
calcium mobilization, platelets
defective, 316
test for, 312
***Candida* septicaemia**
in myeloperoxidase deficiency, 218
organisms in leucocytes, **263**
differential diagnosis, 260, **263**
***Capnocytophaga* sp. septicaemia (dog-bite)**
bacteria in leucocytes, **262**
differential diagnosis, 260, **263**
carbonic anhydrase
in Hb electrophoretic patterns, **31**
cardiolipin, antibodies to
with lupus anticoagulant, 284
cardiopulmonary bypass surgery
coagulation factor deficiencies, 296
disseminated intravascular coagulation, 296
thrombocytopathy, 315
carnitine deficiency
lipid vacuoles in neutrophils (Jordans anomaly), 214
cartilage-hair hypoplasia
and neutropenia, 241
cbl (cellular cobalamin) defects, 38, **39**
cerebrospinal fluid
atypical (reactive) lymphocytes, **115**, **137**
eosinophilia (plastic tubing), **257**
leukaemic lymphoblasts, **115**
medulloblastoma, **189**
normal mesothelial cells, **189**
ceroid lipofuscinosis
see **Batten's disease**
Charcot-Leyden crystals
see **crystals**
Chediak-Higashi
-like granulation, AML, 148, 150, **149**
syndrome, 220
granulocytes, 220, **215**
lymphocytes, 212, **213**
monocytes, 224
platelets, 309, 313, 315
cherry red spot-myoclonus syndrome (neuraminidase deficiency without dysmorphism, sialidosis I), 202, 204, 205, 206
child abuse
APTT prolongation, 286
DIC from brain damage, **293**
prothrombin complex deficiency, 287
self-inflicted, 274, **279**
childhood malignancy
fetal origins, 124
chloramphenicol
marrow damage, 47, **43**
sideroblastic anaemia, 19
chloroacetate esterase cytochemistry
ALL, 126
AML
M2Eo, **149**
M3, **153**
Auer rods, **153**
cholesteryl ester storage disease (adult Wolman's), 202, 204, 205, 228
Christmas disease
see **coagulation factor deficiency**
chromatin, altered
in ALL, 122, **122**
chromomeres
in leucocytes, 257, **259**
chromosome abnormalities
ALL, 126, 127
AML, 146
CML adult, 173
eosinophilic leukaemia, 182
Ewing's sarcoma, 192
fragility, Fanconi's anaemia, 48
juvenile CML, 170
malignant histiocytosis, 198
myelodysplastic syndromes, 178
neuroblastoma, 184
retinoblastoma, 188
rhabdomyosarcoma, 190
by number
t(1;5)MPD with eosinophilia, 182
5q- syndrome, 182
monosomy 7, 174
8p deletion with hereditary spherocytosis, 68
t(9;22)(Ph), 126, 127, 173, **171**
chronic benign (autoimmune) neutropenia of infancy, 245
chronic disease, anaemia of, 18
of obscure cause, **17**
vs iron deficiency, thal minor, 19
chronic lymphocytic leukaemia, 140
chronic mucocutaneous candidiasis
bone marrow hypoplasia, 52
chronic myeloid leukaemias, 170ff., **171**, **175**, **177**, **179**, **181**
CML, adult, 176, **171**
following ALL, 176, **171**
CML, juvenile, 170, **171**
eosinophilic leukaemia, 182
essential thrombocythaemia, 180, **181**
familial myeloproliferative disease, 172
5q-syndrome, 182
monosomy 7 MPD, 174, **175**, **177**
myelodysplastic syndromes, 178
de novo, **179**
post chemotherapy, **181**
polycythaemia vera, 182
t(1;5) MPD with eosinophilia, 182
5q- syndrome, 182
chylomicronaemia (hypertriglyceridaemia), 230
haemolysis in, **101**
hereditary, **231**
in:
ALL, **131**
haemolytic-uraemic syndrome, **231**
infection-associated haemophagocytosis, 267
nephrosis, **231**
leucocyte smudging, spurious leucopenia, 230
citrate excess (in vitro)
prolonged PT+APTT, 276, 287
***Clostridium welchii* sepsis**
bacteria in leucocytes, 260, **262**
differential diagnosis, 260, **263**
haemolysis, 70, **69**
T activation, 74
coagulation factor/s
deficiency
I, *see* **fibrinogen**
II, isolated, 287
II, VII, IX, X
see **prothrombin complex**
V, isolated, 287
platelet dysfunction in, 316
V+VIII, 287
VII, 286
VII+X, 286
VIII, 280
carrier state, detection, 282
inhibitors, 282
IX, 284
X, isolated, 286, 287
X+VII, 286
XI, 285
XII, 285
thrombosis in, 298
XIII, 277, **275**

high MW kininogen, 285
Passovoy defect, 286
prekallikrein, 285
von Willebrand factor
see **von Willebrand factor**
inhibitors
fibrinogen, 288
Factor
II, *see* **lupus anticoagulant**
V, 287
VII, 287
VIII, 282
IX, 284
XII, 285
XIII, 277
lupus type
see **lupus anticoagulant**
minimum levels for normal
haemostasis, 277
tests, 277
mutant F V (activated protein C resistance)
thrombosis, 298
natural inhibitors of
normal values, 279
normal values, 278
coagulation, schema, 281
cobalamin
deficiency, 35ff., **37**, **39**
breast-fed infant of vegan mother, 36, **37**
cellular utilization/metabolism
defects (cbl defects), 38, **39**
ileal disease, 36
intrinsic factor, **35**
congenital absence of or non-functioning, 36, **35**
gastric atrophy (juvenile pernicious anaemia), 36
receptor defect (Imerslund-Gräsbeck), 36, **35**
TCII deficiency, 38, **35**
metabolism, **35**
serum, normal values, 6
coeliac disease
iron deficiency, 16
splenic atrophy, 108
Cohen's syndrome
and neutropenia, 241
colchicine poisoning
granulocyte pyknosis, **223**
cold agglutinin titre
in autoimmune haemolysis, 75
colitis, milk
eosinophilia, 255, 256
iron deficiency, 16, **15**
colony-stimulating factors
abnormal eosinophils, **219**
neutrophilia, 249
toxic neutrophils, 259
common immunophenotype ALL, 116
congenital
coagulation factor deficiencies
see **coagulation factors**
cobalamin deficiency
see **cobalamin**
dyserythropoiesis
see **dyserythropoiesis**
erythroblastopenia
see **erythroblastopenia**
erythropoietic
porphyria (Günther), haemolysis in, 107
protoporphyria, microcytosis in, 22
heart disease
acyanotic
haemostatic abnormalities, 296
cyanotic
asplenia, Ivemark, 108, **109**
coagulation factor deficiencies, 296
polycythaemia, 182
thrombosis, 297
spherocytosis, **69**
splenic atrophy, 108
thrombocytopathy, 296
thrombocytopenia, 296
fragmentation haemolysis, 80, 311
leukaemia, 124, **161**
microcytic anaemia with iron overload, 20
myelodysplasia, 178
thrombotic disorders
see **thrombosis**
Coombs test
see **antiglobulin test**
copper
deficiency
megaloblastosis, sideroblastosis, 247
neutropenia, 247
intoxication
spherocytosis, 70
cow's milk
allergy, 255, 256
enteropathy, iron deficiency from, 16, **15**
C-reactive protein
in:
microcytic anaemias, 19
neonatal sepsis, 258
crenation, 90, **81**, **89**, **91**
Crohn's disease
see **inflammatory bowel disease**
cryohaemolysis, hypertonic
in spherocytosis, 68, **67**
cryohydrocytosis, 96
cryptantigen exposure (T activation)
DAT-negative haemolysis, 65(T3.6), 74
in:
haemolytic-uraemic syndrome, 80, **81**
infection, 99
crystals, blood, marrow, 236
Auer rods
see **Auer rods**
Charcot-Leyden, 236
basophils, AML, **151**
bone marrow macrophages
AML, **151**
benign eosinophilia, **237**
monosomy 7 MPD, 174
bone marrow necrosis, ALL, **129**
eosinophils
AML, myelodysplasia, **149**, **179**
normal eosinophils, **237**
neutrophils, AML, **151**
cystine, 236, **237**
fat, neutral, **237**
Gaucher-like, **227**
HbC, 28, **28**
hydroxyapatite, Michaelis-Gutmann bodies, **219**
orotic acid, 56
starch, **237**
tyrosine, 236
unidentified
bone marrow, mannosidosis, **237**
eosinophils, genetic anomaly, 220, **221**
monocytes, Letterer-Siwe disease, **197**
curvilinear bodies
Batten's disease, late infantile, **205**
Cushing's disease
bruising, 278
cyanosis
cytochrome reductase deficiency, 30
HbM's, 30
under-oxygenation, 30
cyanotic congenital heart disease
see **congenital heart disease**
cyclic neutropenia, 240
harbinger of
ALL, 240
myeloproliferative disease, 176, **177**
cyclo-oxygenase (platelet), 317
deficiency and thrombocytopathy, 316
cyclosporin
and:
haemolytic-uraemic syndrome, 292
platelet hyperreactivity, thrombosis, 299
cystic fibrosis
acanthocytosis, hypobetalipoproteinaemia, **89**
atypical, with
marrow hypoplasia, 50, **49**
neutropenia, **243**
iron deficiency, 16
cystinosis, 236, **237**
cytochemistry
see specific stains and diseases
cytochrome b reductase deficiency
methaemoglobinaemia, 30
cytogenetics
see **chromosome abnormalities**
cytomegalovirus infection
atypical lymphocytosis, 252
benign lymphoblastosis, 136, 144
disseminated intravascular coagulation, 292
haemolysis, 98
immune thrombocytopenia, 306
multinucleate cells in marrow, 156, **157**
myelomonocytosis, **157**
paraproteinaemia, **157**
promyelocytic hyperplasia, 156, **157**
cytopenias
preceding ALL, 134, **135**
see also **pancytopenia**
cytotoxics
bone marrow aplasia, 47
dyserythropoiesis, **43**
elliptocytosis, 76
eosinophilia, 256
erythroblastopenia, 53
foamy macrophages, marrow, 230, **231**
haemolytic-uraemic syndrome, 292
lymphopenia, 254
macrocytosis, megaloblastosis, 57
myelodysplastic syndrome, 178, **181**
sideroblastic anaemia, 19
splenic hypofunction, 108, 133
stomatocytosis, 97, **95**
thrombocytopenia, 311
toxic neutrophils, 259

D-dimer test for FDP, 290
D group incompatibility
fetomaternal, 56, 72, 98, **99**
D^u group, maternal
apparent acquisition, fetomaternal haemorrhage, 62
death, leucocytic
see **apoptosis**
defensins
in neutrophil granules, 216

delayed haemorrhagic disease of newborn, 286, **275**
dermatitis
and folate deficiency 38, 40
dermatitis herpetiformis
splenic atrophy in, 108
diabetes insipidus
DIDMOAD constellation, 40
Hand-Schüller-Christian disease, 194
diabetes mellitus
chylomicronaemia, 230
maternal, and disseminated coagulation in neonate, 296
and MPO deficiency, candidiasis in, 218
neutrophilia, 249
platelet hyperreactivity, thrombosis, 298
vessel dysfunction, 278
dialysis, renal
haemolysis, 99
Diamond-Blackfan anaemia, 53, **51**
DIDMOAD constellation (Wolfram's disease)
thiamine-responsive megaloblastosis, 40
di-epoxy butane, chromosome fragility
Fanconi's anaemia, 48
di George syndrome
and lymphopenia, 254
di Guglielmo disease, 162, **163**
dihydrofolate reductase, 35
deficiency, 40
dilutional thrombocytopenia, 312
disseminated intravascular coagulation, 290ff., **293**, **295**
neonatal, due to maternal disease, 296
see also individual causes
dog-bite, septicaemia
see ***Capnocytophaga***
Döhle bodies, 257, 258, **217**, **259**
Döhle-like bodies
Fechtner syndrome, 216, 309
May-Hegglin anomaly, 216, 309, **217**
Sebastian syndrome, 216, 309
Donath-Landsteiner antibody, 72, 74, 75
Down's syndrome
AML M7, 166
macrocytosis, 42
monosomy 7 MPD, **177**
transient abnormal myelopoiesis, 168, **169**
drugs (these are also indexed separately: anticonvulsants, L-asparaginase, aspirin, chloramphenicol, cytotoxics, glue, heparin, quinidine/quinine, steroids, warfarin)
aplastic anaemia, 46, **43**
dyserythropoiesis, 42, **43**
eosinophilia, 256
erythroblastopenia, 56
haemolysis
bite cells, 86, **87**
G6PD deficiency and, 106
haemolytic-uraemic syndrome, 292
Heinz body
G6PD deficiency, 104, **93**
neonatal idiopathic, 84, **85**
immune, 76
pyruvate kinase deficiency and, 104
stomatocytosis, 96, **95**
lupus anticoagulant, 285
lymphopenia, 254
macrocytosis/megaloblastosis, 56
methaemoglobinaemia, 33
neutropenia
immune, 246
non-immune, 248
neutrophilia, 249
sideroblastic anaemia, 19(T2.5), 22
thrombocytopathy, 316
thrombocytopenia
immune, 310
non-immune, 311(T8.31)
thrombosis, 297
drumsticks, nuclear, 222, **223**
Dubin-Johnson syndrome
F VII deficiency, 286
Dubowitz syndrome
bone marrow aplasia, 51
Duffy (Fy^a) group
fetomaternal incompatibility, 72
Duncan's disease (X-linked lymphoproliferative syndrome), 252
atypical lymphocytes, 'tumours' of, **253**
lymphoma, bowel, **253**
dyserythropoiesis, erythroblast damage
AML M6, **163**
β thal major, 30
bone marrow aplasia, 44
chloramphenicol, **43**
congenital, 40
with hereditary elliptocytosis, 78
type I, **41**
type II (HEMPAS), **41**
unclassified, **43**
copper deficiency, 247
cytotoxics, **43**
Fanconi's anaemia, 48
folate, defective cellular uptake of, 40
iron deficiency anaemia, 14
megaloblastic anaemia
see **megaloblastosis**
myelodysplastic syndromes, **179**, **181**
parvovirus, **53**
transient erythroblastopenia of childhood, 54, **53**
dysfibrinogenaemia, 288
thrombosis in, 298
dyskeratosis congenita
aplastic anaemia, neutropenia, 48, **49**
dyspoiesis
erythroblastic
see **dyserythropoiesis**
granulocytic
ALL, bilineage, **117**
Chediak-Higashi syndrome, 220, **215**
chloramphenicol, **43**
copper deficiency, 247
myeloid leukaemias/MDS, **147**, **149**, **151**, **153**, **159**, **171**, **175**, **179**, **181**
neutropenias with abnormal marrow neutrophils, 244
see also **Pelgerization**
megakaryocytic
MDS, myeloid leukaemias, **167**, **175**, **179**
with thrombocytopenia, 303
transient abnormal myelopoiesis of trisomy 21, 168, **169**
transient megakaryocytic dyspoiesis, 170

early precursor B ALL, 116
eccentrocytes (blister cells, hemighosts), 92
favism, **93**
Heinz body haemolysis, idiopathic neonatal, **85**
echinocytes (crenated cells), 90, **81**, **89**, **91**
echovirus
atypical lymphocytes, 252
eclampsia, maternal
and disseminated coagulation in neonate, 296
eczema
and:
eosinophilia, 255
folate deficiency, 40
in:
alopecia, lymphoid hyperplasia, thrombocytopenia syndrome, 308
Job's syndrome, 256
Omenn's syndrome, 250
Wiskott-Aldrich syndrome, 304
Ehlers-Danlos syndrome, **279**
thrombocytopathy, 312
vessel dysfunction, 278
electrolyte flux, erythrocytic, disorders of
hereditary
cryohydrocytosis, 96
hydrocytosis, 96
xerocytosis, 94, **93**
electrophoresis of Hbs, 30, **24**, **25**, **27–29**, **31**
elliptocytosis, 76
hereditary
haemolytic, with spherocytosis, 78, **77**
Melanesian (S.E.Asian), 78, **77**
mild ('common'), 76, **77**
homozygous, 97(T3.21)
with:
acanthocytosis, 78, **77**, **87**
dyserythropoiesis, 78
pyknocytosis, 78
thalassaemia, **27**
pyropoikilocytosis, 78, **79**
endothelial cells
in blood films, **366**
enteropathy/colitis, milk
eosinophilia, 255, 256
iron deficiency, 16, **15**
envenomation
disseminated intravascular coagulation, 296
fragmentation haemolysis, 80
hypofibrinogenaemia, 289(T8.14), **275**
spherocytosis, 70
vessel dysfunction, 278
enzymes, erythrocytic
deficiency, 102, **93**, **103**, **105**
normal values, neonate, 6
see also specific enzymes
eosinopenia
absence of eosinophils, acquired, 218
steroids, 257
eosinophilia
blood/marrow, 255
ALL, 132, **133**
AML
M2, M2Eo, 148, **149**
M4Eo, 158, **159**
Charcot-Leyden crystals in
see **crystals**
CML, 173
drugs, 256
eosinophilic gastroenteropathy, 256
eosinophilic leukaemia, 182
familial, 256, **257**
histiocytosis, 255(T7.19), **197**
hypereosinophilic syndrome, 255(T7.19), 256
ALL, 132, **133**
cardiac valve thrombosis in, **257**
Job's syndrome, 256
Loa loa, **257**
milk protein colitis, 16, 255, 256, **15**
obscure origin, 256

Omenn's syndrome, **251**
paraprotein, serum, in, 256
parasites, 256
plastic tubing, 255
in premature infants, 256
thrombocytopenia, immune, 307
CSF
allergy to plastic tubing, **257**
eosinophilic
gastroenteropathy, 256
granuloma, 194, 195, **197**
leukaemia, 182
eosinophils
absence, acquired, 218
in AML
M2, M2Eo, 148, **149**
M4Eo, 158, **159**
blood, normal values, 8
in Chediak-Higashi disease, 220, **215**
crystals in
Charcot-Leyden
AML, MDS, **149**, **179**
normal eosinophils, **237**
unidentified; genetic anomaly, 220, **221**
granule agglutination, GM-CSF treatment, **219**
granule deficiency, 218
GM-CSF treatment, **219**
infantile free sialic acid storage disease, **219**
with Michaelis-Gutmann bodies, 218, **219**
grey-staining inclusions, 220, **221**
leukaemia of, 182
marrow, normal values, 10
nuclear hypersegmentation, 224
Pelger-Huet anomaly, 222, **223**
peroxidase deficiency, hereditary, 218
see also **eosinopenia, eosinophilia, eosinophilic**
Epstein macrothrombocytopenia, 309
Epstein-Barr virus, 252
benign lymphoblastosis, 136
bone marrow hypoplasia, 46
chronic myelomonocytosis, 172
erythroblastopenia, 56
lymphoma, **139**, **253**
serology, 254
see also **infectious mononucleosis**
erythroblastopenia, 53
drugs, 53
EB virus, 56
fetomaternal D incompatibility, 56
hereditary
Diamond-Blackfan, 53, **51**
PNP deficiency, 56
TCII deficiency, 56
Hodgkin's disease, 56
immune, 56
parvovirus, 54, **55**
preceding ALL, 134
thymoma, 56
transient erythroblastopenia of childhood, 54, **55**
vs Diamond-Blackfan anaemia, 53
erythroblasts
blood, normal values in neonate, 3
with Cabot ring, AML M6, **163**
dysplasia/dyspoiesis
see **dyserythropoiesis**
giant, parvovirus infection, **53**
large, transient erythroblastopenia of childhood, **53**
marrow, normal values, 10
phagocytosis of
ALL, **123**
infection-associated haemophagocytosis, **268**
septicaemia, **265**
vacuolation
chloramphenicol, 47(T2.27), **43**
copper deficiency, 247
Diamond-Blackfan anaemia, 53
Pearson's syndrome, 216, **217**
phenylalanine-restricted diets, 46
erythrocyte/s
antigens
ABH
normal development, 6
i, I
in:
congenital dyserythropoietic anaemias, 42
Diamond-Blackfan anaemia, 53
Fanconi's anaemia, 48
normal development, 6
count, normal values, 3
electrolyte flux, disorders of hereditary
cryohydrocytosis, 96
hydrocytosis, 95, 96
xerocytosis, 94, **93**
enzymes
deficiency, 102, **93**, **103**, **105**
normal values, neonate, 6
see also specific enzymes
in liver disease/obstructive jaundice, 91, **83**, **91**
membrane
protein defects and stomatocytosis, 96
structure, **66**
peculiarities, normal neonate, 2, **5**
pitted (pocked)
asplenia (Ivemark), **109**
normal values, 4
splenic atrophy
collagen disease, **109**
Sβ thal, **29**
protoporphyrin
see **protoporphyrin**
in renal disease, 98, **99**
see also **haemolytic-uraemic syndrome**
sedimentation rate
in:
appendicitis vs non-surgical abdominal pain, 249(T7.11)
neuroblastoma, 184
stippled, 97
lead poisoning, **21**
pyrimidine 5′ nucleotidase deficiency, 97
see also specific morphology, disorder
erythrophagocytosis
by:
lymphoblasts, ALL, **123**
macrophages/monocytes
autoimmune haemolysis, **73**
infection-associated haemophagocytosis, **268**
septicaemia, **265**
monoblasts, AML M5, **161**
neutrophils, autoimmune haemolysis, 74
promyelocytes, CMV infection, **157**
rhabdomyosarcoma cells, 190
erythropoietin
deficiency and anaemia, 64
***Escherichia coli*, septicaemia**
bacteria in leucocytes, 260, **262**
differential diagnosis, 260, **263**
essential thrombocythaemia, 180, **181**
thrombosis in, 297(T8.22)
esterases
see **ANAE, ANBE**
Estren-Dameshek anaemia
and Fanconi's anaemia, 48
Evans syndrome (autoimmune haemolysis + thrombocytopenia), 75(T3.10), 246
Ewing's sarcoma
in marrow, 192, **192**
extracorporeal bypass surgery
coagulation factor deficiencies, 296
thrombocytopathy, 315(T8.36)

F (fetal Hb-containing) cells
haemoglobinopathy, 30
hereditary persistence of fetal Hb, 30
maternal, fetomaternal haemorrhage, 62, **63**
see also **fetal Hb**
Fabry's disease, 204(T6.3), 205, 230
factors, coagulation
see **coagulation factor/s**
familial
eosinophilia, 256, **257**
haemophagocytosis, 267
myeloproliferative disease (Randall), 172
neutrophilia, 248
Fanconi's anaemia, 48, **49**
vs thrombocytopenia-absent radius syndrome, 302
Farber's lipogranulomatosis, 204, 205, 230
fat, neutral
embolism, vessel dysfunction, 278
in marrow, 236, **11**, **231**, **237**
necrosis of, in marrow, 230
favism, 107(T3.26)
blister cells, Heinz bodies, 92, **93**
Fechtner's syndrome
Döhle-like bodies, thrombocytopenia, 216, 309
Felty's syndrome, 246
ferrochelatase deficiency
congenital erythropoietic protoporphyria, 22
congenital microcytic anaemia with iron overload, 22
hereditary sideroblastic anaemia, 20
lead poisoning, 22
fetal
granulopoiesis, lymph node, **171**
haemoglobins, 6
Hb
electrophoretic mobility, **24**, **25**, **27**, **29**, **31**
hereditary persistence of, 30
increase
acquired amegakaryocytic thrombocytopenia, 52
AML, 146
aplastic anaemia, 44
Diamond-Blackfan anaemia, 53
Fanconi's anaemia, 48
haemoglobinopathy, 23, 25, 26, 27
hereditary persistence of fetal Hb, 30
juvenile CML, 172, 173
maternal, fetomaternal haemorrhage, 62, **63**
monosomy 7 MPD, 176
normal values, 6, 7
synthesis in fetus, 6
see also **F cells**
infection, and thrombocytopenia, 300
leukaemia
AML
M5, **161**
M7, 166
marker in ALL, 124, **124**
origins of childhood malignancy, 124
transient abnormal myelopoiesis, 170, **169**
feto-fetal haemorrhage, 62, **63**

fetomaternal
alloimmune thrombocytopenia, 310
blood group incompatibility
ABO, 71
non-ABO, 72, **73**
obscure origin, 70, **73**
Rh, 72, 98, **99**
disseminated intravascular coagulation, 296
erythroblastopenia, 56
haemorrhage
apparent change in maternal D neg to D[u], 62
neonatal anaemia
normocytic, 62, **63**
iron deficiency, 16, **15**
fibrils
normal, marrow, **187**
neurofibrils, neuroblastoma, 184, **187**
fibrin(ogen) degradation products
detection, 290, 291(T8.18)
fibrinogen
deficiency, 288, 289(T8.14, 8.16)
DIC from brain haemorrhage, **293**
snake bite, **275**
spurious, 276
high, artefact, 276
fibrin(ogen)olysis, 288, 289 (T8.14, 8.15)
defective, and thrombosis, 297(T8.22), 298
Fitzgerald trait (high MW kininogen deficiency), 285
5q- syndrome, 182
Fletcher trait (pre-kallikrein deficiency), 285
foamy macrophages
see **macrophages, foamy**
folate
deficiency, 38, **35**
cellular uptake/metabolism, defective, 38, 50
dermatitis, eczema, 38, 40
dietary, 38
dihydrofolate reductase deficiency, 40, **35**
haemolytic disorders, 40
prematurity, 40, **37**
malabsorption
due to anticonvulsants, 38, 57
global, 38
hereditary folate malabsorption, 38
metabolism, **35**
normal values, 6
fragmentation haemolysis, 80
cardiac valve disease, 80
haemolytic-uraemic syndrome
see **haemolytic-uraemic syndrome**
hereditary pyropoikilocytosis, 78, **79**
liver disease, **91**
selenium deficiency, **101**
thrombotic thrombocytopenic purpura, 80
free sialic acid storage disorders
see **sialic acid**
fructose 1–6 diphosphatase deficiency
thrombocytopathy, **275**
fucosidosis, 202(T6.2), 204(T6.3), 205, 206, 228(T6.13)

galactosialidosis, 202(T6.2), 204(T6.3), 205, 206, 213(T6.6), 228(T6.13)
Gardner-Diamond syndrome (auto-erythrocyte sensitization), 278(T8.3)
Gasser
lymphocytes, 208, **209**
'reticulum' cells, 209, 234, **235**
Gaucher
cells, 224, **227**
disease, 204(T6.3), 205, 225
Gaucher-like cells, 226
ALL, 132, **133**, **227**
Shwachman's syndrome, **227**
G-CSF
see **colony stimulating factors**
gene rearrangements
ALL, AML, 128
gestational thrombocytopenia
and thrombocytopenia in neonate, 310
Gilbert's syndrome
and F VII deficiency, 286
Glanzmann's thrombasthenia, 313(T8.35). 314, **315**
globin chains, Hb
α, inclusions of, congenital dyserythropoiesis I, **41**
synthesis, 6
glucose-6-phosphatase deficiency (glycogenosis I)
thrombocytopathy, 312(T8.32)
glucose-6-phosphate dehydrogenase, 103
deficiency, 106, **93**
glucose phosphate isomerase, 103
deficiency and haemolysis, 104(T3.25)
glue-sniffing
aplastic anaemia, 47(T2.28)
glutathione, 103
depletion and haemolysis, 102
glycogenosis I
neutropenia, 242(T7.5)
thrombocytopathy, 312(T8.32)
glycogenosis II, 202(T6.2), 205, 208
glycoproteins, platelet membrane
see **platelets**
GM-CSF
abnormal eosinophils, **219**
neutrophilia, 249(T7.10)
G_{M1} gangliosidosis
I (infantile), 202(T6.2), 204(T6.3), 205, 206, 228(T6.13)
II (late infantile), 204(T6.3), 205, 232
Gower 1,2 haemoglobins, 6
graft vs host disease
bone marrow aplasia, 50
eosinophilia, 255
lymphopenia, 254
splenic atrophy, 108
transfusion-associated, 50
granular osmiophilic deposits, lymphocytes
infantile Batten's disease, 204
granulocytes
see **basophils, eosinophils, neutrophils**
Greaves macrothrombocytopenia, 304
grey-platelet syndrome, 313(T8.35), 314, **315**
Günther's disease (congential erythropoietic porphyria), 107

haemangioma
and intravascular coagulation, 292, **293**
placental, and intravascular coagulation in neonate, 294
haematocrit
normal values, 3
haematogones
in normal marrow, 10, **11**
haemochromatosis, neonatal
lipid vacuoles in neutrophils, 214, **217**
haemodialysis
haemolysis, 98
neutropenia, 240
haemoglobin
abnormal, transient megakaryocytic dyspoiesis, 170
A2, **31**
in haemoglobinopathies, 23, 25, 26, 27, 30, **24**, **27**, **28**, **29**
normal values, 7
synthesis in fetus, 6
α globin chains, inclusions of
β thal major, 30
congenital dyserythropoiesis I, 40, **41**
unstable Hb, 32
Bart's, **31**
in α thalassaemias, 26, 27(T2.11), **27**
hydrops, 26, **25**
normal values, 6
Bristol, 32
C, **31**
crystals, 28, **28**
disorders, 26, 27, **28**, **29**
concentration, normal values, 3
Constant Spring, 26(T2.11)
D, **31**
Dβ thal, **25**
E, **31**
disorders, 26(T2.12), 27, **28**
F
see **fetal Hb**
Geneva, 32
Gower, 6
H, 30, **27**
disease, 25, 26(T2.11)
disease and mental retardation/dysmorphism, 23
Hammersmith, 32
Köln, 32, **31**
Lepore, 26(T2.11), 29(T2.14), **31**
Ms, 30
Portland, 6, **31**
S, **31**
disorders, 26(T2.12), 27, **29**
structural variants, 26, 27, **25**, **28**, **29**, **31**
synthesis in fetus, 6
unstable, 32, **31**
haemoglobinopathy, 22ff., **24**, **25**, **27**, **28**, **29**, **31**
see also **haemoglobin, thalassaemias**
haemoglobins
electrophoretic mobility, 30, **24**, **25**, **27**, **28**, **29**, **31**
synthesis in fetus, 6
unstable, 32, **31**
haemoglobinuria, 107
Donath-Landsteiner haemolysis, 74
PNH, 50
haemolysins
in:
anaemia of infection, 98
clostridial sepsis, **69**
haemolysis, haemolytic anaemias, 64ff.
disseminated intravascular coagulation in, 296
erythrocyte morphology of value in diagnosis, 65
in infection, 75, 98, **69**, **81**
investigation, 65(T3.4)
with normal or nondescript erythrocyte morphology, 98
see also specific morphology/disorder
haemolytic-uraemic syndrome, 80, 292, **81**, **293**
chylomicronaemia, **231**
haemostatic changes, 286, 292, 293
pneumococcus-associated, 80, **81**
relation to TTP, 80
haemophagocytic lymphohistiocytosis
see **haemophagocytosis**
haemophagocytosis
familial, 267
idiopathic, **268**

infection-associated, 194, 267, **268**
see also **erythrophagocytosis**
haemophilia A, 280
carrier state, detection, 282
F VIII inhibitors, 282
haemophilia B (Christmas), 284
F IX:
inhibitors, 284
loss in urine, nephrosis, 284
***Haemophilus influenzae*, septicaemia**
bacteria in leucocytes, 260, **262**
differential diagnosis, 260, **263**
haemorrhage
feto-fetal, 62, **63**
feto-maternal
apparent change in maternal group D neg to D[u], 62
neonatal anaemia
normocytic, 62, **63**
iron deficiency, 16, **15**
intracranial, causing DIC, **293**
iron deficiency anaemia, 16, 17, **15**
neonatal, causes, 62
haemorrhagic disease of newborn, 286
delayed, 286, **275**
haemosiderin
bone marrow, normal, 10
leucocytes
from frequent transfusions, **223**
neonatal haemochromatosis, 214
sputum, idiopathic pulmonary haemosiderosis, 16, **15**
urine, 16, 64
haemolysis, enzyme deficiency, **105**
haemosiderosis, idiopathic pulmonary
iron deficiency anaemia, 16, **15**
haemostatic defects
screen for, 276
Hagberg-Santavuori (infantile Batten's) disease
granular osmiophilic deposits, lymphocytes, 204
Hageman trait (F XII deficiency), 285
thrombosis in, 298
Hallervordern-Spatz disease, 86, **87**
acanthocytosis, **87**
sea-blue histiocytes, marrow, 232(T6.15)
Ham's (acid haemolysis) test
congenital dyserythropoietic anaemias, 42(T2.23)
PNH, 42, 52
'hand-mirror' ALL, **119**
Hand-Schüller-Christian disease, 194
haptoglobin, serum
in haemolytic disorders, 64
normal values, 8
heart disease, congenital
see **congenital heart disease**
heart valve disease/surgical repair
fragmentation haemolysis, 80, 311
thrombocytopenia, 296
see also **congenital heart disease**
heat-stroke
botryoid nuclei in neutrophils, 224
Heinz body haemolysis
G6PD deficiency, favism, 106, **93**
with methaemoglobinaemia, **85**
neonatal, 84, **85**
oxidant exposure, 84
unstable Hb, 32, **31**
vitamin C excess, 100
hemighosts (blister cells, eccentrocytes), 92
favism, **93**
idiopathic neonatal Heinz body haemolysis, **85**
HEMPAS, 40, **41**
Henoch-Schönlein purpura
bleeding in, **279**
heparin
coagulation tests, changes, 285
cofactor II, normal values, 279
-induced thrombocytopenia, 310
-like glycosaminoglycans, septicaemia, 292
hepatitis viruses, infection
bone marrow hypoplasia, 46, **45**
immune thrombocytopenia, 306
hereditary
deficiency of eosinophil peroxidase, 218
deficiency of neutrophil/monocyte peroxidase, 218
dyserythropoietic anaemias
see **dyserythropoiesis**
elliptocytosis
see **elliptocytosis**
folate malabsorption, 38
giant neutrophils, 222, **223**
hydrocytosis, 94, 96
orotic aciduria, 56
persistence of fetal Hb, 30
pyropoikilocytosis, 78, **79**
sideroblasts anaemias
see **sideroblastic anaemias**
spherocytosis
see **spherocytosis**
xerocytosis, 94, **93**
Hermansky-Pudlak syndrome, 232
Hernández syndrome
and neutropenia, 241(T7.4)
herpes simplex, neonatal
apoptosis of leucocytes, **264**
disseminated intravascular coagulation, 292
haemolysis, 98
heterophile antibodies
see **Paul Bunnell test**
hexokinase, **103**
deficiency and haemolysis, 104(T3.25)
high MW kininogen, **281**
deficiency, 285
histiocytes, ear-lobe blood
chronic bacteraemia, 266, **266**
histiocytes, sea-blue, 232
foamy
Niemann-Pick B and C, **229**, **233**
granular sea-blue
ALL, **233**
Niemann-Pick B, **233**
histiocytosis, 194
eosinophilic granuloma, **195**, **197**
Hand-Schüller-Christian disease, 194
infection-associated haemophagocytosis, 194, 267, **268**
Langerhans cell, 194, **195**, **197**
vs infection-associated haemophagocytosis, 268
Letterer-Siwe disease, 194, **195**
crystals in monocytes, **197**
malignant, 198, **198**
non-Langerhans, 196, **197**
reactive, 194
sinus histiocytosis with massive lymphadenopathy (Rosai-Dorfman), 198
Histoplasma
in:
blood leucocytes, **263**
bone marrow, **267**
HIV infection
bone marrow hypoplasia, 46
cobalamin deficiency, microsporidiosis of bowel, 36
Histoplasma in leucocytes, **263**
immune thrombocytopenia, 306, 308(T8.28)
lupus anticoagulant, 285(T7.18)
lymphopenia, 254
neutropenia, 241(T7.1)
tuberculosis, bacteria in leucocytes, **262**
Hodgkin's disease
anaemia of chronic disease, 19(T2.4)
autoimmune:
haemolysis, 75(T3.10)
lymphopenia, 254
thrombocytopenia, 306(T8.27)
eosinophilia, 255
erythroblastopenia, 56
in bone marrow, 140, **140**
homocystinuria
F VII deficiency, 286
thrombosis, 298
Howell-Jolly bodies
asplenia/splenic atrophy, 108, **109**
normal neonate, 4, **5**
HTLV I infection
and lymphocytosis, 250
Hunter MPS, 209, 210, **211**
Gasser lymphocytes, **209**
Hurler MPS, 209, 210, **211**
Gasser
lymphocytes, **209**
reticulum cells, marrow, **235**
Hurler-Scheie MPS, 209, 210, **211**
hydrocytosis, hereditary, 94, 96
hydrops fetalis
Hb Bart's, 25, **25**
parvovirus infection and, 54
hydroxyapatite crystals
in macrophages, Michaelis-Gutmann bodies, **219**
hypercholesterolaemia, familial, 230
foam cells in marrow, 230(T6.14)
hyperchylomicronaemia
see **chylomicronaemia**
hypereosinophilic syndrome, 255(T7.19), 256
ALL, 132, **133**
cardiac valve thrombosis in, **257**
hyperfibrinolysis
see **fibrin(ogen)olysis**
hyperostosis, infantile cortical
and thrombosis, 297(T8.22)
hyperphagocytic marrow macrophages
fucosidosis, 228(T6.13)
with hypogranular eosinophils and Michaelis-Gutmann bodies, 218, **219**
with neutropenia, 248
hypersegmentation, nuclear
eosinophils, 224
neutrophils, 222
hereditary giant neutrophils, 222, **223**
iron deficiency, 14
Lightsey anomaly (neutropenia with gigantism and multinuclearity of marrow neutrophils), 245
MDS, myeloid leukaemias, **175**, **179**, **181**
megaloblastosis, benign, 34, **39**
toxic states, **259**
hypersplenism
neutropenia, 248
pancytopenia, 44(T2.24)
thrombocytopenia, 312
hyperthyroidism
and thrombocytopenia, 306(T8.27)
hypertonic cryohaemolysis
in spherocytosis, 68, **67**
hypobetalipoproteinaemia
and acanthocytosis, 86(T3.17), 88, **15**, **89**

hypofibrinogenaemia
see **fibrinogen deficiency**
hypogammaglobulinaemia
see **immunodeficiency**
hypophosphataemia
spherocytosis in, 70
hypoplasia/aplasia, marrow
see **aplastic/hypoplastic anaemia**
hypoprothrombinaemia
see **prothrombin complex deficiency**
hypothalamic failure
in protein C deficiency, 294
hypothyroidism
acanthocytosis, 86(T3.17), 88, **89**
macrocytosis, 40
hypoxia
and DIC/thrombosis, 291(T8.20), 299

i, I antigens
in:
congenital dyserythropoietic anaemias, 42
Diamond-Blackfan anaemia, 53
Fanconi's anaemia, 48
juvenile chronic myeloid leukaemia, 173
normal development of, 6
I cell disease (mucolipidosis II), 202(T6.2), 204(T6.3), 205, 206
ichthyosis and neutral lipid storage disease, 214
idiopathic thrombocytopenic purpura, 308
vs post-viral thrombocytopenia, 308
Imerslund-Gräsbeck syndrome (intrinsic factor receptor defect), 36, **35**
immunodeficiency
autoimmune haemolysis, 75(T3.10)
eosinophilia, 255, 256
lymphopenia, 254
neutropenia, 241(T7.4), 242(T7.5)
see also specific disorders
immunoglobulin gene rearrangements
ALL, AML, 128
immunoglobulin, intravenous
and immune haemolysis, 75
immunophenotype, leukaemias
see specific leukaemias
inclusions
of erythrocytes
see **erythrophagocytosis**
intranuclear
CMV infection, 156, **157**
in leucocytes
see individual leucocytes
of virus-like particles, ALL, 122, **123**
incoagulable blood, 290
incompatibility, blood group, and haemolysis
blood transfusion, 72
disseminated intravascular coagulation in, 296
Jk[a], delayed haemolysis, 72
bone marrow transplant, ABO, 72
fetomaternal
ABO, 71
non-ABO, 72, **73**
obscure origin, 70, **73**
Rh, 72, 98, **99**
liver transplant, ABO, 72
ineffective haemopoiesis
see **dyserythropoiesis, dyspoiesis**
infantile cortical hyperostosis
thrombocytosis and thrombosis, 297(T8.22)
infantile genetic agranulocytosis (Kostmann), 242, **243**
infantile pyknocytosis, 82, **83**
infection
anaemia, 98
apoptosis of leucocytes, 264, **264**, **265**
appendicitis vs non-surgical abdominal pain
haematology of, 248, 249
-associated haemophagocytosis, 194, 267, **268**
bacteria in leucocytes, septicaemia, 260, **261**, **262**
differential diagnosis, 260, **263**
bacterial vs viral infection
leucocyte changes in, 258(T7.22)
bone marrow aplasia, 46, **45**
disseminated intravascular coagulation, 292, **293**
eosinophilia, 255
haemolysis, 75, 98, **69**, **81**
histiocytes, ear-lobe blood, 266, **266**
lupus anticoagulant, 285
lymphocytosis, 251
lymphopenia, 254
monocytes, phagocytic (bacteria, cell inclusions), 257(T7.20), 265, **261**, **262**, **265**
monocytosis, 265
neonatal sepsis
haematological scoring system for diagnosis, 258
C reactive protein in, 258
neutropenia, 240
neutrophilia, 248
thrombocytopenia
see **thrombocytopenia**
thrombocytosis, 180(T5.8, 5.9)
toxic changes in leucocytes, 257ff., **259**, **264**
vessel dysfunction, 278(T8.3)
see also **virus infection**, specific viruses/bacteria
infection-associated haemophagocytosis, 194, 267, **268**
infectious lymphocytosis, 250
infectious mononucleosis, 252
apoptosis, 264, **253**
atypical lymphocytes, **253**, **265**
immune thrombocytopenia, 306
phagocytic monocytes, **265**
see also **X-linked lymphoproliferative disorder**
inflammatory bowel disease (Crohn's disease, ulcerative colitis)
anaemia of chronic disease, 19
autoimmune
haemolysis, 75(T3.10)
lymphopenia, 254
thrombocytopenia, 306(T8.27)
bite cells (sulpha drugs), **87**
eosinophilia, 255(T7.19)
neutrophilia, 249(T7.10)
splenic atrophy, 108(T3.28)
toxic change in neutrophils, 259(T7.25)
inhibitors to coagulation factors
see **coagulation factor/s**
integrin adhesion molecules, deficiency
neutrophilia, 248
intralipid
see **intravenous lipid alimentation**
intravascular coagulation
see **disseminated intravascular coagulation**
intravenous
anti A/B/D material
immune spherocytosis, 75
immunoglobulin
immune spherocytosis, 75
lipid alimentation
chylomicronaemia, 230
spherocytosis, 70
thrombocytopenia, 311(T8.31)
intrinsic factor, **35**
deficiency, juvenile pernicious anaemia, 36
receptor defect (Imerslund-Gräsbeck), 36
intussusception
atypical lymphocytes in, 252(T7.14)
iron
binding capacity
see **transferrin**
deficiency anaemia, 14ff., **15**
combined with:
anaemia of chronic disease, 18
lead poisoning, 16
loss in urine
see **haemosiderin**
malabsorption, specific for iron, 16
marrow, normal, 10
overload
blood transfusions, **223**
congenital microcytic anaemia with, 22
haemochromatosis, 214, **217**
serum
in:
anaemia of chronic disease, 19
iron deficiency anaemia, 19
thalassaemia minor, 19
normal values, 7
irritable hip
atypical lymphocytes in, 252(T7.14)
iso-agglutinins, blood group
anti A,B
normal development, 6
in Wiskott-Aldrich syndrome, 304
isovaleric (organic) acidaemia
neutropenia, thrombocytopenia, 242(T7.5)
Ivemark syndrome, 108, **109**

jaundice, obstructive
erythrocyte changes, 91(T3.18), **83**, **91**
Job's syndrome
and eosinophilia, 255(T7.19), 256
Jordans anomaly (lipid vacuoles in neutrophils), 214
neonatal haemochromatosis, **217**
juvenile chronic myeloid leukaemia, 170, **171**

kala-azar
Leishmania in marrow, **267**
Kasabach-Merritt syndrome, 292, **293**
Kawasaki disease
atypical lymphocytes, 252(T7.14)
neutrophilia, 248(T7.10)
thrombosis/disseminated coagulation, 291(T8.20), 297(T8.22)
toxic neutrophils, 259(T7.25)
Kell blood group
fetomaternal incompatibility, 72
Kidd (Jk[a]) blood group
delayed haemolysis from incompatible transfusion, 72
kidney, transplantation
disseminated coagulation in, 291(T8.20)
Klebsiella pneumoniae **septicaemia**
bacteria in leucocytes, **262**
differential diagnosis, 260(T7.26), **263**
erythrophagocytosis, 265
Kostmann's neutropenia, 242, **243**

Lactobacillus **sp. septicaemia**
bacteria in leucocytes, **262**
differential diagnosis, 260(T7.26), **263**
lactoferrin
in neutrophil granules, 216

Langerhans cell histiocytosis, 194, **195**, **197**
vs infection-associated haemophagocytosis, 268
Langerhans cells
vs monocytes/macrophages, 194
large granular lymphocytes
see **lymphocytes**
lazy leucocyte syndrome, 244
lead poisoning, 22
combined with iron deficiency, 16
sideroblastic anaemia, **21**
stippled erythrocytes, **21**
lecithin:cholesterol acyltransferase deficiency, 204(T6.3), 232
foamy macrophages, marrow, 230(T6.14)
sea-blue histiocytes, marrow, 232
target cells, anaemia, 82
leishmaniasis (kala-azar)
Leishmania in marrow, **267**
Lesch-Nyhan syndrome
megaloblastosis, 58
Letterer-Siwe disease, 194, **195**
see also **histiocytosis**
leucocytes
see individual types
leucoerythroblastic anaemias
ALL, 133(T4.6), **131**
CMV infection, **157**
juvenile CML, 173(T5.6)
neuroblastoma, 184
osteopetrosis, 56, **57**
tuberculosis, 249(T7.10)
see also **leukaemoid reactions**
leukaemia
congenital, 124, **161**
fetal origins of, 124
see also specific types
leukaemoid reactions, 144(T5.1)
resembling:
ALL, 136, **137**
AML
M0, 144, **169**
M2, 150
M3, 156, **157**
M4, 158, **157**
M7, 168, **169**
CML
adult, 196, 300
juvenile, 172
Levine-Critchley syndrome (normolipaemic chorea-acanthocytosis), 88
acanthocytosis, 86(T3.17)
Lightsey anomaly (neutropenia with gigantism and multinuclearity of marrow neutrophils), 244
lineage switch at leukaemia relapse, 134
ALL
→AML M5a, **161**
→bilineage ALL, **117**
→CML adult, 176, **171**
AML M2 Neut→M2 Baso, **151**
lipofuscinosis, neuronal
see **Batten's disease**
Listeria
and haemolysis, 98
liver
disease
dysfibrinogenaemia, 288
erythrocytes in, 90(T3.18), **83**, **91**
haemostasis, 291(T8.19)
vs disseminated intravascular coagulation, 290
hypofibrinogenaemia, 288
neutrophilia, 249(T7.10)
thrombosis, 298
transplantation
alloimmune haemolysis, 72
hepatic artery thrombosis, **297**
Loa loa
eosinophilia, **257**
Löffler syndrome, 255(T7.19)
and eosinophilia, 256
lupus
anticoagulants, 284
with purpura fulminans, 295
syndrome, neonatal (maternal SLE), 246
see also **systemic lupus erythematosus**
lymphangiectasia
bone marrow, anaemia in, 56, **57**
intestinal, lymphopenia in, 255
lymphoblastosis, benign, 136, **137**
lymphoblasts
leukaemic
see **acute lymphoblastic leukaemia**
normal
blood, 8, **9**
bone marrow, 10, **11**
see also **lymphoblastosis, benign**
lymphocytes
apoptosis, viral infection, **264**
atypical (reactive), 252, **253**
adenovirus infection, **137**
apoptosis, **253**
appendicitis vs non-surgical abdominal pain, 249(T7.11)
blastic, **137**
in CSF, **115**, **137**
increase, causes, 252
infectious mononucleosis, **253**
measles, 252, **253**
phagocytosed by monocytes, **265**
azurophil granules, normal, **263**
'black-granuled', 212, **213**
Chediak-Higashi syndrome, 212, **213**
curvilinear bodies, late infantile Batten's disease, 204, **205**
decrease, 254
Gasser (metachromatic granulation), 208, **209**
granular osmiophilic deposits, infantile Batten's disease, 204
grey-staining inclusions, 220, **221**
immature
normal:
blood, 8, **9**
bone marrow, 10, **11**
increase
see **lymphocytosis**
in infantile free sialic acid storage disease, 207, **207**, **215**
large granular, 8
normal values, **9**
normal values
blood, 8, **9**
bone marrow, 10
vacuolated, 202ff.
infantile free sialic acid storage disease, **207**, **215**
Spielmeyer-Vogt type Batten's disease, **203**
Wolman's disease, **203**
lymphocytosis (of normal lymphocytes), 250
infectious lymphocytosis, 250
Omenn's syndrome, **251**
eosinophilia in, 255(T7.19), **251**
pertussis, 250, **251**, **279**
T lymphocytosis with neutropenia, 247
unexplained, 250
lymphoma
Hodgkin's
immune thrombocytopenia, 306(T8.27)
in bone marrow, 140, **140**
non-Hodgkin
haemophagocytosis, 267
immune thrombocytopenia, 306(T8.27)
in:
blood, **131**
bone marrow, 138, **115**, **139**
bowel, X-linked lymphoproliferative disease, 253
lupus anticoagulant, 285
lymphopenia, 254

macrocytosis, macrocytic anaemias, 32ff.
normal for age, 2, 3
of obscure cause, **59**
spurious, 32
see also specific causes
macrophages, blood
in toxic states, 257(T7.20), 265, **265**
see also **monocytes, phagocytic**
macrophages, marrow
abnormal, types of, 224(T6.12)
Auer rods in, **153**
with blue-staining vacuoles, neuraminidase deficiency, 230(T6.14)
crystals in
see **crystals**
foamy, 226ff.
ALL (cytotoxics, infection), **231**
chylomicronaemia, 230, **231**
immune thrombocytopenia, 306
infection-associated haemophagocytosis, 267, **268**
Niemann-Pick
B, 228, **229**, **233**
C, 228, **229**
rhabdomyosarcoma, **191**
Wolman's, **231**
foamy blue, Niemann-Pick B, C, 232, **229**, **233**
Gasser 'reticulum' cells, 209, 234, **235**
haemophagocytosis, infection-associated, 267, **268**
Histoplasma in, **267**
hyperphagocytic
fucosidosis, 204(T6.3), 228(T6.13)
with hypogranular eosinophils and Michaelis-Gutmann bodies , 218, **219**
with neutropenia, 248
in infection, toxic changes, 257(T7.20)
Leishmania in, **267**
organisms in, **267**
sea-blue
see **histiocytes, sea-blue**
striated sky-blue
G_{M1} gangliosidosis II, 232
macrophages/monocytes
vs Langerhans cells, 194
macropolycytes
hereditary giant neutrophils, 222, **223**
as toxic change, **259**
macrothrombocytopenias, 309, **303**
see also individual disorders
malabsorption
global, and
cobalamin deficiency, 35
folate deficiency, 38
iron deficiency, 16, 17
vitamin K deficiency, 287(T8.13)

malabsorption (*contd*)
specific for
cobalamin
Imerslund-Gräsbeck, 36, **35**
folate
anticonvulsants, 38
hereditary, 38
iron, 16
malaria
atypical lymphocytes, 252(T7.14)
disseminated coagulation, 292
immune
haemolysis, 74
thrombocytopenia, 307
malignancy
chylomicronaemia, 230
disseminated coagulation, 291(T8.20)
fetal origins of, 124
non-haemopoietic
in:
blood, **193**
bone marrow, general features, 183
see also specific malignancies
malignant histiocytosis, 198, **198**
malnutrition
and:
acanthocytosis, cystic fibrosis, **89**
splenic hypofunction, 108(T3.28)
mannosidosis, 202(T6.2), 204, 205, 228(T6.13), **203**
crystals, marrow, **237**
plasma cells, vacuolated, **213**
marathon running
stomatocytosis, 97
Marfan's syndrome
thrombocytopathy, 312
vessel dysfunction, 278
Maroteaux-Lamy MPS, 209, 210
Alder anomaly, **215**
marrow
see **bone marrow**
marrow-pancreas syndromes
cystic fibrosis, atypical
with:
marrow hypoplasia, 50, **49**
neutropenia, **243**
Pearson's, 48(T2.29), 216
ringed sideroblastosis, **217**
vacuolation of precursor cells, **217**
Shwachman
bone marrow aplasia, 241(T7.4)
Gaucher-like cells, **227**
mast cells
aberrant, AML M2, **149**
grey-staining inclusions, 220
normal, **235**
May-Hegglin anomaly
Döhle-like bodies, 216, **217**
thrombocytopenia, 302, 313(T8.34, 8.35), **303**
MCH
normal values, 3
McLeod phenotype
acanthocytosis, 88
MCV
normal values, 3
measles (rubeola)
apoptosis of lymphocytes, **264**
atypical lymphocytes, 252, **253**
bone marrow hypoplasia, 46
immune thrombocytopenia, 306
see also **virus infection, lupus anticoagulant**
Meckel's diverticulum, 16
Mediterranean
macrothrombocytopenia, 309
stomatocytosis, 96
medulloblastoma, 188
in cerebrospinal fluid, **189**
megakaryocytes
absence
see **amegakaryocytic thrombocytopenia**
deficiency
outline, 310(T8.25)
spurious, 300
dysplasia
AML M7, 166, **167**
essential thrombocythaemia, 180, **181**
inherited syndromes, 302(T8.25), **303**
monosomy 7 MPD, **175**
myelodysplastic syndromes, **179**
transient abnormal myelopoiesis, 168, **169**
transient megakaryocytic dyspoiesis, 170
megaloblastosis, megaloblastic anaemias, 32ff.
AML M6, 162, **163**
causes, 33(T2.17)
cobalamin deficiency
see **cobalamin**
congenital dyserythropoietic anaemia I, 43(T2.23)
copper deficiency, 247
drugs, 57
folate deficiency
see **folate**
investigation, 34
reversal of after treatment, sequence of changes, 34
thrombocytopenia in, 302(T8.26)
Melanesian (S.E.Asian) ovalocytosis, 78, **77**
melanoma, disseminated
cells in blood, **193**
meningococcus
see ***Neisseria meningitidis***
Mentzer variant of myelokathexis, 244
mesenteric adenitis
atypical lymphocytes in, 252(T7.14)
mesothelial cells, normal
in cerebrospinal fluid, **189**
metachromasia
see **toluidine blue**
methaemoglobinaemia
cytochrome reductase deficiency, 30
drugs, 33
G6PD deficiency, 104
HbMs, 30
neonatal Heinz body haemolysis, **85**
methylmalonic acid, 35
methylmalonic acidaemia, 242(T7.5)
neutropenia, thrombocytopenia, 242(T7.5)
Michaelis-Gutmann bodies, 218, **219**
microcytosis, microcytic anaemias
causes, 14
of obscure cause, **17**
see also specific causes
microsporidia
bowel infestation and cobalamin deficiency, 36
milk protein colitis
eosinophilia, 255, 256
iron deficiency, 16, **15**
monocytes
bacteria in, septicaemia, **261**, **262**
bilirubin in, **225**
chromomeres, **259**
crystals, Letterer-Siwe disease, **197**
Döhle-like bodies, May-Hegglin anomaly, **217**
dyspoietic
AML
M4Eo, **159**
M5, **160**, **161**
JCML, **171**
erythrophagocytosis
autoimmune haemolysis, **73**
septicaemia, **265**
grey-staining inclusions, 220
in infection, 257(T7.20), 265, **259**, **261**, **262**, **265**
leucocytes within, viral/bacterial infection, **265**
in May-Hegglin anomaly, **217**
monocytes/macrophages vs Langerhans cells, 194
in mucopolysaccharidosis, **225**
myeloperoxidase deficiency, 218
normal values, blood, 8
phagocytic, for
bacteria, cells, 265, **261**, **262**, **265**
erythrocytes
autoimmune haemolysis, **73**
septicaemia, **265**
toxic changes
see **monocytes in infection**
vacuolation, 224, **265**
monocytosis
infection, 265
monosomy 7
in AML, 146(T5.2), **149**
ataxia-pancytopenia-monosomy 7 syndrome, 51
MPD, 174, **175**, **177**
Montreal macrothrombocytopenia, 309
Morquio MPS
see **mucopolysaccharidosis**
motorneurone disease
and acanthocytosis, 88
mucolipidosis I
see **neuraminidase deficiency**
mucolipidosis II (I cell disease), 202(T6.2), 204(T6.3), 205, 206
mucolipidosis III (pseudo-Hurler polydystrophy), 202(T6.2), 205, 212(T6.6)
mucopolysaccharidosis/es (MPS), 209ff.
Alder granulation, Maroteaux-Lamy MPS, 214, **215**
Hunter (MPS II), 209, 210, **211**
Gasser lymphocytes, **209**
Hurler (MPS IH), 209, 210, **211**
Gasser
lymphocytes, **209**
reticulum cells, **235**
Hurler-Scheie (MPS IHS), 209, 210, **211**
lymphocytes, Gasser, 208, 209, **209**
Maroteaux-Lamy (MPS VI), 209, 211
Alder granulation, **215**
Gasser lymphocytes, **209**
monocytes in, **225**
Morquio (MPS IV), 209, 214, **211**
neutrophils, coarse granules, 214, **215**
mucosulphatidosis,
see **mucosulphatidosis**
osteoblasts in, **235**
plasma cells, Buhot, 209, 212, **213**
reticulum cells, Gasser, 209, 234, **235**
Sanfilippo (MPS III), 209, 210, **211**
Buhot plasma cells, **213**
Gasser
lymphocytes, **209**
reticulum cells, **235**
Scheie (MPS IS), 209, 210
Sly (MPS VII), 209, 210
mucosulphatidosis (multiple sulphatase deficiency), 209, 212
Alder granulation, 215(T6.8)
multinucleated cells

cytomegalovirus infection, 156, **157**
histiocytes, blood, **266**
histiocytosis, bone marrow, **197**
Hodgkin's disease, **140**
melanoma, **193**
necrobiotic, ALL, 132, **133**
rhabdomyosarcoma, **191**
multiple sulphatase deficiency
see **mucosulphatidosis**
mumps
immune thrombocytopenia, 306
neonatal, and disseminated intravascular coagulation, 292
muramidase (lysozyme)
in
AML
M4, 156
M5, 160
CML juvenile, 170
monosomy 7 MPD, 174
mycobacteria
see **tuberculosis**
mycoplasma infection
atypical lymphocytes, 252(T7.14)
autoimmune haemolysis, 75(T3.10)
neutrophil agglutination, **73**
myelodysplastic syndromes (refractory anaemias), 178
de novo, **179**
post chemotherapy, **181**
see also **chronic myeloid leukaemias**
myelofibrosis, 170(T5.4)
ALL, 130, **131**
AML M7, 166, **167**
grey-platelet syndrome, 314
histiocytosis, 196
monosomy 7 MPD, 174, **177**
neuroblastoma, 184
rhabdomyosarcoma, **191**
myelokathexis (neutropenia with abundant, degenerate neutrophils in marrow), 244
myelomonocytosis, chronic
CML, juvenile
see **chronic myeloid leukaemias**
EBV infection and, 172
familial myeloproliferative disease (Randall), 172
myeloperoxidase cytochemistry
in
ALL, 114
AML
M1, **145**
M2, 146
M5, 160
M7, 166
myeloperoxidase deficiency
eosinophils, 218
neutrophils and monocytes, 218
myeloproliferative disease
familial (Randall), 172
see also **chronic myeloid leukaemias**
myocardial infarction
mural thrombosis, **299**

Najean-Lecompte thrombocytopenia, 304
N-CAM (UJ13A) monoclonal antibody
in neuroblastoma, 184, **187**
necrosis, bone marrow
ALL, 128, **129**
necrotizing enterocolitis
cryptantigen exposure, 75
disseminated intravascular coagulation, 291(T8.20)
toxic neutrophils, 259
***Neisseria meningitidis*, septicaemia**
bacteria in leucocytes, 260(T7.26, 7.27), **261**
disseminated intravascular coagulation, **293**
purpura fulminans, 294
neonate/neonatal
anaemia
see individual types of anaemia
lupus syndrome, 246
neutropenia
see **alloimmune, autoimmune**
normal blood, values/morphology
see **normal blood**
sepsis
haematological scoring system for diagnosis, 258
C reactive protein in, 258
thrombosis
see **thrombosis**
viral infection and
disseminated intravascular coagulation, 292
haemolysis, 98
nephrosis
chylomicronaemia, 230
loss in urine of
AT III, 298
factor
IX, 284
XI, 285
XII, 285
haemosiderin, 16, 64
plasminogen, 298
protein C, 294
platelet hyperreactivity, 298
thrombosis, 298
neuraminidase deficiency, primary, 202(T6.2), 204(T6.3), 205, 206, 212(T6.6), 228(T6.13), 230(T6.14)
neuroblastoma, bone marrow, 184, **185–187**
differential diagnosis, 188
disseminated intravascular coagulation, 291(T8.20)
neurofibrils
neuroblastoma, 184, **187**
neuronal lipofuscinosis
see **Batten's disease**
neutropenia (isolated), 240ff.
with abnormal granule structure, **243**
ALL following, 240, 247
alloimmune
see **alloimmune neutropenia**
autoimmune
see **autoimmune neutropenia**
bacterial infection, 240
with binucleate, tetraploid marrow neutrophils (Mamlok), 244
after blood transfusion, 244
bone marrow transplant, 246
burns, 240
cartilage-hair hypoplasia, 241(T7.4)
Chediak-Higashi syndrome, 220, **213**, **215**
chronic benign, 245
Cohen's syndrome, 241(T7.4)
copper deficiency, 247
cyclic, 240
harbinger of
ALL, 240
myeloproliferative disease, 176, **177**
drugs
immune, 246, 247
non-immune, 248
dyskeratosis congenita, 48, **49**
Fanconi syndrome, 48, **49**
Felty's syndrome, 246
with gigantism and multinuclearity of marrow neutrophils (Lightsey), 244
glycogenosis I, 242(T7.5)
Hernández syndrome, 241(T7.4)
immune
alloimmune
see **alloimmune neutropenia**
autoimmune
see **autoimmune neutropenia**
drugs, 246, 247
with immune haemolysis/thrombocytopenia (Evans), 75(T3.10), 246
immunodeficiency and, 242(T7.5)
infantile genetic (Kostmann), 242, **243**
infection, 240, 246, 258(T7.22)
apoptosis in, **264**
inherited, outline, 241, 242 (T7.3–7.5)
investigation, 241
Kostmann's, 242, **243**
lazy leucocyte syndrome, 244
Mentzer variant of myelokathexis, 244
monosomy 7 MPD following, 176, **177**
myelokathexis, 244
neonatal lupus (maternal SLE), 246
organic acidaemias, 242(T7.5)
parvovirus infection, 246
reticular dysgenesis, 242(T7.5)
Shwachman syndrome, 50
SLE, 246
spurious, 240
T lymphocytosis with neutropenia, 247
viral infection, 240, 246
apoptosis in, **264**
neutrophilia (benign), 248
appendicitis vs non-surgical abdominal pain, 248, 249
familial, 248
infection, 248
leukaemoid reactions
see **leukamoid reactions**
pertussis, 250, **251**
spurious, 248
Sweet's syndrome, 248
neutrophil/s
Acinetobacter in, septicaemia, **262**
actin microfilaments, inclusions of, 220
Aerococcus in, septicaemia, **261**
agglutination, mycoplasma infection, **73**
Alder granulation
see **Alder anomaly**
alkaline phosphatase, 173(T5.6), 257(T7.20)
antibodies to
see **alloimmune, autoimmune neutropenia**
apoptosis
see **apoptosis**
Auer rods in, AML, **147**, **153**
azurophil granulation, coarse, Morquio MPS, 214, **215**
bacteria in, septicaemia, 260, **261**, **262**
differential diagnosis, 260, **263**
binucleate tetraploid marrow neutrophils and monocytes with neutropenia (Mamlok), 244
botryoid nuclei, heat stroke, 224
Candida in, septicaemia, **263**
Capnocytophaga in, septicaemia, **262**
Charcot-Leyden crystals in, AML, **151**
Chediak-Higashi
-like granulation, AML, 148, 150, **149**
syndrome, 220, **215**
chromomeres in, 257(T7.20), **259**

neutrophil/s *(contd)*
Clostridium in, septicaemia, **262**
in colchicine poisoning, **223**
cytoplasmic anomalies, 215
degranulation
see granulation deficient, below
degenerate, in marrow, with neutropenia (myelo-kathexis), 244
Döhle bodies, 257, 258, **217**, **259**
Döhle-like bodies
Fechtner syndrome, 216, 309
May-Hegglin anomaly, 216, 309, **217**
Sebastian anomaly, 216, 309
drumsticks, nuclear, **223**
dyspoiesis
ALL,
bilineage, **117**
Ph positive, **171**
myeloid leukaemias/MDS, **147**, **149**, **151**, **153**, **155**, **159**, **163**, **171**, **175**, **177**, **179**, **181**
erythrophagocytosis, autoimmune haemolysis, 74
Escherichia coli in, septicaemia, **262**
fetal granulopoiesis, lymph node, **171**
giant
see macropolycytes, below
gigantism and multinuclearity of marrow neutrophils with neutropenia (Lightsey), 244
granulation
abnormal
AML, **147**, **149**, **151**, **153**, **155**
Chediak-Higashi, 220, **215**
Chediak-Higashi-like, AML, 148, 150, **149**
Morquio MPS, 214, **215**
with neutropenia and pancreatic fibrosis, **243**
toxic, 257(T7.20), 258, **259**
deficient, 218
monosomy 7 MPD, **177**
toxic states, 257(T7.20), 258(7.21), **259**
grey-staining inclusions, 220, **221**
Haemophilus influenzae in, septicaemia, **262**
haemosiderin in,
from frequent transfusions, **223**
neonatal haemochromatosis, 214
Histoplasma in, **263**
hypersegmentation,
see **hypersegmentation**
in infection
toxic changes, 257(T7.20), 258, **259**
inclusions, unidentified
AML
M2, **149**
M3, **155**
grey-staining inclusion body syndromes, 220, **221**
MDS, **179**
Jordans anomaly (lipid vacuolation), 214, **217**
Klebsiella in, septicaemia, **262**
macropolycytes
hereditary, 222, **223**
toxic change, **259**
Mamlok anomaly
see binucleate, above
in Maroteaux-Lamy MPS, **215**
May-Hegglin anomaly, 216, **217**
Mentzer variant of myelokathexis, 244
in Morquio MPS, 214, **215**
myelokathexis, 244
myeloperoxidase deficiency, 218
and spurious neutropenia, 240
Neisseria meningitidis in, septicaemia, **261**
normal values, 8
nucleus
anomalies, 222
appendages, normal, **263**
drumsticks, **223**
hypersegmentation
see **hypersegmentation**
tags, excessive, trisomy 13, 222, **223**
in Pearson's syndrome, 216, **217**
Pelger-Huet anomaly, 222, **223**
Pelgerization
see **Pelgerization**
peroxidase deficiency, 218
phagocytic
bacteria
see **bacteria**, specific organisms
erythrocytes, autoimmune haemolysis, 74
toxic states, 257(T7.20)
specific granule deficiency, 216
Staphylococcus aureus in, septicaemia, **261**
streptococci in, septicaemia, **261**
Streptococcus pneumoniae in, septicaemia, **261**
toxic changes, 257–259, **259**
vacuolation
chloramphenicol, **43**
copper deficiency, 246
galactosialidosis, 206
lipid (Jordans anomaly), 214, **217**
Pearson's syndrome, 216, **217**
toxic states, 257–259, **259**
Nezelof's syndrome
and lymphopenia, 255
Niemann-Pick disease
general: 202(T6.2), 204(T6.3), 205, 228 (T6.13), 232(T6.15)
type A, 208
foamy macrophages, 228(T6.13), **229**
type B, 228
foamy macrophages, 228(T6.13), **229**
plasma cell vacuolation, **213**
sea-blue cells, marrow, **233**
type C, 228
foamy macrophages, blue foam cells, 228(T6.13), **229**
non-Hodgkin lymphoma
see **lymphoma**
non-Langerhans histiocytosis, 194(T5.15), 195(T5.16), 196, **197**
normal blood, values/morphology
coagulation factors, 278
coagulation factors, natural inhibitors, 279
cobalamin, serum, 6
eosinophils, 8
erythroblasts, neonate, 3
erythrocyte/s
antigens, ABH, i, I, 6
count, 3
folate, 6
morphology in neonate, 4, 5(T1.1), **5**
pitted (pocked), 4
folate, serum/erythrocytes, 6
haematocrit, 3
haptoglobin, serum, 8
HbA2, 7
Hb concentration, 3
HbF, 7
iso-agglutinins, blood group, 6
lymphoblasts, 8, **9**
lymphocytes, 9, **9**
MCH, 3
MCV, 3
monocytes, 8
neutrophils, 8
pitted (pocked) erythrocytes, 4
platelet count, neonatal, 280
reticulocytes, 3
normal bone marrow
see **bone marrow**
normal cerebrospinal fluid
mesothelial cells, **189**
normocytic anaemias
outline, 62
see also specific causes
normolipaemic chorea-acanthocytosis (Levine-Critchley), 88
nucleus/nuclear
degeneration, of part nucleus, ALL, **122**
demarcations, ALL, 124, **124**
drumsticks, female neutrophil, **223**
hypersegmentation, granulocytes
see **hypersegmentation**
tags in granulocytes, trisomy 13, 222, **223**
nutrition, total parenteral
chylomicronaemia, 230
spherocytosis, 70
thrombocytopenia, 311(T8.31)

oil red O cytochemistry
ALL, 126, **127**
malignant histiocytosis, **198**
neonatal haemochromatosis, neutrophils, **217**
Wolman's disease
lymphocytes, **203**
macrophages, **231**
Omenn's syndrome, 250
eosinophilia, **251**
lymphocytosis, **251**
organic acidaemias
neutropenia, thrombocytopenia, 242(T7.5)
orotic aciduria, hereditary
megaloblastosis, 56
osmotic fragility
in hereditary spherocytosis, 68
osteoblasts, bone marrow
Hurler MPS, **235**
infantile sialic acid storage disease, **235**
normal, **185**
osteogenesis imperfecta, 278(T8.3), 312(T8.32)
osteopetrosis (Albers-Schönberg), 56, **57**
ovalo-stomatocytosis, S.E.Asian (Melanesian), 78, **77**
oxygen affinity
of unstable/abnormal Hb's, 32

pancreas-marrow syndromes
see **marrow-pancreas syndromes**
pancytopenia
outline, 44
preceding overt ALL, 134, **135**
panhypoplasia, marrow
see **aplastic/hypoplastic anaemia**
paraproteinaemia, serum
CMV infection, **157**
eosinophilia, idiopathic, 256
parasites
and eosinophilia, 255, 256, **257**
parietal cell autoantibodies
immune thrombocytopenia, 306
juvenile pernicious anaemia, 36(T2.21)
paroxysmal nocturnal haemoglobinuria, 50, 52
parvovirus B19 infection, 54
bone marrow hypoplasia, 46
erythroblasts, inclusions in, 252
giant pronormoblasts, **55**

transient erythroblastopenia of childhood, 54
PAS cytochemistry
ALL, 124, **125**
AML
M3, **153**
M4Eo, **159**
M6, **163**
blue foam cells, Niemann-Pick C, **229**
essential thrombocythaemia, **181**
Ewing's sarcoma, **192**
Gaucher-like cells, treated ALL, **227**
Michaelis-Gutmann bodies, **219**
myelodysplastic syndrome, megakaryocytes, **179**
neuroblastoma, 188(T5.12)
rhabdomyosarcoma, 190
sea-blue cells, 232
Passovoy defect, 286
Paul-Bunnell test, 254
Pearson's marrow-pancreas syndrome, 216
ringed sideroblastosis, **217**
vacuolation of precursor cells, **217**
Pelger-Huet anomaly, 222, **223**
Pelgerization, 222
ALL, bilineage, **117**
Ph positive, **171**
colchicine poisoning, **223**
inherited specific granule deficiency, 216
myeloid leukaemias, **147**, **163**, **171**
toxic states, **259**
peroxidase deficiency
eosinophils, 218
neutrophils+monocytes, 218
pertussis, 250
lymphocytosis, **251**
subconjunctival haemorrhage, **279**
Ph chromosome, 126, 127, 173, **171**
phagocytosis
of:
bacteria
see **bacteria**, specific organisms
erythrocytes
see **erythrophagocytosis**
haemopoietic cells
see **haemophagocytosis**
by:
leucocytes, infection, 251(T7.20), 260, 265ff., **261–263**, **265–268**
leukaemic lymphoblasts, **123**
monoblasts, AML M5 variant, **161**
rhabdomyosarcoma cells, 190
phocomelia
and amegakaryocytic thrombocytopenia, 302
phosphofructokinase, 103
deficiency and haemolysis, 104(T3.25)
phototherapy
thrombocytopathy, 317(T8.38)
thrombocytopenia, 311(T8.31)
pica
iron deficiency anaemia, 16
lead poisoning, 16, 22
'pincer cell'
variant of hereditary spherocytosis, **67**
Pink test
in hereditary spherocytosis, 68
pitted (pocked) erythrocytes
see **erythrocytes, pitted**
placenta
neonatal intravascular coagulation from
abruptio placentae, 296
haemangioma, 294
plasma cells
metachromatic inclusions in (Buhot), 212, **213**
normal values, marrow, 10
vacuolation, 212, **213**
plasminogen, 281
deficiency, and thrombosis, 298
plastic tubing
eosinophilia, 256, **257**
platelet/s
aggregations, 313(T8.35), 317(T8.37)
α granule deficiency (grey platelet), 313(T8.35), 314, **315**
antibody
ITP, 308
post-viral thrombocytopenia, 307
arachidonic acid, **317**
impaired release of, 316
calcium mobilization
defective, 316
investigation, 312(T8.33)
count, normal neonate, 280
cyclo-oxygenase, **317**
drug inhibition, 316, 317
dense body deficiency, 313(T8.35), 314, 315
dysfunction
see **thrombocytopathy**
glycoproteins, **301**
defective
Ia, 314
Ib-IX, Bernard-Soulier, 313
IIb-IIIa
Glanzmann, 314
other, 316
V, Bernard-Soulier, 313
hyperreactivity, and thrombosis, 297(T8.22), 298
refractoriness to transfusions of, 311
release defects (thromboxane synthesis/receptor), 314ff.
vs storage pool deficiency, 313(T8.35)
satellitism, 276(T8.1), **285**
storage pool disease, 314
thromboxane synthesis/receptor defects
see release defects, above
plumbism
see **lead poisoning**
pneumococcus
see ***Streptococcus***
poikilocytosis, bizarre
causes, 97
polycythaemia
outline, 182
vera, 182
thrombosis in, 297(T8.22)
porphyria
congenital erythropoietic
porphyria (Günther), haemolysis, 107
protoporphyria, microcytosis, 22
Portland Hb, 6(T1.8)
post-viral thrombocytopenia
see **autoimmune thrombocytopenia**
Pr antibody
autoimmune haemolysis, 75(T3.10), **73**
pre-B ALL, 116(T4.1)
pre-kallikrein, 281
deficiency (Fletcher trait), 285
prematurity/premature infants
anaemia, 64
eosinophilia, 256
Heinz body haemolysis, 84, **85**
normal values, Hb, erythroblasts, erythrocytes, 3
pronormoblasts, giant
parvovirus infection, 54, **55**
propionic acidaemia
neutropenia, thrombocytopenia, 242(T7.5)
protein C
deficiency, 294
purpura fulminans, 294
normal values, 279
protein deficiency
and anaemia, 64, **89**
protein S
deficiency, 294
purpura fulminans, 294, **295**
normal values, 279
protein 3, 66
deficiency and stomatocytosis, 96
protein 4.1, 66
in hereditary spherocytosis, 66
protein 4.2, 66
in hereditary
spherocytosis, 96
stomatocytosis, 96
prothrombin complex, 281
concentrates and thrombosis, 297(T8.22)
deficiency, 286
artefact, 276
delayed haemorrhagic disease of newborn, 286, **275**
minimum levels for normal haemostasis, 277
normal values, 278, 280
prothrombin time
normal, 278
prolonged
artefact, 276
F VII deficiency, 286
+prolonged APTT, 286(T8.12)
shortened, 276
protoporphyria, congenital erythropoietic, microcytosis, 22
protoporphyrin, free erythrocytic
in:
anaemia of chronic disease, 19(T2.3)
erythropoietic protoporphyria, 22
hereditary sideroblastic anaemia, 21(T2.6)
iron deficiency anaemia, 19(T2.3)
lead poisoning, 22
pseudotumour cerebri (benign intracranial hypertension)
dysfibrinogenaemia, 288
pseudo-von Willebrand's disease (platelet type)
see **von Willebrand's disease**
pseudoxanthoma elasticum
bleeding in, 278(T8.3)
puddling of Hb, 92
hereditary xerocytosis, 94, **93**
pulmonary haemosiderosis, idiopathic
iron deficiency anaemia, 16, **15**
punctate basophilia
see **erythrocytes, stippled**
purine nucleoside phosphorylase deficiency
autoimmune haemolysis, 75(T3.10)
erythroblastopenia, 56
purpura fulminans, 294, **295**
due to:
protein C deficiency, 294
protein S deficiency, 294
pyknocytosis, 82
Heinz body haemolysis, 84, **85**
infantile, **82**, **83**
normal, 4, **5**
unstable Hbs, **31**
vitamin excess, **101**

pyrimidine 5′ nucleotidase, **97**
deficiency
and haemolysis, 97
in lead poisoning, 22
pyropoikilocytosis, hereditary, 78, **79**
pyruvate kinase, **103**
deficiency and haemolysis, 104(T3.25), **105**

quinidine/quinine
haemolytic-uraemic syndrome, 247
immune
neutropenia, 247
thrombocytopenia, 247, 310

Randall's (familial myeloproliferative) disease, 172
reactive lymphocytes
see **lymphocytes, atypical**
red cell/s
see **erythrocyte/s**
Reed-Sternberg cells
in bone marrow, **140**
refractory anaemias
see **myelodysplastic syndromes**
relapse, ALL, 134
as AML M5, **161**
as CML adult type, **171**
renal disease
anaemia, 98
chronic disease, non-specific erythrocyte changes, **99**
haemolytic-uraemic syndrome
see **haemolytic-uraemic syndrome**
protein C deficiency, 294
thrombocytopathy, 316
thrombocytopenia, 311
thrombotic thrombocytopenic purpura, 80
residual disease, ALL, 134
reticular dysgenesis
lymphopenia, neutropenia, 242(T7.5)
reticulocytes
in haemolytic disorders, 64
normal values, 2, 3
retinoblastoma
in bone marrow, 188, **186**
with non-Hodgkin lymphoma, **139**
rhabdomyosarcoma
in bone marrow, 190, **191**
Rh blood group
fetomaternal incompatibility, 72, 98, **99**
disseminated intravascular coagulation, 296
immune haemolysis from infused anti A/B/D, 75
incompatible transfusion, 72
null, mod, 96, **95**
rheumatoid arthritis
anaemia of chronic disease, 19
eosinophilia, 255(T7.19)
erythroblastopenia (immune), 53(T2.32), 56
haemolysis, 75(T3.10)
lupus anticoagulant, 285
with neutropenia and splenomegaly (Felty), 246
neutrophilia, 249(T7.10)
sideroblastic anaemia, 22
splenic atrophy, 108(T3.28)
thrombocytopenia, 306(T8.27)
thrombocytosis, 180(T5.9)
toxic neutrophils, 259(T7.25)
Reider lymphocytes, 250
Rosai-Dorfman disease (sinus histiocytosis with massive lymphadenopathy), 198
rosette formation, bone marrow
Ewing's sarcoma, **192**
neuroblastoma, 184, **186**
normal marrow, rosette-like knots, **186**
retinoblastoma, **186**
Rotor syndrome
and F VII deficiency, 286
rubella
atypical lymphocytes, 252
immune thrombocytopenia, 306
neonatal, and:
disseminated intravascular coagulation, 292
haemolysis, 99

Sanfilippo MPS
see **mucopolysaccharidosis**
scarlet fever (scarlatina)
atypical lymphocytes, 252(T7.14)
screening tests
for haemostatic defects, 276
scurvy
anaemia, 40
bleeding, 278, **279**
sea-blue histiocytes
see **histiocytes**
S.E.Asian (Melanesian) ovalostomatocytosis, 78, **77**
Sebastian platelet syndrome, 216, 309
Sekel syndrome
bone marrow aplasia, 51
selenium deficiency
haemolysis, **101**
self-inflicted bruising, 274, **279**
septicaemia (bacterial)
anaemia, 98, **69**, **81**
apotosis of leucocytes, **264**
bacteria in leucocytes, 260, **261**, **262**
differential diagnosis, 260, **263**
see also individual organisms
disseminated intravascular coagulation, 292, **293**
haemostasis in, 292
histiocytes, blood, **266**
neutropenia, 240
phagocytic monocytes, **265**
purpura fulminans, 294
thrombocytopenia, immune, 307
toxic change in leucocytes, 257ff., **259**
vessel dysfunction, 278(T8.3)
severe combined immunodeficiency
lymphopenia, 254
Shwachman's syndrome
bone marrow hypoplasia, 50
Gaucher-like cells, **227**
sialidosis I (neuraminidase deficiency without dysmorphism, cherry-red spot-myoclonus), 202(T6.2), 204(T6.3), 205, 206, 230(T6.14)
sialidosis II (neuraminidase deficiency, dysmorphic, childhood onset), 202(T6.2), 204(T6.3), 205, 206, 228(T6.13)
sickle cells/Hb, 26, 27(T2.13), **29**, **31**
thrombosis, 297(T8.22)
sideroblastic anaemias, 20
cellular cobalamin (cbl) defects, 36(T2.21), **39**
copper deficiency, 247
hereditary, 20, **21**
lead poisoning, 22, **21**
Pearson's syndrome, 216, **217**
thiamine responsive (Wolfram), 40
sinus histiocytosis with massive lymphadenopathy (Rosai-Dorfman), 198
Sly MPS, 209, 210
smudge cells
in:
ALL, 130, **131**
chylomicronaemia, 230
spurious neutropenia, 230
snake bite
disseminated intravascular coagulation, 296
fragmentation haemolysis, 80(T3.13)
hypofibrinogenaemia, **275**
spherocytosis, 70
spectrin, **66**
defects, hereditary spherocytosis, 66
spherocytes/spherocytosis, 64ff.
alloimmune
see **alloimmune haemolysis**
anti A/B/D material, infusion of, 75
autoimmune
see **autoimmune haemolysis**
burns, 68, **69**
Cl. welchii septicaemia, 70, **69**
copper intoxication, 70
cryptantigen exposure (T activation), 74
cyanotic congenital heart disease, 70, **69**
drug-immune, 76
envenomation, 70
enzyme deficiency, 65(T3.6), 104
hereditary, 66ff., **67**
with acanthocytosis, 66, **67**
'pincer-cell' variant, **67**
hypophosphataemia, 70
infection, non-immune spherocytosis, 70, **69**
intravenous:
Ig, anti A/B/D material, 75
lipid alimentation, 70
normal, 4, **5**
obstructive jaundice/liver failure, 90(T3.18)
spiculated (spur cells, whiskered spherocytes)
see **spiculated cells**
T activation, 74
total parenteral nutrition, 70
spiculated (spur) cells, (whiskered spherocytes), 90
enzyme deficiency, 104, **105**
obstructive jaundice/liver failure, **91**
renal disease, **99**
Spielmeyer-Vogt disease
see **Batten's disease**
spleen absence/atrophy, 108, **109**
in collagen disease, **109**
Ivemark syndrome, 108, **109**
sickle cell disorders, 28, **29**
neutrophilia, 249(T7.10)
spur (spiculated) cells
see **spiculated cells**
spurious results
see **artefact**
Staphylococcus aureus
septicaemia
bacteria in leucocytes, 260(T7.27), **261**
differential diagnosis, 260(T7.26), **263**
in skin squames, **263**
starch
in films of marrow aspirates, **237**
steroids
and:
chylomicronaemia, 230
eosinopenia, 257
foamy macrophages, marrow, 230(T6.14)
lymphopenia, 254(T7.18)
neutrophilia, 249
thrombocytopenia, 311(T8.31)

Stewart's syndrome
- macrothrombocytopenia, stomatocytosis, 96

stippled erythrocytes, 97
- lead poisoning, **21**
- pyrimidine 5′ nucleotidase deficiency, 97

stomatocytosis, 94ff.
- drugs, 97, **95**
- Rh null, mod, 97, **95**

storage pool disease (platelet), 314ff.
- deficiency of
  - α granules (grey platelet), 313(T8.35), 316, **315**
  - dense bodies, 313(T8.35), 314, 315
- release defects (thromboxane synthesis/receptor), 314ff.

Stormorken macrothrombocytopenia, 309

Streptococcus
- in leucocytes, septicaemia, 260(T7.27), **261**
- *see also* ***Streptococcus pneumoniae***

Streptococcus pneumoniae
- cryptantigen exposure
  - haemolysis/haemolytic-uraemic syndrome, 74, 80, **81**
- purpura fulminans, 294
- septicaemia
  - bacteria in leucocytes, 260(T7.27), **261**
    - differential diagnosis, 260(T7.26), **263**

striated sky-blue cells
- G_{M1} gangliosidosis II, 232

sucrose lysis
- in:
  - congenital dyserythropoietic anaemias, 42(T2.23)
  - PNH, 52

sudan black B cytochemistry
- lymphoblasts, ALL, 116(T4.2), 124, **117**
- macrophages, marrow, 228(T6.13), 230(T6.14), **229**
- sea-blue histiocytes, marrow, 232

Sweet's syndrome (acute febrile neutrophilic dermatosis), 248

'Swiss cheese' macrothrombocytopenia, 309, 313(T8.34)

syphylis, congenital
- haemolysis, 98

systemic lupus erythematosus
- apoptosis of leucocytes, **264**
- autoimmune
  - haemolysis, 75(T3.10)
  - neutropenia, 246
  - thrombocytopenia, 308
- bone marrow hypoplasia, 52
- chylomicronaemia, 230
- eosinophilia, 255(T7.19)
- erythroblastopenia, 53(T2.32), 56
- haemophagocytosis, 267
- lupus anticoagulant, 284
- lymphopenia, 254(T7.18)
- neonatal lupus syndrome (maternal SLE), 246
- neutrophilia, 249(T7.10)
- splenic atrophy, 108(T3.28)
- toxic neutrophils, 259(T7.25)
- von Willebrand disease, acquired, 284

t(1;5) MPD with eosinophilia, 182

T activation
- *see* **cryptantigen exposure**

T cell
- ALL, 116(T4.1), 132
- receptor gene rearrangements, 128

T lymphocytosis with neutropenia, 247

Tangier disease, 96
- foamy macrophages, marrow, 228(T6.13)
- stomatocytosis, 96

target cells, 82
- biliary obstruction, **83**
- Hb:
  - C disorders, 26(T2.12), 27(T2.13), **28**
  - E disorders, 26(T2.12), **28**
  - S disorders, 26(T2.12), 27(T2.13), **29**
- thalassaemias, **24, 25, 83**

telangiectasia, hereditary haemorrhagic
- bleeding, 17(T2.2)

thalassaemias, 22ff.
- alpha, 25, **25, 27, 83**
  - with mental retardation/dysmorphism, 23
- beta, 23, 26, 27, **24**
  - acquired, monosomy 7 MPD, 174
- Cβ thal, 27
- Constant Spring, 26
- delta-beta (high F thal), 28(T2.14)
- delta-beta fusion (Lepore), 26, 28(T2.14), **31**
- Eβ thal, 27, 28(T2.14)
- gamma-delta-beta, 26
- with G6PD deficiency, **93**
- high F (δβ), 26, 28(T2.14)
- intermedia, origins of, 28(T2.14)
- investigation for, 23
- vs iron deficiency, 19(T2.3)
- Sβ thal, 27, **29**
- thal changes in unstable Hb, 32
- *see also* **haemoglobin, haemoglobins**

thiamin-responsive megaloblastosis, 40

thrombin clotting time
- normal, 278
- prolonged, 288ff.
  - artefact, 276

thrombocythaemia, essential, 180, **181**
- vs reactive thrombocytosis, 180
- thrombosis, 297(T8.22)

thrombocytopathy, 309, 312ff.
- in normal neonate, 280
- *see also* individual disorders

thrombocytopenia
- (many individual disorders are indexed separately)
- absent radius syndrome, 300, **301**
- alloimmune
  - *see* **alloimmune**
- amegakaryocytic
  - *see* **amegakaryocytic thrombocytopenia**
- autoimmune
  - *see* **autoimmune**
- dilutional, 312
- drug-induced
  - immune, 310
  - non-immune, 311(T8.31)
- familial, outline, 309
- gestational, 310
- heparin-induced, 310
- hypersplenism, 312
- idiopathic (immune), 308
  - maternal, and neonatal thrombocytopenia, 310
- immune, 304ff.
  - alloimmune,
    - *see* **alloimmune**
  - autoimmune
    - *see* **autoimmune**
  - drugs, 310
  - immune diseases with, 308
  - with immune haemolysis/neutropenia, 308
  - passive acquisition from mother, 310
- ineffective thrombopoiesis, 302, **303**
- infection
  - immune
    - bacterial, 307
    - post-viral, 306, 308(T8.28), **305**
      - vs ITP, 308(T8.28)
  - non-immune, 300, 311
- investigation, 301
- neonatal
  - alloimmune, 310
  - fetal infection, 300
  - passive acquisition from mother, 310
- non-immune damage, 311
- outline, 301(T8.23)
- post-viral, 306, **305**
  - with:
    - autoimmune haemolysis, 307
    - parietal cell, thyroid auto-antibodies, 307
  - vs ITP, 308
- spurious, 276, **285**
- thrombopoietin deficiency, 304
- von Willebrand's disease, 283

thrombocytosis
- reactive, 180
  - vs essential thrombocythaemia, 180
- spurious, 276, **285**

thrombopoiesis, ineffective, 302, **303**
- *see also* individual causes

thrombopoietin deficiency
- and thrombocytopenia, 304

thrombosis, thrombotic states, 296ff.
- neonatal, 299, **299**
  - and maternal disease, 296
- post liver transplant, 298, **297**
- *see also* individual causes, **disseminated intravascular coagulation**

thrombotic thrombocytopenia purpura, 80

thromboxane, platelet, **290**
- synthesis/receptor defects, 314ff.
  - vs storage pool deficiency, 313(T8.35)

thymoma
- bone marrow hypoplasia, 52
- erythroblastopenia, 56

thymus
- absence, di George syndrome, 254
- transplantation and autoimmune thrombocytopenia, 306(T8.27)

thyroid autoantibodies
- in:
  - immune thrombocytopenia, 307
  - juvenile pernicious anaemia, 36

tissue plasminogen activator, 289(T8.15), **281**
- deficiency, and thrombosis, 298

toluidine blue, metachromasia
- AML M3 variant, **155**
- mucopolysaccharidosis
  - Buhot plasma cells, **213**
  - Gasser lymphocytes, **209**
  - Gasser reticulum cells, **235**
  - monocytes, **225**

total parenteral nutrition
- chylomicronaemia, 230
- spherocytosis, 70
- thrombocytopenia, 311(T8.31)

toxic changes in leucocytes, 257ff., **259**

Toxocara canis
- eosinophilia, 255(T7.19)

toxoplasmosis
- atypical lymphocytes in, 252(T7.14)
- in bone marrow, **267**
- haemolysis, 98

transcobalamin II, **35**
- deficiency
  - erythroblastopenia, 56

transcobalamin II (*contd*)
deficiency (*contd*)
lymphopenia, 254(T7.18)
megaloblastosis, 36(T2.21), 38
in neutrophil granules, 216
transferrin
congenital deficiency, 18
in:
anaemia of chronic disease, 19(T2.3)
hereditary sideroblastic anaemia, 20
iron deficiency anaemia, 19, 20
thalassaemia minor, 19
normal values, 7
receptor, antibody to and microcytic anaemia, 18
transfusion, blood
alloimmune neutropenia, 245
graft-vs-host disease, 50
haemophagocytosis, 266
incompatible
see **incompatibility**
massive, and
coagulation factor deficiencies, 287
thrombocytopenia, 312
platelets, refractoriness to, 311
transient
abnormal myelopoiesis of trisomy 21, 168, **169**
CML-like reaction, thrombocytopenia-absent radius syndrome, 300
erythroblastopenia of childhood, 54, **55**
vs Diamond-Blackfan anaemia, 53
megakaryocytic dyspoiesis, 170
see also **leukaemoid reactions**
transplant
see **bone marrow, kidney, liver, thymus**
trauma
haemostatic abnormalities, 291(T8.20), 296
self-inflicted, 274, **279**
triose phosphate isomerase, 103
deficiency and haemolysis, 104(T3.25)
triploidy
macrocytosis, 42
trisomy 13
excessive nuclear tags, 222, **223**
trisomy 18
amegakaryocytic thrombocytopenia, 302
macrocytosis, 42
trisomy 21
in AML, 146(T5.2)
and:
AML M7, 166
macrocytosis, 42
transient abnormal myelopoiesis, 168, **169**
tuberculosis
anaemia of chronic disease, 19
in bone marrow, **267**
mycobacteria in blood leucocytes, HIV infection, **262**
tumour lysis syndrome
ALL, 130, **131**
disseminated intravascular coagulation in, 291(T8.20)
typhoid
atypical lymphocytes in, 252(T7.14)
tyrosinosis, 236
dysfibrinogenaemia, 288

ulcerative colitis
see **inflammatory bowel disease**
unstable haemoglobins, 32, **31**
uraemia
see **renal disease**

vacuolation
see individual cell types
varicella
bone marrow destruction, 46, **45**
immune
protein S deficiency, 294
thrombocytopenia, 306
purpura fulminans, 294, **295**
veganism, strict
cobalamin deficiency in breast-fed infant, 36, **37**
venepuncture
frequent, iron deficiency in, 16
venom, snake etc
see **envenomation**
vessel dysfunction/vasculitis
bleeding in, 278
allergic, **279**
Ehlers-Danlos syndrome, **279**
Henoch-Schönlein purpura, **279**
scurvy, **279**
disseminated intravascular coagulation in, 297(T8.22)
virus/infection
in AML M5, 160, **160**
anaemia, 75(T3.10), 98, **81**
apoptosis of leucocytes, **253**, **264**
atypical lymphocytes
see **lymphocytes**
vs bacterial infection, leucocyte changes, 258
bone marrow aplasia, 46, **45**
disseminated intravascular coagulation, 292
erythroblastopenia, 54, **55**
erythroblasts, giant, 54, **55**
haemolysis, 75(T3.10), 98, **81**
infection-associated haemophagocytosis, 194, 267, **268**
in intussusception, 252(T7.14)
in irritable hip, 252(T7.14)
leukaemoid reactions
see **leukaemoid reactions**
lupus anticoagulant, 284
lymphoblastosis, benign, 136, **137**
lymphocytosis (of normal lymphocytes), 250
lymphoma, **139**, **253**
lymphopenia, 254(T7.18)
megakaryocyte deficiency, 300, 306
in mesenteric adenitis, 252(T7.14)
multinucleate cells, **157**
neutropenia, 240, 246
neutrophilia, 248
phagocytic monocytes, **265**
protein S, autoantibody to, 294
purpura fulminans, 294, **295**
spherocytosis, 75(T3.10), **81**
thrombocytopenia
immune, 306
non-immune, 311
transient erythroblastopenia, 54
virus-like particles, ALL, 122, **123**
see also specific viruses
vitamin
B_1, deficiency
thiamine-responsive megaloblastosis, 40
B_{12}
see **cobalamin**
C
deficiency
anaemia, 40
bleeding, **279**
excess, and haemolysis, 100, **101**
E, deficiency, and haemolysis, 82, 100
K, deficiency
with protein C, S deficiency, 286
prothrombin complex deficiency, 286, **275**
see also individual disorders
von Willebrand factor, 273, 283, **301**
von Willebrand's disease, 282ff., 313
types, 283

warfarin
coumarin-induced prothrombin complex deficiency, 287(T8.13)
skin necrosis, in protein C deficiency, 294
Wegener's granulomatosis
thrombosis, 297(T8.22)
whiskered spherocytes
see **spiculated cells**
Williams trait (high MW kininogen deficiency), 285
Wilms tumour
acquired von Willebrand's disease, 284
mucoid deposit in blood film, **193**
Wiskott-Aldrich syndrome, 304
autoimmune haemolysis, 75(T3.10)
thrombocytopenia, **305**
Wolfram's syndrome (thiamine-responsive megaloblastosis), 40
Wolman's disease, 204(T6.3), 205, 207, **203**
foamy macrophages, 226(T6.13), **231**
lymphocyte vacuolation, 202(T6.2), **203**
see also **cholesteryl ester storage disease (adult Wolman's)**
Woronets trait
acanthocytosis, 86
WT syndrome
and bone marrow aplasia, 51(T2.31)

xerocytosis, hereditary, 94, **93**
X-linked a/hypogammaglobulinaemia
haemolysis, 75(T3.10)
neutropenia, 242(T7.5)
X-linked lymphoproliferative disorder, 252, **253**
bone marrow hypoplasia, 46

zinc deficiency
stomatocytosis, 95(T3.20)